CHRONIC LYMPHOCYTIC LEUKEMIA

Edited by **Pablo Oppezzo**

Chronic Lymphocytic Leukemia
Edited by Pablo Oppezzo

Published by InTech

Janeza Trdine 9, 51000 Rijeka, Croatia

Publishing Process Manager Marko Rebrovic

Technical Editor Teodora Smiljanic

Cover Designer InTech Design Team

Additional hard copies can be obtained from orders@intechopen.com

Chronic Lymphocytic Leukemia, Edited by Pablo Oppezzo
p. cm.
978-953-307-881-6

For EU product safety concerns:
IN TECH d.o.o., Prolaz Marije Krucifikse Kozulić 3, 51000 Rijeka, Croatia, info@intechopen.com or visit our website at intechopen.com.

Meet the editor

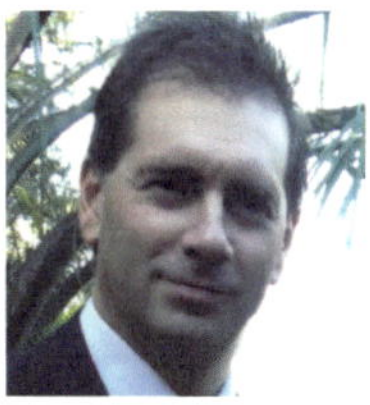

Dr Pablo Oppezzo received his MSc in Molecular and Cellular Biology from PEDECIBA (Uruguay) in 1999. In 2004, he received his PhD in Immunology from the University Paris VI, and did post-doctoral work at the Biochemical Structural Unit at the Pasteur Institute of Paris. In 2006 he obtained a position as Principal Investigator of Recombinant Protein Unit at Institut Pasteur de Montevideo, Uruguay. Dr Pablo Oppezzo is now the Head of the Recombinant Protein Unit and Professor in the Immunology department at the School of Medicine, Republic University (UdelaR), Uruguay. Dr Oppezzo's research focuses on the mechanisms involved in the origins of haematopoietic B-cell malignancies, specifically the study of the mutagenic action of the enzyme Activation-Induced cytidine deaminase. In the last years, he contributed to elucidate the mechanism of somatic hypermutation and class switch recombination process in Chronic Lymphocytic Leukemia and to identify new prognosis markers for this disease.

Contents

Preface

Chronic lymphocytic leukemia (CLL) follows an extremely variable course with survival ranging from months to decades. Recently, there has been major progress in the identification of molecular and cellular markers that may predict the tendency for disease progression in CLL patients. In particular, the mutational profile of Ig genes and some cytogenetic abnormalities have been found to be important predictors of prognosis in CLL. However, this progress has raised new questions about the biology, prognosis and management of the disease, some of which are addressed here.

CLL is characterized by accumulation of CD5 positive monoclonal B cells in primary and secondary lymphoid tissues. It is described as the most common leukemia in the occidental world (4.4-5.4/100.000) [1], whereas it is rare in Asian populations [2]. The existence of mature neoplastic lymphocytes with an abnormally long life span has been a hallmark of this disease but recent data show that the proliferative rates of CLL cells can be higher than previously expected indicating that CLL B cells have a dynamic kinetic behavior [3]. As most circulating CLL B cells are in the G_0 / early G_1 phase of the cell cycle, it was long thought that CLL clones hardly proliferate and die infrequently. However, circulating leukemic cells in the peripheral blood are the tip of the iceberg. Clearly the most significant pathophysiological events occur in tissues where leukemic cells: **a)** are activated by exposure to antigens, although it is still unclear where and how this exposure takes place, **b)** proliferate in specific niches, (the so-called pseudofollicular proliferation centres) which are not detected in any B-cell malignancy other than CLL, and **c)** receive the proper T-cell help and interact with stromal cells that favour cell proliferation and accumulation. These observations turn the attention towards the occurrence of different sub-populations inside the tumoral clone in which a homeostatic balance exists in patients with stable lymphocyte counts and good clinical course or an imbalance in patients with rising lymphocyte counts and poor outcome [4]. Different cellular subsets in CLL could receive survival signals from specific microenvironments increasing their proliferative potential and consequently leading to a more aggressive disease.

The standard clinical procedures to estimate prognosis are the clinical staging systems developed by Rai and Binet [5,6]. These systems define early (Rai 0, Binet A), intermediate (Rai I/II, Binet B) and advanced (Rai III-V, Binet C) stage disease. However, the high heterogeneity of this disease among individual patients does not allow us to predict how the disease will evolve. In order to refine outcome prediction for individual patients, there has been intensive work to identify additional clinical and/or biological factors of potential prognostic relevance. Among them, the genetic characteristics of the CLL clone are undoubtedly the most relevant. Molecular genetics of CLL can be divided into two major issues: **1)** mutation status of the variable VH genes of immunoglobulin's (Ig), which could be related to the cellular origin of CLL and **2)** Genomic aberrations, some of which are involved in the progression and/or refractoriness to treatment.

Since B-CLL cells express the CD5 protein on their surface membrane, it was assumed that these cells would behave similarly to CD5 positive B cells in mice (B1a B cell subset) and would not accumulate significant numbers of immunoglobulins (Ig) V gene mutations. However, it was not the case and we now know that somatic mutations do occur in a significant proportion of B-CLL cases. [7]. The presence of these mutations denotes subgroups of patients with markedly different clinical course and outcomes. This important scientific observation has been correlated with a clinical relevant application, since absence of mutations in IgVH is associated with a short survival (unmutated patients -Um-), whereas the presence of mutations in this region is linked with a good prognosis (mutated patients -Mut-) [8]. The biased use of certain IgVH genes and the existence of similarities among Ig rearrangements raise the possibility that an antigenic stimulation could support the malignant cell growth.

The other genetic parameter shown to be of pathogenic and clinical relevance in CLL is the presence of genomic aberrations in the leukemic clone. In contrast with what is observed in other B cell malignancies, which typically exhibit balanced chromosomal translocations, the most frequent abnormalities in CLL are mutations, deletions or trisomies. Döhner *et al.* demonstrated in a series of 325 CLL patients that chromosomal aberrations can be detected in interphase cells by fluorescence *in situ* hybridization (FISH) in 82% of cases [9]. The most frequent alterations are 13q deletions, observed in 55% of patients, followed by trisomy 12 (18%) and the 11q deletion (16%). The 17p deletion involving the p53 protein is observed less frequently (7%). Interestingly, the presence of a 17p or 11q deletion is associated with poor prognosis and predominates among advanced stages of the disease and among patients displaying Um VH genes, whereas the 13q deletion or a normal karyotype are associated with good prognosis, early disease and Mut VH genes. Based in these studies it is clear that VH mutation status and genomic aberrations are among the strongest currently available parameters and are of independent value to predict outcome in CLL.

Despite a common gene expression signature Mut and Um CLL cases differentially express more than 100 genes [10]. Among them, over-expression of genes encoding zeta-chain-associated protein (ZAP-70), lipoprotein lipase (LPL), BCL-7a, dystrophin and gravin are observed in the aggressive Um cases, while stable mutated cases over-express Wnt3, CTLA-4, NRIP1 nuclear receptor gene, ADAM and the transcription factor TCF7 [11]. In addition some evidence indicates that particular IgVH genes, such as VH1-69 and VH3-21, might be associated to differential gene expression. These results suggest that indolent Mut and aggressive Um CLLs constitute two variants of the same disease. The reasons accounting for the striking differences in clinical outcome between these two variants remain unsolved.

CLL is not only the prototype of B cell chronic lymphoid malignancies, but has also become an interesting model that offers biologists and clinicians the opportunity of interaction towards a common goal: to translate the exciting developments of basic sciences into effective new approaches to patients´ benefit.

Many reasons account for this growing interest. First, both ethnic disparity and strong familial tendency provide compelling evidence for a CLL genetic susceptibility. Second, the CLL has numerous features that cause uncertainties about its cellular origin. Third, CLL is a dynamic process which results from cells that proliferate and die, often at appreciable rates [3].This evidence suggests that the crosstalk with accessory cells in specialized tissue microenvironments, such as the bone marrow and secondary lymphoid organs, favours disease progression by promoting malignant B-cell growth and drug resistance. Therefore, understanding the crosstalk between malignant B-cells and their milieu could give us new keys on the cellular and molecular biology of CLL that can finally lead to novel strategies in the treatment of this disease. Fourth, very recently, and with the aim to increase our knowledge on CLL biology, it has been described some animal models capable to reproduce or mimic a real human CLL disease Fifth, we must take into account that CLL has a considerable clinical heterogeneity. Some patients present aggressive disease and poor prognosis, others have an indolent course and a virtually normal life expectancy. Thus, the establishment of a prognosis marker able to predict the evolution in order to stratify patients constituted one of the major achievements, in the last years.

Finally, CLL serves as a model to understand how micro-environmental stimuli, antigenic drive and epigenetic deregulation are combined in cancer pathogenesis.

"Chronic Lymphocytic Leukemia" will provide a comprehensive overview of the disease from the basic mechanisms underlying CLL origin and progression, its epidemiology, pathophysiology, classification and clinical presentation.

Space dictates that this review will be limited in scope. However, we hope to provide the reader with enough insight and information to serve as a source for knowledge and inspiration for hemato-oncologists, molecular immunologist and/or clinical researchers.

Pablo Oppezzo, PhD,
Recombinant Protein Unit, Institut Pasteur de Montevideo,
Uruguay

References

[1] Zenger V. et al. (2004) *Chronic Lymphocitic Leukemia*, Humana Press

[2] Tamura, K. et al. (2001) Chronic lymphocytic leukemia (CLL) is rare, but the proportion of T-CLL is high in Japan. *Eur J Haematol* 67 (3), 152-157

[3] Chiorazzi, N. (2007) Cell proliferation and death: forgotten features of chronic lymphocytic leukemia B cells. *Best Pract Res Clin Haematol* 20 (3), 399-413

[4] Caligaris-Cappio, F. (2011) Inflammation, the microenvironment and chronic lymphocytic leukemia. *Haematologica* 96 (3), 353-355

[5] Binet, J.L. et al. (1981) A new prognostic classification of chronic lymphocytic leukemia derived from a multivariate survival analysis. *Cancer* 48 (1), 198-206

[6] Rai, K.R. et al. (1975) Clinical staging of chronic lymphocytic leukemia. *Blood* 46 (2), 219-234

[7] Schroeder, H.W., Jr. and Dighiero, G. (1994) The pathogenesis of chronic lymphocytic leukemia: analysis of the antibody repertoire. *Immunol Today* 15 (6), 288-294

[8] Damle, R.N. et al. (1999) Ig V gene mutation status and CD38 expression as novel prognostic indicators in chronic lymphocytic leukemia. *Blood* 94 (6), 1840-1847

[9] Dohner, H. et al. (2000) Genomic aberrations and survival in chronic lymphocytic leukemia. *N Engl J Med* 343 (26), 1910-1916

[10] Klein, U. et al. (2001) Gene expression profiling of B cell chronic lymphocytic leukemia reveals a homogeneous phenotype related to memory B cells. *J Exp Med* 194 (11), 1625-1638

[11] Oppezzo, P. et al. (2005) The LPL/ADAM29 expression ratio is a novel prognosis indicator in chronic lymphocytic leukemia. *Blood* 106 (2), 650-657

Part 1

Introduction

1

Selected Topics in Chronic Lymphocytic Leukemia Pathogenesis

Sergio Bianchi[1,2], Guillermo Dighiero[1] and Otto Pritsch[1,3]
[1]*Institut Pasteur de Montevideo,*
[2]*Depto. de Fisiopatología, Facultad de Medicina,Universidad de la República*
[3]*Depto. de Inmunobiología, Facultad de Medicina, Universidad de la República*
Uruguay

1. Introduction

Chronic lymphocytic leukemia (CLL) is the most common form of leukemia in Western countries mainly affecting individuals older than 50 years. It follows an extremely variable course, with survival ranging from months to decades. Available treatments often induce remissions, though almost all patients relapse and CLL remains an incurable disease [1]. However, recent advances in molecular biology have enabled us to better understand the disease physiopathology and together with the development of new therapeutic agents have made the management of the disease more rational and more effective.

2. Epidemiology

The annual incidence of CLL varies with the age and sex structure of the population. Whereas in the USA it has been estimated at 3.5 per 100,000 (males 5.0: females 2.5) [2], in the UK estimates of 6.15 per 100,000 have been reported [3]. However, since in a majority of patients diagnosis is established because of an incidental blood count performed for irrelevant reasons and because of increasing life expectancies, the prevalence should augment in the future. The median age for diagnosis is 70 for males and 74 for females. Caucasian populations have a clearly higher incidence when compared to Japanese and Chinese population, even among patients having migrated to the USA, which suggests that genetic influences are stronger than environmental factors in the pathogenesis of the disease. The nature of this genetic predisposition remains unknown as yet.

CLL may rarely occur in families [4, 5]. First-degree relatives of patients are three times more likely also to have CLL or another lymphoid neoplasm than the general population [6]. Using a four color flow-cytometric assay, Rawstron et al discovered that 3.5% of normal individuals over the age of 40 have a population of monoclonal lymphocytes (MBL) with the immune phenotypic characteristics of CLL cells in their blood at levels below the 3.5×10^9/L [7], and that in first degree relatives of patients with familial CLL the prevalence of such cells is between 13.5% and 18% [8, 9]. The relationship of this subclinical CLL with the full blown disease is a matter of intense investigation in several laboratories. MBL has been proposed as a precursor state of CLL, since MBL clones often carry typical CLL genetic lesions and may represent pre-malignant cells. In approximately 2% of the cases, MBL progresses to CLL, and there is evidence that CLL is generally preceded by MBL [10, 11].

3. Selected topics in CLL pathogenesis

Clinical course of CLL is variable. Recently, progress has been made in the identification of biological markers that could predict disease progression. Particularly, the expression of unmutated Ig genes, some cytogenetic abnormalities like 17p and 11q deletions and the expression of the zeta-associated protein 70 (ZAP-70) are associated to a poor prognosis. A major scientific goal is to find a biomolecular explanation for CLL prognosis heterogeneity that can provide clues in the understanding of disease etiology and pathogenic mechanisms which favor the onset of the disease, as well as its progression and evolution into aggressive variants (Richter's lymphoma or prolymphocytoid leukemia) [12]. Given the important advances operated during recent years in CLL understanding, a full review of these topics is not possible within the space confines of this article. Hence, we will concentrate in 3 major topics: the genetic abnormalities, the B cell receptor and the balance between proliferation and apoptosis.

3.1 Genetic abnormalities

The nature of genetic predisposition for CLL remains unknown. None of the reported genetic aberrations is constant and it is presently unclear whether they constitute initial events or occur during evolution. In contrast with what is observed in other B cell malignancies, which typically exhibit balanced chromosomal translocations, in CLL the most frequent abnormalities are mutations, deletions or trisomies. Reciprocal balanced chromosomal translocations involving the heavy and light chain are very rare in CLL as compared to B-NHL [13, 14, 15], and aberrant somatic hypermutation, frequently present in DLBCL, is not observed in CLL [16]. This is consistent with the concept that CLL B-cells have non-active mechanisms involved in Ig class switch recombination and somatic hypermutation [15]. Thus, the transformation of the CLL precursor is likely to occur after the antigen-driven B-cell maturation. In the case of hairy cell leukemia, which correspond to an antigen-experienced post-GC B cells [15, 17], there is also a lack of reciprocal balanced chromosome translocations [18, 19]. Overall, these tumor malignancies form a group of B-cell tumors that originate from the transformation of antigen-experienced B cells.

Progress in cytogenetic techniques and the advent of fluorescence in situ hybridization (FISH) allowed important progress in this field. Döhner et al demonstrated in a series of 325 CLL patients that chromosomal aberrations can be detected in 82% of cases [13]. In these conditions, 13q deletions are observed in 55% of patients, followed by trisomy 12 (18%) and the 11q deletion (16%). A deletion on chromosome 17p including a monoallelic deletion of TP53 tumor suppressor gene, and very frequently mutations in the remaining allele [20] is less frequently seen (7%)

Deletions in 11q22-q23, typically involve the ataxia telangiectasia (ATM) gene [20] which causes a genomic instability that prevent correct DNA-damage reparation, allow the accumulation of mutations and thus may contribute to CLL pathogenesis. Interestingly, the presence of a 17p or 11q deletion is associated with poor prognosis and predominates among advanced stages of the disease and among patients displaying unmutated VH genes, whereas the 13q deletion or a normal karyotype are associated with good prognosis, early disease and mutated VH genes. The genetic lesions associated with deletions of the short arm of chromosome 17 (del17p13) encoding the p53 tumor suppressor gene and the long arm of chromosome 11 (del11q23) encoding the ataxia telangectasia mutated (ATM), a kinase that regulates p53 gene, result in a loss of function of the p53 gene. p53 is an anti-oncogene which, when strand breaks occur in DNA, triggers apoptosis or cell-cycle arrest. By controlling the repair or elimination of cells with damaged DNA, p53 maintains the integrity of the genome and prevents clonal progression. Many cytotoxic drugs require this pathway to be intact for them to be effective. Defects on this pathway constitute the strongest independent predictor for resistance to standard therapy [21, 22].

The pathogenic implications of trisomy 12 in CLL remain unresolved [23]. It is proposed that a putative proto-oncogen (CLLU1) may have an elevated gene dosage due to trisomy.

The most frequent chromosomal abnormality in CLL is deletion of 13q14, being monoallelic in 76% of cases, and biallelic in 24% [13, 14, 24]. This deletion, also detected in MBL [11] occurs at a much lower frequency in multiple myeloma, DLBCL, mature T-cell lymphomas, and in several solid tumors [25-29]. A minimal deleted region (MDR) has been defined in a large number of CLL cases with monoallelic 13q14 deletion. This region contains the long non-coding RNA deleted in leukemia (DLEU)-2, and the first exon of the DLEU1 gene [30, 31]. Two microRNAs (miR-15a and miR-16-1) were present within intron 4 of DLEU2 [32, 33] and are expressed by using DLEU2 promoter region. It has been also reported that downregulation of DLEU2 and miR-15a/16-1 expression in CLL cases without 13q14 deletion [32], could be explained by suppressive epigenetic mechanisms [34]. Overall, the available data suggested that DLEU2 and/or miR-15a/16-1 are candidate tumor suppressor genes. *In vitro* assays were performed by introducing DLEU2 mRNA into a 13q14-homozygous deleted cell, but failed to produce any effects on cell death or proliferation [35].

Micro-RNAs (miRNAs) play an important role in the regulation of gene expression. Using a microarray methodology, Calin et al demonstrated significant differences in miRNA expression between CLL B cells and normal CD5+ cells. Particularly, they could substantiate the absence of two miRNA (miR15 and miR16) associated to a mutated profile of Ig genes and with deletions in the 13q14 region [36]. Fulci et al [37] also found an overexpression of miR-150, miR-223 and miR-29b, and miR-29c in the *IgVH* mutated CLL compared to the *IgVH* unmutated cases. Marton et al confirmed these findings and found a significant downexpression of MiRs 181, let-7a and MiR 22 [38].

By using biostatistical algorithms it was possible to identify miR-15a/16-1 binding sites in a number of mRNAs encoding gene products involved in regulating proliferation and apoptosis [37-44]. In summary, miR-15a/16-1 are clearly involved in critical cellular processes, and their disruption may contribute to lymphomagenesis.

Two transgenic mice were developed in order to analyze the human 13q14-MDR region. The first model mimicked the MDR, and the second contained a deletion of miR-15a/16-1. Both mouse lines developed mostly indolent clonal lymphoproliferative diseases with low penetrance.

Interestingly, the IGVH-CDR3 expressed by clonal lymphoproliferative B-cells were highly similar (BCR stereotypy), suggesting that an antigen-driven process could be involved in the clonal proliferation of specific tumor cell precursors.

Transgenic mice overexpressing the TCL1 proto-oncogene develop lymphoproliferations similar to those arising in MDR and miR-15a/16-1-deleted mice [45, 46]. TCL1 mRNA expression is upregulated in most human CLL cases but the underlying mechanism is not known as yet [47, 48].

In summary, the DLEU2/miR-15a/16-1 tumor suppressor locus plays a role in regulating the expansion of the mature B-cell pool, by preventing the entry into G0/G1-S transition. The impairment of this cell cycle control in MDR-deleted cells may allow them to proliferate after BCR stimulation by foreign or self antigens.

In these conditions, a model for the pathogenesis of CLL with 13q14 deletion based on the presumptive cellular origin of the tumor cell precursor can be proposed.

The putative CLL precursor could be an antigen-experienced CD27+ B cell, expanded either in the course of a GC B-cell T-dependent or T-independent response by chronic antigen-stimulation through extrinsic or autoantigens. Over time, genetic abnormalities may accumulate in the genome of these chronically stimulated B cells and lead to the outgrow of clones with MBL phenotype. Additional genetic aberrations may be incorporated in the course of proliferation leading to the oncogenic hit that transform these precursor in bona fide CLL cells.

Despite clinical and molecular differences, global gene expression profile analysis demonstrated that all CLL show a homogeneous gene expression profile irrespective of their IgV mutational status and differing from other lymphoid cancers, which suggests a common cellular precursor [49, 50]. These analyses in addition revealed that the gene expression profile of all CLL is related to that of antigen-experienced B cells, which in the human are defined by expression of the CD27 cell surface antigen, and that include classical memory B cells and marginal zone B cells which can be somatically mutated or unmutated [51, 52].

However, despite sharing a common signature CLLs expressing mutated and unmutated *IgVH* genes differentially express more than 100 genes. Among these, over-expression of genes encoding zeta-chain-associated protein 70 (ZAP-70), lipoprotein lipase (LPL), BCL-7a, dystrophin and gravin are observed in the aggressive unmutated cases, while stable mutated cases over-express *Wnt3, CTLA-4, NRIP1* nuclear receptor gene, *ADAM29* and the transcription factor *TCF7* [53]. These results suggest that indolent mutated and aggressive unmutated CLLs constitute two variants of the same disease. The reasons accounting for these striking differences in clinical outcomes of these two variants remain unsolved.

Genome-wide association studies have detected some loci influencing CLL risk [54, 55] and a recent whole-genome sequencing study identified 46 somatic mutations plus four recurrent mutations in the genes NOTCH1, XPO1, MYD88 and KLHL6 [56].

3.2 B-cell receptor (BCR) characteristics in CLL

Three main phenotypic features define B-CLL: the predominant population shares B-cell markers (CD19, CD21, and CD23) with the CD5 antigen, in the absence of other pan-T-cell markers; the B cells are monoclonal with regard to expression of either *k* or λ light chains and the B cells characteristically express surface immunoglobulin (slg), CD79b, CD20 and CD22 with low density. These characteristics are generally adequate for a precise diagnosis of CLL, and they also distinguish CLL from other disorders such as prolymphocytic leukemia, hairy-cell leukemia, mantle-cell lymphoma and other lymphomas that can mimic CLL [57-59].

The BCR is a multimeric complex formed by the assembly of surface immunoglobulin (SIg) and the noncovalently bound heterodimer Igα/Igβ (CD79a/CD79b). Low expression of the BCR is the hallmark of the B-CLL lymphocyte [60, 61].

The mechanisms accounting for poor expression of the BCR in CLL remain elusive. There is no evidence of genetic defects in the BCR components [62, 63] and in contrast with their poor expression at the membrane level, transcription and intra-cellular synthesis of BCR components are normal [63, 64]. However, they cannot be assembled and transported from the endoplasmic reticulum to the cell surface because of a folding and glycosolation defect of the mu and CD79a chains though not of the CD79b chain. The poor expression of the CD22 molecule in B-CLL cells, was also found to result as a consequence of a folding defect occurring in its α chain [65].

One unsolved issue concerns the role of the clonal B-cell receptor (BCR) in disease progression. Despite the fact that low expression of the BCR correlates with reduced induction of protein tyrosine kinase activity and defective intracellular calcium mobilization and tyrosine phosphorylation [66] this receptor conserves the capacity of antigen recognition and signaling, controlling thereby key behaviors of tumor cell, like proliferation and cell survival. Individual patients have different responses to IgM ligation which are related to *VH* gene status. In a majority of cases, CLL cells expressing unmutated *IgVH* genes showed a better response than cases expressing mutated *IgVH* genes [67].

The vast majority of B-CLL cells express a CD5+ and IgM/IgD mantle zone-like phenotype of naive cells, which, in normal conditions express unmutated Ig genes [68]. However, 50%-70% of CLL harbor somatic mutations of *IgVH* genes [69] as if they had matured in a lymphoid follicle. Interestingly, the presence or absence of somatic mutations is associated with the use of particular *IgVH* genes. For instance, alleles of the *V1-69* [70] gene and the *V4-39* gene display an unmutated profile [71].

Two reports demonstrated that the clinical behavior of CLL is related to the mutational status of immunoglobulin (Ig) genes [72, 73]. CLLs with mutated Ig genes display a good prognosis and those with unmutated Ig genes a poor prognosis. This observation has been extensively confirmed [74, 75] and it is well established that the mutational status of *Ig* genes constitutes a strong prognostic indicator in CLL. The mutational profile of *Ig* genes delineates prognostic groups within all Binet's stages [76]. Interestingly, the rearrangement of a specific *IgVH* gene, *V3-21*, has been associated with poor prognosis whether mutated or not [77].

Evidence for the notion that CLL is a tumor of antigen experienced B cells comes from the structure of the rearranged IgV genes. Analyses of large panels of CLL cases revealed that certain IgV gene family members, which could be hypermutated or unmutated, were expressed significantly more frequently in CLL than would be expected from their expression in the IgV gene repertoire of normal B cells [69]. Of note, it was confirmed that the CLL-characteristic IgV gene repertoire does not simply reflect its known restriction during the aging process. These findings suggest that all CLL express restricted sets of

BCRs, and led to the conclusion that many if not all CLL originate from the malignant transformation of B cells previously stimulated by antigen. This concept was virtually proven to be true when it emerged that more than 20% of CLL cases from unrelated patients can have extremely similar, sometimes even identical antigen receptors [78–82]. The use of almost identical BCRs in 1.3% of CLLs provided compelling evidence that the Igs expressed by CLL B cells are highly selected. It would be statistically unexpected to find 2 cases with such similar BCRs in 1 million patients [83]. This finding, known as BCR 'stereotypy', occurs at various levels, including IgV gene usage, VD-J junctional regions (heavy chain complementarity determining region-3; CDR3), and combination of certain heavy chain CDR3s with light chain CDR3s [84].

These results strongly suggest that a common antigen epitope is recognized by these highly homologous molecules. Concerning the epitope recognized, it has been shown that unmutated CLL cells express highly polyreactive antibodies while most mutated ones do not [85, 86]. Indeed, 'CLL antigens' have recently been identified which represent autoantigens derived from cells normally destined for apoptosis; some of the recognized epitopes appear to be highly similar to microbial antigens [87–89]. While signaling through the BCR, either in a tonic or antigen-mediated fashion, is generally assumed to play a role in the pathogenesis of B-cell lymphomas with few exceptions (i.e. Hodgkin lymphoma which expresses 'crippled' BCRs) [90], the BCR stereotypy unique for CLL demonstrate that antigen as such seems to have a decisive role in the etiology of this disease.

Results from microarray and flow cytometric studies have revealed the unexpected expression among tumoral CLL cells, of molecules involved in cell activation like the zeta associated protein 70 (ZAP-70), the CD38 molecule, the activation induced cytidine deaminase (AID) and the lipoprotein lipase (LPL).

Thus, high levels of ZAP-70, usually found in T and NK cells but not in normal circulating B cells, are detected in the majority of unmutated CLLs [50]. CLL B cells that express ZAP-70 are more likely to respond to IgM cross-linking with increased tyrosine phosphorylation and calcium flux than ZAP-70 negative CLL B cells. This effect could occur because following BCR ligation ZAP-70 undergoes tyrosine phosphorylation and becomes associated with surface immunoglobulin and CD79b [91] and/or because ZAP-70 mediates inhibition events that terminate the signalling response [92] and/or because ZAP-70 expression is associated with advantageous survival responses [93]. Altogether, expression of ZAP-70 in CLL allows more effective IgM signaling in CLL B cells, which might be responsible for a more aggressive course. The apparently anomalous expression of ZAP-70 in CLL cells is not completely explained. Recent data revealed that ZAP-70 is expressed at initial stages of B cell maturation and in other B-cell malignancies, like acute lymphoblatic leukemia [94].

Another unexpected molecule expressed by a subset of CLL B cells is CD38. This molecule is present during B-cell development when cell-to-cell interactions are crucial to development [95]. Examples include an early bone marrow precursor cell, cells in the germinal center and plasma cells [96]. In CLL, expression of this molecule predominates among those with unmutated *IgVH* genes and is associated to poor prognosis [97].

Interestingly, the activation induced cytidine deaminase (AID), a B cell-restricted enzyme, required for somatic mutation and isotype switching, is upregulated in unmutated CLL cells

[98-100]. While there is evidence that AID expression could be confined to a small proportion of the clone [101], it appears to be functional, since unmutated CLL cases can generate isotype-switched transcripts and proteins and mutations in the pre-switch μ region [98]. Upregulation of AID may be associated with loss of target specificity resulting in mutations in non-immunoglobulin genes such as *BCL-6, MYC, PAX-5 and RHOH* which are associated with more aggressive disease [102, 103].

In a previous work from our group, we reported that expression of the lipoprotein lipase (LPL) gene at the RNA level was clearly associated to an unmutated profile of Ig genes and a clinical poor outcome in CLL [104]. LPL is normally produced by parenchymal cells in several tissues, with the largest expression found in adipose tissue, cardiac and skeletal muscle and lactating mammary gland. In addition, LPL can augment interaction between cells where it has been shown to form a bridge between monocyte and endothelial cell surface heparan sulfate-proteoglycans. However, LPL expression has never been previously reported in the case of normal B cells. For this reason, its infidel expression in CLL B cells, constitutes a suitable marker to study disease prognosis.

3.3 The balance between proliferation and apoptosis in CLL

CLL can be defined as a low-grade B-cell tumor with antigen experienced monoclonal CD5+ B cells that, having escaped programmed cell death and undergone cell cycle arrest in the G0/G1 phase [105], relentlessly accumulate in lymphoid organs (lymph nodes, spleen and bone marrow) and circulate into the peripheral blood. This leukemic B cell accumulation results from a complex balance between activation of cell proliferation and inhibition of apoptotic death. Interestingly, circulating CLL B-lymphocytes are quiescent cells in the G0/G1 phase of cell cycle. Thus, CLL B cells are characterized by high expression of the anti-apoptotic BCL-2 protein in the absence of specific translocations and by high expression of the $p27^{kip}$ protein, which blocks progression into cell cycle. Given the key role of this protein in cell cycle progression, its over-expression in CLL cells could account for the accumulation of B cells in early phases of the cell cycle. In addition, other members of the BCL-2 family such as anti-apoptotic proteins BCL-XL, BAG-1 and MCL-1 are over-expressed, while pro-apoptotic proteins like BAX and BCL-XS are under-expressed [106, 107]. Taken together, these data suggest that CLL is a disease resulting from accumulation rather than from proliferation.

As opposed to *in vivo* results, apoptosis occurs after *in vitro* culture, which suggests a role of the microenvironment in CLL cell survival [108, 109]. In agreement with this hypothesis are results indicating that apoptosis *in vitro* is prevented by exposure to interleukin-4 (IL-4) as well as by stimulation via surface CD40 [109].

Most scientific work focusing in CLL uses circulating leukemic cell samples obtained from peripheral blood. However, it is reasonably to propose that the most important physiopathological events presumably occur in tissues [110] where leukemic cells: (i) are activated by antigen - BCR stimulation; (ii) are regulated and expanded by T-cell signals; (iii) proliferate in pseudofollicular centers, and (iv) interact with stromal cells that favor cell accumulation.

In vivo, inhibition of apoptosis may occur in pseudo-follicles observed in the lymph nodes and in the cell clusters described in the bone marrow [111]. These pseudo-follicles include in close contact with proliferating B cells increased numbers of CD4-T cells expressing CD40L. These activated CD4-T cells could be recruited by tumor B cells since they constitutively express the T cell-attracting chemokines CCL17 and 22 [112, 113]. CLL lymphocyte localization depends on sequential engagement of adhesion molecules and chemokine receptors (CXCR3, CXCR4, and CXCR5) that may direct leukemic cell chemotaxis *in vitro* [110]. In addition, CLL cell apoptosis can be prevented by interactions with stromal and nurse-like cells [114].

The interaction between CD38 and CD31 also favors the survival of leukemic cells [115]. Furthermore, interleukin-4 and CXCL13/SDF-1 might expand CLL clones by up-regulating the expression of anti-apoptotic genes including *BCL2*, *SURVIVIN*, and *MCL1*. These findings suggest that different subsets of T-cell may influence malignant B-cell to proliferate and that different stromal and accessory cells may favors prolonged survival and accumulation [110].

Toll-like receptors (TLR), concomitantly with the BCR, may also play a role in the co-stimulation of CLL cells [116]. Antigen stimulation and inflammation signals could be involved in the initial steps and in the progression of different B-cell chronic lymphoid malignancies. It has been recently reported that an inflammatory microenvironment, including TLR signaling, is at the basis of the CLL cell survival support provided by stromal accessory cells. CCL2 was reported to be induced in monocytes by the presence of CLL cells *in vitro* and increased levels of CCL2 were also detected in serum from CLL patients [117]. CCL2 binds to the chemokine receptors CCR2 and CCR4 [118], has chemotactic activity for monocytes and basophils, recruits memory T cells and dendritic cells to the sites of inflammation, and has also been implicated in the migration and localization of follicular lymphoma cells [119]. Taken together, these results could be in agreement with a model of selective survival of clones which would receive survival signals in these particular sites.

By using a non-radioactive, stable isotopic labelling method to measure CLL kinetics, Messmer et al showed that B-CLL is not a static process that results simply from accumulation of long-lived lymphocytes, but a disease where a dynamic process in which cells proliferate and die, often at appreciable levels ranging from 0.08% to 1.7% of the clone [120]. This finding is in conflict with the dogma that CLL is a disease characterized almost exclusively by cell accumulation due to a defect in apoptosis. It is clear that most, if not all, proliferative events occur in the tissues where leukemic cells are able to exploit microenvironment interactions in order to avoid apoptosis and acquire tumoral growing conditions. This mechanism may compensate for the clonal decrease that could occur in the periphery by apoptosis and depending on its importance could play a major role in the regulation of the tumor burden.

4. Conclusions

Considerable progress has been achieved in recent years in the comprehension of CLL pathogenesis. We are starting to understand which genes, molecules and accessory cell subsets are involved in CLL cell/microenvironment interactions and what roles they play. However, we still have to elucidate the molecular mechanisms through which these cells promote the accumulation of leukemic cells. Particularly, the role of cytokines, chemokines and chemokine receptors in shaping a supportive microenvironment is still poorly understood as well as the respective role of stromal cells and different T cell subsets.

The BCR appears to play a major role in CLL pathogenesis. However, we cannot provide a plausible explanation of the mechanisms leading to its poor expression at the membrane level and why the mutational profile of Ig genes plays such a major role in CLL prognosis.

Considerable progress has been achieved in the identification of the genetic lesions involved in CLL, particularly in the case of the 13q deletion, for which transgenic mouse models have provided important information on its role in CLL pathogenesis. However, the definitive role of these genetic lesions in CLL pathogenesis remains elusive as yet.

Space dictates that this review be limited in scope. We are aware that there are many other aspects of this fascinating disease which we have not covered.

5. References

[1] Dighiero, G. and Hamblin, T.J. (2008) Chronic lymphocytic leukaemia. Lancet 371, 1017-1029

[2] National Cancer Institute. (2007) SEER cancer statistics review 1975-2001. http://seer.cancer.gov/csr/1975_2001/

[3] Cartwright, R.A., et al. (1987) Chronic lymphocytic leukaemia: case control epidemiological study in Yorkshire. Br J Haematol 56, 79-82

[4] Linet M.S., et al. (1989) Familial cancer history and chronic lymphocytic leukemia: a case-control study. Am J Epidemiol 130, 655-664

[5] Sellick, G.S., et al. (2006) Familial chronic lymphocytic leukemia. Semin Oncol 33, 195-201

[6] Cuttner J. (1992) Increased incidence of hematologic malignancies in first degree relatives of patients with chronic lymphocytic leukemia. Cancer Invest 10, 103-109

[7] Rawstron A.C., et al. (2002) Monoclonal B lymphocytes with the characteristics of "indolent" chronic lymphocytic leukemia are present in 3 • 5% of adults with normal blood counts. Blood 100, 635-639.

[8] Rawstron A.C., et al. (2002) Inherited predisposition to CLL is detectable as subclinical monoclonal B-lymphocyte expansion. Blood 100, 2289-2290

[9] Marti G.E., et al. (2003) B-cell monoclonal lymphocytosis and B-cell abnormalities in the setting of familial B-cell chronic lymphocytic leukemia. Cytometry B Clin Cytom 52, 1-12

[10] Landgren O., et al. (2009) B cell clones as early markers for chronic lymphocytic leukemia. N Engl J Med. 360, 659-667

[11] Rawstron A.C., et al. (2008) Monoclonal B-cell lymphocytosis and chronic lymphocytic leukemia. N Engl J Med 359, 575–583

[12] Rossi D. and Gaidano G. (2009) Richter syndrome: molecular insights and clinical perspectives. Hematol Oncol 27, 1–10

[13] Döhner H., et al. (2000) Genomic aberrations and survival in chronic lymphocytic leukemia. N Engl J Med 343, 1910–1916

[14] Döhner H, et al. (1999) Chromosome aberrations in B-cell chronic lymphocytic leukemia: reassessment based on molecular cytogenetic analysis. J Mol Med 77:266–281

[15] Klein U., and Dalla-Favera R. (2010) New insights into the pathogenesis of chronic lymphocytic leukemia. Semin Cancer Biol. 20, 377-383
[16] Pasqualucci L., et al. (2001) Hypermutation of multiple proto-oncogenes in B-cell diffuse large-cell lymphomas. Nature 412, 341-346
[17] Basso K., et al. (2004) Gene expression profiling of hairy cell leukemia reveals a phenotype related to memory B cells with altered expression of chemokine and adhesion receptors. J Exp Med 199, 59–68
[18] Haglund U., et al. (1994) Hairy cell leukemia is characterized by clonal chromosome abnormalities clustered to specific regions. Blood 83, 2637–2645
[19] Sambani C., et al. (2001) Clonal chromosome rearrangements in hairy cell leukemia: personal experience and review of literature. Cancer Genet Cytogenet 129, 138–144
[20] Zenz T., et al. (2010) From pathogenesis to treatment of chronic lymphocytic leukaemia. Nat Rev Cancer 10, 37–50
[21] Lin K., et al. (2002) Relationship between p53 dysfunction, CD38 expression, and IgV(H) mutation in chronic lymphocytic leukemia. Blood 100, 1404-1409
[22] Austen B., et al. (2005) Mutations in the ATM gene lead to impaired overall and treatment-free survival that is independent of IGVH mutation status in patients with B-CLL. Blood 106, 3175-3182
[23] Winkler D., et al. (2005) Protein expression analysis of chromosome 12 candidate genes in chronic lymphocytic leukemia (CLL). Leukemia 19, 1211–1215
[24] Kalachikov S., et al. (1997) Cloning and gene mapping of the chromosome 13q14 region deleted in chronic lymphocytic leukemia. Genomics 42, 369–377
[25] Avet-Loiseau H., et al. (1999) Monosomy 13 is associated with the transition of monoclonal gammopathy of undetermined significance to multiple myeloma. Intergroupe Francophone du Myelome. Blood 94, 2583–2589
[26] Cigudosa J.C., et al. (1998) Characterization of non random chromosomal gains and losses in multiple myeloma by comparative genomic hybridization. Blood 91, 3007–3010
[27] Liu Y., et al. (1995) 13q deletions in lymphoid malignancies. Blood 86, 1911–1915
[28] Stilgenbauer S., et al. (1998) Expressed sequences as candidates for a novel tumor suppressor gene at band 13q14 in B-cell chronic lymphocytic leukemia and mantle cell lymphoma. Oncogene 16, 1891–1897
[29] Rosenwald A., et al. (1999) A biological role for deletions in chromosomal band 13q14 in mantle cell and peripheral t-cell lymphomas? Genes Chromosomes Cancer 26, 210–214
[30] Liu Y., et al. (1997) Cloning of two candidate tumor suppressor genes within a 10 kb region on chromosome 13q14, frequently deleted in chronic lymphocytic leukemia. Oncogene 15, 2463–2473
[31] Migliazza A., et al. (2001) Nucleotide sequence, transcription map, and mutation analysis of the 13q14 chromosomal region deleted in B-cell chronic lymphocytic leukemia. Blood 97, 2098–2104
[32] Calin G.A., et al. (2002) Frequent deletions and down-regulation of micro- RNA genes miR15 and miR16 at 13q14 in chronic lymphocytic leukemia. Proc Natl Acad Sci USA 99, 15524–15529.

[33] Lagos-Quintana M., et al. (2001) Identification of novel genes coding for small expressed RNAs. Science 294, 853–858
[34] Mertens D., et al. (2002) Down-regulation of candidate tumor suppressor genes within chromosome band 13q14.3 is independent of the DNA methylation pattern in B-cell chronic lymphocytic leukemia. Blood 99, 4116–4121
[35] Klein U., et al. (2010) The DLEU2/miR-15a/16-1 cluster controls B cell proliferation and its deletion leads to chronic lymphocytic leukemia. Cancer Cell 17, 28–40
[36] Calin G.A., et al. (2004) MicroRNA profiling reveals distinct signatures in B cell chronic lymphocytic leukemias. Proc Natl Acad Sci USA 101, 11755-11760
[37] Fulci V., et al. (2007) Quantitative technologies establish a novel microRNA profile of chronic lymphocytic leukemia. Blood 109, 4944-4951
[38] Marton S., et al. (2008) Small RNAs analysis in CLL reveals a deregulation of miRNA expression and novel miRNA candidates of putative relevance in CLL pathogenesis. Leukemia 22, 330-338
[39] Cimmino A., et al. (2005) miR-15 and miR-16 induce apoptosis by targeting BCL2. Proc Natl Acad Sci USA 102, 13944–13949
[40] Raveche E.S., et al. (2007) Abnormal microRNA-16 locus with synteny to human 13q14 linked to CLL in NZB mice. Blood 109, 5079–5086
[41] Linsley P.S., et al. (2007) Transcripts targeted by the microRNA-16 family cooperatively regulate cell cycle progression. Mol Cell Biol 27, 2240–2252
[42] Bandi N., et al. (2009) miR-15a and miR-16 are implicated in cell cycle regulation in a Rb-dependent manner and are frequently deleted or down-regulated in non-small cell lung cancer. Cancer Res 69, 5553–5559
[43] Liu Q., et al. (2008) miR-16 family induces cell cycle arrest by regulating multiple cell cycle genes. Nucleic Acids Res 36, 5391–5404
[44] Zhao H., et al. (2009) The c-myb proto-oncogene and microRNA-15a comprise an active autoregulatory feedback loop in human hematopoietic cells. Blood, 113, 505–516
[45] Bichi R., et al. (2002) Human chronic lymphocytic leukemia modeled in mouse by targeted TCL1 expression. Proc Natl Acad Sci USA 99, 6955–6960
[46] Yan X.J., et al. (2006) B cell receptors in TCL1 transgenic mice resemble those of aggressive, treatment resistant human chronic lymphocytic leukemia. Proc Natl Acad Sci USA 103, 11713–11718
[47] Herling M., et al. (2006) TCL1 shows a regulated expression pattern in chronic lymphocytic leukemia that correlates with molecular subtypes and proliferative state. Leukemia 20, 280–285
[48] Pekarsky Y., et al. (2006) Tcl1 expression in chronic lymphocytic leukemia is regulated by miR-29 and miR-181. Cancer Res 66, 11590–11593
[49] Klein U., et al. (2001) Gene expression profiling of B cell chronic lymphocytic leukemia reveals a homogeneous phenotype related to memory B cells. J Exp Med 194, 1625–1638
[50] Rosenwald A., et al. (2001) Relation of gene expression phenotype to immunoglobulin mutation genotype in B cell chronic lymphocytic leukemia. J Exp Med 194, 1639–1647

[51] Klein U. et al. (1998) Somatic hypermutation in normal and transformed human B cells. Immunol Rev 162, 261–280
[52] Tangye S.G., et al. (1998) Identification of functional human splenic memory B cells by expression of CD148 and CD27. J Exp Med 188, 1691–1703
[53] Vasconcelos Y. et al. (2005) Gene expression profiling of chronic lymphocytic leukemia can discriminate cases with stable disease and mutated Ig genes from those with progressive disease and unmutated Ig genes. Leukemia 19, 2002–2005
[54] Sellick G.S., et al. (2007) A high-density SNP genome-wide linkage search of 206 families identifies susceptibility loci for chronic lymphocytic leukemia. Blood 110, 3326-3333
[55] Crowther-Swanepoel D., et al. (2010) Common variants at 2q37.3, 8q24,21, 15q21,3 and 16q24.1 influence chronic lymphocytic leukemia risk. Nat Genet 42, 132-136
[56] Puente X.S., et al. (2011) Whole-genome sequencing identifies recurrent mutations in chronic lymphocytic leukaemia. Nature 475, 101-105
[57] Moreau E.J., et al. (1997) Improvement of the chronic lymphocytic leukemia scoring system with the monoclonal antibody SN8 (CD79b). Am J Clin Pathol. 108, 378-382
[58] Ternynck T., et al. (1974) Comparison of normal and CLL lymphocyte surface Ig determinants using peroxidase-labeled antibodies. I. Detection and quantitation of light chain determinants. Blood 43, 789-795
[59] Dighiero G. et al. (1976). Comparison of normal and chronic lymphocytic leukemia lymphocyte surface Ig determinants using peroxidase-labeled antibodies. II. quantification of light chain determinants in atypical lymphocytic leukemia. Blood 48, 559-566
[60] Vuillier F., et al. (2005) Lower levels of surface B-cell-receptor expression in chronic lymphocytic leukemia are associated with glycosylation and folding defects of the mu and CD79a chains. Blood 105, 2933–2940
[61] Thompson A.A., et al. (1997) Aberrations of the B-cell receptor B29 (CD79b) gene in chronic lymphocytic leukemia. Blood 90, 1387–1394
[62] Payelle-Brogard B., et al. (1999) Analysis of the B-cell receptor B29 (CD79b) gene in familial chronic lymphocytic leukemia. Blood 94, 3516–3522
[63] Alfarano A., et al. (1999) An alternatively spliced form of CD79b gene may account for altered B-cell receptor expression in B-chronic lymphocytic leukemia. Blood 93, 2327–2335
[64] Payelle-Brogard B, et al. (2002) Defective assembly of the B-cell receptor chains accounts for its low expression in B-chronic lymphocytic leukaemia. Br J Haematol 118, 976–985
[65] Payelle-Brogard B., et al. (2006) Abnormal levels of the alpha chain of the CD22 adhesion molecule may account for low CD22 surface expression in chronic lymphocytic leukemia. Leukemia 20, 877–878
[66] Michel F., et al. (1993) Defective calcium response in B-chronic lymphocytic leukemia cells: alteration of early protein tyrosine phosphorylation and of the mechanism responsible for cell calcium influx. J Immunol 150, 3624–3633

[67] Lanham S., et al. (2003) Differential signaling via surface IgM is associated with VH gene mutational status and CD38 expression in chronic lymphocytic leukemia. Blood 101, 1087-1093
[68] Pascual V., et al. (1994) Analysis of somatic mutation in five B cell subsets of human tonsil. J Exp Med 180, 329-339
[69] Schroeder H.W. Jr. and Dighiero G. (1994) The pathogenesis of chronic lymphocytic leukemia: analysis of the antibody repertoire. Immunol Today 15, 288-294
[70] Kipps T.J. and Carson D.A. (1993) Autoantibodies in chronic lymphocytic leukemia and related systemic autoimmune diseases. Blood 81, 2475-2487
[71] Chiorazzi N. and Ferrarini M. (2003) B cell chronic lymphocytic leukemia: lessons learned from studies of the B cell antigen receptor. Annu Rev Immunol 21, 841-894
[72] Hamblin T.J., et al. (1999) Unmutated Ig V(H) genes are associated with a more aggressive form of chronic lymphocytic leukemia Blood 94, 1848-1854
[73] Damle R.N., et al. (1999) Ig V gene mutation status and CD38 expression as novel prognostic indicators in chronic lymphocytic leukemia. Blood 94, 1840-1847
[74] Maloum K., et al. (2000) Expression of unmutated VH genes is a detrimental prognostic factor in chronic lymphocytic leukemia. Blood 96, 377-379.
[75] Oscier D.G., et al. (2002) Multivariate analysis of prognostic factors in CLL: clinical stage, IGVH gene mutational status, and loss or mutation of the p53 gene are independent prognostic factors. Blood 100, 1177-1184
[76] Dighiero G. (2003) Unsolved issues in CLL biology and management. Leukemia 17, 2385-2391
[77] Tobin G., et al. (2002) Somatically mutated Ig V(H)3-21 genes characterize a new subset of chronic lymphocytic leukemia. Blood 99, 2262-2264
[78] Messmer B.T., et al. (2004) Multiple distinct sets of stereotyped antigen receptors indicate a role for antigen in promoting chronic lymphocytic leukemia. J Exp Med 200, 519-525
[79] Tobin G., et al. (2003) Chronic lymphocytic leukemias utilizing the VH3-21 gene display highly restricted Vlambda2-14 gene use and homologous CDR3s: implicating recognition of a common antigen epitope. Blood 101:4952-4957
[80] Tobin G., et al. (2004) Subsets with restricted immunoglobulin gene rearrangement features indicate a role for antigen selection in the development of chronic lymphocytic leukemia. Blood 104, 2879-2885
[81] Stamatopoulos K., et al. (2007) Over 20% of patients with chronic lymphocytic leukemia carry stereotyped receptors: Pathogenetic implications and clinical correlations. Blood 109, 259-270
[82] Murray F., et al. (2008) Stereotyped patterns of somatic hypermutation in subsets of patients with chronic lymphocytic leukemia: implications for the role of antigen selection in leukemogenesis. Blood 111, 1524-1533
[83] Widhopf G.F., et al. (2004) Chronic lymphocytic leukemia B cells of more than 1% of patients express virtually identical immunoglobulins. Blood 104, 2499-2504
[84] Ghia P., el al. (2008) Microenvironmental influences in chronic lymphocytic leukaemia: the role of antigen stimulation. J Intern Med 264, 549-562

[85] Pritsch O., et al. (1993) V gene usage by seven hybrids derived from CD5+ B-cell chronic lymphocytic leukemia and displaying autoantibody activity. Blood 82, 3103-3112

[86] Herve M., et al. (2005) Unmutated and mutated chronic lymphocytic leukemias derive from self-reactive B cell precursors despite expressing different antibody reactivity. J Clin Invest 115, 1636–1643

[87] Chu C.C., et al. (2008) Chronic lymphocytic leukemia antibodies with a common stereotypic rearrangement recognize non muscle myosin heavy chain IIA. Blood 112, 5122–5129

[88] Catera R., et al. (2008) Chronic lymphocytic leukemia cells recognize conserved epitopes associated with apoptosis and oxidation. Mol Med 14, 665–674

[89] Lanemo Myhrinder A., et al. (2008) A new perspective: molecular motifs on oxidized LDL, apoptotic cells, and bacteria are targets for chronic lymphocytic leukemia antibodies. Blood 111, 3838–3848

[90] Küppers R. (2005) Mechanisms of B-cell lymphoma pathogenesis. Nat Rev Cancer 5, 251–262

[91] Chen L., et al. (2005) ZAP-70 directly enhances IgM signaling in chronic lymphocytic leukemia. Blood 105, 2036–2041

[92] Gobessi S., et al. (2007) ZAP-70 enhances B-cell-receptor signaling despite absent or inefficient tyrosine kinase activation in chronic lymphocytic leukemia and lymphoma B cells. Blood 109, 2032–2039

[93] Richardson S.J., et al. (2006) ZAP-70 expression is associated with enhanced ability to respond to migratory and survival signals in B-cell chronic lymphocytic leukemia (B-CLL). Blood 107, 3584–3592

[94] Crespo M., et al. (2006) ZAP-70 expression in normal pro/pre B cells, mature B cells, and in B cell acute lymphoblastic leukemia. Clin Cancer Res 12, 726–734

[95] Malavasi F., et al. (1994) Human CD38: a glycoprotein in search of a function. Immunol Today 15, 95–97.

[96] Deaglio S., et al. (2001) Human CD38: a (r)evolutionary story of enzymes and receptors. Leuk Res 25, 1–12

[97] Damle R.N., et al. (1999) Ig V gene mutation status and CD38 expression as novel prognostic indicators in chronic lymphocytic leukemia. Blood 94, 1840-1847

[98] Oppezzo P., et al. (2003) Chronic lymphocytic leukemia B cells expressing AID display dissociation between class switch recombination and somatic hypermutation. Blood 101, 4029–32

[99] Oppezzo P., et al. (2005) Different isoforms of BSAP regulate expression of AID in normal and chronic lymphocytic leukemia B cells. Blood 105, 2495–2503

[100] McCarthy H., et al. (2003) High expression of activation-induced cytidine deaminase (AID) and splice variants is a distinctive feature of poor prognosis chronic lymphocytic leukemia. Blood 101, 4903–4908

[101] Albesiano E., et al. (2003) Activation induced cytidine deaminase in chronic lymphocytic leukemia B cells: expression as multiple forms in a dynamic, variably sized fraction of the clone. Blood 102, 375–382

[102] Sahota S.S., et al. (2000) Somatic mutation of bcl-6 genes can occur in the absence of V(H) mutations in chronic lymphocytic leukemia. Blood 95, 3534–3540

[103] Reiniger L., et al. (2006) Richter's and prolymphocytic transformation of chronic lymphocytic leukemia are associated with high mRNA expression of activation-induced cytidine deaminase and aberrant somatic hypermutation. Leukemia 20, 1089–1095

[104] Oppezzo P., et al. (2005) The LPL/ADAM29 expression ratio is a novel prognosis indicator in chronic lymphocytic leukemia. Blood 106, 650-657

[105] Caligaris-Cappio F., and Hamblin T.J. (1999) B-cell chronic lymphocytic leukemia: a bird of a different feather. J Clin Oncol 17, 399–408

[106] Dyer M.J.S., et al. (1994) BCL2 translocations in leukemias of mature B cells. Blood 83, 3682–3688

[107] Vrhovac R., et al. (1998) Prognostic significance of the cell cycle inhibitor p27Kip1 in chronic B-cell lymphocytic leukemia. Blood 91, 4694–4700

[108] Lagneaux L., et al. (1993) Excessive production of transforming growth factor-beta by bone marrow stromal cells in B-cell chronic lymphocytic leukemia inhibits growth of hematopoietic precursors and interleukin-6 production. Blood 82, 2379–2385

[109] Caligaris-Cappio F. (2003) Role of the microenvironment in chronic lymphocytic leukaemia. Br J Haematol 123, 380–388

[110] Caligaris-Cappio F. and Ghia P. (2008) Novel insights in chronic lymphocytic leukemia: are we getting closer to understanding the pathogenesis of the disease? J Clin Oncol 26, 4497-4503

[111] [111] Caligaris-Cappio, F. (2003) Role of the microenvironment in chronic lymphocytic leukaemia. Br J Haematol 123, 380–388.

[112] Granziero L., et al. (2001) Survivin is expressed on CD40 stimulation and interfaces proliferation and apoptosis in B-cell chronic lymphocytic leukemia. Blood 97, 2777–2783

[113] Stevenson F.K. and Caligaris-Cappio F. (2004) Chronic lymphocytic leukemia: revelations from the B-cell receptor. Blood 103, 4389–4395

[114] Muzio M., et al. (2009) Expression and function of toll like receptors in chronic lymphocytic leukaemia cells. Br J Haematol 144, 507-516

[115] Deaglio S., et al. (2007) CD38/CD19: a lipid raft-dependent signaling complex in human B cells. Blood 109, 5390-5398

[116] Burger J.A., et al. (2009) High level expression of the T-cell chemokines CCL3 and CCL4 by chronic lymphocytic leukemia B cells in nurselike cell cocultures and after BCR stimulation. Blood 113, 3050-3058.

[117] Schulz A., et al. (2011) Inflammatory cytokines and signaling pathways are associated with survival of primary chronic lymphocytic leukemia cells in vitro: a dominant role of CCL2. Haematologica 96, 408-416.

[118] Xu L.L., et al. (1996) Human recombinant monocyte chemotactic protein and other C-C chemokines bind and induce directional migration of dendritic cells in vitro. J Leukoc Biol. 60, 365-371

[119] Husson H., et al. (2001) MCP-1 modulates chemotaxis by follicular lymphoma cells. Br J Haematol 115, 554-562

[120] Messmer B.T., et al. (2005) In vivo measurements document the dynamic cellular kinetics of chronic lymphocytic leukemia B cells. J Clin Invest 115, 755-764

Part 2

CLL Biology and Microenvironment

2

Microenvironment Interactions in Chronic Lymphocytic Leukemia: A Delicate Equilibrium Linking the Quiescent and the Proliferative Pool

F. Palacios[1], C. Abreu[1], P. Moreno[1],
M. Giordano[2], R. Gamberale[2] and P. Oppezzo[1,3]
[1]*Recombinant Protein Unit, Institut Pasteur de Montevideo,*
[2]*Department of Immunology, Institute for Hematologic Research, National Academy of Medicine, Buenos Aires,*
[3]*Department of Immunobiology, Faculty of Medicine, University of the Republic, Montevideo,*
Uruguay

1. Introduction

Chronic lymphocytic leukemia (CLL) is the commonest form of leukemia in Europe and North America, and mainly, though not exclusively, affects older individuals. It has a very variable course, with survival ranging from months to decades [1]. It is a neoplastic disorder, characterized by progressive accumulation of monoclonal B lymphocytes, expressing CD5 and CD23 molecules and low amounts of surface membrane Ig and CD79b molecules [2]. About one-third of patients never requires treatment, has a long survival and dies of causes unrelated to CLL; in another third an initial indolent phase is followed by progression of the disease; the remaining third of patients has aggressive disease at the onset and requires early treatment [3]

Accumulation of mature B-cells that have escaped programmed cell death and undergone cell-cycle arrest in the G0/G1 phase is the hallmark of CLL [4]. In this leukemia elevated levels of the cyclin negative regulator $p27^{Kip1}$ protein are found in a majority of patients [5]. Given the key role of this protein in cell cycle progression, the over-expression of $p27^{Kip1}$ could account for the accumulation of CLL B-cells in early phases of the cell cycle. Furthermore, it has been postulated that the survival advantage of CLL lymphocytes is also due to aberrant over-expression of antiapoptotic Bcl-2 family proteins in general [6] and Bcl-2 and Mcl-1 proteins in particular [7]. Other members of the Bcl-2 family, such as anti-apoptotic proteins BCL-XL and BAG1 are overexpressed in CLL B-cells whereas proapoptotic proteins, such as BAX and BCL-XS, are underexpressed [4]. These antiapoptotic proteins sequester pro-apoptotic counterparts and a balance between both determines the fate of a cell. Additionally, the most consistent cytogenetic lesion in CLL is chromosomal deletions of 13q14, resulting in loss of microRNAs, miR-15a and miR-16-1. Expression of these microRNAs has been founded inversely correlated to Bcl-2 expression and thus, suggested that translocation 13q14 is associated to survival of CLL B-cells [8]. These observations establish anti-apoptotic Bcl-2 family proteins as key survival factors for CLL [9].

High expression of cyclin cell cycle negative regulator $p27^{Kip1}$, antiapoptotic molecules such as Bcl-2 or Mcl-1, and a characteristic non activated phenotype of CLL B- lymphocytes (low surface immunoglobulin (Ig) expression and absence of activated lymphocyte molecules) led to the assumption that CLL disease is a leukemia resulting from accumulation rather than from proliferation. However this traditional view that CLL is a disease deriving from an inherent defect in apoptosis has being called into question [10]. Recent studies suggest that CLL is a dynamic process, comprising leukemic cells that multiply and die at measurable rates. Furthermore, since CLL cells do not appear to be inherently immortal, patient´s compromise does not occur from passive accumulation, but from active generation of subclones that over time develop dangerous genetic abnormalities which further change the birth/death ratios [10,11].

These observations have turned the attention towards the occurrence of different sub-populations inside the tumoral clone. It is clear that most, if not all, proliferative events occur in tissues where leukemic cells are able to exploit microenvironment interactions in order to avoid apoptosis and acquire tumoral growing conditions [12]. This concept is supported by reports showing that, despite their monoclonal origin, there are different subpopulations within clonal CLL B-cells [13,14 and 15].

These works which underline the presence of a proliferative B-cell subset within the tumoral clone, furnish new strength to the hypothesis that the microenvironment plays a central role in the maintenance and progression of this disease. Thus, upregulation of antiapoptotic proteins such as Survivin [16], Mcl-1, Bcl-2, as well as specific chemokines and cytokines in CLL (reviewed in [17]), like CCL2 [18], CCL3/CCL4 [19,20] CXCR4–CXCL12 [21], and IL-4 [22] among others, support a process of activation and reinforcement of the malignant cells by the microenvironment. These key interactions provide survival signals to the leukemic cells leading to the progression and treatment resistance of the tumoral clone. Therefore, the development and design of therapeutic agents with the goal of disrupting the crosstalk between malignant B cells and their microenvironment is an attractive novel strategy in the treatment of CLL, a heterogeneous disease that as yet remains incurable.

In this chapter we will compile the available evidence related to the main B-cell/microenvironment interactions responsible to maintain a CLL proliferative subset. We will discuss the present knowledge about the proliferative B-cell subsets and how they are preserved within the tumoral CLL clone.

2. Role of the microenvironment in CLL-B cell survival

All the physiological processes during which B-cells encounter their antigen (Ag) occur in specific anatomical sites so-called "specialized microenvironments". Germinal centers are the typical immunological picture of these activation places. In this environment B-cell stimulation is totally dependent on complex supportive interactions with both Ag-specific and Ag-non-specific accessory populations. T cells and a variety of different types of adherent cells, generally defined as 'stromal cells', are the main elements of this microenvironment.

In CLL disease, the proliferating compartment is represented by focal aggregates of proliferating prolymphocytes and para-immunoblasts that give rise to the called pseudo-follicles or proliferation centres [23]. Pseudo-follicles are the histological CLL hallmark in lymph nodes (LN), splenic white pulp and bone marrow (BM) where they appear as vaguely nodular areas never surrounded by a mantle zone. These areas are usually infiltrated with an important number of CLL B-cells that after interaction with T-cells and/or stromal/follicular dendritic cells, are able to express the proliferation marker Ki-67 and the progression disease molecules such as CD38 [24] and CD49d [25].

The general observation that CLL B-cells rapidly dye by apoptosis after culture in the absence of accessory cells strongly indicate that CLL B-cells maintain their capacity to respond to selected external stimuli that confer to leukemic cells a growth advantage and an extended survival. Furthermore, numerous *in-vitro* evidence indicate a predominant role of the microenvironment in CLL cell survival [26].

T lymphocytes, the bone marrow stromal cells, and the follicular dendritic cells are involved in the natural history of the disease and appear to be major players in delivering key signals for the proliferation of tumoral clone and disease progression [27]. The exposure of malignant cell subclones to microenvironmental stimuli results in increased proliferation, a prerequisite for the occurrence of new genetic abnormalities that lead to the development of a more aggressive disease.

The pattern of tissue infiltration by CLL cells may be variable. More frequently, malignant cells are seen only or predominantly in the peripheral blood (PB) and the BM. In some instances a vast LN involvement is observed together with a modest PB involvement. These clinical observations point to the existence of mechanisms that selectively control the trafficking and homing of malignant lymphocytes to distinct microenvironments. One such mechanism might be accounted by chemokines and chemokine receptors. Recent data indicate that CLL cells may express specific sets of chemokine receptors and/or respond to specific chemokines produced by microenvironmental elements that selectively attract individual cells to explicit anatomical sites [17].

Chemokines constitute a growing family of chemotactic cytokines that are generally involved in leukocyte migration. According to a current classification based on their function, they are subdivided into three different groups: (1) the homeostatic chemokines regulating lymphocyte migration and homing processes under physiological conditions, (2) the inducible chemokines expressed during inflammation and (3) an overlapping group involved in both processes. Their expression can be induced by various stimuli, including growth factors and inflammatory cytokines. Besides these general aspects, chemokines are also associated to a variety of pathological processes. During tumourigenesis, they are known to play a crucial role informing and modifying the tumour stroma by inducing the infiltration of various hematopoietic cells (e.g.macrophages, natural killer (NK) cells, eosinophils, B and T lymphocytes) as well as fibroblasts and endothelial cells. They also contribute to the neovascularisation, the growth and the spreading of tumours [17].

2.1 Role of T-cells in the CLL microenvironment

The peripheral T-cell repertoire in CLL is significantly altered with a marked increase in oligoclonality in both CD4 and CD8 positive cells [28]. A multitude of *in-vitro* findings indicate that T lymphocytes are attractive candidates to play a role in the inhibition of the malignant B-cell apoptosis and to favour disease progression [29,30]. The weight of evidence points to a dialogue between malignant CLL B-cells and $CD4^{pos}$ T-cells, based upon bidirectional interactions that are regulated by adhesion molecules and chemokines and translate into the production of several cytokines by both cell types (reviewed by [26]). T-cell cytokines, including IL-4, IFN-γ, and IL-2 inhibit CLL B-cell apoptosis by upregulating Bcl-2 protein, reinforcing the concept that the ability of CLL cell to avoid apoptosis may be strongly influenced by external stimuli provided by the microenvironment [26].

Within pseudofollicular proliferation centers, proliferating leukemic lymphocytes are in contact with numerous CD3^{pos} T-cells, most of which are CD4^{pos}, and express CD40L, which can support the growth of CLL B-cells through CD40 ligation. CD40 is a member of the tumour necrosis factor (TNF) receptor superfamily that is expressed by B-cells, dendritic cells and monocytes [31]. The stimulation of CD40 and interleukin 4 (IL-4) rescues CLL B-cells from apoptosis and induces their proliferation [32]. Moreover, CD40 crosslinking on CLL B-cells induces up-regulation of CD80 and CD54 and turns nonimmunogenic CLL cells into effective T-cell stimulators [33]. Later studies of Granziero *et al.* have shown that this proliferative CLL B-cells activated through CD40 also express survivin, a member of the family protein of inhibitor of apoptosis, (IAPs) [16]. This protein is the only IAP whose expression is induced in CLL B-cells by CD40L. The survivin positive cells have an extended survival, an increased proliferative rate and retain Bcl-2 positivity.

It is unclear why and how CD4^{pos} T-cells that gather in CLL pseudo-follicles are activated. Under normal circumstances, CD4^{pos} T-cells that cooperate with B lymphocytes in primary follicles recognize the antigenic peptide in the context of MHC-II class molecules (peptide MHCII binds to T cell receptor, TCR). This interaction results in the transient up-regulation of CD40L. However, T-cells in CLL patients exhibit defective immunological synapse formation which may account for the defects in T-cell helper function seen in earlier studies [30]. Whatever causes their activation, CD40L^{pos} T-cells are in close physical contact with CD40^{pos} CLL within proliferation centers [24]; hence the physiological stimulus provided by CD40L is available to malignant B-cells. Subsequent research has shown that these activated CD4^{pos} T-cells tend to assemble in pseudo-follicles attracted by the chemokines, CCL17 and CCL22 [22] and CCL3 and CCL4 [19,20] produced by proliferating CLL B-cells themselves, (Figure 1A).

In regard to CCL17 and CCL22, it is interesting that leukemic cells purified from LN and BM, but not from PB, constitutively express mRNA for both of them. The CD40-crosslinking of PB CLL cells induces the expression of these chemokines at RNA level [22]. Of them, CCL22 is released and is capable of attracting activated CD4^{pos} /CD40L^{pos} T-cells, while CCL17 is released only when IL-4 is added to the *in-vitro* system [16] (Figure 1A).

3. Role of stromal cells in the CLL microenvironment

T cells are not the only active responsible partners for leukemic B-cells. A number of adherent accessory cells present in different microenvironments are gaining increasing attention in the last years in the CLL progression. It has been convincingly demonstrated that a direct physical contact between BM stromal cells and leukaemic cells extends the survival of CLL B-cell [34]. Stromal cells are key regulators of normal B lymphopoiesis. However, even if they are known to provide binding sites and growth factors to developing B-cells, the precise nature of ligand–receptor interactions are not fully known. The interest has been initially focused upon adhesion molecules. *In-vitro*, it has been shown that malignant CLL B-cells interact with BM stromal cells via β1 and β2 integrins [34]. This binding rescues CLL cells from apoptosis and extends their lifespan, suggesting a potential mechanism for the preferential *in-vivo* accumulation and survival of CLL cells within the BM.

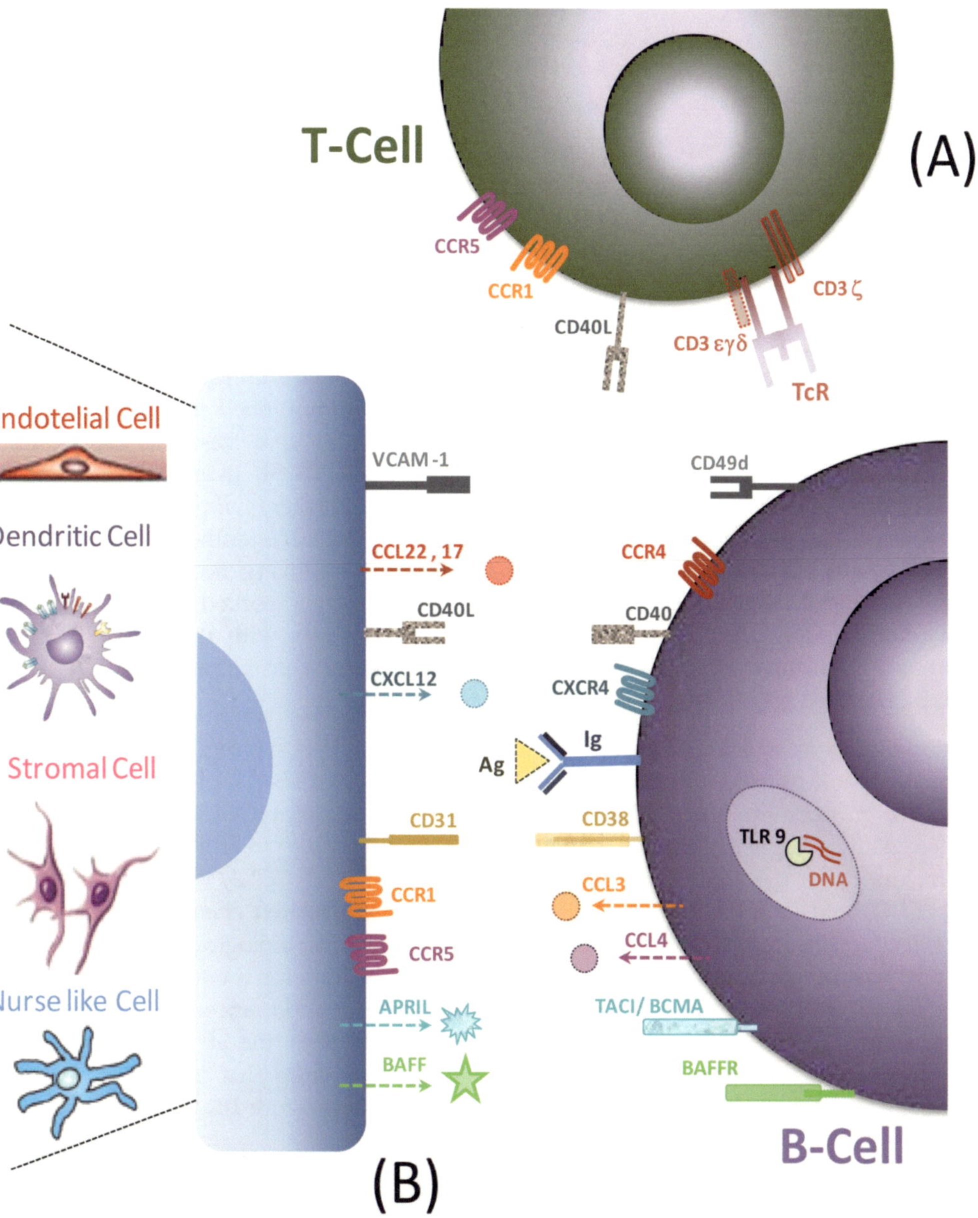

Fig. 1. The microenvironment stimuli on CLL B-cells . Main signaling interactions regulating the survival and the proliferation of leukemic clone. A) T-cells signals to CLL B-cells. B) Endothelial, dendritic and nurse like cells signals to CLL B-cells.

The PB of CLL patients has been shown to contain cells that *in-vitro* can differentiate into adherent nurse-like cells, endowed with the capacity of protecting the attached leukaemic B-cells from spontaneous apoptosis [21]. Blood-derived nurse cells protect CLL B-cells from apoptosis by utilizing a mechanism dependent on SDF-1 (CXCL12), a CXC chemokine that is constitutively secreted by BM stromal cells and regulates B lymphopoiesis upon binding its receptor CXCR4 (CD184). CXCR4 is consistently over expressed by CLL B-cells [21]. In this sense, a recent work of Vaisitti et al., clearly shows that CD38 synergizes with the CXCR4 pathway supporting the working hypothesis that migration is a central step in disease progression and that expression of CD38 is correlated to this expression [35].

Using gene expression profiles comparing $CD38^{pos}/CD49d^{pos}$ versus $CD38^{neg}/CD49d^{neg}$ CLL B-cells, Zucchetto *et al.* [19] showed an over expression of the CCL3 and CCL4 chemokines in leukemic cells from the $CD38^{pos}/CD49d^{pos}$ subset. CCL3 and CCL4 are up-regulated by CD38 engagement in $CD38^{pos}/CD49d^{pos}$ CLL B-cells and also CCL3 was found to be expressed by CLL B-cells from bone marrow biopsies (BMB) of $CD38^{pos}/CD49d^{pos}$ but not $CD38^{neg}/CD49d^{neg}$ cases. High levels of CCR1 and, to a lesser extent, CCR5, the receptors for CCL3 and CCL4, were found in CLL-derived monocyte-macrophages. Consistently, CCL3 induced monocyte migration and CD68+ macrophage infiltration was particularly high in BMB from $CD38^{pos}/CD49d^{pos}$ CLL B-cells. Conditioned media from CCL3-stimulated macrophages induced endothelial cells to express vascular cell adhesion molecule-1 (VCAM1), the CD49d ligand, likely through TNF-α over production. These effects were apparent in BMB from $CD38^{pos}/CD49d^{pos}$ CLL, where lymphoid infiltrates were characterized by a prominent meshwork of VCAM-1+ stromal/endothelial cells. It appears that the CD31/CD38/ZAP-70 axis may represent a point of convergence of proliferative and migratory signals. CD38/CD31 interactions are followed by a marked upregulation of the semaphorin family member CD100, which in turn interacts with the plexin B1 ligand expressed by stromal cells and contributes to further sustain proliferation and survival of CLL B-cells [36].

Underlying the role of stromal cells in the CLL survival signals, a recent work of Zuchetto et al., show that T-cells do not emerge as relevant players in CCL3/CCL4-driven dynamics in CLL BM microenvironment. Rather, this work proposes that CCL3/CCL4 chemokines preferentially target monocytes/macrophages, which are recruited by this/these chemokine/s, in the context of microenvironmental sites of CCL3/CLL4-producing CLL [19]. CCL3 and CCL4 are small (8–10 kDa), structurally related chemokines that, under normal conditions, are secreted by mature hematopoietic cells. Biologically, CCL3 and CCL4 have overlapping effects and act as potent chemoattractants for monocyte, macrophages, dendritic, T, and natural killer cells [37]. Highlighting the importance of the expression of these chemokines in CLL progression, a recent work of Sivina *et al.*, proposes CCL3 chemokine as a novel prognostic marker in CLL, suggesting that its evaluation might become useful for risk-assessment in patients with CLL [38] (Figure 1B).

Leukemic CLL B-cells are not only exposed to signals delivered by accessory, non-malignant cells in the lymphoid tissues, but they are also capable of sensing pathogen associated molecular patterns through a variety of membrane or cytosolic receptors. Toll-like receptors (TLR) are probably the best characterized. TLR7 and TLR9, which recognize single stranded RNA and bacterial DNA respectively, are virtually always expressed (Figure 1). Other evidence which reinforces the importance of the microenvironment on the survival of B-cells came from Decker *et al.* These authors have been shown that stimulation of CLL B-cells with an analog of bacterial DNA (CpG -ODN) induces the expression of cyclin D2 and cyclin D3 and reduces the expression of p27-kip1 associated with cell cycling. Both cyclins were associated with cdk4, which is the catalytic partner of D-type cyclins in normal B cells. Moreover, immune complexes consisting of cyclin D2-cdk4 or cyclin D3-cdk4 were both functional and phosphorylated the RB protein *in-vitro* [39].

Finally, not only signals delivered by stromal cells appear to be essential in the microenvironment crosstalk with the leukemic B lymphocyte. Cytokine array and enzyme-linked immunosorbent assay studies revealed increased expression of soluble CD14 by monocytes in the presence of CLL B-cells. This work shows that monocytes help in the survival of CLL B-cells by secreting soluble CD14, which induces nuclear factor κ β activation in these cells [40].

Overall, these data provide a link between microenvironmental factors and the proliferation/apoptosis dilemma of CLL B-cells. CLL is now revealing itself to be an environment-dependent hematological malignancy. This idea could be in agreement with a model of selective survival of certain clonal submembers, which would receive survival signals in these particular lymphoid sites.

3.1 Other microenvironment soluble factors involved in CLL progression

Several works in the last years, display the importance of soluble factor regulating the balance between stability and progression of this disease. It is known that CLL B-cells themselves can secrete pro-angiogenic factors such as vascular endothelial growth factor (VEGF) and angiopoietin (Ang) which are involved in the formation of new blood vessels. These newly formed vessels are characterized by increased permeability, and thus contribute to disease dissemination [12]. CLL B-cells can also express receptors for some of these pro-angiogenetic factors, including VEGF receptors VEGFR1 and 2 as well as the Ang-receptor. Signaling through these receptors significantly prolongs cell survival [41]. Additionally, it has been described that thioredoxin (Trx) is expressed in LN of CLL patients and that this expression can increase the CLL survival clone. In this work, the authors found that adding Trx at CLL B-cells increased in a dose-dependent fashion the release of TNF-α, which has been suggested to be an autocrine growth factor for these cells. Secretion of TNF-α maintained Bcl-2, and diminish the apoptosis in the CLL B-cells. [42].

4. Proliferative pool in CLL

It is well established that CLL is a heterogeneous disease: some patients experience a slowly progressive clinical course, but most will eventually enter an advanced phase requiring repeated treatment. Different groups have suggested that cytoskeletal organization, cellular adhesion and the migratory potential of the leukemic clone regulate tissue distribution of CLL cells, possibly influencing a patient's outcome [43,44]. This highlights the significance of topographical issues in disease progression and provides convincing evidence that CLL B-cells with enhanced motility are associated with aggressive disease. Independent confirmation of these results comes from data generated in patients, showing that a significant proportion of the leukemic clone proliferates and that proliferation occurs predominantly in lymphoid organs.

Messmer and col. clearly demonstrate that a proliferative compartment exists in CLL, [11] although major part probably resides in the solid tissues [14]. Further, it is self-evident that the accumulated CLL B-cells in the PB are constantly nourished by an upstream proliferation cell compartment. It is reasonable to assume that the balance between the two compartments may be at the bases of the highly variable clinical course of CLL, which may behave as a stable and indolent monoclonal lymphocytosis, or as an aggressive disease.

At present, two proliferative subsets related to disease progression has been described in CLL. Chiorazzi´s group proposed that the subset CD38 positive/Ki67 positive CLL B-cells could be a proliferative pool in this disease [14]. Additionally a recent work of Palacios *et al.*, also describe a proliferative subset in UM CLL patients characterized by the presence of active class switch recombination process and anomalous expression of the Activation-Induced cytidine Deaminase (AID) enzyme [15].

4.1 Proliferative CD38 positive CLL B-cells

Despite the large number of surface markers described in the CLL, the expression of CD38 and its association with the disease has been intensively studied. CD38 is accepted as a dependable marker of unfavorable prognosis and as an indicator of activation and possibly proliferation of CLL cells at the time of analysis. Leukemic clones with higher numbers of CD38 positive cells are more responsive to BCR signaling and are characterized by enhanced migration. *In-vitro* activation through CD38 drives CLL proliferation and chemotaxis, via activation of a signaling pathway that includes ZAP-70 and ERK1/2. *In-vivo* interaction of CD38 with CD31, its cognate receptor, have an important role in cell-cell interactions activating survival pathways in normal and leukemic lymphocytes [45].

An important work of Chiorazzi´s group highlights the cell-cycling status of CLL cells, focusing on those leukemic cells expressing CD38 [14]. In order to going deeper in this area Pepper *et al.* extended these observations by comparing gene profile of $CD38^{pos}$ and $CD38^{neg}$ CLL B-cells of a single patients. The results showed that $CD38^{pos}$ CLL cells possess a distinct gene expression profile compared with their $CD38^{neg}$ sub-clones. $CD38^{pos}$ CLL B-cells relatively overexpress vascular endothelial growth factor (VEGF), which is associated with increased expression of the anti-apoptotic protein Mcl-1 [13]. Detailed characterization of the proliferating CLL B-cell convincingly demonstrated a close association between CD38 expression and increased percentages of Ki-67 and ZAP-70 positive cells, suggesting that $CD38^{pos}$ clonal members are more highly activated and prone to enter the cell cycle than their negative counterpart [13].

However, further studies of the same laboratory failed to establish a strong correlation between the percentage of $CD38^{pos}$ proliferating cells in CLL clones and survival and disease progression [46]. The fact that CD38 is expressed in a high percentage of tumoral cells in UM patients indicate that $CD38^{pos}$ leukemic cells constitute a heterogeneous population including a small fraction of cells with an increased proliferative potential. Results from Messmer *et al.* show that leukemic CLL proliferating rates range from 0.08% to 1.7% [11] suggesting that not all CD38 positive cells, are proliferating.

The scenario outlined by these data indicates that the CD38pos cells subpopulation involve a discrete and small subset of cells, also CD38 positive, that have recently exited a solid tissue, and have received freshly proliferation signals.

4.2 Proliferative AID positive CLL B-cells

Recent evidences from our group outline the importance of another cellular subset, characterized by an anomalous expression of the mutagenic molecule AID in a proliferative leukemic clone [15]. This protein is a B cell–restricted enzyme, induced principally through the contact of T and B-cells via CD40-CD40L interactions, despite that recent works also show that the innate immune response via TLR receptor is able to trigger their expression [47]. The physiological expression of this enzyme is responsible for somatic hypermutation (HMS) and class switch recombination (CSR) process in B lymphocytes [48]. However, the mutational activity of AID identifies this enzyme as the first genome mutator in humans with oncogenic potential [49]. Supporting this view, different works report that constitutive AID expression is associated with a loss in the target specificity and with lymphoproliferative disorders [49,50].

In the CLL disease we have reported that AID is anomalous expressed in the PB of some patients with UM VH genes, active CSR and clinical poor outcome [51]. Despite expression of a functional AID as assessed by an active CSR and mutations induced in the preswitch region, CLL B-cells in these patients did not succeed to achieve the SHM process [52]. Although clonal CSR has been described in CLL B-cells long ago [53,54] and different works have shown that this process occurs principally in patients with UM disease [52,55], the origin and the biologic implications of this subpopulation in the physiopathology of CLL remain elusive.

Because AID expression in CLL is associated with ongoing CSR in patients with UM disease, we investigated the relation of AID expression, CSR process, and microenvironment activation in the PB of CLL patients with different clinical profiles. Our results show that high expression of AID is almost exclusively restricted to the subpopulation of tumoral B-cells having an active CSR process (IgGpos CLL B-cells). This subset expresses high levels of proliferation and antiapoptotic molecules such as Ki-67, c-*Myc*, and Bcl-2. In addition, this particular subset of leukemic cells display high levels of CD49d and CCL3/CCL4 chemokines, as well as a decreased expression of cell cycle inhibitor p27-kip1 compared with their quiescent counterpart IgM B-cells. Finally, the presence of this subpopulation in patients with UM CLL is closely related to an aggressive course of the disease [15]. Additionally to this, over-expression of anti-apoptotic and proliferative molecules as well as expression of molecules implicated in the microenvironment interactions has also been established. Thus, this tumoral CLL subset appears to be a hallmark of a recent contact with an activated microenvironment exclusively found in UM CLL patients with a poor clinical outcome [15].

It is difficult to determine the precise role of these highly proliferating activated tumoral B-cells. Since the presence of this subset is clearly associated to poor prognosis, it might have an adjuvant role in the maintenance of the CLL proliferative pool. However, given their increased proliferative potential they should normally outnumber the IgMpos cells and this is not the case. Thus, we could assume that these cells should undergo apoptosis once leaving the pseudo-follicles. A recent work suggesting a link between AID expression and B-cell apoptosis in GC favour this view [56]. In these conditions, the IgG^{pos} subset could reflect the existence of an active microenvironment leading to permanent stimulation of the IgM^{pos} pool, which would be turn on the CSR machinery maintaining this IgG^{pos} subset in the PB. Alternatively, an adjuvant role in the maintenance of the CLL IgM proliferative pool by this subset could be considered. Recently, evidence indicates that outside the GC, there is a fraction of AID^{pos} B-cells subset of interfollicular large B-lymphocyte and in the thymic medullae of tonsils [57]. Interestingly, these AID positive B-cells ongoing CSR form prominent cytoplasmic extensions, lending them to a "dendritic cell-like" appearance [57]. In this respect, unpublished results from our laboratory indicate that *in-vitro* stimulation with CD40L/IL-4 not only induces B-cells to proliferate, but also activates lymphocytes to adopt a morphological aspect of "pseudo-dendritic" cells expressing B-cell markers. If the stimulation through CD40L or other stimulation molecules are able to induce these "pseudo-dendritic" cells to become efficient antigen presenting cells remains elusive yet. Whatever the case, the hypothesis that in the UM subgroup stimulation of BCR takes place by an unknown auto-antigen [27,58] and that this is responsible for consecutives stimulations sustaining survival/expansion signals in the tumoral clone, results an interesting issue highlighted by these results.

In this context, we hypothesize that the survival signals of this AID^{pos} CLL B-cells subset could be constitutively triggered by the recognition of an autoantigen present in LN and/or BM (figure 2). In order to explain, why an active AID^{pos} tumor clone is unable to carry out the SHM process, we propose that an unidentified cofactor of AID is absent in the AID^{pos}, UM CLL subset. The correct expression of both, AID and its cofactor, enables the leukemic clone to achieve the SHM process. Once mutated, the clone loses its ability to recognize the autoantigen and, consequently it loses the possibility to receive pro-survival and proliferative signals (figure 2 panel A). In contrast, the expression of AID in the absence of its cofactor prevents BCR mutations, allowing a persistent interaction of the leukemic cells with the autoantigen (figure 2 panel B). The positive signaling through the BCR together with pro-survival and proliferative factors from the microenvironment leads to the accumulation of CLL B-cells and the progression of the disease. The high proliferation rate, the over-expression of AID and other factors, could favor DNA translocations and oncogenic mutations finally associated with progressive and refractory disease (figure 2 panel B).

Inhibition of apoptosis may occur *in-vivo* in pseudo-follicles observed in the lymph nodes, and in the cell clusters described in the bone marrow. These pseudo-follicles include proliferating B-cells in close contact with increased numbers of CD4 T-cells expressing CD40L, which is necessary for AID expression. These activated CD4 T-cells could be recruited by tumor B-cells through the expression of T cell–attracting chemokines such as CCL17 and CCL22 [22] and/or CCL3 and CCL4 [20]. Besides this, the CD38 and CD49d proteins appear to be important additional players interacting with nurse-like cells, stromal, and endothelial cells to complete the activation pathway within the proliferative centers [19]. Overall, these observations favor the view that certain cellular subsets in CLL could receive survival signals in the specific microenvironments, increasing their proliferative potential and consequently associated with a more aggressive disease.

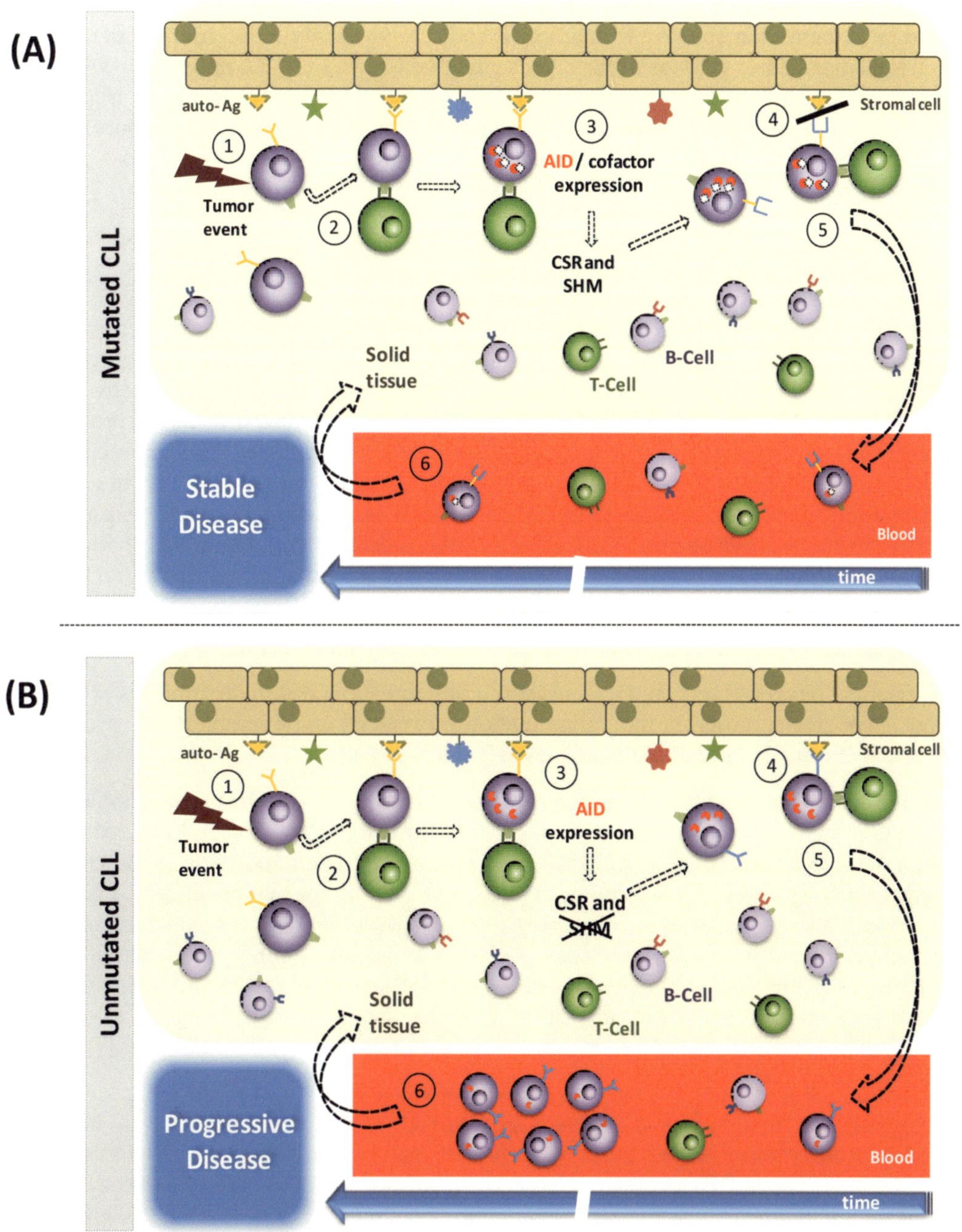

Fig. 2. Anomalous AID expression in UM CLL patients: potential role of autoantigen in the progression diseases.

The survival signals of the proliferative AID^{pos} CLL B-cells subset could be constitutively triggered by the recognition of an autoantigen (auto-Ag) present in LN and/or BM.

In the mutated cases we propose that after an unknown tumor event (1), the tumoral B-cell could be recognize an auto-Ag through BCR and receive collaboration from other cells such as T follicular helper cells or antigen-presenting cell (APC) (2). At this level proliferation centers could be initiated and after this activation the tumor clone might trigger AID expression and its unknown partners in order to achieve SHM and CSR (3) Once mutated the VDJ regions of BCR, the leukemic clone loses its ability to recognize the auto-Ag (4) and, consequently also loses the possibility to receive survival and proliferative signals.

In UM patients, panel B, tumor event occurs in a B-cell (1), BCR of this leukemic cell recognizes the auto-Ag and is induced to proliferate with the help of another T-cells or APC. (2) The leukemic clone expresses AID and their partners, but not the specific cofactor necessary to achieve a correct SHM process (3). Constitutive AID expression in this scenario only is able to trigger CSR, but it cannot mutate the VDJ region of BCR (4). This persistent activation of the leukemic clone leads to the existence of this proliferative subset IgG^{pos}/AID^{pos}. The increasing number of these leukemic, switched cells in the proliferative centers leds to the leukemic cells extravasation to peripheral blood (5). These circulating cells might home to solid tissues eventually and thus, they would receive proliferation/survival signals again (6). Cycles of these last two events overtime, produce an increase in the number of proliferating AID^{pos} CLL B-cells (detectable in peripheral blood), which is considered as a hallmark of a proliferative and progressive leukemia.

5. Inflammation role in an activated CLL microenvironment

The relationship between antigen stimulation/inflammation and the natural history of CLL is not surprising considering that inflammation is involved in the initiation and progression of several chronic lymphoid malignancies of B-cell type [59].

Chronic inflammation and CLL are inter-related in many aspects. The malfunctioning of the immune system helps the first few cancer cells to establish into a full-fledged CLL. In comparison to normal B-cells, leukemic cells are rescued from apoptosis by bone-marrow stromal cells, signifying the selectivity of microenvironment for malignant cells. Compelling evidences show us that CLL progression is originated in an inflammatory microenvironment in which many cells (T-cells, stromal cells, monocytes, macrophage and dendritic cells) are all able to delivered survival signals supporting the tumoral clone. These microenvironmental responses are often brought about by the interplay of different chemokines, cytokines, transcriptional factors or post-translational modifications [9].

The inflammatory chemokines are expressed in inflamed tissues and signal for recruitment of neutrophils. On the other hand, homeostatic chemokines produced constitutively in distinct tissue microenvironments to sustain traffic of mature lymphocytes in lymphoid and nonlymphoid tissues [17]. Despite the protective function it has on the CLL B-cells through apoptosis inhibition this factor also allows the spontaneous migration of malignant cells towards BM stromal cells, suggesting that CLL B-cells may utilize this mechanism to infiltrate the BM [21]. SDF-1 and other chemokines such as CCL3 and CCL4 secreted proteins, appear to form a pro-survival circuitry by regulating leukocyte trafficking, extravagating into sites of tissue inflammation and maintaining extended lymphocyte survival [19].

Cytokines are signaling key mediators of inflammation or an immune response, involved in accelerating inflammation and also are present in high levels in CLL patients. They are classified as pro-inflammatory (IL1, IL6, IL15, IL17, IL23 and TNF-α [61,62]), or anti-inflammatory (IL4, IL10, IL13, transforming growth factor(TGFβ) and TNF-α depending on their function in tumorigenesis [60]). Another work, recently performed by Schulz *et al.* [61] touch upon the issue of inflammatory cytokines and signaling pathways associated with CLL survival. Consistent with this possibility inflamatory cytokines genes are upregulated in this work. Among these genes chemokine (C-C motif) ligand 2 (CCL2) was shown to be induced in monocytes by the presence of CLL cells *in- vitro*.

In addition to chemokines and cytokines, the key mediators of inflammation-induced cancer include activation of transcription factors. There are a wide range of transcriptional factors that bind to the promoter region of target genes and activate transcription of these oncogenes. Aberrant expression of the transcription factors like MYC, STAT and NF-kB are associated to inflammatory immune response but also in carcinogenesis and poor prognosis in CLL [62].

The fact that inflammatory receptors such as Toll-like receptors (TLR) can be engaged concomitantly with the BCR, it becomes reasonable to presume that TLR may also play a role in BCR co-stimulation of CLL cells. Indeed, bacterial lipopeptides protect CLL cells from spontaneous apoptosis mediated by TLR signaling [63]. On the other hand, post-translational modifications may affect the activity and longevity of the proteins anti- and pro-apoptotic proteins in an inflammatory microenvironment. Bcl-2 protein undergoes phosphorylation at sites Thr56, Thr69, Ser70, Thr74 and Ser87 in response to different stimuli [64]. Taken together, the extracellular signals from cytokines and chemokines, the contribution of transcriptional factors and post-translational modifications on anti-apoptotic proteins ultimately form a complex network to deliver microenvironmental support to the malignant cells [9].

6. Conclusion

Important progress resulting in high levels of clinical and even molecular remissions has been recently achieved in CLL treatment. However, CLL remains an incurable disease. Compelling evidence suggests that crosstalk with accessory cells in specialized tissue microenvironments, such as the BM and secondary lymphoid organs, favours disease progression by promoting malignant B-cell growth and drug resistance. We are starting to understand which genes, molecules and accessory cells are involved in CLL B-cell/microenvironment interactions and what roles they play. Nevertheless, we need a more proper knowledge about the signals received and/or transmitted by CLL B-lymphocyte, interacting with T lymphocytes, and/or with stromal, endothelial, dendritic and nurse-like cells in the particular CLL microenvironment. Therefore, understanding the crosstalk between malignant B-cells and their milieu could give us new keys in the cellular and molecular biology of CLL that can finally lead to novel strategies in the treatment of this disease.

7. References

[1] Dighiero, G. and Hamblin, T.J. (2008) Chronic lymphocytic leukaemia. *Lancet* 371 (9617), 1017-1029

[2] Dighiero, G. (2003) Unsolved issues in CLL biology and management. *Leukemia* 17 (12), 2385-2391

[3] Vasconcelos, Y. et al. (2003) Binet's staging system and VH genes are independent but complementary prognostic indicators in chronic lymphocytic leukemia. *J Clin Oncol* 21 (21), 3928-3932

[4] Caligaris-Cappio, F. and Hamblin, T.J. (1999) B-cell chronic lymphocytic leukemia: a bird of a different feather. *J Clin Oncol* 17 (1), 399-408

[5] Vrhovac, R. et al. (1998) Prognostic significance of the cell cycle inhibitor p27Kip1 in chronic B-cell lymphocytic leukemia. *Blood* 91 (12), 4694-4700

[6] Krajewski, S. et al. (1995) Immunohistochemical analysis of Mcl-1 protein in human tissues. Differential regulation of Mcl-1 and Bcl-2 protein production suggests a unique role for Mcl-1 in control of programmed cell death in vivo. *Am J Pathol* 146 (6), 1309-1319

[7] Opferman, J.T. et al. (2003) Development and maintenance of B and T lymphocytes requires antiapoptotic MCL-1. *Nature* 426 (6967), 671-676

[8] Cimmino, A. et al. (2005) miR-15 and miR-16 induce apoptosis by targeting BCL2. *Proc Natl Acad Sci U S A* 102 (39), 13944-13949

[9] Chen, L.S. et al. (2010) Inflammation and survival pathways: chronic lymphocytic leukemia as a model system. *Biochem Pharmacol* 80 (12), 1936-1945

[10] Chiorazzi, N. (2007) Cell proliferation and death: forgotten features of chronic lymphocytic leukemia B cells. *Best Pract Res Clin Haematol* 20 (3), 399-413

[11] Messmer, B.T. et al. (2005) In vivo measurements document the dynamic cellular kinetics of chronic lymphocytic leukemia B cells. *J Clin Invest* 115 (3), 755-764

[12] Deaglio, S. and Malavasi, F. (2009) Chronic lymphocytic leukemia microenvironment: shifting the balance from apoptosis to proliferation. *Haematologica* 94 (6), 752-756

[13] Pepper, C. et al. (2007) Highly purified CD38+ and CD38- sub-clones derived from the same chronic lymphocytic leukemia patient have distinct gene expression signatures despite their monoclonal origin. *Leukemia* 21 (4), 687-696

[14] Damle, R.N. et al. (2007) CD38 expression labels an activated subset within chronic lymphocytic leukemia clones enriched in proliferating B cells. *Blood* 110 (9), 3352-3359

[15] Palacios, F. et al. (2010) High expression of AID and active class switch recombination might account for a more aggressive disease in unmutated CLL patients: link with an activated microenvironment in CLL disease. *Blood* 115 (22), 4488-4496

[16] Granziero, L. et al. (2001) Survivin is expressed on CD40 stimulation and interfaces proliferation and apoptosis in B-cell chronic lymphocytic leukemia. *Blood* 97 (9), 2777-2783

[17] Burger, J.A. (2010) Chemokines and chemokine receptors in chronic lymphocytic leukemia (CLL): from understanding the basics towards therapeutic targeting. *Semin Cancer Biol* 20 (6), 424-430

[18] Schulz, A. et al. (2010) Inflammatory cytokines and signaling pathways are associated with survival of primary chronic lymphocytic leukemia cells in vitro: a dominant role of CCL2. *Haematologica*

[19] Zucchetto, A. et al. (2009) CD38/CD31, the CCL3 and CCL4 chemokines, and CD49d/vascular cell adhesion molecule-1 are interchained by sequential events sustaining chronic lymphocytic leukemia cell survival. *Cancer Res* 69 (9), 4001-4009

[20] Burger, J.A. et al. (2009) High-level expression of the T-cell chemokines CCL3 and CCL4 by chronic lymphocytic leukemia B cells in nurselike cell cocultures and after BCR stimulation. *Blood* 113 (13), 3050-3058

[21] Burger, J.A. et al. (2000) Blood-derived nurse-like cells protect chronic lymphocytic leukemia B cells from spontaneous apoptosis through stromal cell-derived factor-1. *Blood* 96 (8), 2655-2663

[22] Ghia, P. et al. (2002) Chronic lymphocytic leukemia B cells are endowed with the capacity to attract CD4+, CD40L+ T cells by producing CCL22. *Eur J Immunol* 32 (5), 1403-1413
[23] Lennert, K. et al. (1978) Malignant Lymphomas Other than Hodgkin's Disease. *Springer-Verlag*, 119-129
[24] Patten, P.E. et al. (2008) CD38 expression in chronic lymphocytic leukemia is regulated by the tumor microenvironment. *Blood* 111 (10), 5173-5181
[25] Gattei, V. et al. (2008) Relevance of CD49d protein expression as overall survival and progressive disease prognosticator in chronic lymphocytic leukemia. *Blood* 111 (2), 865-873
[26] Caligaris-Cappio, F. (2003) Role of the microenvironment in chronic lymphocytic leukaemia. *Br J Haematol* 123 (3), 380-388
[27] Ghia, P. et al. (2008) Microenvironmental influences in chronic lymphocytic leukaemia: the role of antigen stimulation. *J Intern Med* 264 (6), 549-562
[28] Rezvany, M.R. et al. (2003) Leukemia-associated monoclonal and oligoclonal TCR-BV use in patients with B-cell chronic lymphocytic leukemia. *Blood* 101 (3), 1063-1070
[29] Borge, M. et al. (2010) CXCL12-induced chemotaxis is impaired in T cells from ZAP-70-chronic lymphocytic leukemia patients. *Haematologica*
[30] Ramsay, A.G. et al. (2008) Chronic lymphocytic leukemia T cells show impaired immunological synapse formation that can be reversed with an immunomodulating drug. *J Clin Invest* 118 (7), 2427-2437
[31] Grewal, I.S. and Flavell, R.A. (1998) CD40 and CD154 in cell-mediated immunity. *Annu Rev Immunol* 16, 111-135
[32] Kitada, S. et al. (1999) Bryostatin and CD40-ligand enhance apoptosis resistance and induce expression of cell survival genes in B-cell chronic lymphocytic leukaemia. *Br J Haematol* 106 (4), 995-1004
[33] Ranheim, E.A. and Kipps, T.J. (1993) Activated T cells induce expression of B7/BB1 on normal or leukemic B cells through a CD40-dependent signal. *J Exp Med* 177 (4), 925-935
[34] Lagneaux, L. et al. (1998) Chronic lymphocytic leukemic B cells but not normal B cells are rescued from apoptosis by contact with normal bone marrow stromal cells. *Blood* 91 (7), 2387-2396
[35] Vaisitti, T. et al. (2010) CD38 increases CXCL12-mediated signals and homing of chronic lymphocytic leukemia cells. *Leukemia*
[36] Deaglio, S. et al. (2008) CD38 at the junction between prognostic marker and therapeutic target. *Trends Mol Med* 14 (5), 210-218
[37] Menten, P. et al. (2002) Macrophage inflammatory protein-1. *Cytokine Growth Factor Rev* 13 (6), 455-481
[38] Sivina, M. et al. (2010) CCL3 (MIP-1{alpha}) plasma levels and the risk for disease progression in chronic lymphocytic leukemia (CLL). *Blood*
[39] Decker, T. et al. (2002) Cell cycle progression of chronic lymphocytic leukemia cells is controlled by cyclin D2, cyclin D3, cyclin-dependent kinase (cdk) 4 and the cdk inhibitor p27. *Leukemia* 16 (3), 327-334
[40] Seiffert, M. et al. (2010) Soluble CD14 is a novel monocyte-derived survival factor for chronic lymphocytic leukemia cells, which is induced by CLL cells in vitro and present at abnormally high levels in vivo. *Blood* 116 (20), 4223-4230
[41] Letilovic, T. et al. (2006) Role of angiogenesis in chronic lymphocytic leukemia. *Cancer* 107 (5), 925-934
[42] Nilsson, J. et al. (2000) Thioredoxin prolongs survival of B-type chronic lymphocytic leukemia cells. *Blood* 95 (4), 1420-1426

[43] Stamatopoulos, B. et al. (2009) Gene expression profiling reveals differences in microenvironment interaction between patients with chronic lymphocytic leukemia expressing high versus low ZAP70 mRNA. *Haematologica* 94 (6), 790-799

[44] Scielzo, C. et al. (2010) HS1 has a central role in the trafficking and homing of leukemic B cells. *Blood* 116 (18), 3537-3546

[45] Malavasi, F. et al. (2011) CD38 and chronic lymphocytic leukemia: a decade later. *Blood*

[46] Calissano, C. et al. (2009) In vivo intra- and inter-clonal kinetic heterogeneity in B-cell chronic lymphocytic leukemia. *Blood*

[47] Glaum, M.C. et al. (2008) Toll-like receptor 7-induced naive human B-cell differentiation and immunoglobulin production. *J Allergy Clin Immunol*

[48] Kinoshita, K. and Honjo, T. (2001) Linking class-switch recombination with somatic hypermutation. *Nat Rev Mol Cell Biol* 2 (7), 493-503.

[49] Okazaki, I.M. et al. (2003) Constitutive expression of AID leads to tumorigenesis. *J Exp Med* 197 (9), 1173-1181.

[50] Perez-Duran, P. et al. (2007) Oncogenic events triggered by AID, the adverse effect of antibody diversification. *Carcinogenesis* 28 (12), 2427-2433

[51] Oppezzo, P. et al. (2005) Different isoforms of BSAP regulate expression of AID in normal and chronic lymphocytic leukemia B cells. *Blood* 105 (6), 2495-2503

[52] Oppezzo, P. et al. (2003) Chronic lymphocytic leukemia B cells expressing AID display a dissociation between class switch recombination and somatic hypermutation. *Blood* 9, 9

[53] Kimby, E. et al. (1985) Surface immunoglobulin pattern of the leukaemic cell population in chronic lymphocytic leukaemia (CLL) in relation to disease activity. *Hematol Oncol* 3 (4), 261-269

[54] Sthoeger, Z.M. et al. (1989) Production of autoantibodies by CD5-expressing B lymphocytes from patients with chronic lymphocytic leukemia. *Journal of Experimental Medicine* 169 (1), 255-268

[55] Efremov, D.G. et al. (1996) IgM-producing chronic lymphocytic leukemia cells undergo immunoglobulin isotype-switching without acquiring somatic mutations. *J Clin Invest* 98 (2), 290-298.

[56] Zaheen, A. et al. (2009) AID constrains germinal center size by rendering B cells susceptible to apoptosis. *Blood*

[57] Moldenhauer, G. et al. (2006) AID expression identifies interfollicular large B cells as putative precursors of mature B-cell malignancies. *Blood* 107 (6), 2470-2473

[58] Potter, K.N. et al. (2006) Structural and functional features of the B-cell receptor in IgG-positive chronic lymphocytic leukemia. *Clin Cancer Res* 12 (6), 1672-1679

[59] Caligaris-Cappio, F. (2011) Inflammation, the microenvironment and chronic lymphocytic leukemia. *Haematologica* 96 (3), 353-355

[60] Zenz, T. et al. (2010) From pathogenesis to treatment of chronic lymphocytic leukaemia. *Nat Rev Cancer* 10 (1), 37-50

[61] Schulz, A. et al. (2011) Inflammatory cytokines and signaling pathways are associated with survival of primary chronic lymphocytic leukemia cells in vitro: a dominant role of CCL2. *Haematologica* 96 (3), 408-416

[62] Hazan-Halevy, I. et al. (2010) STAT3 is constitutively phosphorylated on serine 727 residues, binds DNA, and activates transcription in CLL cells. *Blood* 115 (14), 2852-2863

[63] Muzio, M. et al. (2009) Expression and function of toll like receptors in chronic lymphocytic leukaemia cells. *Br J Haematol* 144 (4), 507-516

[64] Willimott, S. and Wagner, S.D. (2010) Post-transcriptional and post-translational regulation of Bcl2. *Biochem Soc Trans* 38 (6), 1571-1575

3

Dysregulation of Apoptosis and Proliferation in CLL Cells

Marcin Wójtowicz and Dariusz Wołowiec
Regional Hospital in Opole, Wroclaw Medical University
Poland

1. Introduction

It is well established, that the appearance of chronic lymphocytic leukemia (CLL), the most frequent form of leukemia in adults, in the developed countries, is mainly due to the gradual accumulation of malignant clone originated from CD5/CD19/CD23 positive lymphocytes. This accumulation results from a dysregulation between proliferation and apoptosis of neoplastic cells. In normal lymphocytes these processes are in equilibrium, so that total number of these cells in the organism remains stable. It has been known for two decades that the accumulation of leukemic lymphocytes in CLL is a consequence of defects of programmed cell death, but also, to some extent, of their dysregulated proliferative activity, as shown by the blockade of certain CLL lymphocytes in G_1 cell cycle phase (Decker et al., 2002). The aim of this chapter is to discuss essential abnormalities of CLL cells apoptosis and proliferation which contribute to the development of the disease and may determine its clinical course. However it must be remembered, that significant majority of experimental data concerning survival and apoptosis of CLL cells, especially regarding cytokines, come from in vitro studies, thus it is difficult to apply them directly to in vivo situation.

Numerous studies allowed to establish, that leukemic cells both circulating in the blood and residing in lymphoid organs survive in vivo for a very long time, counted in months, due to inhibition of their programmed death, but they undergo rapid, spontaneous apoptosis in a few days when cultured in in vitro conditions (Collins et al., 1989). It is then plausible that the prolonged in vivo lifespan is due to the prosurvival influence of microenvironmental factors, in particular to the interactions of malignant lymphocytes with stromal cells (Munk-Pedersen & Reed, 2004; Deaglio & Malavasi, 2009), and probably to the B cell receptor engagement by antigens (Ghia et al., 2008; Burger et al., 2009a). The removal of CLL cells from microenvironment to in vitro culture deprives them of indispensable stimuli and leads to their rapid apoptosis. Several subpopulations of accessory stromal cells have been individualized in the connective tissue. Monocyte-derived CD68+ nurse-like cells, mesenchymal stromal cells and follicular dendritic cells seem to play a particularly important role in this process (Burger et al., 2009b).

1.1 Trafficking and homing of CLL cells in microenvironment

Interaction between chemokine receptor CXCR4 and its ligand CXCL12, formerly known as stromal cell-derived factor-1 (SDF-1), plays a crucial role in the homing of malignant lymphocytes within host niches of the microenvironment (Burger & Kipps, 2006). Stromal cells and nurse-like cells constitutively secrete CXCL12, what is essential for retention of hematopoietic stem cells, physiologically expressing CXCR4, inside bone marrow. CLL cells, which usually strongly express CXCR4 independently from the type of the disease, make use of CXCR4/CXCL12 axis to remain in a favourable environment (Broxmeyer et al., 2005). Analogous mechanism acts through receptor CXCR5, present in high density on leukemic lymphocytes and ligand CXCL13 synthesized by nurse-like cells in lymphatic nodes and a spleen (Burkle et al., 2007). CLL cells also overexpress CCR7, a receptor interacting with chemokines CCL19 and CCL21. The intensity of this ligation is additionally regulated by atypical, non-signalling receptors CRAM and CCX-CKR (Catusse et al., 2010) and correlates with infiltration of lymphatic nodes, a process which requires a cooperation of α4 integrin (Till et al., 2002). Higher expression of CCR7 has been related to more advanced stage of the disease and the presence of lymphadenopathy (Ghobrial et al., 2004). The role of another chemokine receptor, CXCR3, is relatively poorly understood. Its expression on malignant lymphocytes considerably varies between patients but remains stable over time in individual cases, and surprisingly - lower level of CXCR3 is strongly associated with Rai stages III and IV, diffuse pattern of the bone marrow infiltration and shorter overall survival (Ocana et al., 2007). Another mechanism involved in the adhesion of CLL cells to components of microenvironment concerns integrins - glycoproteins composed of α and β subunits, mediating cell-to-cell and cell-to-matrix junction. The $\alpha_4\beta_1$ integrin called VLA-4 or CD49d is variously expressed on malignant lymphocytes and acts as a receptor for fibronectin and vascular cell adhesion molecule-1 (VCAM-1 or CD106), cooperating with chemokine receptors in adhesion of these cells to stromal cells and extracellular matrix. Moreover, high expression of VLA-4 correlates with more advanced stage of the disease and shorter overall survival, revealing value as an independent negative prognostic factor (Gattei et al., 2008).

1.2 Reversible influence of CLL cells on the microenvironment

Malignant clone of CLL cells not only uses microenvironmental stimuli, but also influences neighbouring tissues in order to increase attained benefits. Communication between neoplastic lymphocytes and their microenvironment may be executed by microvesicles - detached fragments of malignant cells cytoplasm surrounded by a cell membrane, which are able to fuse nearby cells carrying there numerous proteins and lipids thus exerting impact profitable for a growth and progression of leukemia. A particular mechanism described in CLL concerns transmission of agents stimulating stromal cells to produce vascular endothelial growth factor (VEGF), what leads to enhanced angiogenesis in the bone marrow (Ghosh et al., 2010). Malignant lymphocytes can also actively attract accessory cells, particularly T lymphocytes and monocytes, thus accumulating them in microenvironment, what modifies local immune response in favour of the neoplasm progression. Main factors secreted by CLL cells for this purpose are chemokines CCL3 and CCL4, synthesized after B-cell receptor stimulation (Sivina et al., 2011), and CCL22, produced after CD40 ligation (Ghia et al., 2002).

2. Apoptosis

Processes leading to a programmed cell death can be initiated by either intracellular or extracellular signals. Accordingly, two pathways of apoptosis are distinguished: intrinsic, otherwise called "mitochondrial" and extrinsic, triggered by death receptors signalling.

A wide range of intracellular factors, like DNA damage leading to expression of p53 protein, hypoxia, or growth factors deficiency activate an intrinsic pathway influencing the transcription of Bcl-2 family proteins what leads to an increased release of cytochrome c from mitochondria to cytosol. Thereafter, cytochrome c together with Apaf-1 (apoptotic protease activating factor 1), inactive procaspase-9 and dATP form a complex called apoptosome, which activates caspase-9. This enzymatic complex launches caspase cascade, what causes nuclear condensation, DNA fragmentation, membrane blebbing and finally leads to the cell death. A protein named apoptosis inducing factor (AIF), released from mitochondrion in the same circumstances as cytochrome c, enters the nucleus and results in a cell death without cooperation of caspases. An extrinsic pathway of apoptosis is initiated by activation of several membrane receptors including Fas and TNFαR by their respective ligands. Activated receptors trigger caspase cascade via protein called Fas associated death domain (FADD), which contains domain activating procaspase-8, what leads to cell death.

2.1 Intracellular pathways of apoptosis

Human lymphocytes, as all eukaryotic cells, are equipped with a complicated machinery serving to execute an extracellular or intracellular suicide signal in response to various situations which necessitate cell its death, e.g. unrepairable DNA damage, penetration of a virus into a cell, or neoplastic transformation. Numerous anomalies disturbing this machinery were described in CLL lymphocytes. Those anomalies result in ineffective apoptosis of malignant cells and consequently in their gradual accumulation in blood and lymphoid tissue, thus influencing a clinical course of the disease.

2.1.1 Bcl-2 protein family

The Bcl-2 family is a very conservative class of proteins, detected in a wide range of eukaryotic organisms, from simple nematodes, like Caenorhabditis elegans, to mammalians. Its fundamental role is to control the mitochondrial pathway of apoptosis, by regulation of the permeability of mitochondrial membranes. Bcl-2 and Bcl-xL are principal antiapoptotic proteins of this family. They are located in the outer mitochondrial membrane where they inhibit the release of the cytochrome c from intermembrane space and the creation of the apoptosome, so that the activation of caspase-9 is impaired. As a result of prosurvival activity of Bcl-2 and Bcl-xL, caspase cascade is not activated and cells are protected from apoptosis. Mcl-1 is another important prosurvival protein in this group, structurally different from previous ones, localized predominantly in endoplasmic reticulum and nuclear membrane, interfering with other Bcl-2 agents and inhibiting the cytochrome c release. Proapoptotic members of Bcl-2 family can be divided into two subgroups, depending on number of repeated homological domains called "BH" in their structure: "multidomains" (Bax, Bak, Bok), possessing four domains called BH1, BH2, BH3, BH4, and "BH3-only" (Bim, Bad, Bid, Puma and Noxa). Those proteins can be activated by various signals, like growth factors deprivation, or p53 induced by DNA damage e.g. after radiation or cytotoxic therapy. They deactivate Bcl-2 and Bcl-xL, and support cytochrome c release, thus promoting caspase dependent programmed cells death. In some situations Bid undergoes activation by Fas receptor-induced cleavage and by caspase-8, then it promotes cytochrome c release and triggers the caspases cascade. Therefore it connects both apoptotic pathways: intrinsic and extrinsic one. (Packham & Stevenson, 2005)

Numerous abnormalities of Bcl-2 family proteins expression were observed in CLL cells and it is generally accepted, that shifted balance between different members of that family towards antiapoptotic ones plays a crucial role in prolonging of neoplastic cells in vivo survival. Relatively high expression of Bcl-2 probably because of hypomethylation of its gene were detected in cytoplasm of malignant lymphocytes (Hanada et al., 1993; Robertson et al., 1996). An elevated Bcl-2/Bax ratio was found to be related to chemoresistance and worse prognosis in this disease (Aguilar-Santelises et al., 1996; Molica et al., 1998; Thomas et al., 2000). Yet another observation proves an importance of high Bcl-2 and low Bax levels in programmed cell death inhibition: CLL cells which underwent apoptosis induced by an external factor, e.g. resveratrol, revealed remarkably decreased Bcl-2/Bax ratio (Podhorecka et al., 2011). Increased proteosomal degradation of Bax is considered as a cause of its lower expression (Agraval et al., 2008). Data concerning clinical significance of a decreased Bax level as the only disturbance are somewhat controversial, since some studies suggest its negative prognostic role (Bannerji et al., 2003), while some other ones do not confirm it (Faderl et al., 2002). Increased expression of prosurvival protein Mcl-1 was detected in approximately half of CLL cases, what is thought to inhibit apoptosis and hamper the therapeutic effect of chlorambucil as well as fludarabine (Kitada et al., 1998; Pepper et al., 2008), and rituximab (Awan et al., 2009). Moreover, low expression of MCL-1 gene was correlated with prolonged overall survival in the disease (Veronese et al., 2008). Some other observations suggest that upregulated expression of Mcl-1 plays a crucial role in a protective influence of microenvironmental factors on leukemic cells (Pedersen et al., 2002). Less is known about other Bcl-2 family members. It was shown that simultaneous deficiency of Bax and Bak proteins was related to cells resistance to majority of proapoptotic signals (Wei et al., 2001). Noxa, a protein inducing programmed cells death, is paradoxically excessively expressed in CLL lymphocytes (Mackus et al., 2005). Significance of that phenomenon remains unclear, but it was suggested, that leukemic cells in lymphatic nodes expressed low levels of Noxa, due to proliferative stimuli of microenvironment. In the absence of these signals in circulation Noxa becomes upregulated, but not strongly enough to overcome an apoptosis blockade of highly expressed Bcl-2 (Smit et al., 2007).

2.1.2 Role of p53 in activation of apoptosis

One physiological defense mechanism, aimed at the genome integrity protection, is based on induction of apoptosis when cellular DNA damage becomes irreparable. A key role in that phenomenon is played by p53, a transcription factor which expression is induced by DNA damage. This factor stimulates the expression of $p21^{Cip1/WAF1}$ – universal inhibitor of cyclin-dependent kinases - cyclin complexes, which blocks the cell cycle progression and allows the cell to repair the genetic material. When this repair cannot be completed, p53 enhances the transcription of genes encoding Bax, Puma and Noxa – proapoptotic members of Bcl-2 family, thus initiating the mitochondrial pathway of programmed cell death (Vousden & Lu, 2002). In addition, recent studies suggest, that p53 acts not only as a transcription factor, but is also able to induce apoptosis through direct binding to Bcl-2 protein, deactivating it, what subsequently activates Bax, Puma and triggers caspase cascade (Chipuk et al., 2004; Steele et al., 2008). Approximately 10% to 15% of CLL patients reveal structural aberrations or point mutations in locus 17p13, containing TP53 (gene encoding p53), what results in an improper function of this protein and defective apoptosis of leukemic cells in response to alkylating agents and purine analogues. Those disturbances have a profound influence on the clinical picture of CLL. The presence of 17p deletion or TP53 mutations is associated with higher clinical stage of the disease, shorter treatment-free survival (Dohner et al., 2000), more aggressive clinical course, shorter progression-free and overall survival (Rossi et al., 2009). It should be mentioned, that double-strand DNA breaks activate p53 through phosphorylation and dephosphorylation of single aminoacids of its chain by ATM protein (Johnson et al., 2009). That is why the inactivation of ATM gene, located in locus 11q22.3 to 11q23.1, leads to p53 functional deficiency. Therefore ATM mutations, resulting mainly from 11q22 - q23 deletions and detected in about 20% of CLL patients, are also considered as negative prognostic factors in the disease, although of lesser importance than 17p aberrations and TP53 mutations (Dohner et al., 2000; Austen et al., 2005).

2.1.3 NF-κB signal transduction pathway

Transcription factor called nuclear factor kappa-B (NF-κB) is a homo- or heterodimeric protein composed of subunits belonging to Rel family, which contains following members identified so far: RelA, RelB, c-Rel, p50 and p52. In the inactive state NF-κB is sequestrated in the cytosol by binding to one of its specific inhibitors: IκB-α, IκB-β, IκB-γ, IκB-ε, Bcl-3, p100 or p105, called collectively "IκB" (Zheng et al., 2011). Activation of NF-κB pathway starts by the interaction of a specific ligand with a receptor activator of NF-κB (RANK), which belongs to a family of TNF-α receptors. Numerous factors can induce NK-κB: tumor necrosis factor α (TNF-α), interleukin 1β (IL-1β), osteoprotegerin, ionizing radiation, oxidative stress, or bacterial endotoxins (Vallabhapurapu & Karin, 2009). Stimulated RANK activates a group of kinases called IKK, which phosphorylate IκB liberating it from NF-κB. RANK is also able to activate NF-κB through a specific NF-κB inducing kinase (NIK). When activated, NF-κB enters the nucleus, where it induces the expression of numerous important antiapoptotic genes encoding such proteins as: prosurvival members of Bcl-2 family (Bcl-2, Bcl-xL), cellular inhibitors of apoptosis (IAP family) deactivating caspases, FLICE-like inhibitory protein (FLIP) blocking Fas-associated death domain (FADD), or TNF receptor-associated factor (TRAF), mediating antiapoptotic signals (Fan et al., 2008).

CLL malignant cells show higher constitutive activation of NF-κB than normal lymphocytes (Furman et al., 2000). The impulses such as: CD40 ligation, induction of B-cell receptor (BCR), IL-4, BAFF (B-cell activating factor) or APRIL (a proliferation inducing ligand) were reported to stimulate NF-κB in CLL cells and to antagonize physiological pathways of a programmed cell death. NF-κB expression was reported to show individual variations and may correlate with tumor burden and lymphocytes doubling count, confirming the importance of this signalling pathway in the development and progression of the disease (Hewamana et al., 2008). Currently it is generally accepted that NF-κB is one of the most important transducers of external stimuli, keeping CLL cells alive with blocked apoptosis (Cuni et al., 2004).

2.1.4 PI3K/Akt survival pathway

It is commonly acknowledged that cells need a permanent stimulation with appropriate growth factors to survive. A signalling cascade of the phosphatidylinositide 3'-OH kinase (PI3K) and Akt kinase is thought to be, at least partially, responsible for transduction of prosurvival extracellular stimuli. Their binding to membrane ligands results in displacement of PI3K to the inner surface of a cell membrane. PI3K phosphorylates membrane phosphoinositides, which recruit Akt from cytosol to plasma membrane and change its conformation into more accessible as a substrate for specific 3-phosphoinositide-dependent protein kinases (PDK-1 and PDK-2). Thereafter PDKs activate Akt by phosphorylation. Five targets of Akt antiapoptotic action on intracellular machinery of a programmed cell death were identified. The first one is Bad – proapoptotic member of Bcl-2 family. Akt phosphorylates Bad inactivating it, thus preventing interaction between Bad and Bcl-xL. Bcl-xL liberated from Bad performs its physiological prosurvival role of blocking cytochrome c release from mitochondria. The second one is caspase-9 – an important link between apoptosome and effector caspase-3. Akt inactivates it and thus interrupts caspase cascade. The third site of Akt's influence on apoptosis is its activating action on IKKs – kinases inducing antiapoptotic pathway of NF-κB, as described above in appropriate section of this chapter. The fourth target of Akt is so called Forkhead family of transcription factors, which regulates expression of several genes important for apoptosis, including Fas ligand gene. Akt inactivates Forkhead family members by phosphorylation, thus reducing their proapoptotic effect (Datta et al., 1999). XIAP (X-linked inhibitor of apoptosis protein), one of most potent inhibitors of caspases, is the fifth target of Akt. XIAP phosphorylated by Akt becomes more resistant to ubiquitination and proteolytic degradation, therefore its prosurvival influence becomes prolonged (Dan et al., 2004).

Stimulation with microenvironmental, non-malignant, bystander cells results in a high activity of PI3K/Akt pathway in CLL lymphocytes. Those prosurvival signals reach leukemic cells through various membrane receptors, like B-cell receptor, CD40 (Cuni et al., 2004), or, described recently, CD160 – membrane protein not present in normal B lymphocytes, but expressed on leukemic ones, which has the property of activating PI3K/Akt pathway (Liu et al., 2010). It is supposed, that enhanced activity of Bcl-xL and NF-κB is the most important way of Akt's influence on cell apoptosis in CLL. Additionally, recent studies suggest that sustained activation of Akt results also in increased expression of Mcl-1 in leukemic cells, what shifts the balance between members of Bcl-2 family towards the prosurvival ones (Longo et al., 2008).

2.1.5 Ambiguous role of JNK in apoptosis

The c-Jun N-terminal protein kinase (JNK) belongs to the family of the mitogen activated protein kinase (MAPK) and is involved in a regulation of cellular apoptosis, responding to a variety of extracellular signals. Despite extensive studies published so far, the exact role of JNK in apoptosis remains unclear. Some studies suggested its proapoptotic function (Davis, 2000), some other showed its antiapoptotic activity (Yu et al., 2004), and other ones did not prove any impact at all of this factor on the programmed cell death (Lin, 2003). Probably a real effect of JNK on apoptosis depends on the type of investigated cells and stimuli tested. FasL and TNF-α may activate JNK and lead to the suppression of Bcl-2 and subsequently inhibition of the apoptosis. Some studies suggest that prior inhibition of NF-κB may be required for this antiapoptotic action of JNK (Liu & Lin, 2005). Moreover, studies performed on pro-B hematopoietic cells displayed a suppression of a programmed cell death via inactivation of Bad – proapoptotic member of Bcl-2 family – through its phosphorylation by JNK in response to interleukin-3 stimulation (Yu et al., 2004). As it was presented in one study, B-cell receptor stimulation probably did not reveal any effect on the activity of JNK pathway in CLL cells (Petlickovski et al., 2005).

2.1.6 Caspase cascade

Majority of pathways transducing extra- and intracellular proapoptotic signals converge toward caspases, a family of cysteine proteases, main executors of apoptotic processes. These proteins localize in cytosol as inactive zymogens and after induction of apoptosis they form a proteolytic chain of consecutively activated enzymes, which is called a caspase cascade. Generally, two classes of caspases are distinguished: initiator and effector ones. Initiator caspases (caspase-8, 9, 10 and 12) transduce signals from apoptotic pathways, cleave and activate effector ones (caspase-3, 6 and 7) (Riedl & Shi, 2004). The intrinsic pathway of apoptosis leads to the formation of apoptosome, which is, as already mentioned, a complex containing Apaf-1, cytochrome c liberated from mitochondria, procaspase-9 and dATP. Apoptosome activates caspase-9 which subsequently activates effector caspase-3 and caspase-6. Induction of the extrinsic pathway results in caspase-8 and caspase-10 activation through FADD, thereafter both initiator caspases mentioned above activate the effector caspase-3. Afterwards caspase-3 activates downstream effector caspase-7. Finally, main effector caspase-3, in cooperation with caspase-6 and 7, cleaves a variety of proteins, like laminA, actin, gas2, what causes cell shrinkage and membrane blebbing. Additionally, caspase-3 inactivates ICAD (inhibitor of CAD), what liberates CAD (caspase activated DNAse) and results in DNA fragmentation and nuclear chromatin condensation. All these processes finally lead to cell death (Logue & Martin, 2008).

The function of caspase cascade is controlled by a group of cysteine proteases, called IAP (inhibitor of apoptosis), containing XIAP, IAP1, IAP2, survivin and livin. They bind and potently inhibit caspase-3, 7 and 9, stopping the cascade regardless of pathway of induction - intrinsic or extrinsic one (Deveraux & Reed, 1999). The activity of IAP family proteins may increase in response to stimulation by various antiapoptotic signals which serve as effectors of specific pathways. For example, one of antiapoptotic activities of Akt is mediated through XIAP, since Akt phosphorylates XIAP, making it more resistant to proteasome-mediated degradation (Dan et al., 2004). FLIP (FLICE-like inhibitory protein), existing in two variants: c-FLIP$_S$ and c-FLIP$_L$, represents another control point of caspases activation. It contains a fragment interacting with death domain motif of FADD and simultaneously prevents activation of caspase-8 and 10, thus blocking Fas receptor signalling pathway and inhibiting programmed cell death (Irmler et al., 1997). However a physiological function of c-FLIP$_L$ is not fully explained, since recent reports suggested its role in activation of caspase-8 (Boatright et al., 2004).

CLL cells do not differ significantly from normal lymphocytes regarding to the expression of caspase family proteins. Nevertheless, as apoptosis inhibition is thought to be principal mechanism of malignant lymphocytes accumulation, so efforts to induce caspase-dependent programmed cell death are evident therapeutic direction. Indeed, caspase activation may be used as a surrogate biomarker of successful induction of apoptosis in leukemic cells by various chemotherapeutic drugs. A choice of caspase-3 activity assessment for this purpose is quite obvious, in view of central effector role of this protein in execution of death signals deriving from variety of pathways. Starting from the oldest drugs, chlorambucil is thought to induce expression of caspase-3 and apoptosis in CLL cells (Brajuskovic et al., 2004). The same phenomenon is observed for newer chemotherapeutics, like fludarabine (Stoetzer et al., 1999) and a monoclonal antibody anti-CD20 - rituximab (Byrd et al., 2002). Alemtuzumab, a monoclonal antibody anti-CD52, another immunochemotherapeutic agent used in CLL treatment, was not reported to involve caspases pathway, but induces apoptosis through a non-classical, caspase-independent pathway (Mone et al., 2006). The latter mechanism may also represent another possible mode of action of rituximab (Stanglmaier et al., 2004).

2.1.7 Caspase-independent programmed cell death

More than ten years ago an observation was published that cells were capable to undergo apoptosis even when caspases expression was suppressed. This finding pointed out to the existence of caspase-independent mechanisms leading to a programmed cell death (Susin et al., 2000). However regardless of numerous studies, caspase-independent cell death still remains poorly understood. Currently apoptosis is classified into three subtypes. Type I, named "classical apoptosis", is the best explored one and covers all processes triggering caspase cascade, therefore it is often called "caspase-dependent". Each signalling pathway described earlier in this chapter belongs to type I of apoptosis. Type II of programmed cell death is related to increased permeability of mitochondrial membrane, analogically to intrinsic pathway of classical apoptosis activation (Kim et al., 2005). Proteins released from mitochondrial intermembrane space activate proapoptotic factors other than caspases, like calpains, cathepsins and other proteases (Constantinou et al., 2009). AIF (apoptosis inducing factor) is the best known among them, it is released from mitochondrion, then enters nucleus and initiates chromatin condensation and DNA fragmentation. Morphologically this type of apoptosis is characterized by large vacuolization of cytoplasm due to appearance of autophagosomes (Tait & Green, 2008). Type III of apoptosis is less explored; it resembles cellular necrosis and is defined strictly morphologically, with absence of visible nuclear chromatin condensation (Bras et al., 2007).

There are only single reports concerning caspase-independent apoptosis observed in CLL lymphocytes. The mechanism reported so far is triggered by membrane glycoprotein CD47, thrombospondin-1-binding member of the immunoglobulin superfamily. Activation of CD47 by appropriate ligand leads to activation of serpases which afterwards damage cytoskeletal protein called F-actin. Improper function of F-actin results in cell shrinkage secondary to cytoskeletal damage, and in translocation of Drp1 (dynamin related protein-1) from cytosol to mitochondria, where it disrupts the electron transport chain, therefore lowering ATP levels (Barbier et al., 2009). As a result of described mechanisms, disturbances in cell architecture and mitochondrial function, but no pronounced chromatin condensation are detected in cells undergoing the caspase-independent apoptosis. CLL lymphocytes can undergo the caspase-independent programmed cell death even when the classical apoptosis is disrupted. It raises hope for discovering new agents able to overcome chemoresistancy to classical drugs. Further studies on that phenomenon are thus very promising from a clinical point of view.

2.2 Membrane receptors

All metazoan cells receive numerous external stimuli determining their fate depending on momentary requirements of physiological balance in the organism, keeping them alive, or pushing onto a path of a programmed death. These signals are transmitted into cells through a multitude of receptors, among which a superfamily of TNF (tumor necrosis factor) receptor is one of the most important. Depending on structure and signalling properties, members of TNF receptors family are generally classified into three large groups (Dempsey et al., 2003).

The first one contains: Fas receptor (FasR or CD95), TNF-α receptor 1 (TNF-R1 or CD120a), death receptor 3 binding to TWEAK (DR3, TRAMP or LARD), death receptors 4 and 5 binding to TRAIL (DR4 and DR5). All these proteins possess a characteristic death domain in their cytoplasmic tail. After activation of receptors by external ligands their death domains interact with corresponding transmitter proteins - FasR, DR4 and DR5 with Fas-associated death domain (FADD), while TNF-R1 and DR3 with TNFR-associated death domain (TRADD). In the next step the caspase cascade is triggered through a caspase-8 activation and the cell undergoes apoptosis (Kischkel et al., 2000).

The second group of TNF receptors superfamily contains: TNF-α receptor 2 (TNF-R2 or CD120b), CD40, CD27, CD30, B-cell activating factor receptor (BAFFR), TACI and BCMA (receptors recognizing both: BAFF and APRIL - a proliferation inducing ligand), lymphotoxin-β receptor (LT-βR or CD18), OX40 (CD134), TNF-α receptor 2 related protein (TNFR2-RP or TNFRIII), receptor activator of NF-κB (RANK), receptor expressed in lymphoid tissues (RELT), herpes virus entry mediator (HVEM), and others, not detected on B lymphocytes, like LIGHT receptor (LIGHTR), TROY/Taj, p75 neurotrophin receptor (p75NGFR), ectodysplasin-A receptor (EDAR), fibroblast growth factor inducible 14 (Fn14), or glucocorticoid-induced tumor necrosis factor receptor (GITR) (Darnay et al., 1999). Cytoplasmic tails of these receptors contain various numbers of TIM (TRAF interacting motifs) - protein sequences reacting with members of TRAF family (TNF receptor-associated factor). Activated TRAFs form expanded complexes with TNF receptors, IAPs and RIPs (the death domain kinase receptor interacting protein) mediating antiapoptotic signals through induction of numerous prosurvival pathways, like NF-κB, PI3K/Akt, JNK, ERK (extracellular signal regulated kinase) and others (Xie et al., 2008). Therefore activation of TNF family receptors of the second group induces inhibition of apoptosis, what brings us to an interesting conclusion, that TNF-α can act in two ways - not only proapoptotically, through TNF-R1, but also antiapoptotically, through TNF-R2 (Ihnatko & Kubes, 2008).

A class of proteins unable to transduce stimuli into intracellular signalling pathways forms the third group of TNF receptor family members. Decoy receptor 1 (DcR1 or TRAIL-R3), decoy receptor 2 (DcR2 or TRAIL-R4), decoy receptor 3 (DcR3) and TNF receptor superfamily members 22 and 23 (TNFRSF22 and TNFRSF23) belong to that group. They probably compete with other TNF receptors for their ligands, therefore impeding their activation and induction of intracellular signalling pathways (Falschlehner et al., 2007).

Available data concerning aberrations of the TNF receptors superfamily expression and function in CLL lymphocytes are scanty, but some interesting observations were published. Fas receptor is distinctly downregulated on leukemic cells (Laytragoon-Lewin et al., 1998) and attempts of its upregulation by various factors in vitro are not as efficient as in normal B cells (De Fanis et al., 2003). Nevertheless, this is unlikely to be the cause of their resistance to Fas-mediated apoptosis, because eliciting high FasR expression on a surface of CLL lymphocytes does not restore their susceptibility to that way of a programmed cell death (Romano et al., 2005). Moreover it seems that the expression of FasR on leukemic cells does not have prognostic significance to clinical course of the disease (Hjalmar et al., 2002). CD40 is strongly expressed both on CLL cells and normal B lymphocytes, without significant difference between them. Activation of CD40 on leukemic cells by its specific ligand CD40L (otherwise called CD154) induces expression of proapoptotic FasR, but at the same time it strongly activates prosurvival NF-κB pathway. As a result, antiapoptotic effect of CD40 activation prevails in CLL cells (von Bergwelt-Baildon et al., 2004). In addition it has been observed that ligation of CD40 reduces the efficacy of apoptosis induction by fludarabine in CLL lymphocytes in vitro (Romano et al., 1998). CD27 is considered as a marker of memory B cells and, when activated by CD70, it leads to plasma cell differentiation (Agematsu et al., 2000). Its expression on a surface of CLL cells does not differ significantly from normal lymphocytes, but serum levels of soluble CD27 are higher in CLL patients than control healthy subjects and correlate with some unfavourable prognostic factors, like high lymphocyte count, advanced clinical stage or high serum levels of β_2-microglobulin (Molica et al., 1998). Antigen CD30 is typical of Hodgkin lymphoma and hairy cell leukemia variant, but in contrast to normal lymphocytes, it is also detectable at low density on CLL cells. TNF-R1 is expressed neither on malignant nor on normal B lymphocytes, while TNF-R2 is detected on both, although without significant differences between them (Trentin et al., 1997).

Not only TNF superfamily receptors regulate the survival of malignant lymphocytes. CD38 is a glycoprotein mediating cell to cell interactions and acting as an adhesion molecule, with a reliable negative prognostic value for CLL patients. In vitro observations show that activation of CD38 by its ligand CD31 induces proliferation and differentiation of CLL cells and impairs their apoptosis by influence on the expression of numerous proteins of Bcl-2 family, like Bax, Bim, Puma or Mcl-1 (Deaglio et al., 2010). Similar effect is exerted by CD100 activation with plexin-B1. Since nurse-like cells from lymphoid tissue produce both ligands - CD31 and plexin B1, this phenomenon evidences the importance of environmental factors for CLL cells viability (Deaglio et al., 2005).

2.3 Influence of chemokines on the survival of CLL cells

Trafficking and homing of leukemic cells in a favourable microenvironment gives them an opportunity to benefit from a set of prosurvival factors secreted there. CXCL12, belonging to CXC chemokines and improving leukemic lymphocytes viability through induction of mitogen-activated protein kinases (MAPK or ERK 1/2) is one of them (Burger et al., 2000). However survival of CLL cells cultured in vitro together with nurse-like cells is significantly longer than those cultured only with a solution of CXCL12 (Burger et al., 2000), so it is supposed, that other substances produced by nurse-like cells influences the viability of malignant lymphocytes. Currently it is thought, that this role is played by two members of TNF superfamily: APRIL (a proliferation inducing ligand) and BAFF (B-cell activating factor of a TNF family), otherwise called BLyS (B lymphocyte stimulator). They are important survival and maturation factors of normal B lymphocytes (Mackay et al., 2003), probably influencing the expression of Bcl-2 family members (Craxton et al., 2005). After secretion by nurse-like cells, they support CLL cells survival in a paracrine manner, independently from CXCL12, through activation of NF-κB pathway, inhibiting both: spontaneous and drug-induced apoptosis (Nishio et al., 2005). Moreover, neoplastic lymphocytes also express BAFF and APRIL, probably enhancing their own viability in an autocrine way (Kern et al., 2004).

A number of studies conducted in vitro showed an influence of interleukins on a programmed cell death and survival of malignant CLL cells. Interleukin 1, nonspecific inflammatory mediator and lymphocytes activating factor, protects leukemic lymphocytes from apoptosis, spontaneous as well as induced by glucocorticosteroids (Jewell et al., 1995). Interleukin 2, the principal growth factor for T lymphocytes, inhibits the apoptosis of CLL cells by enhancing Mcl-1, Bcl-xL and survivin expression. Activated lymphocytes respond to this interleukin stronger then resting ones. Interestingly, at the same time interleukin 2 reduces the expression of Bcl-2, but global result of its activity on CLL lymphocytes remains prosurvival (Decker et al., 2010). Interleukin 4, produced by T helper cells, activates normal B lymphocytes and suppresses the apoptosis of leukemic cells through upregulation of Bcl-2 expression (Panayiotidis et al., 1993). Interleukin 5, a growth factor involved in hematopoiesis, which principal function is to stimulate the eosinophils maturation, increases spontaneous apoptosis rate of malignant lymphocytes in vitro in an unknown way, without influence on Bcl-2 expression (Mainou-Fowler et al., 1994). Interleukin 6 is an important factor of growth and differentiation of B lymphocytes. It is thought to inhibit the programmed CLL cells death by increasing the Bcl-2 levels. Moreover, higher expression of interleukin 6 correlates with more advanced stage of the disease and higher serum concentration of β_2-microglobulin (Lai et al., 2002). Physiological function of interleukin 8 is the induction of chemotaxis. In malignant lymphocytes it upregulates expression of Bcl-2, thus preventing their apoptosis. It is produced mainly by macrophages, but also CLL cells release it into the serum, thus exerting regulatory function on their own clone in an autocrine manner. Approximately a quarter of all CLL patients express abnormally high levels of interleukin 8, what correlates with a higher risk of the disease progression independently from an initial tumor burden (Molica et al., 1999). Interleukin 10 is overexpressed in malignant cells of some CLL patients and correlates with an aggressive course of the disease and short overall survival (Fayad et al., 2001). This probably results from its impact on neoplastic lymphocytes cell cycle, because inhibition of interleukin 10 transcription leads to the enhanced apoptosis of the cells of a murine CLL model (Yen Chong et al., 2001). Interleukin 13, another cytokine involved in B lymphocytes activation, impedes leukemic cells apoptosis induced by interleukin 2 in vitro (Chaouchi et al., 1996). Interleukin 24 triggers apoptosis in CLL cells recruited to the cell cycle, by the inactivation of STAT3 kinase thus stabilizing expression of p53 (Sainz-Perez et al., 2008).

3. Cell proliferation

As mentioned at the beginning, CLL is traditionally considered as a result of inhibition of in vivo apoptosis. A wide variety of disturbances in CLL lymphocytes apoptosis was a subject of earlier sections of this chapter. There are numerous additional evidences supporting this opinion through demonstration of a weak proliferative potential of CLL cells. Low DNA content assessed by flow cytometry, low expression of Ki-67 and PCNA (proliferating cell nuclear antigen) – proteins associated with a nuclear proliferation, finally low rates of BrdU (bromodeoxyuridine) or 3H-thymidine incorporation – assays estimating the extent of DNA synthesis, are similar as in quiescent lymphocytes, what suggests arrest of leukemic cells in G_0 phase of a cell cycle (Caligaris-Cappio & Hamblin, 1999). However there have been several studies published in recent years, supporting the hypothesis, that malignant clone of CLL comprises cells which are recruited to a proliferation cycle but arrested in its G_1 phase (Damle et al., 2010), and that a small but significant fraction of all leukemic cells proliferates with measurable birth rates (Chiorazzi, 2007).

3.1 Proliferation centers

Numerous studies showed that proliferation rate of CLL lymphocytes is not the same in each organ and compartment, but cells with higher birth rate accumulate in specific structures of a bone marrow and lymphatic nodes called pseudofollicles or proliferation centers, composed of lymphocytes, prolymphocytes and paraimmunoblasts of a neoplastic clone, with accompanying follicular dendritic cells, mesenchymal stromal cells and CD4-positive T lymphocytes, where CLL cells have optimal microenvironmental conditions for growth and dividing (Caligaris-Cappio & Ghia, 2008). Malignant cells in those areas are characterized by a higher expression of Ki-67, CD71, CD38, MUM1/IRF-4 and coexpression of survivin and Bcl-2, factors typically associated with proliferation (Soma et al., 2006). Features of proliferation centers have a clear influence on the course of the disease. Patients with larger, confluent pseudofollicles estimated histopathologically in lymphatic nodes, with higher mitotic index and higher Ki-67 expression measured in these areas, more often suffer from the aggressive form of the disease and have significantly shorter overall survival (Gine et al., 2010). Furthermore it is suggested, that pseudofollicles accumulate CLL cells with genetic alterations (Balogh et al., 2011). Estimation of proliferation centers in bone marrow is possible rather in early stages of the disease, because in more advanced stages trephine biopsy often reveals diffuse pattern of a bone marrow infiltration, another well known negative prognostic factor in CLL, with faded structure of pseudofollicles (Mauro et al., 1994).

3.2 Cell cycle regulatory proteins

The important evidences in favour of CLL cells recruitment to a cell cycle were obtained from investigations concerning family of serine-threonine kinases called cyclin dependent kinases (cdk). Their appearance in cytosol and activation in precisely fixed phases of a cell-division cycle by junction with regulatory subunits called cyclins is crucial for a proper course of DNA replication and mitosis. In the beginning of G_1 phase cdk4 and cdk6 bind to cyclin D and phosphorylate the retinoblastoma protein (pRb), what activates transcription factors of E2F family and initiates transcription of proteins participating in DNA replication. Thereafter the association of cdk2 with cyclin E is fundamental for beginning of S phase (Sanchez & Dynlacht, 2005). It is reported, that significant number of malignant lymphocytes express several cyclins and cdks normally present in early G_1 cell cycle phase. The increased levels of cdk4 and cyclin E were observed in CLL cells (Wołowiec et al., 1995; Korz et al., 2002) and higher expression of cdk4 was associated with presence of 17p or 11q deletions (Winkler et al., 2010). Aberrations of cellular content of cyclin D were also reported in leukemic lymphocytes. There are three known subtypes of this cyclin - D1, D2 and D3. Cyclin D3 is definitely overexpressed in CLL cells, what is confirmed by detection of its mRNA (Paul et al., 2005), as well as by the detection of its protein (Wołowiec et al., 2001). Studies concerning cyclin D2 are more discordant, with observations confirming the overexpression of the protein's mRNA (Delmer et al., 1995) and denying it (Paul et al., 2005), while intracellular content of cyclin D2 is elevated comparing to normal B lymphocytes (Wołowiec et al., 2001). Even cyclin E, appearing later in G_1 phase than cyclin D, is detectable in a significant subset of leukemic cells derived from peripheral blood (Decker et al., 2004) and from lymphatic nodes (Obermann et al., 2007). Expression of minichromosome maintenance protein 2 (Mcm-2) is a novel marker of cycling cells since this protein is detectable from the beginning of G_1 phase, earlier than Ki-67 expression. A significant subpopulation of CLL lymphocytes are Mcm-2 positive and Ki-67 negative, what brings additional evidence for their arrest rather in early G_1, than G_0 cell cycle phase (Obermann et al., 2007). Protein $p27^{Kip1}$ is an inhibitor of the majority of known cdk - cyclin complexes, thus regarded as an important antiproliferative factor. CLL cells were demonstrated to express it in higher quantity than normal B lymphocytes and some studies suggested the relationship between higher $p27^{Kip1}$ expression and impaired in vitro apoptosis of leukemic cells, although mechanism of this protein antiapoptotic activity in these cells remained unknown (Vrhovac et al., 1998). Other observations carried out on early and intermediate stage patients did not confirm this connection, nevertheless they revealed negative prognostic significance of high $p27^{Kip1}$ expression in CLL, contrary to the majority of non-hematological malignancies (Wołowiec et al., 2009).

3.3 Telomeres length and DNA synthesis in vivo

Investigations concerning telomeres brought another rationale for proliferation activity of CLL cells. Physiologically DNA composes long, repetitive sequences at the end of every chromosome: these structures are named telomeres. Their function is to protect cells from loss of information-coding segments of DNA during replication, when erosion of a genetic material on chromosomes ends takes place. After replication, an enzyme called telomerase restores lost fragments of telomeres, but only partially, what leads to gradual shortening of telomeres as a part of physiological aging. Therefore telomerase activation and shortening in telomeres length calculated proportionally to age are helpful markers of a cell proliferation (O'Sullivan & Karlseder, 2010). CLL lymphocytes are characterized by shorter telomeres and higher telomerase activity than normal B lymphocytes, what indicates on a greater number of their divisions in the past (Damle et al., 2004). Additionally, shorter telomeres are associated with genetic aberrations of defavourable prognostic signification, mainly unmutated status of the immunoglobulin heavy chain variable gene (Roos et al., 2008), and correlate with shorter progression-free and overall survival of CLL patients (Sellmann et al., 2011). These observations lead to a possible conclusion, that shorter lymphocyte doubling time - well known marker of the aggressive course of the disease - results from higher proliferation rate of neoplastic cells.

Recently designed technique measuring incorporation of deuterium (^2H) from heavy water (^2H_2O), or deuterated glucose into deoxyribose molecules allows to calculate DNA synthesis and proliferation rate of dividing cells in vivo with much higher sensitivity than classic methods like Ki-67 expression or 3H-thymidine incorporation (Busch et al., 2007). Used in CLL, this technique also revealed that malignant cells have measurable birth rates (Messmer et al., 2005), and that among whole population of CLL lymphocytes, those expressing CD38 have significantly higher proliferation rate comparing to CD38-negative cells (Calissano et al., 2009).

4. Summary and therapeutic implications

Although more and more is known about numerous anomalies of CLL cells apoptosis and proliferation, our knowledge still remains incomplete. Decades of research proved the crucial role of these disturbances in the appearance and clinical course of the disease, raising hope, that their pharmaceutical corrections may evoke normal apoptosis of malignant cells, thus restraining CLL progression. Indeed, a lot of molecules, which influence signalling pathways regulating programmed cell death, are currently investigated towards their usefulness in a treatment of the disease (Robak, 2010). Nevertheless, a tremendous heterogeneity of CLL clinical course suggests significant differences of apoptosis and proliferation anomalies among individual patients, so probably no universal drug, efficient in every case, should be expected.

5. References

Agematsu, K.; Hokibara, S.; Nagumo, H. & Komiyama, A. (2000). CD27: a memory N-cell marker. *Immunology Today*, Vol. 21, No. 5, (May 2000), pp. 204-206, ISSN 0167-5699.

Agraval, S.; Liu, F.; Wiseman, C.; Shirali, S.; Liu, H.; Lillington, D.; Du, M.; Syndercombe-Coutr, D.; Newland, A.; Gribben, J. & Jia, L. (2008). Increased proteosomal degradation of Bax is a common feature of poor prognosis chronic lymphocytic leukemia. *Blood*, Vol. 111, No. 5, (March 2008), pp. 2790-2796, ISSN 0006-4971.

Aguilar-Santelises, M.; Rottenberg, M.; Lewin, N.; Mellstedt, H. & Jondal, M. (1996). Bcl-2, Bax and p53 expression in B-CLL in relation to in vitro survival and clinical progression. *International Journal of Cancer*, Vol. 62, No. 2, (April 1996), pp. 114-119, ISSN 0020-7136.

Austen, B.; Powell, J.; Alvi, A.; Edwards, I.; Hooper, L.; Starczynski, J.; Taylor, M.; Fegan, C.; Moss, P. & Stankovic, T. (2005). Mutations in the ATM gene lead to impaired overall and treatment-free survival that is independent of IGVH mutation status in patients with B-CLL. *Blood*, Vol. 106, No. 9, (November 2005), pp. 3175-3182, ISSN 0006-4971.

Awan, F.; Kay, N.; Davis, M.; Wu, W.; Geyer, S.; Leung, N.; Jelinek, D.; Tschumper, R.; Secreto, C.; Lin, T.; Grever, M.; Shanafelt, T.; Zent, C.; Call, T.; Heerema, N.; Lozansky, G.; Byrd, J. & Lucas, D. (2009). Mcl-1 expresion predicts progression-free survival in chronic lymphocytic leukemia patients treated with pentostatin, cyclophosphamide, and rituximab. *Blood*, Vo. 113, No. 3, (January 2009), pp. 535-537, ISSN 0006-4971.

Balogh, Z.; Reiniger, L.; Rajnai, H.; Csomor, J.; Szepesi, A.; Balogh, A.; Deak, L.; Gagyi, E.; Bodor, C. & Matolcsy, A. (2011). High rate of neoplastic cells with genetic abnormalities in proliferation centers of chronic lymphocytic leukemia. *Leukemia and Lymphoma*, Vol. 52, No. 6, (June 2011), pp. 1080-1084, ISSN 1042-8194.

Bannerji, R.; Kitada, S.; Flinn, I.; Pearson, M.; Young, D.; Reed, J. & Byrd, J. (2003). Apoptotic-Regulatory and Complement-Protecting Protein Expression in Chronic Lymphocytic Leukemia: Relationship to In Vivo Rituximab Resistance. *Journal of Clinical Oncology*, Vol. 21, No. 8, (April 2003), pp. 1466-1471, ISSN 0732-183X.

Barbier, S.; Chatre, L.; Bras, M.; Sancho, P.; Roue, S.; Virely, C.; Yuste, V.; Baudet, S.; Rubio, M.; Esquerda, J.; Sarfati, M.; Merle-Beral, H. & Susin, S. (2009). Caspase-independent type III programmed cell death in chronic lymphocytic leukemia: the key role of the F-actin cytoskeleton. *Haematologica*, Vol. 94, No. 4, (April 2009), pp. 507-517, ISSN 0390-6078.

Boatright, K.; Deis, C.; Denault, J.; Sutherlin, D. & Salvesen, G. (2004). Activation of caspases-8 and -10 by $FLIP_L$. *Biochemical Journal*, Vol. 382, No. 2, (September 2004), pp. 651-657, ISSN 0264-6021.

Brajuskovic, G.; Vukosavic-Orolicki, S.; Cerovic, S.; Knezevic-Usaj, S.; Peric, P.; Marjanovic, S.; Dimitrijevic, J.; Romac, S. & Skaro-Milic, A. (2004). The expression of caspase 3 in chronic lymphocytic leukemia. *Archive of Oncology*, Vol. 12, Suppl. 1, (May 2004), p. 65, ISSN 1450-9520.

Bras, M.; Yuste, V.; Roue, G.; Barbier, S.; Sancho, P.; Virely, C.; Rubio, M.; Baudet, S.; Esquerda, J.; Merle-Beral, H.; Sarfati, M. & Susin, S. (2007). Drp1 Mediates Caspase-Independent Type III Cell Death in Normal and Leukemic Cells. *Molecular and Cellular Biology*, Vol. 27, No. 20, (October 2007), pp. 7073-7088, ISSN 0270-7306.

Broxmeyer, H.; Orschell, C.; Clapp, D.; Hangoc, G.; Cooper, S.; Plett, P.; Liles, W.; Li, X.; Graham-Evans, B.; Campbell, T.; Calandra, G.; Bridger, G.; Dale, D. & Srour, E. (2005). Rapid mobilization of murine and human hematopoietic stem and progenitor cells with AMD3100, a CXCR4 antagonist. *Journal of Experimental Medicine*, Vol. 201, No. 8, (April 2005), pp. 1307-1318, ISSN 0022-1007.

Burger, J.; Tsukada, N.; Burger, M.; Zvaifler, N.; Dell'Aquila, M. & Kipps, T. (2000). Blood-derived nurse-like cells protect chronic lymphocytic leukemia B cells from spontaneous apoptosis through stromal cell-derived factor-1. *Blood*, Vol. 96, No. 8, (October 2000), pp. 2655-2663, ISSN 0006-4971.

Burger, J. & Kipps, T. (2006). CXCR4: a key receptor in the crosstalk between tumor cells and their microenvironment. *Blood*, Vol. 107, No. 5, (March 2006), pp. 1761-1767, ISSN 0006-4971.

Burger, J.; Quiroga, M.; Hartmann, E.; Burkle, A.; Wierda, W.; Keating, M. & Rosenwald, A. (2009a). High-level expression of the T-cell chemokines CCL3 and CCL4 by chronic lymphocytic leukemia B cells in nurselike cell cocultures and after BCR stimulation. *Blood*, Vo. 113, No. 13, (March 2009), pp. 3050-3058, ISSN 0006-4971.

Burger, J.; Ghia, P.; Rosenwald, A. & Calligaris-Cappio, F. (2009b). The microenvironment in mature B-cell malignancies: a target for new treatment strategies. *Blood*, Vol. 114, No. 16, (October 2009), pp. 3367-3375, ISSN 0006-4971.

Burkle, A.; Niedermeier, M.; Schmitt-Graff, A.; Wierda, W.; Keating, M. & Burger, J. (2007). Overexpression of the CXCR5 chemokine receptor, and its ligand, CXCL13 in B-cell chronic lymphocytic leukemia. *Blood*, Vol. 110, No. 9, (November 2007), pp. 2216-3325, ISSN 0006-4971.

Busch, R.; Neese, R.; Awada, M.; Hayes, G. & Hellerstein, M. (2007). Measurement of cell proliferation by heavy water labeling. *Nature Protocols*, Vol. 2, No. 12, (December 2007), pp. 3045-3057, ISSN 1754-2189.

Byrd, J.; Kitada, S.; Flinn, I.; Aron, J.; Pearson, M.; Lucas, D. & Reed, J. (2002). The mechanism of tumor clearance by rituximab in vivo in patients with B-cell chronic lymphicytic leukemia: evidence of caspase activation and apoptosis induction. *Blood*, Vol. 99, No. 3, (February 2002), pp. 1038-1043, ISSN 0006-4971.

Caligaris-Cappio, F. & Hamblin, T. (1999). B-cell chronic lymphocytic leukemia: a bird of a different feather. *Journal of Clinical Oncology*, Vol. 17, No. 1, (January 1999), pp. 399-408, ISSN 0732-183X.

Caligaris-Cappio, F. & Ghia, P. (2008). Novel Insights in Chronic Lymphocytic Leukemia: Are We Getting Closer to Understanding the Pathogenesis of the Disease? *Journal of Clinical Oncology*, Vol. 26, No. 27, (September 2008), pp. 4497-4503, ISSN 0732-183X.

Calissano, C.; Damle, R.; Hayes, G.; Murphy, E.; Hellerstein, M.; Moreno, C.; Sison, C.; Kaufman, M.; Kolitz, J.; Allen, S.; Rai, K. & Chiorazzi, N. (2009). In vivo intraclonal and interclonal kinetic heterogeneity in B-cell chronic lymphocytic leukemia. *Blood*, Vol. 114; No. 23, (November 2009), pp. 4832-4842, ISSN 0006-4971.

Catusse, J.; Leick, M.; Groch, M.; Clark, D.; Buchner, M.; Zirlik, K. & Burger, M. (2010). Role of the atypical chemoattractant receptor CRAM in regulating CCL19 induced CCR7 responses in B-cell chronic lymphocytic leukemia. *Molecular Cancer*, Vol. 9, No. 297, (November 2010), pp. 1-12, ISSN 1476-4598.

Chaouchi, N.; Wallon, C.; Goujard, C.; Tertian, G.; Rudent, A.; Caput, D.; Ferrera, P.; Minty, A.; Vazquez, A. & Delfraissy, J. (1996). Interleukin-13 Inhibits Interleukin-2-Induced Proliferation and Protects Chronic Lymphocytic Leukemia B Cells From In Vitro Apoptosis. *Blood*, Vol. 87, No. 3 (February 1996), pp. 1022-1029. ISSN 0006-4971.

Chiorazzi N. (2007). Cell proliferation and death: forgotten features of chronic lymphocytic leukemia B cells. *Best Practice & Research: Clinical Haematology*, Vol. 20, No. 3, (September 2007), pp. 399-413, ISSN 1521-6926.

Chipuk, J.; Kuwana, T.; Bouchier-Hayes, L.; Droin, N.; Newmeyer, D.; Schuler, M. & Green, D. (2004). Direct activation of Bax by p53 mediates mitochondrial membrane permeabilisation and apoptosis. *Science*, Vol. 303, No. 5660, (February 2004), pp. 1010-1014, ISSN 0036-8075.

Collins, R.; Verschuer, L.; Harmon, B.; Prentice, R.; Pope, J. & Kerr, J. (1989). Spontaneous programmed death (apoptosis) of B-chronic lymphocytic leukaemia cells following their culture in vitro. *British Journal of Haematology*, Vol. 71, No. 3, (March 1989), pp. 343-350, ISSN 0007-1048.

Constantinou, C.; Papas, K. & Constantinou, A. (2009). Caspase-independent pathways of programmed cell death: the unraveling of new targets of cancer therapy? *Current Cancer Drug Targets*, Vol. 9, No. 6, (September 2009), pp. 717-728, ISSN 1568-0096.

Craxton, A.; Draves, K.; Gruppi, A. & Clark, E. (2005). BAFF regulates B cell survival by downregulating the BH3-only family member Bim via the ERK pathway. *Journal of Experimental Medicine*, Vol. 202, No. 10, (November 2005), pp. 1363-1374, ISSN 0022-1007.

Cuni, S.; Perez-Aciego, P.; Perez-Chacon, G.; Vargas, J.; Sanchez, A.; Martin-Saavedra, F.; Ballester, S.; Garcia-Marco, J.; Jorda, J. & Durantez, A. (2004). A sustained activation of PI3K/NF-κB pathway is critical for the survival of chronic lymphocytic leukemia B cells. *Leukemia*, Vol. 18, No. 8, (August 2004), pp. 1391-1400, ISSN 0887-6924.

Damle, R.; Batliwalla, F.; Ghiotto, F.; Valetto, A.; Albesiano, E.; Sison, C.; Allen, S.; Kolitz, J.; Vinciguerra, V.; Kudalkar, P.; Wasil, T.; Rai, K.; Ferrarini, M.; Gregersen, P. & Chiorazzi, N. (2004). Telomere length and telomerase activity delineate distinctive replicative features of the B-CLL subgroups defined by immunoglobulin V gene mutations. *Blood*, Vol. 103, No. 2, (January 2004), pp. 375-382, ISSN 0006-4971.

Damle, R.; Calissano, C. & Chiorazzi, N. (2010). Chronic lymphocytic leukemia: a disease of activated monoclonal B cells. *Best Practice & Research Clinical Haematology*, Vol. 23, No. 1, (March 2010), pp. 33-45, ISSN 1521-6926.

Dan, H.; Sun, M.; Kaneko, S.; Feldman, R.; Nicosia, S.; Wang, H.; Tsang, B. & Cheng, J. (2004). Akt Phosphorylation and Stabilization of X-linked Inhibitor of Apoptosis Protein (XIAP). *Journal of Biological Chemistry*, Vol. 279, No. 7, (February 2004), pp. 5405-5412, ISSN 0021-9258.

Darnay, B.; Ni, J.; Moore, P. & Aggarwal, B. (1999). Activation of NF-κB by RANK Requires Tumor Necrosis Factor Receptor-associated Factor (TRAF) 6 and NF-κB-inducing Kinase. *Journal of Biologic Chemistry*, Vol. 274, No. 12, (March 1999), pp. 7724-7731, ISSN 0021-9258.

Datta, S.; Brunet, A. & Greenberg, M. (1999). Cellular survival: a play in three Akts. *Genes & Development*, Vol. 13, No. 22, (November 1999), pp. 2905-2927, ISSN 0890-9369.

Davis, R. (2000). Signal transduction by the JNK group of MAP kinases. *Cell*, Vol. 103, No. 2, (October 2000), pp. 239-252, ISSN 0092-8674.

De Fanis, U.; Romano, C.; Dalla Mora, L.; Sellitto, A.; Guastafierro, S.; Tirelli, A.; Bresciano, E.; Giunta, R. & Lucivero, G. (2003). Differences in constitutive and activation-induced expression of CD69 and CD95 between normal and chronic lymphocytic leukemia B cells. *Oncology Reports*, Vol. 10, No. 3, (May - June 2003), pp. 653-658, ISSN 1021-335X.

Deaglio, S.; Vaisitti, T.; Bergui, L.; Bonello, L.; Horenstein, A.; Tamagnone, L.; Boumsell, L. & Malavasi, F. (2005). CD38 and CD100 lead a network of surface receptors relaying positive signals for B-CLL growth and survival. *Blood*, Vol. 105, No. 8, (April 2005), pp. 3042-3050, ISSN 0006-4971.

Deaglio, S. & Malavasi, F. (2009). Chronic lymphocytic leukemia microenvironment: shifting the balance from apoptosis to proliferation. *Haematologica*, Vol. 94, No. 6, (June 2009), pp. 752-756, ISSN 0390-6078.

Deaglio, S.; Aydin, S.; Grand, M.; Vaisitti, T.; Bergui, L.; D'Arena, G.; Chiorino, G. & Malavasi, F. (2010). CD38/CD31 Interactions Activate Genetic Pathways Leading to Proliferation and Migration in Chronic Lymphocytic Leukemia Cells. *Molecular Medicine*, Vol. 16, No. 3-4, (March - April 2010), pp. 87-91, ISSN 1076-1551.

Decker, T.; Schneller, F.; Hipp, S.; Miething, C.; Jahn, T.; Duyster, J. & Peschel, C. (2002). Cell cycle progression of chronic lymphocytic leukemia cells is controlled by cyclin D2, cyclin D3, cyclin-dependent kinase (cdk) 4 and the cdk inhibitor p27. *Leukemia*, Vol. 16, No. 3, (March 2002), pp. 327-334, ISSN 0887-6924.

Decker, T.; Hipp, S.; Hahntow, I.; Schneller, F. & Peschel, C. (2004). Expression of cyclin E in resting and activated B-chronic lymphocytic leukaemia cells: cyclin E/cdk2 as a potential therapeutic target. *British Journal of Haematology*, Vol. 125; No. 2, (April 2004), pp. 141-148, ISSN 0007-1048.

Decker, T.; Bogner, C.; Oelsner, M.; Peschel, C. & Ringshausen, I. (2010). Antiapoptotic effect of interleukin-2 (IL-2) in B-CLL cells with low and high affinity IL-2 receptors. *Annals of Hematology*, Vol. 89, No. 11, (November 2010), pp. 1125-1132, ISSN 0939-5555.

Delmer, A.; Ajchenbaum-Cymbalista, F.; Tang, R.; Ramond, S.; Faussat, A.; Marie, J. & Zittoun, R. (1995). Overexpression of Cyclin D2 in Chronic B-Cell Malignancies. *Blood*, Vol. 85, No. 10, (May 1995), pp. 2870-2876, ISSN 0006-4971.

Dempsey, P.; Doyle, S.; He, J. & Cheng, G. (2003). The signalling adaptors and pathways activated by TNF superfamily. *Cytokine & Growth Factor Reviews*, Vol. 14, No. 3-4, (June-August 2003), pp. 193-209, ISSN 1359-6101.

Deveraux, Q. & Reed, J. (1999). IAP family proteins - suppressors of apoptosis. *Genes & Development*, Vol. 13, No. 3, (February 1999), pp. 239-252, ISSN 0890-9369.

Dohner, H.; Stilgenbauer, S.; Benner, A.; Leupolt, E.; Krober, A.; Bullinger, L.; Dohner, K.; Bentz, M. & Lichter, P. (2000). Genomic aberrations and survival in chronic lymphocytic leukemia. *New England Journal of Medicine*, Vol. 343, No. 26, (December 2000), pp. 1910-1916, ISSN 0028-4793.

Faderl, S.; Keating, M.; Do, K.; Liang, S.; Kantarijan, H.; O'Brien, S.; Garcia-Manero, G.; Manshouri, T. & Albitar, M. (2002). Expression profile of 11 proteins and their prognostic significance in patients with chronic lymphocytic leukemia (CLL). *Leukemia*, Vol. 16, No. 6, (June 2002), pp. 1045-1052, ISSN 0887-6924.

Falschlehner, C.; Emmerich, C.; Gerlach, B. & Walczak, H. (2007). TRAIL signalling: decisions between life and death. *International Journal of Biochemistry & Cell Biology*, Vol. 39, No. 7-8, (July-August 2007), pp. 1462-1475, ISSN 1357-2725.

Fan, Y.; Dutta, J.; Gupta, N.; Fan, G. & Gelinas, C. (2008). Regulation of programmed cell death by NF-kappaB and its role in tumorigenesis and therapy, In: *Programmed Cell Death in Cancer Progression and Therapy*, R. Khosravi-Far & E. White (Ed.), Vol. 615, pp. 223-250, Springer, ISBN 978-1-4020-6553-8, New York, NY, USA.

Fayad, L.; Keating, M.; Reuben, J.; O'Brien, S.; Lee, B.; Lerner, S. & Kurzrock, r. (2001). Interleukin-6 and interleukin-10 levels in chronic lymphocytic leukemia: correlation with phenotypic characteristics and outcome. *Blood*, Vol. 97, No. 1, (January 2001), pp. 256-263, ISSN 0006-4971.

Furman, R.; Asgary, Z.; Mascarenhas, J.; Liou, H. & Schattner, E. (2000). Modulation of NF-κB Activity and Apoptosis in Chronic Lymphocytic Leukemia B Cells. *Journal of Immunology*, Vol. 164, No. 4, (February 2000), pp. 2200-2206, ISSN 0022-1767.

Gattei, V.; Bulian, P.; Del Principe, M.; Zuchetto, A.; Maurillo, L.; Buccisano, F.; Bomben, R.; Dal-Bo, M.; Luciano, F.; Rossi, F.; Degan, M.; Amadori, S. & Del Poeta, G. (2008). Relevance of CD49d protein expression as overall survival and progressive disease prognosticator in chronic lymphocytic leukemia. *Blood*, Vol. 111, No. 2, (January 2008), pp. 865-873, ISSN 0006-4971.

Ghia, P.; Strola, G.; Granziero, L.; Geuna, M.; Guida, G.; Sallusto, F.; Ruffing, N.; Montagna, L.; Piccoli, P.; Chilosi, M. & Caligaris-Caprio, F. (2002). Chronic lymphocytic leukemia B cells are endowed with the capacity to attract CD4+, CD40L+ T cells by producing CCL22. *European Journal of Immunology*, Vol. 32, No. 5, (May 2002), pp. 1403-1413, ISSN 0014-2980.

Ghia, P.; Chiorazzi, N. & Stamatopoulos, K. (2008). Microenvironment influences in chronic lymphocytic leukemia: the role of antigen stimulation. *Journal of Internal Medicine*, Vol. 264, No. 6, (December 2008), pp. 549-562, ISSN 1365-2796.

Ghobrial, I.; Bone, N.; Stenson, M.; Novak, A.; Hedin, K.; Kay, N. & Ansell, S. (2004). Expression of the Chemokine Receptors CXCR4 and CCR7 and Disease Progression in B-Cell Chronic Lymphocytic Leukemia/Small Lymphocytic Lymphoma. *Mayo Clinic Proceedings*, Vol. 79, No. 3, (March 2004), pp. 318-325, ISSN 0025-6196.

Ghosh, A.; Secreto, C.; Knox, T.; Ding, W.; Mukhopadhyay, D. & Kay, N. (2010). Circulating microvesicles in B-cell chronic lymphocytic leukemia can stimulate marrow stromal cells: implications for disease progression. *Blood*, Vol. 115, No. 9, (March 2010), pp. 1755-1764, ISSN 0006-4971.

Gine, E.; Martinez, A.; Villamor, N.; Lopez-Guillermo, A.; Camos, M.; Martinez, D.; Esteve, J.; Calvo, X.; Muntanola, A.; Abrisqueta, P.; Rozman, M.; Rozman, C.; Bosch, F.; Campo, E. & Montserrat, E. (2010). Expanded and highly active proliferation centers identify a histological subtype of chronic lymphocytic leukemia ("accelerated" chronic lymphocytic leukemia) with aggressive clinical behavior. *Haematologica*, Vol. 95, No. 9, (September 2010), pp. 1526-1533, ISSN 0390-6078.

Hanada, M.; Delia, D.; Aiello, A.; Stadtmauer, E. & Reed, J.C. (1993). bcl-2 Gene Hypomethylation and High-Level Expression in B-Cell Chronic Lymphocytic Leukemia. *Blood*, Vol. 82, No. 6, (September 1993), pp. 1820-1828, ISSN 0006-4971.

Hewamana, S.; Alghazal, S.; Lin, T.; Clement, M.; Jenkins, C.; Guzman, M.; Jordan, C.; Neelakantan, S.; Crooks, P.; Burnett, A.; Pratt, G.; Fegan, C.; Rowntree, C.; Brennan, P. & Pepper, C. (2008). The NF-κB subunit Rel A is associated with in vitro survival and clinical disease progression in chronic lymphocytic leukemia and represents a promising therapeutic target. *Blood*, Vol. 111, No. 9, (May 2008), pp. 4681-4689, ISSN 0006-4971.

Hjalmar, V.; Hast, R. & Kimby, E. (2002). Cell surface expression of CD25, CD54, and CD95 on B- and T-cells in chronic lymphocytic leukemia in relation to trisomy 12, atypical morphology and clinical course. *European Journal of Haematology*, Vol. 68, No. 3, (March 2002), pp. 127-134, ISSN 0902-4441.

Ihnatko, R. & Kubes, M. (2007). THF signaling: early events and phosphorylation. *General Physiology and Biophysics*, Vol. 26, No. 3, (September 2007), pp. 159-167, ISSN 0231-5882.

Irmler, M.; Thome, M.; Hahne, M.; Schneider, P.; Hofmann, K.; Steiner, V.; Bodmer, J.; Schroter, M.; Burns, K.; Mattmann, C.; Rimoldi, D.; French, L. & Tschopp, J. (1997). Inhibition of death receptor signals by cellular FLIP. *Nature*, Vol. 388, No. 6638, (July 1997), pp. 190-195, ISSN 0028-0836.

Jewell, A.; Lydyard, P.; Worman, C.; Giles, F. & Goldstone, A. (1995). Growth factors can protect B-chronic lymphocytic leukaemia cells against programmed cell death without stimulating proliferation. *Leukemia and Lymphoma*, Vol. 18, No. 1-2, (June 1995), pp. 159-162, ISSN 1042-8194.

Johnson, G.; Sherrington, P.; Carter, A.; Lin, K.; Liloglou, T.; Field, J. & Pettitt, A. (2009). A Novel Type of p53 Pathway Dysfunction in Chronic Lymphocytic Leukemia Resulting from Two Interacting Single Nucleotide Polymorphism within the p21 Gene. *Cancer Research*, Vol. 69, No. 12, (June 2009), pp. 5210-5217, ISSN 0008-5472.

Kern, C.; Cornuel, J.; Billard, C.; Tang, R.; Rouillard, D.; Stenou, V.; Defrance, T.; Ajchenbaum-Cymbalista, F.; Simonin, P.; Feldblum, S. & Kolb, J. (2004).

Involvement of BAFF and APRIL in the resistance to apoptosis of B-CLL through an autocrine pathway. *Blood*, Vol. 103, No. 2, (January 2004), pp. 679-688, ISSN 0006-4971.

Kim, R.; Emi, M. & Tanabe, K. (2005). Caspase-dependent and –independent cell death pathways after DNA damage (Review). *Oncology Reports*, Vol. 14, No. 3, (September 2005), pp. 595-599, ISSN 1021-335X.

Kischkel, F.; Lawrence, D.; Chuntharapai, A.; Schow, P.; Kim, K. & Ashkenazi, A. (2000). Apo2L/TRAIL-dependent recruitment of endogenous FADD and caspase-8 to death receptors 4 and 5. *Immunity*, Vol. 12, No. 6, (June 2000), pp. 611-620, ISSN 1074-7613.

Kitada, S.; Andersen, J.; Akar, S.; Zapata, J.; Takayama, S.; Krajewski, S.; Wang, H.; Zhang, X.; Bullrich, F.; Croce, C.; Rai, K.; Hines, J. & Reed, J. (1998). Expression of Apoptosis-Regulating Proteins in Chronic Lymphocytic Leukemia: Correlations With In Vitro and In Vivo Chemoresposes. *Blood*, Vol. 91, No. 9, (May 1998), pp. 3379-3389, ISSN 0006-4971.

Korz, C.; Pscherer, A.; Benner, A.; Mertens, D.; Schaffner, C.; Leupolt, E.; Dohner, H.; Stilgenbauer, S. & Lichter, P. (2002). Evidence for distinct pathomechanisms in B-cell chronic lymphocytic leukemia and mantle cell lymphoma by quantitative expression analysis of cell cycle and apoptosis-associates genes. *Blood*, Vol. 99, No. 12, (June 2002), pp. 4554-4561, ISSN 0006-4971.

Lai, R.; O'Brien, S.; Maushouri, T.; Rogers, A.; Kantarjian, H.; Keating, M. & Albitar, M. (2002). Prognostic value of plasma interleukin-6 levels in patients with chronic lymphocytic leukemia. *Cancer*, Vol. 95, No. 5, (September 2002), pp. 1071-1075, ISSN 1476-4598.

Laytragoon-Lewin, N.; Duhony, E., Bai, X. & Mellstedt, H. (1998). Downregulation of the CD95 receptor and defect CD40-mediated signal transduction in B-chronic lymphocytic leukemia cells. *European Journal of Haematology*, Vol. 61, No. 4, (October 1998), pp. 266-271, ISSN 0902-4441.

Lin, A. (2003). Activation of the JNK signaling pathway: breaking brake on apoptosis. *BioEssays*, Vol. 25, No. 1, (January 2003), pp. 17-24, ISSN 0265-9247.

Liu, F.; Giustiniani, J.; Farren, T.; Jia, L.; Bensussan, A.; Gribben, J. & Agrawal, S. (2010). CD160 signaling mediates PI3K-dependent survival and growth signals in chronic lymphocytic leukemia. *Blood*, Vol. 115, No. 15, (April 2010), pp. 3079-3088, ISSN 0006-4971.

Liu, J. & Lin, A. (2005). Role of JNK activation in apoptosis: A double-edged sword. *Cell Research*, Vol. 15, No. 1, (January 2005), pp. 36-42, ISSN 1001-0602.

Logue, S. & Martin, S. (2008). Caspase activation cascades in apoptosis. *Biochemical Society Transactions*, Vol. 36, No. 1 (February 2008), pp. 1-9, ISSN 0300-5127.

Longo, P.; Laurenti, L.; Gobessi, S.; Sica, S.; Leone, G. & Efremov, D. (2008). The Akt/Mcl-1 pathway plays a prominent role in mediating antiapoptotic signals downstream of the B-cell receptor in chronic lymphocytic leukemia B cells. *Blood*, Vol. 111, No. 2, (January 2008), pp. 846-855, ISSN 0006-4971.

Mackay, F.; Schneider, P.; Rennert, P. & Browning, J. (2003). BAFF AND APRIL: A Tutorial on B Cell Survival. *Annual Review of Immunology,* Vol. 21, No. 1, (April 2003), pp. 231-264, ISSN 0732-0582.

Mackus, W.; Kater, A.; Grummels, A.; Evers, L.; Hooijbrink, B.; Kramer, M.; Castro, J.; Kipps, T.; van Lier, R.; van Oers, M. & Eldering, E. (2005). Chronic lymphocytic leukemia cells display p53-dependent drug-induced Puma upregulation. *Leukemia,* Vol. 19, No. 3, (March 2005), pp. 427-434, ISSN 0887-6924.

Mainou-Fowler, T.; Craig, V.; Copplestone, J.; Hamon, D. & Prentice, A. (1994). Interleukin-5 (IL-5) Increases Spontaneous Apoptosis of B-Cell Chronic Lymphocytic Leukemia Cells In Vitro Independently of bcl-2 Expression, and Is Inhibited by IL-4. *Blood,* Vol. 84, No. 7, (October 1994), pp. 2297-2304, ISSN 0006-4971.

Mauro, F.; De Rossi, G.; Burgio, V.; Caruso, R.; Giannarelli, D.; Monarca, B.; Romani, C.; Baroni, C. & Mandelli, F. (1994). Prognostic value of bone marrow histology in chronic lymphocytic leukaemia. A study of 335 untreated cases from a single institution. *Haematologica,* Vol. 79, No. 4, (July-August 1994), pp. 334-341, ISSN 0390-6078.

Messmer, B.; Messmer, D.; Allen, S.; Kolitz, J.; Kudalkar, P.; Cesar, D.; Murphy, E.; Koduru, P.; Ferrarini, M.; Zupo, S.; Cutrona, G.; Damle, R.; Wasil, T.; Rai, K.; Hellerstein, M. & Chiorazzi, N. (2005). In vivo measurements document the dynamic cellular kinetics of chronic lymphocytic leukemia B cells. *Journal of Clinical Investigation,* Vol. 115, No. 3, (March 2005), pp. 755-764, ISSN 0021-9738.

Molica, S.; Vitelli, G.; Levato, D.; Crispino, G.; Dell'Olio, M.; Dattilo, A.; Matera, R.; Gandolfo, G. & Musto, P. (1998). CD27 in B-cell chronic lymphocytic leukemia. Cellular expression, serum release and correlation with other soluble molecules belonging to nerve factor receptors (NGFr) superfamily. *Haematologica,* Vol. 83, No. 5, (May 1998), pp. 398-402, ISSN 0390-6078.

Molica, S.; Dattilo, A.; Giulino, C.; Levato, D. & Levato, L. Increased bcl-2/bax ratio in B-cell chronic lymphocytic leukemia is associated with a progressive pattern of disease. *Haematologica,* Vol. 83, No. 12, (December 1998), pp. 1122-1124, ISSN 0390-6078.

Molica, S.; Vitelli, G.; Levato, D.; Levato, L.; Dattilo, A. & Gandolfo, G. (1999). Clinico-biological implications on increased serum levels of interleukin-8 in B-cell chronic lymphocytic leukemia. *Haematologica,* Vol. 84, No. 3, (March 1999), pp. 208-211, ISSN 0390-6078.

Mone, A.; Cheney, C.; Banks, A.; Tridandapani, S.; Mehter, N.; Guster, S.; Lin, T.; Eisenbeis, C, Young, D & Byrd, J. (2006). Alemtuzumab induces caspase-independent cell death in human chronic lymphocytic leukemia cells through a lipid draft-dependent mechanism. *Leukemia,* Vol. 20, No. 2, (February 2006), pp. 272-279, ISSN 0887-6924.

Munk-Pedersen, I. & Reed, J. (2004). Microenvironmental interactions and survival of CLL B-cells. *Leukemia and Lymphoma,* Vol. 45, No. 12, (December 2004), pp. 2365-2372, ISSN 1042-8194.

Nishio, M.; Endo, T.; Tsukada, N.; Ohata, J.; Kitada, S.; Reed, J.; Zvaifler, N. & Kipps, T. (2005). Nurselike cells express BAFF and APRIL, which can promote survival of chronic lymphocytic leukemia cells via a paracrine pathway distinct from that of SDF-1α. *Blood*, Vol. 106, No. 3 (August 2005), pp. 1012-1020, ISSN 0006-4971.

Obermann, E.; Went, P.; Tzankov, A.; Pileri, S.; Hofstaedter, F.; Marienhagen, J.; Stoehr, R. & Dirnhofer, S. (2007). Cell cycle phase distribution analysis in chronic lymphocytic leukaemia: a significant number of cells reside in early G1-phase. *Journal of Clinical Pathology*, Vol. 60, No. 7, (July 2007), pp. 794-797, ISSN 0021-9746.

Ocana, E.; Delgado-Perez, L.; Campos-Caro, A.; Munoz, J.; Paz, A.; Franco, R. & Brieva, J. (2007). The prognostic role of CXCR3 expression by chronic lymphocytic leukemia B cells. *Haematologica*, Vol. 92, No. 3, (March 2007), pp. 349-356, ISSN 0390-6078.

O'Sullivan, R. & Karlseder, J. (2010). Telomeres: protecting chromosomes against genome instability. *Nature Reviews Molecular Cell Biology*, Vol. 11, No. 3, (March 2010), pp. 171-181, ISSN 1471-0072.

Packham, G. & Stevenson, F. (2005). Bodyguards and assassins: Bcl-2 family proteins and apoptosis control in chronic lymphocytic leukaemia. *Immunology*, Vol. 114, No. 4, (April 2005), pp. 441-449, ISSN 0019-2805.

Panayiotidis, P.; Ganeshaguru, K.; Jabbars, A. & Hoffbrand, V. (1993). Interleukin 4 inhibits apoptotic cell death and loss of the bcl 2 protein in B-chronic lymphocytic leukaemia cells in vitro. *British Journal of Haematology*, Vol. 85, No. 3, (November 1993), pp. 439-445, ISSN 0007-1048.

Paul, J.; Henson, E.; Mai, S.; Muchinski, F.; Cheang, M.; Gibson, S. & Johnston, J. (2005). Cyclin D expresion in chronic lymphocytic leukemia. *Leukemia and Lymphoma*, Vol. 46, No. 9, (September 2005), pp. 1275-1285, ISSN 1042-8194.

Pedersen, I.; Kitada, S.; Leoni, L.; Zapata, J.; Karras, J.; Tsukada, N.; Kipps, T.; Choi, Y.; Bennett, F. & Reed, J. (2002). Protection of CLL B cells by a follicular dendritic cell line is dependent on induction of Mcl-1. *Blood*, Vol. 100, No. 5, (September 2002), pp. 1795-1801, ISSN 0006-4971.

Pepper, C.; Lin, T.; Pratt, G.; Hewamana, S.; Brennan, P.; Hiller, L.; Hills, R.; Ward, R.; Starczynski, J.; Austen, B.; Hooper, L.; Stankovic, T. & Fegan, C. (2008). Mcl-1 expression has in vitro and in vivo significance in chronic lymphocytic leukemia and is associated with other poor prognostic markers. *Blood*, Vol. 112, No. 9, (November 2008), pp. 3807-3817, ISSN 0006-4971.

Petlickovski, A.; Laurenti, L.; Li, X.; Marietti, S.; Chiusolo, P.; Sica, S.; Leone, G. & Efremov, D. (2005). Sustained signaling through the B-cell receptor induces Mcl-1 and promotes survival of chronic lymphocytic leukemia B cells. *Blood*, Vol. 105, No. 12, (June 2005), pp. 4820-4827, ISSN 0006-4971.

Podhorecka, M.; Halicka, D.; Klimek, P.; Kowal, M.; Chocholska, S. & Dmoszyńska, A. (2011). Resveratrol increases rate of apoptosis caused by purine analogues in malignant lymphocytes of chronic lymphocytic leukemia. *Annals of Hematology*, Vol. 90, No. 2, (February 2011), pp. 173-183, ISSN 0939-5555.

Riedl, S. & Shi, Y. (2004). Molecular mechanisms of caspase regulation during apoptosis. *Nature Reviews Molecular Cell Biology*, Vol. 5, No. 11 (November 2004), pp. 897-907, ISSN 1471-0072.

Robak, T. (2010). Application of New Drugs in Chronic Lymphocytic Leukemia. *Mediterranean Journal of Hematology and Infectious Diseases*, Vol. 2, No. 2, (May 2010), e2010011, ISSN 2035-3006.

Robertson, L.; Plunkett, W.; McConnell, K.; Keating, M. & McDonnell, T. (1996). Bcl-2 expression in chronic lymphocytic leukemia and Its correlation with the induction of apoptosis and clinical outcome. *Leukemia*, Vol. 10, No. 3, (March 1996), pp. 456-459, ISSN 0887-6924.

Romano, C.; De Fanis, U.; Sellitto, A.; Chiurazzi, F.; Guastafierro, S.; Giunta, R.; Tirelli, A.; Rotoli, B. & Lucivero, G. (2005). Induction of CD95 upregulation does not render chronic lymphocytic leukemia B-cells susceptible to CD95-mediated apoptosis. *Immunology letters*, Vol. 97, No. 1, (February 2005), pp. 131-139, ISSN 0165-2478.

Romano, M.; Lamberti, A.; Tassone, P.; Alfinito, F.; Constantini, S.; Chiurazzi, F.; Defrance, T.; Bonelli, P.; Turco, M. & Venuta, S. (1998). Triggering of CD40 antigen inhibits fludarabine-induced apoptosis in B chronic lymphocytic leukemia cells. *Blood*, Vol. 92, No. 3, (August 1998), pp. 990-995, ISSN 0006-4971.

Roos, G.; Krober, A.; Grabowski, P.; Kienle, D.; Buhler, A.; Dohner, H.; Rosenquist, R. & Stilgenbauer, S. (2008). Short telomeres are associated with genetic complexity, high-risk genomic aberrations, and short survival in chronic lymphocytic leukemia. *Blood*, Vol. 111, No. 4, (February 2008), pp. 2246-2252, ISSN 0006-4971.

Rossi, D.; Cerri, M.; Deambrogi, C.; Sozzi, E.; Cresta, S.; Rasi, S.; De Paoli, L.; Spina, V.; Gattei, V.; Capello, D.; Forconi, F.; Lauria, F. & Gaidano, G. (2009). The prognostic value of TP53 mutations in chronic lymphocytic leukemia is independent of Del17p13: implications for overall survival and chemorefractoriness. *Clinical Cancer Research*, Vol. 15, No. 3, (February 2009), pp. 995-1004, ISSN 1078-0432.

Sainz-Perez, A.; Gary-Gouy, H.; Gaudin, F.; Maarof, G.; Marfaing-Koka, A.; de Revel, T. & Dalloul, A. (2008). IL-24 induces apoptosis of chronic lymphocytic leukemia B cells engaged into the cell cycle through dephosphorylation of STAT3 and stabilization of p53 expression. *Journal of Immunology*, Vol. 181, No. 9, (November 2008), pp. 6051-6060, ISSN 0022-1767.

Sanchez, I. & Dynlacht, B. (2005). New insights into cyclins, CDKs, and cell cycle control. *Seminars in Cell & Developmental Biology*, Vol. 16, No. 3, (June 2005), pp. 31-321, ISSN 1084-9521.

Sellmann, L.; de Beer, D.; Bartels, M.; Opalka, B.; Nuckel, H.; Duhrsen, U.; Durig, J.; Seifert, M.; Siemer, D.; Kuppers, R.; Baerlocher, G. & Roth, A. (2011). Telomeres and prognosis in patients with chronic lymphocytic leukaemia. *International Journal of Hematology*, Vol. 93, No. 1, (January 2011), pp. 74-82, ISSN 0925-5710.

Sivina, M.; Hartmann, E.; Kipps, T.; Rassenti, L.; Krupnik, D.; Lerner, S.; LaPushin, R.; Xiao, L.; Huang, X.; Werner, L.; Neuberg, D.; Kantarjian, H.; O'Brien, S.; Wierda, W.; Keating, M.; Rosenwald, A. & Burger, J. (2011). CCL3 (MIP-1α) plasma levels and the risk for disease progression in chronic lymphocytic leukemia. *Blood*, Vol. 117, No. 5, (February 2011), pp. 1662-1669, ISSN 0006-4971.

Smit, L.; Hallaert, D.; Spijker, R.; de Goeij, B.; Jaspers, A.; Kater, A.; van Oers, M.; van Noesel, C. & Eldering, E. (2007). Differential Noxa/Mcl-1 balance in peripheral versus lymph node chronic lymphocytic leukemia cells correlates with survival capacity. *Blood*, Vol. 109, No. 4, (February 2007), pp. 1660-1668, ISSN 0006-4971.

Soma, L.; Craig, F. & Swerdlow, S. (2006). the proliferation centre microenvironment and prognostic markers in chronic lymphocytic leukemia/small lymphocytic lymphoma. *Human Pathology*, Vol. 37, No. 2, (February 2006), pp. 152-159, ISSN 0046-8177.

Stanglmaier, M.; Reis, S. & Hallek, M. (2004). Rituximab and alemtuzumab induce a nonclassic, caspase-independent spoptotic pathway in B-lymphoid cell lines and in chronic lymphocytic leukemia cells. *Annals of Hematology*, Vol. 83, No. 10, (October 2004), pp. 634-645, ISSN 0939-5555.

Steele, A.; Prentice, A.; Hoffbrand, A.; Yogashangary, B.; Hart, S.; Nacheva, E.; Howard-Reeves, J.; Duke, V.; Kottaridis, P.; Cwynarski, K.; Vassilev, L. & Wickremasinghe, R. (2008). p53-mediated apoptosis of CLL cells: evidence for a transcription-independent mechanism. *Blood*, Vol. 112, No. 9, (November 2008), pp. 3827-3834, ISSN 0006-4971.

Stoetzer, O.; Pogrebniak, A.; Scholz, M.; Pelka-Fleischer, R.; Gullis, E.; Darsow, M.; Nussler, V. & Wilmanns, W. (1999). Drug-induced apoptosis in chronic lymphocytic leukemia. *Leukemia*, Vol. 13, No. 11, (November 1999), pp. 1873-1880, ISSN 0887-6924.

Susin, S.; Daugas, E.; Ravagnan, L.; Samejima, K.; Zamzami, N.; Loeffler, M.; Constantini, P.; Ferri, K.; Irinopoulou, T.; Prevost, M.; Brothers, G.; Mak, T.; Penninger, J.; Earnshaw, W. & Kroemer, G. (2000). Two Distinct Pathways Leading to Nuclear Apoptosis. *Journal of Experimental Medicine*, Vol. 192, No. 4, (August 2000), pp. 571-580, ISSN 0022-1007.

Tait, S. & Green, D. 2008. Caspase independent cell death: leaving the set without the final cut. *Oncogene*, Vol. 27, No. 50, (October 2008), pp. 6452-6461, ISSN 0950-9232.

Thomas, A.; Pepper, C.; Hoy, T. & Bentley, P. (2000). Bcl-2 and bax expression and chlorambucil-induced apoptosis in the T-cells and leukaemic B-cells of untreated B-cell chronic lymphocytic leukaemia patients. *Leukemia Research*, Vol. 24, No. 10, (October 2000), pp. 813-821, ISSN 0145-2126.

Till, K.; Lin, K.; Zuzel, M. & Cawley, J. (2002). the chemokine receptor CCR7 and α4 integrin are important for migration of chronic lymphocytic leukemia cells into lymph nodes. *Blood*, Vol. 99, No. 8, (April 2002), pp. 2977-2984, ISSN 0006-4971.

Trentin, L.; Zambello, R.; Sancetta, R.; Facco, M.; Carutti, A.; Perin, A.; Siviero, M.; Basso, U.; Bortolin, M.; Adami, F.; Agostini, C. & Semenzato, G. (1997). B Lymphocytes from Patients with Chronic Lymphoproliferative Disorders Are Equipped with Different Costimulatory Molecules. *Cancer Research*, Vol. 57, No. 21, (November 1997), pp. 4940-4947, ISSN 0008-5472.

Vallabhapurapu, S. & Karin, M. (2009). Regulation and Function of NF-κB Transcription Factors in the Immune System. *Annual Review of Immunology*, Vol. 27, No. 1, (April 2009), pp. 693-733, ISSN 0732-0582.

Veronese, L.; Tournilhac, O.; Verrelle, P.; Davi, F.; Dighiero, G.; Chautard, E.; Veyrat-Masson, R.; Kwiatkowski, F.; Goumy, C.; Vago, P.; Travade, P. & Tchirkov, A. (2008). Low MCL-1 mRNA expression correlates with prolonged survival in B-cell chronic lymphocytic leukemia. *Leukemia*, Vol. 22, No. 6, (June 2008), pp. 1291-1293, ISSN 0887-6924.

von Bergwelt-Baildon, M.; Maecker, B.; Schultze, J. & Gribben, J. (2004). CD40 activation: potential for specific immunotherapy in B-CLL. *Annals of Oncology*, Vol. 15, No. 6, (June 2004), pp. 853-857, ISSN 0923-7534.

Vousden, K. & Lu, X. (2002). Live or let die: the cell's response to p53. *Nature Reviews Cancer*, Vol. 2, No. 8, (August 2002), pp. 594-605, ISSN 1474-175X.

Vrhovac, R.; Delmer, A.; Tang, R.; Marie, J.; Zittoun, R. & Ajchenbaum-Cymbalista, F. (1998). Prognostic Significance of the Cell Cycle Inhibitor $p27^{Kip1}$ in Chronic B-Cell Lymphocytic Leukemia. *Blood*, Vol. 91, No. 12, (June 1998), pp. 4694-4700, ISSN 0006-4971.

Wei, M.; Zong, W.; Cheng, E.; Lindsten, T.; Panoutsakopoulou, V.; Ross, A.; Roth, K.; MacGregor, G.; Thompson, C. & Korsmeyer, S. (2001). Proapoptotic BAX and BAK: A Requisite Gateway to Mitochondrial Dysfunction and Death. *Science*, Vol. 292, No. 5517, (April 2001), pp. 727-730, ISSN 0036-8075.

Winkler, D.; Schneider, C.; Zucknick, M.; Bogelein, D.; Schulze, K.; Zenz, T.; Mohr, J.; Philippen, A.; Huber, H.; Buhler, A.; Habermann, A.; Benner, A.; Dohner, H.; Stilgenbauer, S. & Mertens, D. (2010). Protein expression analysis of chronic lymphocytic leukemia defines the effect of genetic aberrations and uncovers a correlation of CDK4, P27 and P53 with hierarchical risk. *Haematologica*, Vol. 95, No. 11, (November 2010), pp. 1880-1888, ISSN 0390-6078.

Wołowiec, D.; Benchaib, M.; Pernas, P.; Deviller, P.; Souchier, C.; Rimokh, R.; Felman, P.; Bryon, P. & Ffrench, M. (1995). Expression of cell cycle regulatory proteins in chronic lymphocytic leukemias. Comparison with non-Hodgkin's lymphomas and non-neoplastic lymphoid tissue. *Leukemia*, Vol. 9, No. 8, (August 1995), pp. 1382-1388, ISSN 0887-6924.

Wołowiec, D.; Ciszak, L.; Kosmaczewska, A.; Boćko, D.; Teodorowska, R.; Frydecka, I. & Kuliczkowski, K. (2001). Cell cycle regulatory proteins and apoptosis in B-cell chronic lymphocytic leukemia. *Haematologica*, Vol. 86, No. 12, (December 2001), pp. 1296-1304, ISSN 0390-6078.

Wołowiec, D.; Wójtowicz, M.; Ciszak, L.; Kosmaczewska, A.; Frydecka, I.; Potoczek, S.; Urbaniak-Kujda, D.; Kapelko-Słowik, K. & Kuliczkowski, K. (2009). High intracellular kontent of cyklin-dependent kinase inhibitor $p27^{Kip1}$ in early- and intermedia te stage B-cell chronic lymphocytic leukemia lymphocytes predicts rapid progression of the disease. *European Journal of Haematology*, Vo. 82, No. 4, (April 2009), pp. 260-266, ISSN 0902-4441.

Xie, P.; Kraus, Z.; Stunz, L. & Bishop, G. (2008). Roles of TRAF molecules in B lymphocyte Function. *Cytokine & Growth Factor Reviews*, Vol. 19, No. 3-4, (June - August 2008), pp. 199-207, ISSN 1359-6101.

Yen Chong, S.; Lin, Y.; Czarneski, J.; Zhang, M.; Coffman, F.; Kashanchi, F. & Raveche, E. (2001). Cell cycle effects of IL-10 on malignant B-1 cells. *Genes and Immunity*, Vol. 2, No. 5, (August 2001), pp. 239-247, ISSN 1466-4879.

Yu, C.; Minemoto, Y.; Zhang, J.; Liu, J.; Tang, F.; Bui, T.; Xiang, J. & Lin, A. (2004). JNK Suppresses Apoptosis via Phosphorylation of the Proapoptotic Bcl-2 Family Protein BAD. *Molecular Cell*, Vol. 13, No. 3, (February 2004), pp. 329-340, ISSN 1097-2765.

Zheng, C.; Yin, Q. & Wu, H. (2011). Structural studies of NF-κB signaling. *Cell Research*, Vol. 21, No. 1, (January 2011), pp. 183-195, ISSN 1001-0602.

4

DNA Damage Response/Signaling and Genome (In)Stability as the New Reliable Biological Parameters Defining Clinical Feature of CLL

Jozo Delic[1], Jean-Brice Marteau[1], Karim Maloum[2], Florence Nguyen-Khac[2], Frédéric Davi[2], Zahia Azgui[2], Véronique Leblond[3], Jacques-Louis Binet[2], Sylvie Chevillard[1] and Hélène Merle-Béral
[1]*Laboratoire de Cancérologie Expérimentale, Institut de Radiobiologie Cellulaire et Moléculaire, Commissariat à l'Energie Atomique et aux Energies Renouvelables (CEA),*
[2]*Services d'Hématologie Biologique, Groupe Hospitalier Pitié-Salpêtrière,*
[3]*Clinique, Groupe Hospitalier Pitié-Salpêtrièr,*
France

1. Introduction

The commonest hematological malignancy chronic lymphocytic leukemia (CLL) is currently incurable with a high incidence of morbidity and mortality (Chiorazzi et al., 2005; Dighiero & Hamblin, 2008; Hallek & Pflug, 2011). Clinically, the disease is diagnosed in most cases accidentally as an indolent form of leukemia but subsequently it may turn rapidly into an aggressive form. Moreover, in a subset of patients, CLL is presented as high-risk progressive form at diagnosis. This heterogeneous clinical course of CLL relies on the variable expression of defined several biological factors which may affect susceptibility to apoptotic cell death upon treatment (Hamblin 2007; Kipps 2007;; Lanasa 2010; Caligaris-Cappio & Chiorazzi 2010; Zenz et al., 2011; Parker & Strout 2011; Fabris et al., 2011). Our understanding of the molecular alterations leading to the leukemogenesis of CLL, even if these appeared already complex, remains still far to be achieved. Current researches by performing new genomic approaches, allowed an identification of new genes recurrently mutated in CLL suggesting their oncogenic role of potential clinical relevance (Fabri et al., 2011; Puente et al., 2011). Two major biological features such as the usage of mutated or unmutated immunoglobulin heavy chain variable region genes (*IGHV*) and the number and the type of chromosomal aberrations, clearly distinguish distinct clinical patients' subgroups (Fais et al., 1998; Damle et al., 1999; Hamblin et al., 1999; Maloum et al., 2000; Zenz et al., 2007; Klein & Dalla-Favera, 2011). While the *IGHV* status may appear in some cases as a more complex and complicated prognostic marker (Ghiotto et al., 2011; Langerak et al., 2011), specific genomic aberrations appear as an accurate "drivers" of the disease and of its clinical characteristics (Zenz et al., 2011). In some high-risk CLL cases, there is an association between these two independent makers of poor prognosis such as the presence of 11q22 deletions in cells with unmutated *IGHV*.

Another biological hallmark of CLL cells, with an evident therapeutic impact, is the aberrantly increased B cell receptor (BCR) signaling. It consists of surface immunoglobulin associated with heterodimer CD79α and CD79β. This aberrant BCR signaling consequently activates the Src family protein tyrosine kinases Lyn and Syk which promotes an activation in cascade of downstream signaling pathways including phosphatidyl-3-kinase (PI3K, see below), which generates phosphatidylinositol-3-phosphate necessary for the activation of the kinase Akt. Simultaneously to PI3K activation, the phospholypase Cγ2 is also activated. This last enzyme is involved in protein kinase C (PKC) activation which is an essential cell surviving factor. Effectively, an activation of PKC leads to an activation of the transcriptional anti-apoptotic factor NF-κB (see later) and to activation of mitogen-activated kinases (MAPKs) such as MEK/ERK, JNK and p38 MAPK as well as mTorc1 inhibitor rapamycin and cyclin-dependent protein kinase. The final consequence of these cascades of events is an anti-apoptotic "attitude" of CLL cells that may present a major source of the identification of novel therapeutic targets (for review see Wickremasinghe et al., 2011 and references within).

Men are more frequently affected by an aggressive form of the disease and develop it at a younger age than women (Mauro et al., 1999; Cartwright et al., 2002). In addition, CLL cells in men more commonly display no mutations in *IGHV* genes that allow, according to gene expression profiling, putting in evidence that male patients may segregate in a distinct CLL subgroup (Haslinger et al., 2004). We have reported that the gene expression profiles may also be discriminating not only between apoptosis resistant and sensitive cells (Vallat et al., 2003), but also according to patients' gender (Marteau et al., 2011).

In addition to not yet fully defined defect in apoptotic death, the homeostatic balance or imbalance in a dynamic interplay between proliferation and cell death may underline the stable (indolent) or progressive forms of CLL, respectively (Messmer et al., 2005; Chiorazzi & Ferrarini, 2011). The mechanisms that induce a switch from indolent to more aggressive form of this malignancy remain unclear. Hence, clinical and biological heterogeneities may allow us to postulate two models of CLL cell origin; single- or multiple-cell origin model (Chiorazzi & Ferrarini, 2011). Although the microarray data suggested the same cell origin for two major subsets of CLL (i.e. CLLs with mutated and CLLs with unmutated *IGHV* genes, Klein et al., 2001; Rosenwald et al. 2001), according to B-cell receptors (BCRs) repertory and signaling capacity as well to the specific *IGHV* usages, a model of two-cell origin would be more appropriated to explain clonal cell expansion and thus an emergence of indolent and aggressive form of disease (Hamblin et al., 2000; Damle et al., 1999; Schroeder & Dighiero, 1994; Fais et al., 1998; Zupo et al., 1996; Lanham et al., 2003; Herve et al., 2005; Colombo et al., 2011). Both of these two models converge to an antigen-experienced lymphocyte(s) according to the membrane phenotype of CLL cells. Because of the possibility that CLL clones may develop and diversify its Ig receptor (with either mutated or unmutated *IGHV* genes), T-cell dependent, droved to the concept of the unique follicular marginal zone B cell origin. In spite of differences in poly- and auto-antigen-binding activities among CLL clones, the analyses of the amino acid sequences of B-cell receptor showed remarkably similarity in some but not all of these clones (Chiorazzi & Ferrarini, 2011), seeding thus a doubt of one-cell origin. However, if the normal B cell counterparts should absolutely be searched, we should consider also the arguments that human marginal zone B cell population is a separate population that develops and diversifies Ig receptor outside T cell-dependent or -independent immune responses (Weill et al., 2009). In addition, considering the possibility of somatic diversification independent of antigen-driven responses and the existence of the subpopulation of circulating "memory" long-lived B cells harbouring a pre-diversified immunoglobulin repertoire in humans, then the concept of CLL cell origin may also radically differ from above hypotheses of two origin models (Weller et al., 2004; Weill & Reynaud, 2005; Weller et al., 2008). Alternatively, irrespectively to normal cellular counterparts, CLL cells may emerge from initially damaged cell in bone marrow which subsequently followed a development and immunoglobulin diversification according to the extend of its initial damage.

Although, the characterizations of several biological markers fit well with the appearance and/or maintenance of progressive disease, none of them are considered in a clinical decision regarding when and by applying which type of treatment the therapy should really start. The current front line therapies for CLL include drugs that directly or indirectly induce DNA damage which ultimately should result in apoptotic cell death.

2. Two classes of CLL cells according to their ability to activate or not DNA damage-induced apoptosis: Clinical relevance?

The aggressive form of disease resistant to front line treatment develops in approximately one third of patients who succumb rapidly due to the lack of effective therapies and/or a lack of prospective tools enabling the predicting treatment response including early relapse. Alkylating agents (i.e. chlorambucil) or purine nucleoside analogues such as fludarabine, mediate cell death of CLL cells through DNA damage, including double strand breaks (DSBs) and p53-dependent apoptosis (Rosenwald et al., 2004; Austen et al., 2007; Amrein et al, 2007; Döhner et al., 1995). Further, fludarabine treatment *in vivo* induces a gene expression response similar to that induced by the *in vitro* exposure of cells to ionizing irradiation (Rosenwald et al., 2004), suggesting the common mechanisms achievable by these two treatments. The loss of functional p53 or a defect in the ataxia telangiectasia protein (ATM) which acts upstream of p53, leads to a more rapid disease progression, is associated with resistance and shortened overall survival times as well as with an appearance of signs of disease complications (i.e. lymphadenopathy, Döhner et al. 1997).

We have reported that ~20% of patients harbor B cells resistant to DNA damage-induced apoptosis, irrespective of p53 status, while the remaining 80% of patients have p53wt-expressing cells sensitive to genotoxic agents (Figure 1). Although p53 deficiency (through point mutations or 17p13 deletions) defines poor disease outcome (Döhner et al., 1995; Grever et al., 2007; Catovsky et al., 2007; Mohr et al., 2011), we hypothesized that specific pathways independent of p53 and/or acting upstream of this tumor suppressor could operate in resistance mechanisms of CLL cells.

This last observation led us to perform a retrospective study to definitely establish: **i**) the relevance of whether an inherent resistance to DNA damage induced-apoptosis underlines poor disease outcome; **ii**) which dynamic biological alterations shepherd otherwise sensitive cells to become resistant and **iii**) whether these biological features of CLL cells should be considered by clinicians in a decision to apply or not the front line treatment (including DNA damaging drugs such as alkylants and base analogues) for patients harboring these cells.

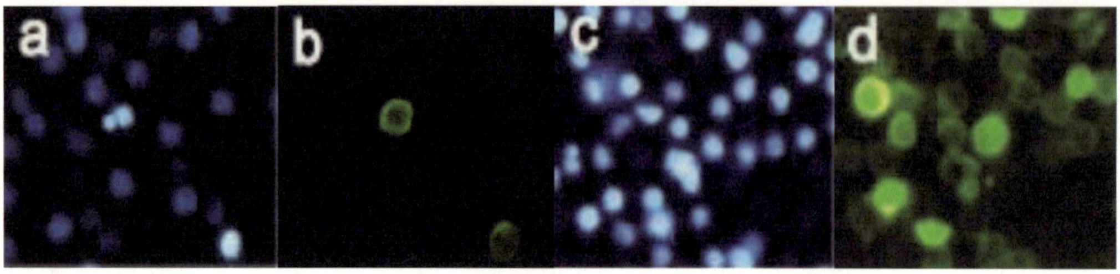

Fig. 1. Fluorescent labeling of apoptotic CLL cells.

Apoptotic cells are revealed by double staining of chromatin-DNA by Hoechst 33342 (a, c) and of phosphatydyl-serine externalization on membrane surface by annexin V-FITC (b, d). Resistant cells (a, b) are clearly distinguished from sensitive cells (c, d) by bright Hoechst staining (a) of annexin V positive cells (b).

A cohort of 308 CLL cases was examined for cell sensitivity/resistance to DNA damage-induced apoptosis and this biological parameter was correlated to the presence/expression of at least another bad prognostic factor described in literature. Together, these biological factors were correlated to the clinical features of each patient covering up to 25 years period.

As shown in Figure 2, 18,8% of CLL cell samples were resistant to DNA damage-induced apoptosis *in vitro* while remaining 82,2% were sensitive. Consistent with data in literature, in this cohort of CLL patients, men appear to be affected more frequently than women. Of note, this gender-dependent ratio appears also to be conserved for the subset of patients' samples resistant to DNA damage-induced apoptosis.

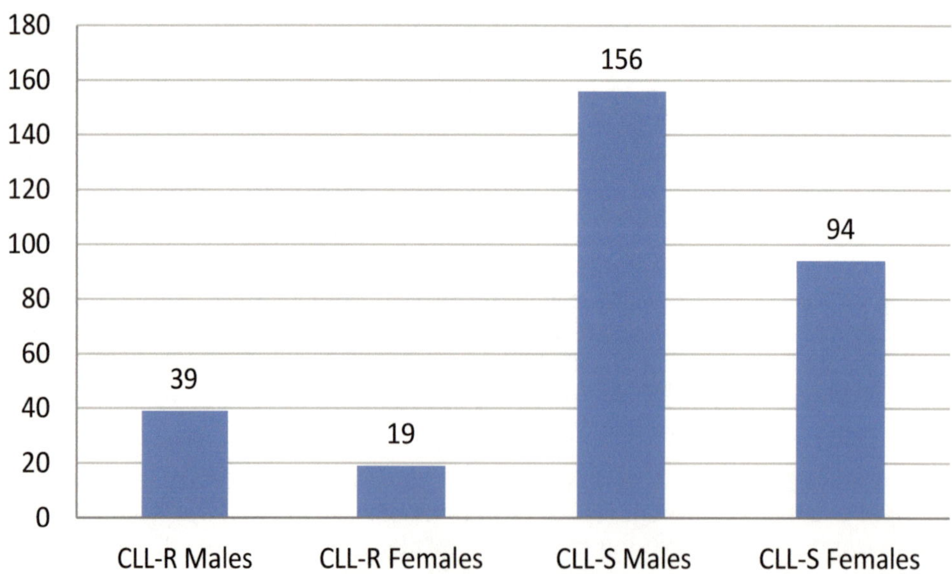

Fig. 2. Incidence of CLL cells resistant (CLL-R) or sensitive (CLL-S) to DNA damage-induced apoptosis *in vitro* in a cohort of 308 patients' samples according to patients' gender.

Percentage of apoptotic cells were determined by fluorescent labeling and microscopic counting at 24h of culture of CLL cells exposed *in vitro* to genotoxic stress (10Gy of γ-rays or 1μM of Neocarcinostatine). Y-axis: number of patients' samples.

After these first observations, our goal was to determine whether and how the presence of at least one biological factor (such as Zap70 and CD38 positivity, elevated level of sCD23, deletions/mutations of *TP53* and *ATM* and/or the presence of other multiple cytogenetic aberrations or complex karyotype), considered to be associated with poor disease outcome ("Bad prognostic factors" in graph 1), the *IGHV* status (graph 2), and the resistance or sensitivity to DNA damage-induced apoptosis (graph 3a, 3b and 3c) may influence overall time survival by comparing the survival curves of two well-defined groups on the basis of these phenotypes from this cohort of CLL patients.

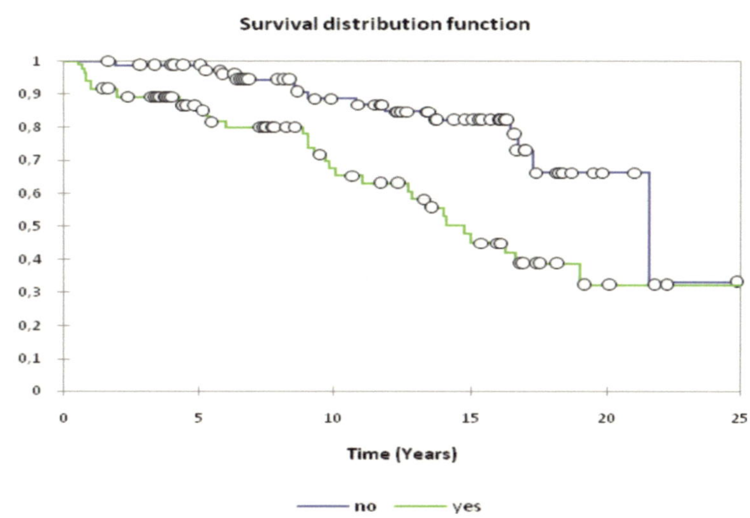

Graph 1. Bad prognostic factors influence on survival time.

50 patients with at least one bad prognostic factor (**yes**) out of 84 have been censured (survival) *vs.* 66 of 80 without bad prognostic factor (**no**). We confirmed that the median survival time was significantly lower for the group of patients harboring malignant B cells with "unfavorable phenotype" than for its counterpart (15.200 ± 1.208 years vs. 18.529 ± 0.757 years). The difference between these two survivor functions is very significant (Log-rank, Wilcoxon and Tarone-ware -tests $p < 0.001$). Thus, the comparison of the two survival curves allows us to confirm that in our cohort, patients with one or more bad prognostic factors have significantly lower survival time than patients without the presence of these factors. These results are in agreement with other studies reported in literature.

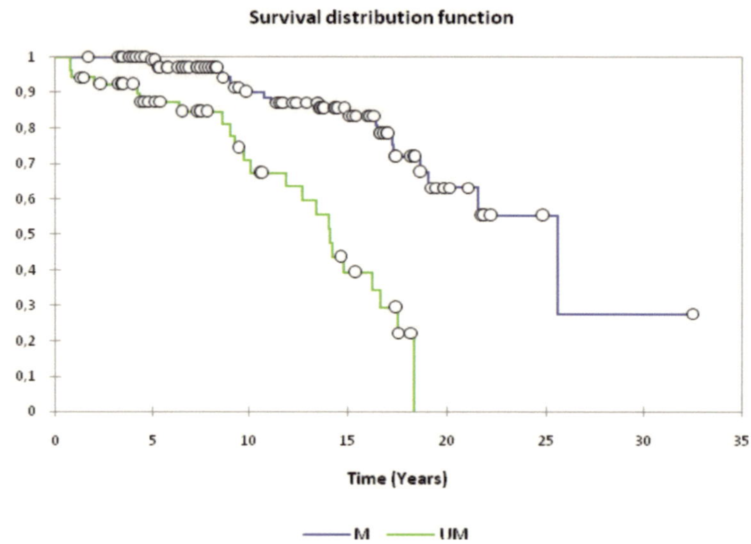

Graph 2. The status of variable regions of heavy chains of immunoglobulin genes (*IGHV*) influence on CLL patients' survival time.

In patients harboring mutated (M) *IGHV* genes, 88 patients from 108 have been censured (survival) and 29 of 52 in the unmutated (UM) group. We notice that the median survival time is a lot lower for the *IGHV* unmutated group than for the *IGHV* mutated group (12.852 ± 0.879 years vs. 21.033 ± 0.876 years). The difference between the two survivor functions is very significant (Log-rank, Wilcoxon and Tarone-ware -tests $p < 0.0001$). The comparison of the two survival curves allows us to conclude and to confirm that the *IGHV* mutated status impacts significantly positively the survival time of patients.

We next addressed the question whether the resistance to DNA damage -induced apoptosis may be a new parameter that also may influence on overall survival of CLL patients and if yes, whether this influence was concomitant to that observed with other bad prognostic factors. For this purpose we designed three comparisons. Two groups of patients' cell samples were selected on the knowledge of their status according to the sensitivity or resistance to DNA damage-induced apoptosis (graph 3a) and then splitted according to the lack (graph 3b) or the presence (graph 3c) of at least one bad prognostic factor (i.e. Zap70, CD38 and sCD23 positivity, UM *IGHV*, *ATM* or *TP53* mutations or deletions or other cytogenetic abnormalities or aberrant karyotype).

In the resistant sub-group, 21 patients out of 58 have been censured (survival) and 203 out of 245 in the sensitive group. We noticed that the median survival time was significantly lower for the resistant group of patients (R) than for the sensitive (S) group of patients (11.562 ± 1.097 years vs. 19.773 ± 0.672 years). The difference between the two survivor functions is very significant (Log-rank, Wilcoxon and Tarone-ware -tests $p < 0.0001$). The comparison of the two survival curves allows us to conclude that the resistance to DNA damage-induced apoptosis *in vitro* negatively impacts in a very significant manner on the survival time of CLL patients.

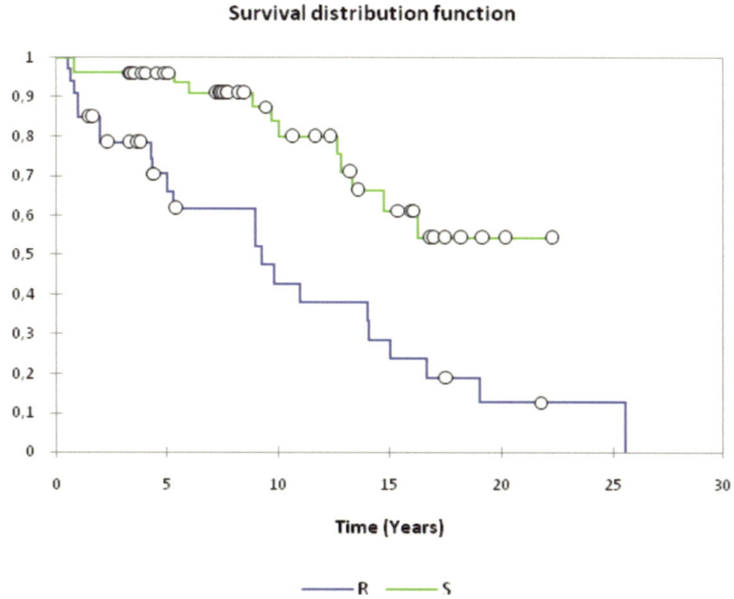
Survival distribution function
1
0,9
0,8
0,7
0,6
0,5
0,4
0,3
0,2
0,1
0
0
5
10
15
20
25
30
Time (Years)
R
S

a

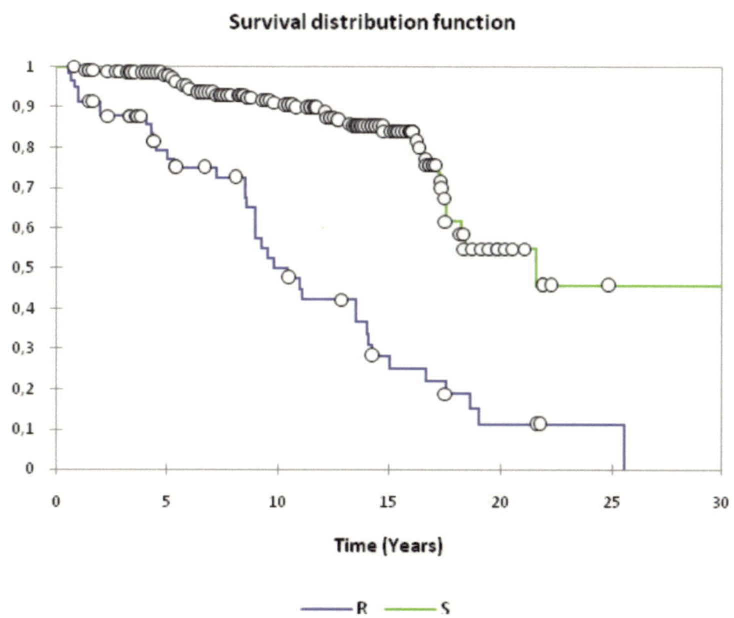
Survival distribution function
1
0,9
0,8
0,7
0,6
0,5
0,4
0,3
0,2
0,1
0
0
5
10
15
20
25
30
Time (Years)
R
S

b

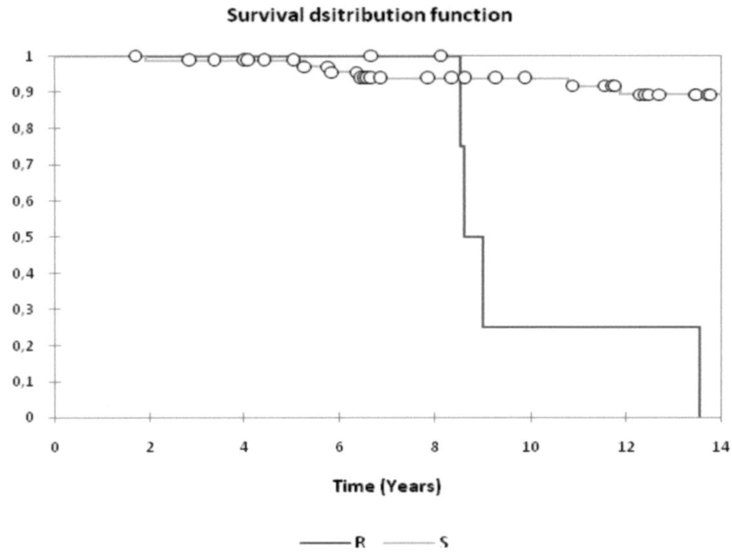

c

Graph 3. a) Survival time in sub-group of patients harboring CLL cells resistant (R) to DNA damage-induced apoptosis vs. sub-group harboring sensitive (S) cells. b) Influence of time survival between patients harboring resistant (R) or sensitive (S) CLL cells with at least one bad pronostic factor expression. c) Influence of time survival between R and S patients without any bad pronostic factor.

When patients have at least one bad pronostic factor (**graph 3b**), the same reduction of overall survival time was observed for the resistant group (11 censored out of 33) i.e. 10.593 ± 1.611 years in contrast to a higher survival time for the sensitive patients (39 censored out of 51) 15.946 ± 1.014 years (Log-rank, Wilcoxon and Tarone-ware –tests, $p < 0.0001$).

In the group of CLL cell samples resistant to radiation induced apoptosis, 2 patients out of 6 have been censured (survival) and 64 of 74 in the sensitive group. We noticed that the median survival time is a much lower for the resistant group (R) group than for the sensitive (S) group (9.92 ± 1.208 years vs. 19.773 ± 0.672 years). The difference between the two survivor functions is very significant (Log-rank, Wilcoxon and Tarone-ware -tests $p < 0.0001$). The comparison of the two survival curves allows us to conclude that the resistance to DNA damage-induced apoptosis negatively impacts the patients' survival time and, despite of the small number of patients without any bad pronostic factor, resistance to DNA damage-induced apoptosis can clearly be considered as a unique independent prognostic factor defining a subset of CLL with poor clinical outcome (**graph 3c**).

In our cohort seven patients (2,2%) clinically evolved during the study and their cells changed the apoptotic status. Effectively, initially sensitive cells became resistant to DNA damage-induced apoptosis *in vitro*. In five patients these changes occurred following front-line treatment because they expressed at least another bad prognostic factor (i.e. UM status of *IGHV*, delTP53, CD38^{+} or Zap70^{+} or presented two chromosomal aberrations). Disease evolved in two other patients who did not received chemotherapy and who did not expressed another bad prognostic factor. Of note, concomitant to this change of the sensitivity toward resistance to activate apoptotic death pathway, increased activity of DNA repair through non-homologous end-joining as well as a shortening of telomeric sequences (see next two paragraphs), have been observed in these evolving cases. These observations let us to speculate that both front-line treatment, when inefficient, may contribute to an emergence of resistant cells and that in patients without an expression of another biological bad prognostic factor, the resistance to DNA damage-induced apoptosis may be a new independent bad prognostic factor for a subset of CLL patients.

Together, data clearly demonstrate that the resistance to DNA damage-induced apoptosis *in vitro* is a parameter reliable of resistant form of disease and that the switching from sensitive to resistant cell status *in vitro* is concomitant to disease progression from indolent to aggressive form. Acquisition of resistant phenotype, critical telomere shortening and NHEJ defect are proposed as events preceding disease switching according to other established parameters (i.e. TP53 and ATM status, chromosomal aberrations, $Zap70^+$, $CD38^+$).

Defining the molecular origin of the underlying mechanisms of cell resistance to DNA damage-induced apoptosis *in vitro* should open new perspectives of clinical use in CLL.

3. Biological features of CLL cells resistant to DNA damage-induced apoptosis

3.1 DNA repair defect?

Our initial observation was that one CLL patient displayed malignant cells sensitive to ionizing irradiation-induced apoptosis *in vitro* while cells from a second patient were completely resistant. These first two cases were confirmed and validated in a large cohort of CLL samples thus allowing us to propose that CLL could be stratified into at least two new subgroups: resistant and sensitive groups. We next asked if this resistance to activate apoptotic death pathway could be due to DNA double strand breaks (DSBs) or to other effects induced by γ-rays. To answer this question we addressed comet assay to measure DNA damage directly in irradiated cells. This assay, performed in alkaline experimental conditions, allows assessing of resting single and double strand breaks directly in interphase nuclei. Surprisingly, an excess of resting DNA damage was established in sensitive rather than in resistant cells 20 min after radiation exposure (Blaise et al., 2001), emphasizing that resistant cells removed DNA damage more rapidly than sensitive cells. To further address DNA damage causality in apoptotic response, we next treated cells with radiomimetic drugs such as neocarcinostatin which is known to specifically induce DNA DSBs without other side effects in cell, or drugs currently used in cancer therapy (topoisomerase I and II inhibitors or fludarabine), also able to induce indirectly DSBs. In this way, we tested whether cell resistance to γ-rays-induced apoptosis would be validated by the same resistance induced by these drugs. Effectively, we reported (Deriano et al., 2005), that these cells were resistant to all tested DNA damaging agents concluding that the resistance to apoptosis should underscore a defect in DNA damage repair/signaling. DNA repair has already been postulated as the mechanism causing drug resistance in CLL (Panasci et al., 2001; rev. Guipaud et al., 2003). First observation of a defective nucleotide excision repair (NER, as the main pathway employed in modified DNA bases clearance after UV exposure or alkylating agent treatments during cancer therapy), occurring in CLL was first reported in 1972 (Huang et al., 1972). Alkylation and interstrand cross-links produced by nitrogen mustards (i.e. chlorambucil) may activate recombinational DNA repair in CLL cells (Bramson et al., 1995). Non-homologous end-joining (NHEJ) was first suspected to play a role in CLL drug resistance through an increased activity of DNA-PK complex (including both, the DNA end-binding activity of heterodimer Ku70/Ku80 and the phosphorylation activity of DNA-PKcs; Muller and Salles, 1997). In consequence, use of wortmanin, an inhibitor of PI3-Kinases along with DNA-PKcs (which is PI3-K like kinase), was able to potentialize cytotoxic effect of chlorambucil in CLL cells (Christodoulopoulos et al., 1998). Also, a DNA-PKcs specific inhibitor Nu7441 combined with drugs inducing DNA DSBs has been pointed as a potential therapy for high risk CLL (Elliott et al., 2011). After genotoxic stress and first cell division, structural chromosomal aberrations (dicentric, acentric or ring chromosomes) occurred more frequently in resistant than in sensitive CLL cells (Blaise et al., 2001), suggesting an accelerated but certainly unfaithful DNA repair. We addressed an *in vitro* assay enabling us to measure the overall activity and fidelity of non-homologous end-joining (NHEJ) DNA repair and the activities of two essential components of NHEJ heterodimer Ku70/Ku80 and DNA-PKcs. Accelerated DNA repair, an increased activity of Ku DNA end-binding as well as an increased kinase activity of DNA-PKcs were observed in resistant cells (Deriano et al., 2005). Moreover, this upregulation of NHEJ was found to be error-prone and thus potentially mutagenic since large DNA deletions occurred at sites of repair (Deriano et al., 2006). The potential impact of such resistance upon the onset of malignancy is likely to be increased by the resulting block on apoptosis induction which may in consequence contribute to the emergence of additional resistant clones from a proliferative pool of mutant cells. Recent reports have shown that drug-induced DSBs in cells in culture *in vitro* (such as CsA or fludarabine) are repaired exclusively by NHEJ (O'Driscol & Jeggo 2009; De Campos-Nebel et al., 2009) which is the main cell cycle-independent repair pathway for this type of DNA damage in mammalian cells (Lieber 2008; Delacote and Lopez, 2008; Mari et al., 2006). According to protein components needed to achieve repair activity, two NHEJ pathways have been found operating in cells (for rev. see Mladenov and Iliakis, 2011); classical NHEJ depending on the activities of at least 7 identified factors (i.e. Ku70, Ku80, DNA-PKcs, Arthemis, XRCC4, Cernunos (also called XRCC4-like factor, XLF) and Ligase IV) and alternative NHEJ which depends on MRN trimmer complex but its repair activity is, obviously, independent of proteins needed for classical pathway (Corneo et al., 2007, Yan et al., 2007; Deriano et al., 2009; Lee-Theilen et al., 2011). This alternative NHEJ was demonstrated to be error-prone and consequently, mutagenic since it uses microhomology pairing and thus nucleotides loss. Whether this pathway may be really involved in initiation of malignant process in humans remain still to be elucidated. An upregulated classical NHEJ was reported to take place in Bloom's syndrome exhibiting high chromosomal instability and cancer susceptibility as well as in myeloid leukemia harboring multiple chromosomal aberrations (Rasool et al., 2003). Defect, also in classical NHEJ, due to ligase IV dysfunction, has been associated with the appearance of radiosensitive leukemia in patients exhibiting developmental delay and immunodeficiency (Riballo et al., 1999; O'Driscoll et al., 2001). ATM deficiency, occurring mainly through point mutations or 11q22 deletions, has been observed in high risk CLLs (Stankovic et al., 1999; Austen et al., 2005). This deficiency causes a defective DNA repair through homologous recombination and consequently, resistance to therapy. One of new concepts to overcome cancer resistance consists in a conversion of one form of DNA damage into another form, that in a cell harboring defective gene involved in DNA damage response, cannot be repaired and inevitably leads to cell death (Helleday et al., 2008). Using this concept, inhibitors of poly (ADP-ribose) polymerase 1 (PARP), a component of the DNA single strand break (SSB) repair complex, may convert unrepaired SSB lesions of DNA into DSBs during DNA replication that require activation of HR repair proteins (i.e. BRCA1/2) for their resolution. If tumor cells defective in *BRCA1/2* were treated with PARP1 inhibitor, they accumulate extensive DNA DSBs and underwent cell death (Bryant et al., 2005; Farmer et al., 2005). Stankovic's group investigated whether this synthetic lethality resulting from inhibition of PARP would also be applicable to *ATM* mutant lymphoid tumors and consequently, may result in their specific killing. They demonstrated a differential *in vitro* and *in vivo* sensitivity of primary and transformed *ATM* mutant CLL and MCL tumor cells to a new clinically tested PARP inhibitor (olaparib) which may be a new promising therapy in high risk CLLs (Weston et al., 2010). Considering a functional overlapping between ATM and XLF (Cernunos) involved in classical NHEJ (Zha et al., 2011), then this strategy would be emphasized from homologous recombination to NHEJ in parallel. Another combined strategy to avoid the fludarabine-resistance of CLL cells uses simultaneously fludarabine and oxaliplatin treatment. In this case, synergistic killing of malignant cells was due to an inhibition of DNA repair by fludarabine that was incorporated into DNA at sites of nucleotide excision repair initiated by oxaliplatin-DNA adducts (Zecevic et al., 2011).

In conclusion, there are now several lines of evidences that aggressive form of CLL displays molecular characteristics of DNA repair defect (i.e. caused by p53 or ATM deficiency or by an upregulation of NHEJ). This new biological feature severely affects overall survival and therapy issues. Taking into account that defect in DNA damage repair and/or signaling contribute to the appearance of genome instability, the results obtained in CLL cells highly suggest that the defect in NHEJ should be a new reliable biological parameter critically impairing efficacy of DNA damaging agent therapies for this subgroup of patients. In consequence, particularly because of a possible mutagenic effect of this type of drugs, the front line treatment should be proscribed for these patients in which malignant cells apparently adhere to the creed of "better wrong than dead" with a deregulated NHEJ that help their illegitimate survival.

3.2 Telomere dysfunction

Telomeres are the capping structures of chromosome ends composed of repeated DNA sequences (~10kb in somatic cells) and a specific complex of associated proteins. Telomeric DNA contain two main domains: a double strand region composed of tandem TTAGGG repeats and a single strand G-rich 3′ overhang (Henderson & Blackburn, 1989). A change in telomere function is one of the mechanisms developed by malignant cells enabling the evolution and maintenance of cancers (Blasco et al., 1997; Stewart & Weinberg, 2006; Cao et al., 2008; Ségal-Bendirdjian & Gilson 2008). The length of telomeric DNA is regulated during cell cycle and couples stress response to cell division and genome integrity (Blasco, 2007; Lansdorp, 2008; Aubert & Lansdorp, 2008). The regulation of telomere length results from the action of telomere lengthening mechanisms, such as the telomerase complex (hTERT, hTR and dyskerin), and of telomere shortening mechanisms, such as replication and recombination. Telomerase activity is regulated in *cis* by the shelterin hexa-protein complex (TRF1, TRF2, hRAP1, POT1, TIN2 and TPP1). Many other proteins involved in DNA replication and repair are also associated in telomeric structure and function (De Lange 2005; Longhese, 2008; Horard & Gilson, 2008). The telomeric nucleoprotein complex ensures chromosome stability and protection. The shortening of telomere sequences upon cell divisions in most somatic cells results in irreversible cell growth arrest called senescence or in apoptosis. Telomere erosion may be critical in tumor suppression as it impairs cell proliferation. To circumvent this, cancer cells have developed molecular strategies to maintain their telomere length by reactivating expression and/or activity of telomerase or by alternative telomere lengthening (ALT) through homologous recombination (Stewart & Weinberg, 2006; Blasco, 2007; Collado et al., 2007; Gilson & Geli, 2007; Lansdorp, 2008). In CLL, telomeric DNA may shorten in a subset of patients in Binet B or C stage compared to patients in A stage. This correlation appears inversed for telomerase activity which increases in B and C stage and decreases for A stage derived cells (Bechter et al., 1998). CLL cells exhibiting unmutated IgVH genes display also short telomeres suggesting both, an increased proliferation history of these resistant cells (Damle et al., 2004) and short telomeres association with the disease of poor prognosis. Effectively, this association of short telomeric DNA sequences further fits with genetic complexity, high-risk genomic aberrations, and short survival in CLL (Roos et al., 2008).

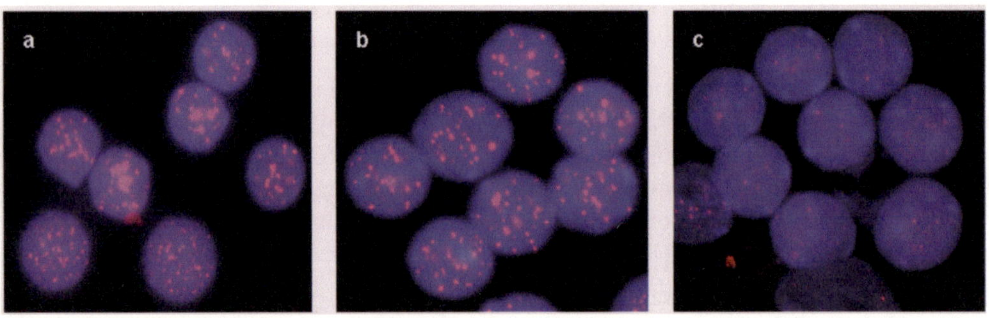

Fig. 3. Telomere labelling in interphase nuclei of CLL cells

Fluorescent *in situ* hybridization with peptide nucleic acid probe (FISH-PNA) was applied to reveal telomeric DNA sequences in interphase nuclei. Interphase nuclei (blue labelling by Hoechst H33342) of CD19+ B cells from healthy donor (**a**), sensitive (**b**) and resistant (**c**) CLL cell samples. Telomere-specific (C3TA2)3 -PNA probe Cy3-labelled (red fluorescence) reveals subtle scattered labelling throughout the nucleus of telomeres in resistant cells (**c**) while sensitive cells (**b**) and normal B cells display very similar brighter and larger spots which may be indicative of longer telomeres and/or of telomeric associations.

Simple FISH-PNA labelling of telomeres in interphase nuclei (Figure 3) show very similar pattern in sensitive CLL cells and in B cells from healthy donors. This labelling in resistant cells was organised in more weaker and discreet spreader spots suggesting that in these cells telomeres are shortened. Effectively, by using Southern blot analysis, we found that CLL cells resistant to DNA damage-induced apoptosis have the mean telomere length below 4 Kb, whereas in sensitive cells telomeric sequences are longer than 6 Kb. Moreover, G-rich 3′ single stranded overhangs that stabilize telomeric structure were found also shortened in resistant cells (Brugat et al., 2010a and 2010b). By chromatin immunoprecipitation assay we further showed that the telomeres of resistant cells are associated with increased levels of Ku70, an essential component of classical NHEJ, as well as with histone H3 lysine 9 trimethylation (3met-H3K9), a hallmark of heterochromatic structures. No difference was observed in the expression of the shelterin components or the hTERT protein complex between resistant and sensitive cell. Together, these results define alterations in telomere structure in resistant forms of CLL that may result from aberrant epigenetic regulation. This altered telomeric structure in resistant cells may confer their recognition as DNA damage since both, DSBs signaling and repair proteins colocalize at these short telomeres (Brugat et al., 2010b). Effectively, in human cells, 5 Kb is considered to be of a critical length since it may induce the DNA damage response and cellular senescence (d'Adda di Fagagna et al., 2003). Thus, we evaluated whether altered telomeres in resistant cells could be revealed by assaying classical DNA damage double-strand break (DSB) signaling and testing for the induction of telomere dysfunction-induced foci (TIF). This hypothesis has been supported by our previous results showing that resistant cells were able to upregulate non-homologous end-joining and in particular, by evidencing an upregulation of the activity of Ku heterodimer DNA end-binding (Deriano et al., 2005). Both, Ku80 and Ku70 have been identified in telomeric complexes, thus emphasizing the deregulation of these factors also at the telomeres in resistant cells. We showed that resistant cells formed TIFs and displayed an increased telomeric concentration of two NHEJ factors Ku70 and phospho-S2056-DNA-PKcs (marker of DSBs). Moreover, these cells display telomeric deletions at one or two chromatids. It is noteworthy that the appearance of these telomeric anomalies in resistant cells is concomitant with the appearance of the multiple chromosomal aberrations and complex karyotypes which are the markers of a poor disease outcome. Thus, in addition to previously identified chromosomal aberrations (i.e. del13q14; del17p13; del11q22; del6q or trisomy12), telomeric deletions appear as new type of chromosomal aberration occurring in cells from patient having aggressive form of disease. It may be speculated that these deletions coincided with extremely short telomeres revealed by a single-molecule telomere length (STELA) method (Lin et al., 2010). This method allows the measurement of individual telomeres without bias in the detection of short telomeres unlike the determination of telomere length by conventional analysis by telomere restriction fragment (Baird et al., 2003). The authors from same group suggested that this critical telomere shortening could results in telomere fusions contributing to disease progression since their frequency increased with advanced disease. When fusion sequences were analyzed, then limited numbers of repeats, subtelomeric deletion, and microhomology (alternative NHEJ), were observed (Lin et al. 2010). Telomeric DNA damage signaling as detected by a recruitment of factors involved in DNA damage, at an early stage of CLL may also be correlated with a down-regulation of two protecting proteins of shelterin complex (TPP1 and TIN2), rather than with shortening of telomeric sequences (Augereau et al., 2011).

Together, it is now widely accepted that mean telomere length may be considered as a reliable prognostic marker for CLL. Moreover, telomere dysfunction appears to precede and/or to evolve in parallel with setting of progressive form of disease suggesting telomere shortening mechanisms to be involved in CLL leukemogenesis (Lin et al., 2010). In agreement with this, in our CLL cohort, 5% of sensitive cases developed the resistance to DNA damage-induced apoptosis *in vitro* and this resistance appeared simultaneously with clinical and biological phenomena such as disease progression, telomeric dysfunction (particularly characterized by TIF signaling and telomere shortening) and an acquisition of second chromosomal aberration (Brugat et al., 2011).

3.3 Epigenetic control and CLL cells resistance to DNA damage-induced apoptosis

The proper gene expression is subjected to epigenetic control through enzymatic modifications of chromatin at both DNA and histone levels. Thus, in addition to DNA code as genetic information, epigenetic modifications are another layer of heritable information controlling gene expression. The stepwise accumulation of genetic alterations and prominent epigenetic abnormalities are tightly coordinated in cancer initiation and maintenance. Effectively, DNA methylation of CpG islands in the promoter regions of specific cancer-relevant genes, which often occur concomitantly with covalent modifications of histones and/or with the appearance of their variants, establishes a direct epigenetic basis for cell transformation. In consequence, cancer cells display genetic lesions (mutations, deletions and translocations) and significant epigenetic changes that convey heritable gene expression profiles critical for tumorigenesis (Ting et al., 2006). With this regard, in addition to transcriptional changes defined by the microarray approach, it has become evident that epigenetic alterations should be integrated into approaches of genome activity in CLL cells. Indeed, molecular profiling in CLL has allowed the identification of new genes for which the expression is dependent on CpG island methylation (Plass et al., 2007). In parallel, global DNA hypomethylation have been reported to take place in CLL (Wahlfors et al., 1992). The evidences of down-regulation of the death-associated protein kinase 1 (DAPK1, involved in apoptotic cell death regulation) gene through promoter CpG methylation in CLL indicate that both genetic and epigenetic factors may define both the sporadic and inherited forms of this disease (Raval et al., 2007).

Thus, altered structural changes of telomeric chromatin regions due to an increased heterochromatinisation (i.e. through 3methylation of histone3-lysine9, Brugat et al., 2010; 2011)), appear to not be restricted to chromosome termini but rather may spread throughout euchromatin to. Effectively, non-coding repetitive DNA sequences (such as Alu sequences, long interspersed nuclear element-1 and satelit-α sequences), have been demonstrated as under-methylated and to be associated with 17p13 deletions in CLL. Moreover, a lower level of satelit-α sequence methylation has been proposed as a new independent prognostic marker associated with shorter therapy-free survival (Fabris et al., 2011).

By using microarray approach (Affymetrix technology), we have established that resistant cells display a specific subset of deregulated genes (Vallat et al., 2003). Intriguingly, we also showed that in male CLL cells resistant to DNA damage-induced apoptosis the global gene expression was down-regulated when compared to sensitive cells, whereas this was not the case in cells derived from female patients. This gene down-regulation was found to be associated with an overall gain of heterochromatin hallmarks (i.e. increase in trimethylated histone 3 lysine 9 (3met-H3K9) and 5-methylcytidine). This approach allowed us to identify *RELB* gene as a discriminatory candidate gene repressed in the male and upregulated in the female resistant cells. Epigenetic control was demonstrated to be involved in *RELB* silencing in male cells through an increase in 3met-H3K9 (Marteau et al., 2010). This finding may be of particular interest because RelB is one of five essential members of NF-κB family of transcriptional factors involved in cellular response to stress and inflammation as well as in cancer development and progression (Hayden and Ghosh, 2008). Another NF-κB member, RelA has already been involved in CLL aggressiveness (Hewamana et al., 2008) suggesting that an imbalance in both canonical and alternative NF-κB pathways may contribute to CLL progression. Considering that NF-κB pathway regulates both apoptosis (after its activation by exogenous stress by reactive oxygen species or DNA damage or by death receptor activation) and early and late B cell differentiation (Mills et al., 2007; Goldmit et al., 2005), then an imbalance in expression of each member of this pathway should be crucial not only in cell response to therapy but also in course of early steps of cell transformation and leukemogenesis of CLL. In this regard, epigenetically up-regulated Aiolos, a member of Ikaros family of transcriptional factors involved in lymphocyte differentiation and lineage specification (rev. Mandel and Grosschedl, 2010; John and Ward, 2011), whose transcriptional regulation is under NF-κB control, may contribute to the resistance of CLL cells to activate apoptotic cell death (Billot et al. 2011).

More recently, emerging evidence imply epigenetic deregulation of microRNAs in carcinogenesis including CLL (Nicoloso et al., 2007). microRNAs are small (22nt) noncoding RNAs that regulate expression of downstream targets by messenger RNA (mRNA) destabilization and translational inhibition resulting in a specific profiling of gene expression. Thus, in cell, a large number of mRNAs are targeted each by multiple miRNAs. Also, a single miRNA can target several hundreds of mRNAs, making microRNAs extremely powerful and dynamic strategy of control of vital cell functions (rev. Subramanyam et al.,2011). Reports in cancer biology underlined general down-regulation of microRNAs. In CLL, microRNAs expression also profile disease prognostic and outcome. Effectively, Calin and co-workers (Calin et al., 2005) ,reported a unique microRNA signature enabling to differentiate the CLL cases with low versus high Zap-70 expression as well as the cases with unmutated from those with mutated IgV(H). Moreover, microRNAs are proposed to underlie the novel model of pathogenesis of indolent subset of CLL through a newly discovered regulation of TP53 (Fabbri et al., 2011). Moreover, microRNAs allowed putting in evidence a novel molecular link between critical chromosomes defects involved in CLL pathology such as interplay between 13q-17p and 17p-11q. In this model, miR-15a/miR-16-1 that regulate the expression level of TP53, are lost by 13q deletions resulting in increased levels of antiapoptotic proteins Bcl2 and Mcl1 and that of TP53. This last pathway remaining intact may explain relatively stable form of disease. Another microRNA, miR-181b, also involved in Mcl1 and Bcl2 regulation, have been associated with disease progression (Visone et al., 2011). In parallel to the loss of microRNAs due to chromosome deletions (at least those by 13q and 11q deletions), they are often down-regulated epigenetically. Effectively, overexpression of PLAG1, a putative oncogene in CLL due to a deregulated microRNAs, and an inactivation of miR-124-1 are another type of examples of epigenetic deregulations (Pallasch et al., 2009; Patz et al., 2010; Wong et al., 2011).

4. Future researches

Although genetic data teach us that CLL is a single disease, the main unsolved biological problem of CLL cells lays on not yet defined cell origin and/or differentiation step when transformation of B cell has been committed. This of course should not been so surprising because our understanding even of normal B cell differentiation remains still far from being complete. While in majority of CLL cases, the disease is preceded by a preleukemic monoclonal B cell lymphocytosis (MBL), the normal counterparts of both CLL and MBL remain unclear. Classical view of CLL resumes it as a mature B cell malignancy in which transformation of cells occurred after V(D)J recombination and germinal center reaction (Chiorazzi and Ferrarini, 2011). New concept of investigation of CLL-initiating cells was open recently by Akashi's group reporting that self-renewing hematopoietic stem cells (HSCs) have already acquired necessary modifications enabling them to develop CLL-like phenotype after xenogeneic transplantation (Kikushige et al., 2011). Depicting the molecular events occurring in HSCs in CLL patients enabling their strict maturation into mono- or oligo-clonal CLL cells phenotype should certainly shed new insights into leukemogenesis of this type of mature B lymphomas. Further, although several biological abnormalities have been established to appear in cells specifying progressive or aggressive disease, none of them were clearly yet involved in causality of evolving of indolent form and/or of directly switching towards aggressive form of disease. Hence, whether DNA repair defect or telomere dysfunction resulting in telomere deletions and/or fusions should be a consequence or a cause of disease progression remain still elusive. This is of crucial importance since depicting causality should shed light on new potential targets in clinical trials and in impeding disease progression. Further, having insights into how the resistance has been developed, should also help our understanding of CLL cell origin. Actually, the refractoriness and/or relapse of front-line (i.e. fludarabine) treated CLL patients with complex karyotype and chromosomal aberrations known to confer poor outcome of disease, may be proved as a major obstacle without favorable therapeutic issues (Badoux et al., 2011). The fact that resistant cells are able to upregulate DNA damage error-prone repair allowed us to speculate that the upsetting of this event may be involved in observed chromosomal and telomeric abnormalities whose appearance in aggressive disease remain still murky. This hypothesis is further strengthened by the progressive feature of these two abnormalities in the course of disease. Our current research targets the molecular origin of how NHEJ could become upregulated in these cells allowing them to survive upon treatment. The molecular ways through which repair of chromatin DNA could be modified are multiples and relay on epigenetic and genetic control. Thus, DNA methylation and hydroxymethylation are not only associated with the control of gene expression (including genes involved in DNA repair), and differentiation but also conditioned the DNA repair; all of these functions which are controlled by the local and global presence of 5-methylcytosines may underlie malignant process (Schär and Fritsch, 2011). Effectively, CLL cells display both local DNA hypermethylation and global hypomethylation (Wahlfors et al., 1992; Plass et al., 2007; Raval et al. 2007; Marteau et al., 2010). While the consequences of global genome hypomethylation on DNA damage repair remain still to be established, local CpG island methylation controls the expression level of nearby genes (such as *DAPK1*, *RELB* or *Aiolos* works cited above). In addition to yet not identified target genes which could be directly or indirectly linked to DNA repair, the expression level of identified transcriptional factors was already suggested to define cell resistance to treatment.

Among other epigenetic modifications affecting vital cell functions, including DNA repair, are post-translational modifications of histones. Thus, following DSBs formation, in their vicinity, histones are modified (mainly through phosphorylation, methylation and acetylation) creating thus a dynamic platform for assembly of DNA repair protein complexes (Greenberg, 2011). The best defined histones modification, directly involved in the promotion of DNA repair is the ATM-dependent phosphorylation of histone variant H2AX at S139 in vicinity of DNA damage (rev. Dickey et al., 2009). This modification is the first and key step involved in the recruitment of other proteins in an ordered dynamic and strikingly hierarchical manner to form so-called DNA repair foci. This formation is achieved by an orchestration of protein-protein interactions which is triggered by a plethora of post-translational modifications such as phosphorylation, acetylation, SUMOylation and ubiquitination. Thus, the formed foci involve protein complexes that should assure not only proper DNA repair but are also coupled with the relaxation of chromatin and the blockage of transcription. Interestingly, H2AX null mice exhibit reduced immunoglobulin class switching but not V(D)J recombination (involving NHEJ). However, in a p53 deficient background, these mice exhibit compromised genomic stability, an increased sensitivity to genotoxic stress and increased cancer susceptibility (Celeste et al., 2002, Celeste et al., 2003). Thus, the cellular level of γ-H2AX and foci formation have been proposed as an indicator of DNA DSBs which could be valuable in monitoring not only a detection of the genotoxic stress but also in monitoring cancer development and progression (rev. Dickey et al., 2009). Remarkably, resistant CLL cells as compared to sensitive, display an increased level of γ-H2AX foci which colocalized at telomeric sequences (Brugat et al., 2010).

Histone methylation involved in an epigenetic control of genome transcription activity also affects DNA repair function. Effectively, dimethyl histone H3 lysine 36 is generated as major event by DSBs induction. This histone modification has been demonstrated to be essential in recruitment of NBS1 and Ku70 to the site of DSB and is followed by an enhanced NHEJ DNA repair (Fnu et al., 2011). Cancer cells often display a plethora of covalent modifications of histones, called "histone onco-modifications" achieved by altered activity of modifying enzymes. These modifications are involved in both development and maintenance of malignant process and which may confer them the resistance to treatment (Füllgrabe et al., 2011). One could notice that the processing of DSBs may also be controlled by enzymes belonging to the family of histone acetyltransferases and deacetylases (HAT and HDAC) which acetylate/deacetylate DNA end-resection factors and participate in this way in DNA damage response and chromosome stability (Robert et al., 2011).

Another way to control the activity of NHEJ repair of DNA in the context of chromatin DNA in human cells involves interaction between Ku70 and ATP-dependent chromatin-remodeling factor (ACF1). This interaction is required for the accumulation of Ku heterodimer at DSBs (Lan et al., 2010).

Finally, protein ubiquitination is another post-translational modification shown to be altered in CLL (Delic et al., 1998; Masdehors et al., 2000; Ma et al., 2008; Sampath et al., 2009), and to be involved in DNA repair (Daigaku et al., 2010; Shanbhag et al., 2010; Larsen et al., 2010; Weitzman et al., 2011; Ramadan and Meerang, 2011). This modification may be of particular interest since it may affect DNA repair through local structural alteration of chromatin (i.e. through histones H2A and H2B and/or chromatin-associating factors' ubiquitination), and directly, through an ubiquitination of the payers involved in DNA repair by NHEJ such as Ku70 or by homologous recombination such as BRCA1 (Gama et al., 2009; Ohta et al., 2011). Phospho-S473-AKT kinase which is activated in many types of human cancers including CLL (Shehata et al., 2010; Hofbauer et al., 2010; Wickremasinghe et al., 2011), is a DNA repair promoting factor through an activation of NHEJ. Moreover, this activity is dependent on the histone ubiquitin ligase RNF 168 (Fraser et al., 2011). Based on an induction of NHEJ in this way by exogenously produced DSBs (irradiation or drugs), it is highly suggestive that this pathway would be involved in resistance mechanisms developed by cancer cells. In agreement with this, in CLL cells decreased phosphorylation of Akt (and other PI3-K family kinases and tensin homolog detected on chromosome 10, PTEN) induces apoptosis in response to fludarabine treatment. A combined inhibition of PI3-K/Akt and recovery of the activity of PTEN has been suggested as a novel concept for CLL therapy (Shehata et al., 2010). A prolonged effect of these kinases may be further strengthen by an over expression of SET oncoprotein which is documented as a potent physiological inhibitor of protein phosphatases 2A (Christensen et al., 2011).

The fact that CLL cells resistant to apoptosis exhibit a constitutive higher activity of Ku heterodimer to bind *in vitro* free ends of DNA (that mimics DSBs), suggest a post-translational modification of Ku70 and/or of Ku80 as well as a presence/absence of enzyme(s) involved in this modification. This hypothesis is supported by the fact that both cells derived from indolent or aggressive form of disease express Ku proteins at same level (protein and mRNA). Proteomic analysis of each subset of CLL cells should help to identify new factors which in turn, would shed light on a NHEJ defect expressed by resistant cells. This knowledge should indicate the new targeted strategies to be developed to improve clinical trials.

5. Conclusion

Biological defects we have identified in CLL cells resistant to DNA damage-induced apoptosis should functionally be interconnected (i.e. DNA repair defect may be impaired by epigenetic modifications; these modifications affect telomere chromatin structure which is also affected by components of DNA repair machinery). Whether and how these defects would be involved in a promotion of observed chromosomal aberrations occurring in majority of aggressive CLL cases, remain still to be demonstrated but their convergence highly suggest a common mechanisms.

Considered together, all biological data we have obtained with CLL cells led us to conclude that:

i. the resistant subset of CLL cells displays a defect in apoptotic pathway triggered by DNA damage *in vitro* and *in vivo*;
ii. resistant cells display a dysfunction of NHEJ DNA repair system (of yet unknown molecular origin) associated with heterochromatinisation of telomeric regions but, heterochromatinisation may also widespread throughout euchromatin regions affecting gene expression;
iii. in some CLL cases, sensitive cells may became resistant to apoptosis and then, telomeric dysfunction drive to an acquisition of new chromosomal abnormality which is associated with an appearance of an additional aberration characteristic of aggressive form of disease.

Since all of these features are hallmarks of cells resistant to DNA damage-induced apoptosis, then a simple and easy-to-perform test of cell susceptibility to activate or not apoptotic death pathway following genotoxic stress *in vitro*, should be useful and highly indicative of whether front line treatment would be appropriated or proscribed for CLL patients.

Future research in this domain should bring further insights into mechanisms of the origin of deregulated NHEJ in this particular subset of CLL. Knowing that during the course of disease progression, biological susceptibility to DNA damage apoptosis *in vitro* simultaneously also evolve (i.e. otherwise sensitive cells become resistant), then this mechanistic knowledge should be certainly of new potential applications in clinic.

6. Acknowledgment

We are grateful to all leukemic benevolent blood donors allowing us to perform the research. We also would like to thank all benevolent healthy blood donors whose samples were used as control. We thank all PhD students and post-doctoral fellows who participated in works cited in main text. Finally, the entire technical staff of the hospital Pitié-Salpêtrière is also warmly thanked; we were enjoyed with the help and cooperation of Colette Barbarat et Isabelle Sevoz. Our work was supported by CEA, Association pour la Recherche sur le Cancer (ARC), Fondation de France (FdF) and Electricité de France (EDF).

7. References

Amrein, L., Loignon, M., Goulet, A.C., Dunn, M., Jean-Claude, B., Aloyz, R. & Panasci L. Chlorambucil cytotoxicity in malignant b lymphocytes is synergistically increased by 2-(morpholin-4-yl)-benzo[h]chomen-4-one (NU7026)-mediated inhibition of DNA double-strand break repair via inhibition of DNA-dependent protein kinase. *Journal of Pharmacology and Experimental Therapeutics,* Vol. 321, No.3, (June 2007), pp. 848-855, PMID: 17351105

Aubert, G. & Lansdorp, P.M. Telomeres and aging. *Physiological Reviews,* Vol. 88, No. 2, (April 2008), pp. 557-579, PMID: 18391173

Augereau, A., T'kint de Roodenbeke, C., Simonet, T., Bauwens, S., Horard, B., Callanan, M., Leroux, D., Jallades, L., Salles, G., Gilson, E. & Poncet, D. Telomeric damage in early stage of chronic lymphocytic leukemia correlates with shelterin dysregulation. *Blood,* 2011 Feb 25. [Epub ahead of print], PMID: 21355086

Austen, B., Skowronska, A., Baker, C., Powell, J.E., Gardiner, A., Oscier, D., Majid, A., Dyer, M., Siebert, R., Taylor, A.M., Moss, P.A. & Stankovic, T. Mutation status of the residual ATM allele is an important determinant of the cellular response to chemotherapy and survival in patients with chronic lymphocytic leukemia containing an 11q deletion. *Journal of Clinical Oncology,* Vol. 25, No. 34, (December 2007), pp. 5448-5457, PMID: 17968022

Austen, B., Powell, J.E., Alvi, A., Edwards, I., Hooper, L., Starczynski, J., Taylor, A.M., Fegan, C., Moss, P. & Stankovic, T. Mutations in the ATM gene lead to impaired overall and treatment-free survival that is independent of IGVH mutation status in patients with B-CLL. *Blood,* Vol. 106, No. 9, (November 2005), pp. 3175-3182, PMID: 16014569

Badoux, X.C., Keating, M.J., Wang, X., O'Brien, S.M., Ferrajoli, A., Faderl, S., Burger, J., Koller, C., Lerner, S., Kantarjian, H. & Wierda, W.G. Cyclophosphamide, fludarabine, rituximab and alemtuzumab (CFAR) as salvage therapy for heavily pre-treated patients with chronic lymphocytic leukemia. *Blood,* 2011 Jun 13. [Epub ahead of print], PMID : 21670470

Baird, D.M., Rowson, J., Wynford-Thomas, D. & Kipling, D. Extensive allelic variation and ultrashort telomeres in senescent human cells. *Nature Genetics,* Vol. 33, No. 2, (February 2003), pp. 203-207, PMID: 12539050

Bechter, O.E., Eisterer, W., Pall, G., Hilbe, W., Kühr, T. & Thaler, J. Telomere length and telomerase activity predict survival in patients with B cell chronic lymphocytic leukemia. *Cancer Research,* Vol.58, No. 21, (November 1998), pp. 4918-4922, PMID: 9810000

Billot, K., Soeur, J., Chereau, F., Arrouss, I., Merle-Béral, H., Huang, M.E., Mazier, D., Baud, V. & Rebollo, A. Deregulation of Aiolos expression in chronic lymphocytic leukemia is associated with epigenetic modifications. *Blood,* Vol. 117, No. 6, (February 2011), pp. 1917-1927, PMID: 21139082

Blaise, R., Alapetite, C., Masdehors, P., Merle-Beral, H., Roulin, C., Delic, J. & Sabatier, L. High levels of chromosome aberrations correlate with impaired in vitro radiation-induced apoptosis and DNA repair in human B-chronic lymphocytic leukaemia cells. *International Journal of Radiation Biology,* Vol. 78, No. 8, (August 2002), pp. 671-679, PMID: 12194750

Blasco, M.A., Lee, H.W., Hande, M.P., Samper, E., Lansdorp, P.M., DePinho, R.A.& Greider, C.W. Telomere shortening and tumor formation by mouse cells lacking telomerase RNA. *Cell,* Vol. 9, No. 1, (October 1997), pp. 25-34, PMID: 9335332

Blasco, M.A. The epigenetic regulation of mammalian telomeres. *Nature Reviews Genet*ics, Vol. 39, No. 4, (April 2007), pp. 299-309, PMID: 17363977

Bramson, J., McQuillan, A., Aubin, R., Alaoui-Jamali, M., Batist, G., Christodoulopoulos, G. & Panasci, L.C. Nitrogen mustard drug resistant B-cell chronic lymphocytic leukemia as an in vivo model for crosslinking agent resistance. *Mutation Research,* Vol. 336, No.3, (May 1995), pp. 269-278, PMID7739615

Brugat, T., Gault, N., Baccelli, I., Maës, J., Roborel de Climens, A., Nguyen-Khac, F., Davi, F., Merle-Béral, H., Gilson, E., Goodhardt, M. & Delic, J. Aberrant telomere structure is characteristic of resistant chronic lymphocytic leukaemia cells. *Leukemia,* Vol. 24, No. 1, (January 2010a), pp. 246-251, PMID: 19847201

Brugat, T., Nguyen-Khac, F., Grelier, A., Merle-Béral, H. & Delic, J. Telomere dysfunction-induced foci arise with the onset of telomeric deletions and complex chromosomal aberrations in resistant chronic lymphocytic leukemia cells. *Blood,* Vol. 116, No. 2, (July 2010b) pp. 239-249, PMID: 20424183

Brugat, T., Nguyen-Khac, F., Merle-Béral, H. & Delic, J. Concomitant telomere shortening, acquisition of multiple chromosomal aberrations and in vitro resistance to apoptosis in a single case of progressive CLL. *Leukemia Research,* Vol. 35, No. 5, (May 2011), pp.e37-40, PMID: 21176960

Bryant, H.E., Schultz, N., Thomas, H.D., Parker, K.M., Flower, D., Lopez, E., Kyle, S., Meuth, M., Curtin, N.J. & Helleday,T. Specific killing of BRCA2-deficient tumours with inhibitors of poly(ADP-ribose) polymerase. *Nature,* Vol. 434, No. 7035, (April 2005), pp. 913-917, PMID: 15829966

Caligaris-Cappio, F. & Chiorazzi, N. Where is the biology of CLL leading us? *Seminars in Cancer Biol*ogy, Vol. 20, No. 6, (December 2010), pp. 361-362, PMID: 21130365

Calin, G.A., Ferracin, M., Cimmino, A., Di Leva, G., Shimizu, M., Wojcik, S.E., Iorio, M.V., Visone, R., Sever, N.I., Fabbri, M., Iuliano, R., Palumbo, T., Pichiorri, F., Roldo, C., Garzon, R., Sevignani, C., Rassenti, L., Alder, H., Volinia, S., Liu, C.G., Kipps, T.J., Negrini, M. & Croce, C.M. A MicroRNA signature associated with prognosis and progression in chronic lymphocytic leukemia. *New England Journal of Medicine,* Vol. 353, No. 17, (October 2005) pp.1793-1801. Erratum in: *New England Journal of Medicine,* Vol. 355, No. 5, (August 2006), pp. 533, PMID: 16251535

Cao, Y., Bryan, T.M. & Reddel, R.R. Increased copy number of the TERT and TERC telomerase subunit genes in cancer cells. *Cancer Science,* Vol. 99, No. 6 (June 2008), pp. 1092-1099, PMID: 1848052

Cartwright, R.A., Gurney, K.A. & Moorman, A.V. Sex ratios and the risks of haematological malignancies. *British Journal of Haematology,* Vol. 118, No. 4 (September 2002), pp. 1071-1077, PMID: 12199787

Catovsky, D., Richards, S., Matutes, E., Oscier, D., Dyer, M.J., Bezares, R.F., Pettitt, A.R., Hamblin, T., Milligan, D.W., Child, J.A., Hamilton, M.S., Dearden, C.E., Smith, A.G., Bosanquet, A.G., Davis, Z., Brito-Babapulle, V., Else, M., Wade, R. & Hillmen, P. Assessment of fludarabine plus cyclophosphamide for patients with chronic lymphocytic leukaemia (the LRF CLL4 Trial): a randomised controlled trial. UK National Cancer Research Institute (NCRI) Haematological Oncology Clinical Studies Group; NCRI Chronic Lymphocytic Leukaemia Working Group. *Lancet,* Vol. 370, No. 9583, (July 2007), pp. 230-2399, PMID: 17658394

Celeste, A., Petersen, S., Romanienko, P.J., Fernandez-Capetillo, O., Chen, H.T., Sedelnikova, O.A., Reina-San-Martin, B., Coppola, V., Meffre, E., Difilippantonio, M.J., Redon, C., Pilch, D.R., Olaru, A., Eckhaus, M., Camerini-Otero, R.D., Tessarollo, L., Livak, F., Manova, K., Bonner, W.M., Nussenzweig, M.C. & Nussenzweig A. Genomic instability in mice lacking histone H2AX. *Science,* Vol. 296, No. 5569, (May 2002), pp. 922-927, PMID : 11934988

Celeste, A., Difilippantonio, S., Difilippantonio, M.J., Fernandez-Capetillo, O., Pilch, D.R., Sedelnikova, O.A., Eckhaus, M., Ried, T., Bonner, WM. & Nussenzweig, A. H2AX haploinsufficiency modifies genomic stability and tumor susceptibility. *Cell,* Vol. 5, No. 7 (July 2003), pp. 675-679, PMID: 12792649

Chiorazzi, N., Rai, K.R. & Ferrarini, M. Chronic Lymphocitic Leukemia. *New England Journal of Medicine,* Vol. 352, No. 8, (February 2005), pp. 804-815, PMID: 15728813

Chiorazzi, N. & Ferrarini, M. Cellular origin(s) of chronic lymphocytic leukemia: cautionary notes and additional considerations and possibilities. *Blood,* Vol. 117, No. 6, (February 2011), pp. 1781-1791, PMID: 21148333

Christensen, D.J., Chen, Y., Oddo, J., Matta, K.M., Neil, J., Davis, E.D., Volkheimer, A.D., Lanasa, M.C., Friedman, D.R., Goodman, B.K., Gockerman, J.P., Diehl, L.F., de Castro, C.M., Moore, J.O., Vitek, M.P. & Weinberg, J.B. SET oncoprotein overexpression in B-cell chronic lymphocytic leukemia and non-Hodgkin's lymphoma: a predictor of aggressive disease and new treatment target. *Blood* 2011 Aug 15. [Epub ahead of print], PMID: 21844565

Christodoulopoulos, G., Muller, C., Salles, B., Kazmi, R. & Panasci, L. Potentiation of chlorambucil cytotoxicity in B-cell chronic lymphocytic leukemia by inhibition of

DNA-dependent protein kinase activity using wortmannin. *Cancer Research*, Vol. 58, No. 9, (May 1998), pp. 1789-1792, PMID: 9581813

Collado, M., Blasco, M.A. & Serrano, M. Cellular senescence in cancer and aging. *Cell*, Vol. 130, No. 2 (July 2007), pp. 223-233, PMID: 17662938

Colombo, M., Cutrona, G., Reverberi, D., Fabris, S., Neri, A., Fabbi, M., Quintana, G., Quarta, G., Ghiotto, F., Fais, F. & Ferrarini, M. Intraclonal cell expansion and selection driven by B cell receptor in Chronic Lymphocytic Leukemia. *Molecular Med*icine 2011 Apr 28. doi: 10.2119/molmed.2011.00047. [Epub ahead of print]

Corneo, B., Wendland, R.L., Deriano, L., Cui, X., Klein, I.A., Wong, S.Y., Arnal, S., Holub, A.J., Weller, G.R., Pancake, B.A., Shah, S., Brandt, V.L., Meek, K. & Roth DB. Rag mutations reveal robust alternative end joining. *Nature*, Vol. 449, No. 7161 (September 2007), pp. 483-486, PMID: 17898768

d'Adda di Fagagna, F., Reaper, P.M., Clay-Farrace, L., Fiegler, H., Carr, P., Von Zglinicki, T., Saretzki, G., Carter, N.P. & Jackson, S.P.A. DNA damage checkpoint response in telomere-initiated senescence. *Nature*, Vol. 426, No. 6963, (November 2003), pp. 194-198, PMID: 14608368

Daigaku, Y., Davies, A.A. & Ulrich, H.D. Ubiquitin-dependent DNA damage bypass is separable from genome replication. *Nature*, Vol. 465, No. 7300 (June 2010), pp. 951-955, PMID: 20453836

Damle, R.N., Wasil, T., Fais, F., Ghiotto, F., Valetto, A., Allen, S.L., Buchbinder, A., Budman, D., Dittmar, K., Kolitz, J., Lichtman, S.M., Schulman, P., Vinciguerra, V.P., Rai, K.R., Ferrarini, M. & Chiorazzi N. Ig V gene mutation status and CD38 expression as novel prognostic indicators in chronic lymphocytic leukemia. *Blood*, Vol. 94, No. 6, (September 1999), pp. 1840-1847, PMID: 10477712

Damle, R.N., Batliwalla, F.M., Ghiotto, F., Valetto, A., Albesiano, E., Sison, C., Allen, S.L., Kolitz, J., Vinciguerra, V.P., Kudalkar, P., Wasil, T., Rai, K.R., Ferrarini, M., Gregersen, P.K. & Chiorazzi, N. Telomere length and telomerase activity delineate distinctive replicative features of the B-CLL subgroups defined by immunoglobulin V gene mutations. *Blood*, Vol. 103, No. 2, (January 2004), pp. 375-382, PMID: 14504108

De Campos-Nebel, M., Larripa, I. & Gonzales-Cid, M. Non-homologous end joining is the responsible pathway for the repair of fludarabine-induced DNA double strand breaks in mammalian cells. *Mutation Research*, Vol. 646, No. 1-2 (November 2008), pp. 8-16, PMID: 18812179

Delacote, F. & Lopez, B.S. Importance of the cell cycle phases for the choice of the appropriate DSB repair pathway, for genome stability maintenance. *Cell Cycle*, Vol. 7, No. 1, (January 2008), pp. 33-38, PMID: 18196958

De Lange, T. Shelterin: the protein complex that shapes and safeguards human telomeres. *Genes & Development*, Vol. 19, No. 18, (September 2005), pp. 2100-2110, PMID: 16166375

Delic, J., Masdehors, P., Omura, S., Cosset, J.M., Dumont, J., Binet, J.L. & Magdelénat H. The proteasome inhibitor lactacystin induces apoptosis and sensitizes chemo- and radioresistant human chronic lymphocytic leukaemia lymphocytes to TNF-alpha-initiated apoptosis. *British Journal of Cancer,* Vol. 77, No. 7, (April 1998), pp. 1103-1107, PMID: 9569046

Deriano, L., Guipaud, O., Merle-Béral, H., Binet, J-L., Ricoul, M., Potocki-Veronese, G., Favaudon, V., Maciorowski, Z., Muller, C., Salles, B., Sabatier, L. & Delic, J. Human chronic lymphocytic leukemia B cells can escape DNA damage-induced apoptosis through the nonhomologous end-joining DNA repair pathway. *Blood,* Vol. 105, No. 12, (June 2005), pp. 4776-4783, PMID: 15718417

Deriano, L., Merle-Béral, H., Guipaud, O., Sabatier, L. & Delic, J. Mutagenicity of non-homologous end joining DNA repair in a resistant subset of human chronic lymphocytic leukaemia B cells. *British Journal of Haematology,* Vol. 133, No. 5 (June 2006), pp. 520-525, PMID: 16681639

Deriano, L., Stracker, T.H., Baker, A., Petrini, J.H. & Roth, D.B. Roles for NBS1 in alternative nonhomologous end-joining of V(D)J recombination intermediates. *Molecular Cell,* 2009, 34 :13-25.

Dickey, J.S., Redon, C.E., Nakamura, A.J., Baird, B.J., Sedelnikova, O.A. & Bonner, W.M. H2AX: functional roles and potential applications. *Chromosoma,* Vol. 118, No. 6, (December 2009), pp. 683-692, PMID: 19651821

Dighiero, G. & Hamblin, T.J. Chronic Lymphocytic Leukemia. *Lancet,* Vol. 371, No. 9617, (March 2008), pp. 1017-1029, PMID: 18358929

Döhner, H., Fischer, K., Bentz, M., Hansen, K., Benner, A., Cabot, G., Diehl, D., Schlenk, R., Coy, J., Stilgenbauer, S., Volkman, M., Galle, P.R., Poustka A.M., Hunstein, W. & Lichter, P. p53 gene deletion predicts for poor survival and non-response to therapy with purine analogs in chronic B-cell leukemias. *Blood,* Vol. 85, No. 6, (June 1995), pp. 1580-1589, PMID: 7888675

Döhner, H., Stilgenbauer, S., James, M.R., Benner, A., Weilguni, T., Bentz, M., Fischer, K., Hunstein, W. & Lichter, P. 11q deletions identify a new subset of B-cell chronic lymphocytic leukemia characterized by extensive nodal involvement and inferior prognosis. *Blood,* Vol. 89, No. 7, (1997 April 1997), pp. 2516-2522, PMID: 9116297

Elliott, S.L., Crawford, C., Mulligan, E., Summerfield, G., Newton, P., Wallis, J., Mainou-Fowler, T., Evans, P., Bedwell, C., Durkacz, B.W. & Willmore, E. Mitoxantrone in combination with an inhibitor of DNA-dependent protein kinase: a potential therapy for high risk B-cell chronic lymphocytic leukaemia. *British Journal Haematol*ogy, Vol. 152, No. 1, (January 2011), pp. 161-171, PMID: 21083655

Fabbri, M., Bottoni, A., Shimizu, M., Spizzo, R., Nicoloso, M.S., Rossi, S., Barbarotto, E., Cimmino, A., Adair, B., Wojcik, S.E., Valeri, N., Calore, F., Sampath, D., Fanini, F., Vannini, I., Musuraca, G., Dell'Aquila, M., Alder, H., Davuluri, R.V., Rassenti, L.Z., Negrini, M., Nakamura, T., Amadori, D., Kay, N.E., Rai, K.R., Keating, M.J., Kipps, T.J., Calin, G.A. & Croce, C.M. Association of a microRNA/TP53 feedback circuitry with pathogenesis and outcome of B-cell chronic lymphocytic leukemia. *The Journal of American Medical Association (JAMA),* Vol. 305, No. 1, (January 2011), pp. 59-67, PMID: 21205967

Fabbri, G., Rasi, S., Rossi, D., Trifonov, V., Khiabanian, H., Ma, J., Grunn, A., Fangazio, M., Capello, D., Monti, S., Cresta, S., Gargiulo, E., Forconi, F., Guarini, A., Arcaini, L., Paulli, M., Laurenti, L., Larocca, L.M., Marasca, R., Gattei, V., Oscier, D., Bertoni, F.,

Mullighan, C.G., Foá, R., Pasqualucci, L., Rabadan, R., Dalla-Favera, R. & Gaidano, G. Analysis of the chronic lymphocytic leukemia coding genome: role of NOTCH1 mutational activation. *Journal of Experimental Medicine,* Vol. 208, No. 7, (July 2011), pp. 1389-1401, PMID: 21670202

Fabris, S., Scarciolla, O., Morabito, F., Cifarelli, R.A., Dininno, C., Cutrona, G., Matis, S., Recchia, A.G., Gentile, M., Ciceri, G., Ferrarini, M., Ciancio, A., Mannarella, C., Neri, A. & Fragasso, A. Multiplex ligation-dependent probe amplification and fluorescence in situ hybridization to detect chromosomal abnormalities in Chronic lymphocytic leukemia: A comparative study. *Genes Chromosomes and Cancer,* Vol. 50, No.5, (September 2011), pp. 726-734, PMID: 21638517

Fabris, S., Bollati, V., Agnelli, L., Morabito, F., Motta, V., Cutrona, G., Matis, S., Grazia Recchia, A., Gigliotti, V., Gentile, M., Deliliers, G.L., Bertazzi, P.A., Ferrarini, M., Neri, A. & Baccarelli A. Biological and clinical relevance of quantitative global methylation of repetitive DNA sequences in chronic lymphocytic leukemia. *Epigenetics,* Vol. 6, No. 2, (February 2011), pp. 188-894, PMID: 20930513

Fais, F., Ghiotto, F., Hashimoto, S., Sellars, B., Valetto, A., Allen, S.L., Schulman, P., Vinciguerra, V.P., Rai, K., Rassenti, L.Z., Kipps, T.J., Dighiero, G., Schroeder, H.W. Jr., Ferrarini, M. & Chiorazzi, N. Chronic lymphocytic leukemia B cells express restricted sets of mutated and unmutated antigen receptors. *Journal of Clinical Investigation,* Vol. 102, No. 8, (October 1998), pp. 1515-1525, PMID: 9788964

Farmer, H., McCabe, N., Lord, C.J., Tutt, A.N., Johnson. D.A., Richardson, T.B., Santarosa, M., Dillon, K.J., Hickson, I., Knights, C., Martin, N.M., Jackson, S.P., Smith, G.C. & Ashworth, A. Targeting the DNA repair defect in BRCA mutant cells as a therapeutic strategy. *Nature,* Vol. 434, No. 7035, (April 2005), pp. 917-921, PMID: 15829967

Fnu, S., Williamson, E.A., De Haro, L.P., Brenneman, M., Wray, J., Shaheen, M., Radhakrishnan, K., Lee, S.H., Nickoloff, J.A. & Hromas, R. Methylation of histone H3 lysine 36 enhances DNA repair by nonhomologous end-joining. *Proceedings of National Academy of Sciences, U S A,* Vol. 108, No. 2, (January 2011), pp. 540-545, PMID: 21187428

Fraser, M., Harding, S.M., Zhao, H., Coackley, C., Durocher, D. & Bristow, R.G. MRE11 promotes AKT phosphorylation in direct response to DNA double-strand breaks. *Cell Cycle,* 2011 Jul 1;10(13). [Epub ahead of print], PMID: 21623170

Füllgrabe, J., Kavanagh, E. & Joseph, B. Histones onco-modifications. *Oncogene.* 2011, April 25. [Epub ahead of print], PMID : 21516126

Gama, V., Gomez, J.A., Mayo, L.D., Jackson, M.W., Danielpour, D., Song, K., Haas, A.L., Laughlin, M.J. & Matsuyama S. Hdm2 is a ubiquitin ligase of Ku70-Akt promotes cell survival by inhibiting Hdm2-dependent Ku70 destabilization. *Cell Death and Differentiation,* Vol. 16, No. 5, (May 2009), pp. 758-769, PMID: 19247369

Ghiotto, F., Marcatili, P., Tenca, C., Calevo, M.G., Yan, X.J., Albesiano, E., Bagnara, D., Colombo, M., Cutrona, G., Chu, C.C., Morabito, F., Bruno, S., Ferrarini, M., Tramontano, A., Fais, F. & Chiorazzi, N. Mutation pattern of paired immunoglobulin heavy and light variable domains in chronic lymphocytic leukemia B-cells. *Molecular Medicine,* (July 2011). doi: 10.2119/molmed.2011.00104. [Epub ahead of print

Gilson, E. & Géli, V. How telomeres are replicated. *Nature Reviews Molecular and Cellular Biology,* Vol. 8, No. 10 (October 2007), pp. 825-838, PMID: 17885666

Goldmit, M., Ji, Y., Skok, J., Roldan, E., Jung, S., Cedar, H. & Bergman, Y. Epigenetic ontogeny of the Igk locus during B cell development. *Nature Immunology,* Vol. 6, No. 2, (February 2005), pp. 198-203, PMID: 15619624

Greenberg, R.A. Histone tails: Directing the chromatin response to DNA damage. *FEBS Letter,* 2011 May 27. [Epub ahead of print], PMID: 21621538

Grever, M.R., Lucas, D.M., Dewald, G.W., Neuberg, D.S., Reed, J.C., Kitada, S., Flinn, I.W., Tallman, M.S., Appelbaum, F.R., Larson, R.A., Paietta, E., Jelinek, D.F., Gribben, J.G. & Byrd, J.C. Comprehensive assessment of genetic and molecular features predicting outcome in patients with chronic lymphocytic leukemia: results from the US Intergroup Phase III Trial E2997. *Journal of Clinical Oncology,* Vol. 25, No. 7, (March 2007), pp. 799-804, PMID: 17283363

Guipaud, O., Deriano, L., Salin, H., Vallat, L., Sabatier, L., Merle-Béral, H. & Delic, J. B-cell chronic lymphocytic leukaemia: a polymorphic family unified by genomic features. *Lancet Oncology,* Vol. 4, No. 8, (August 2003), pp. 505-514, PMID: 12901966

Hallek, M. & Pflug, N. State of the art treatment of chronic lymphocytic leukaemia. *Blood Reviews,* Vol. 25, No. 1 (January 2011), pp. 1-9, PMID21095047

Hamblin, T.J., Davis, Z., Gardiner, A., Oscier, D.G. & Stevenson, F.K. Unmutated Ig V(H) genes are associated with a more aggressive form of chronic lymphocytic leukemia. *Blood,* Vol. 94, No. 6, (September 1999), pp. 1848-1854, PMID: 10477713

Hamblin, T.J., Orchard, J.A., Gardiner, A., Oscier, D.G., Davis, Z. & Stevenson FK. Immunoglobulin V genes and CD38 expression in CLL. *Blood,* Vol. 95, No7, (April 2000), pp. 2455-2457, PMID: 10787241

Hamblin, T.J. Prognostic markers in chronic lymphocytic leukaemia. *Best Practice & Research Clinical Haematology,* Vol. 20, No. 3, (September 2007), pp. 455-468, PMID: 17707833

Haslinger, C., Schweifer, N., Stilgenbauer, S., Döhner, H., Lichter, P., Kraut, N., Stratowa, C. & Abseher, R. Microarray gene expression profiling of B-cell chronic lymphocityc leukemia subgroups defined by genomic aberrations and VH mutation status. *Journal of Clinical Oncology,* Vol. 22, No. 19, (October 2004), pp. 3937-3949, PMID: 15459216

Hayden, M.S. & Ghosh, S. Shared principles in NF-kappaB signaling. *Cell,* Vol. 132, No. 3, (February 2008), pp. 344-362, PMID: 18267068

Helleday, T., Petermann, E., Lundin, C., Hodgson, B. & Sharma, R.A. DNA repair pathways as targets for cancer therapy. *Nature Reviews Cancer,* Vol. 8, No. 3, (March 2008), pp. 193-204, *PMID: 18284484*

Hervé, M., Xu, K., Ng, Y.S., Wardemann, H., Albesiano, E., Messmer, B.T., Chiorazzi, N. & Meffre, E. Unmutated and mutated chronic lymphocytic leukemias derive from self-reactive B cell precursors despite expressing different antibody reactivity. *Journal of Clinical Investigation,* Vol. 115, No. 6, (June 2005), pp. 1636-1643, PMID: 15902303

Henderson, E.R. & Blackburn, E.H. An overhanging 3' terminus is a conserved feature of telomeres. *Molecular and Cellular Biology*, Vol. 9, No. 1, (January 1989), pp. 345-348, PMID: 2927395

Hewamana, S., Alghazal, S., Lin, T.T., Clement, M., Jenkins, C., Guzman, M.L., Jordan, C.T., Neelakantan, S., Crooks, P.A., Burnett, A.K., Pratt, G., Fegan, C., Rowntree, C., Brennan, P. & Pepper C. The NF-kappaB subunit Rel A is associated with in vitro survival and clinical disease progression in chronic lymphocytic leukemia and represents a promising therapeutic target. *Blood*, Vol. 111, No. 9, (May 2008), pp. 4681-4689, PMID: 18227347

Hofbauer, S.W., Piñón, J.D., Brachtl, G., Haginger, L., Wang, W., Jöhrer, K., Tinhofer, I., Hartmann, T.N. & Greil, R. Modifying akt signaling in B-cell chronic lymphocytic leukemia cells. *Cancer Res*earch, Vol. 70, No. 18, (September 2010), pp. 7336-7344, PMID: 20823161

Horard, B. & Gilson, E. Telomeric RNA enters the game. *Nature Cell Biology*, Vol. 10, No. 2, (February 2008), pp. 113-115, PMID: 18246034

Huang, A.T., Kremer, W.B., Laszlo, J. & Setlow, R.B. DNA repair in human leukaemic lymphocytes. *Nature New Biology*, Vol. 240, No. 99, (November 1972), pp. 114-116, PMID: 4509023

John, L.B. & Ward, A.C. The Ikaros gene family: Transcriptional regulators of hematopoiesis and immunity. *Molecular Immunology*, Vol. 48, No. 9-10, (May 2011), pp. 1272-1278, PMID: 21477865

Kikushige, Y., Ishikawa, F., Miyamoto, T., Shima, T., Urata, S., Yoshimoto, G., Mori, Y., Iino, T., Yamauchi, T., Eto, T., Niiro, H., Iwasaki, H., Takenaka, K. & Akashi, K. Self-renewing hematopoietic stem cell is the primary target in pathogenesis of human chronic lymphocytic leukemia. *Cancer Cell*, Vol. 20, No. 2, (August 2011), pp. 246-259, PMID: 21840488

Kipps, T.J. The B-cell receptor and ZAP-70 in chronic lymphocytic leukemia. *Best Practice & Research Clinical Haem*atology, Vol. 20, No. 3 (September 2007), pp. 415-424, PMID: 17707830

Klein, U., Tu, Y., Stolovitzky, G.A., Mattioli, M., Cattoretti, G., Husson, H., Freedman, A., Inghirami, G., Cro, L., Baldini, L., Neri, A., Califano, A. & Dalla-Favera R. Gene expression profiling of B cell chronic lymphocytic leukemia reveals a homogeneous phenotype related to memory B cells. *Journal of Experimental Medicine*, Vol. 194, No. 11, (December 2001), pp. 1625-1638, PMID: 11733577

Klein, U. & Dalla-Favera R. New insights into the pathogenesis of chronic lymphocytic leukemia. *Seminars in Cancer Bio*logy, Vol. 20, No. 6, (December 2010), pp. 377-383, PMID: 21029776

Lan, L., Ui, A.A., Nakajima, S., Hatakeyama, K., Hoshi, M., Watanabe, R., Janicki, S., Ogiwaraa, H., Kohno, T., Kanno, S-I. & Yasui, A. The ACF1 complex is required for DNA double-strand break repair in human cells. *Molecular Cell*, Vol. 40, No. 6, (December 2010), pp. 976-987, PMID: 21172662

Lanasa, M.C. Novel insights into the biology of CLL. *Hematology/ American Society of Hematology Education Program*, 2010; 2010:70-76, PMID: 21239773

Langerak, A.W., Davi, F., Ghia, P., Hadzidimitriou, A., Murray, F., Potter, K.N., Rosenquist, R., Stamatopoulos, K. & Belessi, C. Immunoglobulin sequence analysis and prognostication in CLL: guidelines from the ERIC review board for reliable interpretation of problematic cases. *Leukemia*, Vol., 25, No. 6 (June 2011), pp. 979-984, PMID: 21455216

Lanham S, Hamblin T, Oscier D, Ibbotson R, Stevenson F, Packham G. Differential signaling via surface IgM is associated with VH gene mutational status and CD38 expression in chronic lymphocytic leukemia. *Blood*, Vol. 101, No. 3, (February 2003), pp. 1087-1093, PMID: 12393552

Lansdorp, P.M. Telomeres, stem cells, and haematology. *Blood*, Vol. 111, No. 4, (February 2008), pp. 1759-1766, PMID: 18263784

Larsen, D.H., Poinsignon, C., Gudjonsson, T., Dinant, C., Payne, M.R., Hari, F.J., Danielsen, J.M., Menard, P., Sand, J.C., Stucki, M., Lukas, C., Bartek, J., Andersen, J.S. & Lukas, J. The chromatin-remodeling factor CHD4 coordinates signaling and repair after DNA damage. *Journal of Cell Biology, Vol.* 190, No. 5, (September 2010), pp. 731-740, PMID: 20805324

Lee-Theilen, M., Matthews, A.J., Kelly, D., Zheng, S., Chaudhuri, J. CtIP promotes microhomology-mediated alternative end joining during class-switch recombination. *Nature Structural & Molecular Biology*, Vol. 18, No. 1, (January 2011), pp. 75-79, PMID: 21131982

Lieber, M.R. The mechanism of human nonhomologous DNA end joining. *Journal of Biological Chemistry*, Vol. 283, No. 1, (January 2008), pp. 1-5, PMID: 17999957

Lin, T.T., Letsolo, B.T., Jones, R.E., Rowson, J., Pratt, G., Hewamana, S., Fegan, C., Pepper, C. & Baird, D.M. Telomere dysfunction and fusion during the progression of chronic lymphocytic leukemia: evidence for a telomere crisis. *Blood*, Vol. 116, No. 11, (September 2010), pp. 1899-1907, PMID: 20538793

Longhese, M.P. DNA damage response at functional and dysfunctional telomeres. *Genes & Development*, Vol. 22, No. 2, (January 2008), pp. 125-140, PMID: 18198332

Ma, W., Kantarjian, H., O'Brien, S., Jilani, I., Zhang, X., Estrov, Z., Ferrajoli, A., Keating, M., Giles, F. & Albitar, M. Enzymatic activity of circulating proteasomes correlates with clinical behavior in patients with chronic lymphocytic leukemia. *Cancer*, Vol. 112, No. 6, (March 2008), pp. 1306-1312, PMID: 18224667

Mandel, E.M. & Grosschedl, R. Transcription control of early B cell differentiation. *Current Opinion in Immunology,* Vol. 22, No. 2, (April 2010), pp. 161-167, PMID: 20144854

Mari, P.O., Florea, B.I., Persengiev, S.P., Verkaik, N.S., Brüggenwirth, H.T., Modesti, M., Giglia-Mari, G., Bezstarosti, K., Demmers, J.A., Luider, T.M., Houtsmuller, A.B. & van Gent, D.C. (2006) Dynamic assembly of end-joining complexes requires interaction between Ku70/80 and XRCC4. *Proceedings of National Academy of Sciences, USA*, Vol. 103, No. 49, (December 2006), pp. 18597-18602, PMID: 17124166

Marteau, J-B., Rigaud, O., Brugat, T., Gault, N., Vallat, L., Kruhoffer, M., Orntoft, T.F., Nguyen-Khac, F., Chevillard, S., Merle-Beral, H. & Delic, J. Concomitant heterochromatinisation and down-regulation of gene expression unveils epigenetic silencing of *RELB* in an aggressive subset of chronic lymphocytic leukemia in males. *BMC Med Genomics*, Vol. 3 (November 2010), 3:53, PMID: 21062507

Masdehors, P., Merle-Béral, H., Maloum, K., Omura, S., Magdelénat, H. & Delic J. Deregulation of the ubiquitin system and p53 proteolysis modify the apoptotic response in B-CLL lymphocytes. *Blood,* Vol.96, No. 1, (July 2000), pp. 269-274, PMID: 10891461

Mauro, F.R., Foa, R., Giannarelli, D., Cordone, I., Crescenzi, S., Pescarmona, E., Salla, R., Cerretti, R. & Mandelli, F. Clinical characteristics and outcome of young chronic lymphocytic leukemia patients: a single institution study of 204 cases. *Blood,* Vol. 94, No. 2, (July 1999), pp. 448-454, PMID: 10397712

Messmer, B.T., Messmer, D., Allen, S.L., Kolitz, J.E., Kudalkar, P., Cesar, D., Murphy, E.J., Koduru, P., Ferrarini, M., Zupo, S., Cutrona, G., Damle, R.N., Wasil, T., Rai, K.R., Hellerstein, M.K. & Chiorazzi, N. *In vivo* measurements document the dynamic cellular kinetics of chronic lymphocytic leukemia B cells. *Journal of Clinical Investigation,* Vol. 115, No. 3, (March 2005), pp. 755-764, PMID: 15711642

Mills, D.M., Bonizzi, G. & Karin, M. Rickert RC. Regulation of late B cell differentiation by intrinsic IKKalpha-dependent signals. *Proceedings of National Academy of Sciences, U S A,* Vol. 104, No. 15, (April 2007), pp. 6359-6364, PMID: 17404218

Mladenov, E. & Iliakis, G. Induction and repair of DNA double strand breaks: The increasing spectrum of non-homologous end joining pathway. *Mutation Research,* Vol. 711, No. 1-2, (June 2011), pp. 61-72, PMID: 21329706

Mohr, J., Helfrich, H., Fuge, M., Eldering, E., Bühler, A., Winkler, D., Volden, M., Kater, A.P., Mertens, D., Te Raa, D., Döhner, H., Stilgenbauer, S. & Zenz, T. DNA damage-induced transcriptional program in CLL: biological and diagnostic implications for functional p53 testing. *Blood,* Vol. 117, No. 5, (February 2011), pp. 1622-1632, PMID: 21115975

Muller, C. & Salles, B. Regulation of DNA-dependent protein kinase activity in leukemic cells. *Oncogene,* Vol. 15, No. 19, (November 1997), pp. 2343-2348, PMID: 9393878

Nicoloso, M.S., Kipps, T.J., Croce, C.M. & Calin, G.A. MicroRNAs in the pathogeny of chronic lymphocytic leukaemia. *British Journal of Haematology,* Vol. 139, No. 5, (December 2007), pp. 709-716, PMID: 18021085

O'Driscoll, M., Cerosaletti, K.M., Girard, P.M., Dai, Y., Stumm, M., Kysela, B., Hirsch, B., Gennery, A., Palmer, S.E., Seidel, J., Gatti, R.A., Varon, R., Oettinger, M.A., Neitzel, H., Jeggo, P.A. & Concannon, P. DNA ligase IV mutations identified in patients exhibiting developmental delay and immunodeficiency. *Molecular Cell,* Vol.8, No. 6, (December 2001), pp. 1175-1185, PMID: 11779494

O'Driscoll, M. & Jeggo, P.A. CsA can induce DNA double-strand breaks: implications for BMT regimens particularly for individuals with defective DNA repair. *Bonne Marrow Transplantation,* Vol. 41, No. 11, (June 2008), pp. 983-989, PMID: 18278071

Ohta, T., Sato, K. & Wu, W. The BRCA1 ubiquitin ligase and homologous recombination repair. *FEBS Lett*er, 2011 May 9. [Epub ahead of print], PMID: 21570976

Pallasch, C.P., Patz, M., Park, Y.J., Hagist, S., Eggle, D., Claus, R., Debey-Pascher, S., Schulz, A., Frenzel, L.P., Claasen, J., Kutsch, N., Krause, G., Mayr, C., Rosenwald, A., Plass, C., Schultze, J.L., Hallek, M. & Wendtner, C.M. miRNA deregulation by epigenetic silencing disrupts suppression of the oncogene PLAG1 in chronic lymphocytic leukemia. *Blood,* Vol. 114, No. 15, (October 2009), pp. 3255-3264, PMID: 19692702

Panasci, L. Chlorambucil drug resistance in chronic lymphocytic leukemia: the emerging role of DNA repair. *Clinical Cancer Research,* Vol. 7, No. 3, (March 2001), pp. 454-461, PMID: 11297233

Parker, T.L. & Strout, M.P. Chronic lymphocytic leukemia: prognostic factors and impact on treatment. *Discovery Medicine,* Vol. 11, No. 57, (February 2011), pp. 115-123, PMID: 21356166

Patz, M., Pallasch, C.P.& Wendtner, C.M. Critical role of microRNAs in chronic lymphocytic leukemia: overexpression of the oncogene PLAG1 by deregulated miRNAs. *Leukemia & Lymphoma,* Vol. 51, No. 8, (August 2010), pp. 1379-1381, PMID: 20687796

Plass, C., Byrd, J.C., Raval, A., Tanner, S.M. & de la Chapelle, A. Molecular profiling of chronic lymphocytic leukaemia: genetics meets epigenetics to identify predisposing genes. *British Journal of Haematology,* Vol. 139, No. 5, (December 2007), pp. 744-752, PMID: 18021078

Puente, X.S., Pinyol, M., Quesada, V., Conde, L., Ordóñez, G.R., Villamor, N., Escaramis, G., Jares, P., Beà, S., González-Díaz, M., Bassaganyas, L., Baumann, T., Juan, M., López-Guerra, M., Colomer, D., Tubío, J.M., López, C., Navarro, A., Tornador, C., Aymerich, M., Rozman, M., Hernández, J.M., Puente, D.A., Freije, J.M., Velasco, G., Gutiérrez-Fernández, A., Costa, D., Carrió, A., Guijarro, S., Enjuanes, A., Hernández, L., Yagüe, J., Nicolás, P., Romeo-Casabona, C.M., Himmelbauer, H., Castillo, E., Dohm, JC., de Sanjosé, S., Piris, M.A., de Alava, E., Miguel, J.S., Royo, R., Gelpí, J.L., Torrents, D., Orozco, M., Pisano, D.G., Valencia, A., Guigó, R., Bayés, M., Heath, S., Gut, M., Klatt, P., Marshall, J., Raine, K., Stebbings, L.A., Futreal, P.A., Stratton, M.R., Campbell, P.J., Gut, I., López-Guillermo, A., Estivill, X., Montserrat, E., López-Otín, C. & Campo, E. Whole-genome sequencing identifies recurrent mutations in chronic lymphocytic leukaemia. *Nature,* Vol. 475, No. 7354, (June 2011), pp. 101-105, PMID: 21642962

Ramadan, K. & Meerang, M. Degradation-linked ubiquitin signal and proteasome are integral components of DNA double strand break repair: New perspectives for anti-cancer therapy. *FEBS Letter,* 2011, Apr 28. [Epub ahead of print], PMID: 21536036

Rassool, F.V. DNA double strand breaks (DSB) and non-homologous end joining (NHEJ) pathways in human leukemia. *Cancer Letter, Vol.* 193, No. 1, (April 2003) pp. 1-9, PMID: 12691817

Raval, A., Tanner, S.M., Byrd, J.C., Angerman, E.B., Perko, J.D., Chen, S.S., Hackanson, B., Grever, M.R., Lucas, D.M., Matkovic, J.J., Lin, T.S., Kipps, T.J., Murray, F., Weisenburger, D., Sanger, W., Lynch, J., Watson, P., Jansen, M., Yoshinaga, Y., Rosenquist, R., de Jong, P.J., Coggill, P., Beck, S., Lynch, H., de la Chapelle, A. & Plass C: Downregulation of death-associated protein kinase 1 (DAPK1) in chronic lymphocytic leukemia. *Cell,* Vol. 129, No. 5, (June 2007), pp. 879-890, PMID: 17540169

Riballo, E., Critchlow, S.E., Teo, S.H., Doherty, A.J., Priestley, A., Broughton, B., Kysela, B., Beamish, H., Plowman, N., Arlett, C.F., Lehmann, A.R., Jackson, S.P. & Jeggo, P.A. Identification of a defect in DNA ligase IV in a radiosensitive leukaemia patient. *Current Biology*, Vol. 9, No. 13, (July 1999), pp. 699-702, PMID: 10395545

Robert, T., Vanoli, F., Chiolo, I., Shubassi, G., Bernstein, K.A., Rothstein, R., Botrugno, O.A., Parazzoli, D., Oldani, A., Minucci, S. & Foiani, M. HDACs link the DNA damage response, processing of double-strand breaks and autophagy. *Nature*, Vol. 471, No. 7336, (March 2011), pp. 74-79, PMID: 21368826

Roos, G., Kröber, A., Grabowski, P., Kienle, D., Bühler, A., Döhner, H., Rosenquist, R. & Stilgenbauer, S. Short telomeres are associated with genetic complexity, high-risk genomic aberrations, and short survival in chronic lymphocytic leukemia. *Blood*, Vol. 111, No. 4, (February 2008), pp. 2246-2252, PMID: 18045969

Rosenwald, A., Alizadeh, A.A., Widhopf, G., Simon, R., Davis, R.E., Yu, X., Yang, L., Pickeral, O.K., Rassenti, L.Z., Powell, J., Botstein, D., Byrd, J.C., Grever, M.R., Cheson, B.D., Chiorazzi, N., Wilson, W.H., Kipps, T.J., Brown, P.O. & Staudt, LM. Relation of gene expression phenotype to immunoglobulin mutation genotype in B cell chronic lymphocytic leukemia. *Journal of Experimental Medicine*, Vol. 194, No. 2001, 194:1639-1647, PMID: 11733578

Rosenwald. A., Chuang, E.Y., Davis, R.E., Wiestner, A., Alizadeh, A.A., Arthur, D.C., Mitchell, J.B., Marti, G.E., Fowler, D.H., Wilson, W.H. & Staudt, L.M. Fludarabine treatment of patients with chronic lymphocytic leukemia induces a p53-dependent gene expression response. *Blood, Vol.* 104, No. 5, (September 2004), pp. 1428-1434, PMID: 15138159

Sampath, D., Calin, G.A., Puduvalli, V.K., Gopisetty, G., Taccioli, C., Liu, C.G., Ewald, B., Liu, C., Keating, M.J. & Plunkett W. Specific activation of microRNA106b enables the p73 apoptotic response in chronic lymphocytic leukemia by targeting the ubiquitin ligase Itch for degradation. *Blood*, Vol. 113, No. 16, (April 2009), pp. 3744-3753, PMID: 19096009

Schär, P. & Fritsch, O. DNA repair and the control of DNA methylation. *Progress in Drug* Research Vol. 67, 2011, pp. 51-68, PMID: 21141724

Schroeder, H.W .Jr., & Dighiero, G. The pathogenesis of chronic lymphocytic leukemia: analysis of the antibody repertoire. *Immunology Today*, Vol. 15, No. 6, (June 1994), pp. 288-294, PMID: 7520700

Ségal-Bendirdjian, E. & Gilson, E. Telomeres and telomerase: from basic research to clinical applications. *Biochimie*, Vol. 90, No. 4, (April 2008), pp. 1-4, PMID: 20096746

Shanbhag, N.M., Rafalska-Metcalf, I.U., Balane-Bolivar, C., Janicki, S.M. & Greenberg, R.A. ATM-dependent chromatin changes silence transcription in cis to DNA double-strand breaks. *Cell*, Vol. 141, No. 6, (June 2010), pp. 970-981, PMID: 20550933

Shehata, M., Schnabl, S., Demirtas, D., Hilgarth, M., Hubmann, R., Ponath, E., Badrnya, S., Lehner, C., Hoelbl, A., Duechler, M., Gaiger, A., Zielinski, C., Schwarzmeier, J.D. & Jaeger U. Reconstitution of PTEN activity by CK2 inhibitors and interference with the PI3-K/Akt cascade counteract the antiapoptotic effect of human stromal cells in chronic lymphocytic leukemia. *Blood,* Vol. 116, No. 14, (October 2010), pp. 2513-2521, PMID: 20576813

Stankovic, T., Weber, P., Stewart, G., Bedenham, T., Murray, J., Byrd, P.J., Moss, P.A. & Taylor, A.M. Inactivation of ataxia telangiectasia mutated gene in B-cell chronic lymphocytic leukaemia. *Lancet,* Vol. 353, No. 9146, (January 1999), pp. 26-29, PMID: 10023947

Stewart, S.A. & Weinberg, R.A. Telomeres: cancer to human aging. Annual Reviews Cell and Developmental Biology, Vol. 22, 2006, pp. 531-557, PMID: 16824017

Subramanyam, D. & Blelloch, R. From microRNAs to targets: pathway discovery in cell fate transitions. *Current Opinion in Genetics and Development, Vol.* 2011 May 31. [Epub ahead of print], PMID: 21636265

Ting, A.H., McGarvey, K.M. & Baylin, S.B. The cancer epigenome--components and functional correlates. *Genes & Development,* Vol. 20, No. 23, (December 2006), pp. 3215-3231, PMID: 17158741

Vallat, L., Magdelénat, H., Merle-Béral, H., Masdehors, P., Potocki de Montalk, G., Davi, F., Kruhoffer, M., Sabatier, L., Orntoft, T.F. & Delic J. The resistance of B-CLL cells to DNA damage-induced apoptosis defined by DNA microarrays. *Blood,* Vol. 101, No. 11, (June 2003), pp. 4598-4606, PMID: 12586635

Visone, R., Veronese, A., Rassenti, L.Z., Balatti, V., Pearl, D.K., Acunzo, M., Volinia, S., Taccioli, C., Kipps, T.J.& Croce CM. MiR-181b is a biomarker of disease progression in chronic lymphocytic leukemia. *Blood,* 2011 Jun 2. [Epub ahead of print], PMID: 21636858

Wahlfors, J., Hiltunen, H., Heinonen, K., Hämäläinen, E., Alhonen, L. & Jänne, J. Genomic hypomethylation in human chronic lymphocytic leukemia. *Blood,* Vol. 80, No. 8, (October 1992), pp. 2074-2080, PMID: 138719

Weill, JC. & Reynaud, CA. Do developing B cells need antigen? *Journal of Experimental Medicine,* Vol. 201, No. 1, (January 2005), pp. 7-9, PMID: 15630132

Weill, JC., Weller, S. & Reynaud CA. Human Marginal Zone B Cells. *Annual Review of Immunology,* Vol., 27 (2009), pp. 267-285, PMID: 19302041

Weitzman, M.D., Lilley, C.E. & Chaurushiya MS. Changing the ubiquitin landscape during viral manipulation of the DNA damage response. *FEBS Letter,* 2011 May 5. [Epub ahead of print], PMID: 21549706

Weller, S., Mamani-Matsuda, M., Picard, C., Cordier, C., Lecoeuche, D., Gauthier, F., Weill, JC. & Reynaud, C.A. Somatic diversification in the absence of antigen-driven responses is the hallmark of the IgM+ IgD+ CD27+ B cell repertoire in infants. *Journal of Experimental Medicine,* Vol. 205, No. 6, (June 2008), pp. 1331-1342, PMID: 18519648

Weller, S., Braun, M.C., Tan, B.K., Rosenwald, A., Cordier, C., Conley, M.E., Plebani, A., Kumararatne, D.S., Bonnet, D., Tournilhac, O., Tchernia, G., Steiniger, B., Staudt, L.M., Casanova, J.L., Reynaud, C.A. & Weill, JC. Human blood IgM "memory" B cells are circulating splenic marginal zone B cells harboring a prediversified immunoglobulin repertoire. *Blood,* Vol. 104, No. 12, (December 2004), pp. 3647-3654, PMID: 15191950

Weston, V.J., Oldreive, C.E., Skowronska, A., Oscier, D.G., Pratt, G., Dyer, M.J., Smith, G., Powell, J.E., Rudzki, Z., Kearns, P., Moss, P.A., Taylor, A.M., & Stankovic, T. The PARP inhibitor olaparib induces significant killing of ATM-deficient lymphoid tumor cells in vitro and in vivo. *Blood*, Vol. 116, No. 22, (November 2010), pp. 4578-4587, PMID: 20739657

Wickremasinghe, R., Prentice, A.G. & Steele AJ. Aberrantly activated anti-apoptotic signalling mechanisms in chronic lymphocytic leukaemia cells: clues to the identification of novel therapeutic targets. *British Journal of Haematology*, Vol. 153, No. 5, (June 2011), pp. 545-556, PMID: 21501136

Wong, K.Y., So, C.C., Loong, F., Chung, L.P., Lam, W.W., Liang, R., Li, G.K., Jin, D.Y.& Chim, C.S. Epigenetic Inactivation of the miR-124-1 in Haematological Malignancies. *PLoS One*. April 2011, 6(4):e19027, PMID: 21544199

Yan, C.T., Boboila, C., Souza, E.K., Franco, S., Hickernell, T.R., Murphy, M., Gumaste, S., Geyer, M., Zarrin, A.A., Manis, J.P., Rajewsky, K. & Alt, F.W. IgH class switching and translocations use a robust non-classical end-joining pathway. *Nature*, Vol. 449, No. 7161, (September 2007), pp. 478-482, PMID: 17713479

Zecevic, A., Sampath, D., Ewald, B., Chen, R., Wierda, W. & Pliunkett, W. Killing of chronic lymphocytic leukemia by the combination of fludarabine and oxaliplatin is dependent on the activity of XPF endonuclease. *Clinical Cancer Research*, Vol. 17, No. 14, (July 2011), pp. 4731-4741, PMID: 21632856

Zenz, T., Döhner, H. & Stilgenbauer, S. Genetics and risk-stratified approach to therapy in chronic lymphocytic leukemia. *Best Practice & Research Clinical Haematology*, Vol. 20, No. 3, (September 2007), pp. 439-453, PMID: 17707832

Zenz, T., Mertens, D., Döhner, H. & Stilgenbauer, S. Importance of genetics in chronic lymphocytic leukemia. *Blood Reviews*, Vol. 25, No. 3, (May 2011), pp. 131-137, PMID: 21435757

Zha, S., Guo, C., Boboila, C., Oksenych, V., Cheng, H.L., Zhang, Y., Wesemann, D.R., Yuen, G., Patel, H., Goff, P.H., Dubois, R.L. & Alt FW. ATM damage response and XLF repair factor are functionally redundant in joining DNA breaks. *Nature*, Vol. 469, No. 7329, (Jaanuary 2011), pp. 250-254, PMID: 21160472

Zupo, S., Isnardi, L., Megna, M., Massara, R., Malavasi, F., Dono, M., Cosulich, E.& Ferrarini, M. CD38 expression distinguishes two groups of B-cell chronic lymphocytic leukemias with different responses to anti-IgM antibodies and propensity to apoptosis. *Blood*, Vol. 88, No. 4, (August 1996), pp. 1365-1374, PMID : 8695855

5

Current Knowledge of Microarray Analysis for Gene Expression Profiling in Chronic Lymphocytic Leukemia

Ida Franiak-Pietryga and Marek Mirowski
Department of Pharmaceutical Biochemistry, Medical University of Lodz
Poland

1. Introduction

Chronic lymphocytic leukemia (CLL) is characterised by the accumulation of mature CD5+/CD19+ B-lymphocytes in the blood, bone marrow, lymph nodes and spleen (Caligaris-Cappio & Hamblin, 1999). Although the role of cellular proliferation disorders in CLL may originally have been underestimated, the typical characteristic of the disease is still regarded as a failure of malignant cells to undergo apoptosis (Munk Pedersen & Reed, 2004). CLL is a heterogeneous disease and although it is relatively stable in some patients, it progresses rapidly in others (Caligaris-Cappio & Hamblin, 1999). The mutational status of immunoglobulin heavy chain variable gene segment (*IGHV*) and the expression of CD38 and/or ZAP70 are important prognostic factors of disease so their detection is very useful for stratification of patients into indolent or aggressive subgroups (Hamblin et al., 1999; Krober et al., 2002; Orchard et al., 2004).

However, a more robust approach to subclassifying CLL is to identify the genomic changes in the malignant clone. The heterogeneity of the disease may result from different genetic abnormalities in distinct subclasses of patients. Furthermore, there is a strong relationship between specific genetic aberrations and the clinical course of the disease. On the basis of the mutational status of the variable region of the IGH, CLL can be divided into two subtypes. Somatic hypermutation of *IGHV* occurs in more than half of the patients and is associated with a more indolent clinical course. Additionally, deletions of the long arm of chromosome 13 or 11 and the short arm of chromosome 17, as well as trisomy of chromosome 12, are prognostically most important for the CLL patients. The most common abnormality in CLL, observed in more than 50% patients, is del(13)(q14) and, along with hypermutation of *IGHV*, this is linked with a good prognosis (Damle et al., 1999; Schroeder & Dighiero, 1994).

2. Gene expression profiling

Recent advances in genomics have transformed research on hematologic malignancies by improving molecular approaches to gene networks. New technologies have been designed to meet the need for methods to address the functional significances of nucleotides sequences. Microarrays have emerged as powerful tools for increasing the potential of standard methods through genome-wide biological studies. They have been focused mainly on gene expression profiling (GEP), but also on mutational screening, genotyping of polymorphisms and copy number analyses.

2.1 Contribution of microarray study to comprehension of CLL pathophysiology

DNA microarrays can be used to detect either DNA, as in comparative genomic hybridization, or to detect RNA, usually as complementary DNA (cDNA) after reverse transcription. The process of measuring gene expression via cDNA is called *expression analysis* or *expression profiling* (Schena et al., 1995). Alizadeh et al., (2000) investigated the construction of a commercial cDNA microarray (Lymphochip) for studies of normal and malignant human cells. They examined each stage of lymphocyte differentiation that can be defined by a characteristic gene expression signature. Genes that are coregulated by over hundreds of experimental conditions often encode functionally related proteins. GEP also provide an unprecedented ability to define the molecular and functional relationships between normal and malignant lymphocyte cell populations (Alizadeh & Staudt, 2000).

Using different microarray platforms such as oligonucleotide arrays, cDNA arrays printed on glass slides and on nylon membranes, Wang et al., (2004) found that several genes were consistently differently expressed between CLL and normal B-cell samples. The following 10 genes were shown to be expressed differently in CLL compared with tonsillar B-lymphocytes and plasma cells: *FCER2* (*CD23*), *FGR, TNFRSF1B, CCR7, IL4R, PTPN12, FMOD, TMEM1, CHS1* and *ZNF266* (Zent et al., 2003).

The results of GEP tests on CLL cells indicated that their profile was more closely related to non-proliferating B cells, or memory B cells, than to cells from a naïve germinal centre (GC), mitogenically activated blood cells or CD5+ B cells (Klein et al., 2001). Over the last few years, global GEP has been revised and defined CLL as a tumor of antigen-experienced B cells. These could be marginal zone or memory B cells. Now we know, that CLL results not only from an accumulation of transformed B cells, due to an imbalance between cell generation and cell death rate, but also from a proliferation of B cells in particular microenvironments in the lymphoid tissues and bone marrow (Klein & Dalla-Favera, 2010). Based on these findings, it can be suggest, that the leukemic B cells are more complex mixture than we have hitherto expected. Other genes have been dubbed *CLL signature genes* because they are selectively expressed in CLL and not in normal cells or other types of B-cell malignancy (Rosenwald et al., 2001). The CLL signature includes genes already known to be characteristic for CLL, such as *CD5, IL2Rα (CD25)* and *BCL2,* and genes not previously known to be expressed in CLL, such as *WNT3, TITIN, ROR1* and *MRC-OX2. ROR1* and *MRC-OX2* encode membrane proteins, so they might be useful for decisions concerning treatment with humanised monoclonal antibodies. *WNT3* probably regulates B lymphocyte proliferation (Zent et al., 2003; Reya et al., 2000). A study by Zent et al., (2003) showed that the GEP of CLL lymphocyte is different from multiple myeloma (MM) cells. CLL expressed higher levels of tumour necrosis factor (TNF) and TNF receptor pathway genes (*LTB, TRAF5, TNFRSF9, TNFSF7* and *LITAF).* The *IAP* family gene (*BIRC1*) and the *XIAP* antagonist (*HSXIAPAF1*) were expressed at higher levels only in CLL to MM, similar to *BCL-2* expression.

2.2 Contribution to the identification of new genes that might be considered as prognostic factors

In the last few years, the development of cytogenetics and molecular biology has led to the release of new genetic prognostic markers such as *IGHV* mutational status, genomic aberrations and individual gene mutations.

To determine possible genetic and molecular abnormalities related to early clinical progression in CLL, Fernandez et al., (2008) investigated alterations in genomic and gene expression profiles in a series of samples sequentially obtained at diagnosis in early stage of the disease and at the time of clinical progression before treatment. A group of 58 genes was identified by supervised analysis comparing the initial and progressed samples: 37 were over-expressed while 21 were down-regulated. No significant differences were observed in the expression of these genes in samples from the three CLL cases with stable clinical decease. Functional analysis of the over-expressed genes showed that they are involved in different pathways, including cell cycle and cell growth (*MCM4, RAPGEF2, OGG1, ESCO1, ESR1, ACTL6A, CENPJ, ATG5*) and ion regulation (*MYLC2PL, ADRB1, TRPV5, TMCO3*). Interestingly, 6 of the 21 down-regulated genes were considered negative regulators of integrin-mediated cell adhesion and motility (*PRAM1, CDC42EP4, COL4A2, PLCB2, RAPGEF1, FLNA*). These findings suggest that in early stage CLL, clinical progression is associated with inactivation of tumour suppressor genes and modulation of the expression of a small number of genes that are inhibitors of cell adhesion and motility.

Ferrer et al., (2004) performed gene expression profiling on 31 CLL cases and investigated the *HV* gene mutation status by nucleotide sequencing. The array data showed that the greatest differences between the unmutated (20 cases) and the mutated (11 cases) groups were observed in the expression of such genes as: *ZAP70, RAF1, PAX5, TCF1, CD44, SF1, S100A12, NUP214, DAF, GLVR1, MKK6, AF4, CX3CR1, NAFTC1* and *HEX*. *ZAP70* was significantly more highly expressed in the *IGHV*-unmutated CLL group, whereas all the other genes were more highly expressed in the *IGHV*-mutated cases. This study confirmed that *ZAP70* expression can predict the *HV* mutation status and suggested that *RAF1, PAX5* and other differentially expressed genes may be good markers for differentiating between these two groups and can serve as prognostic markers.

2.2.1 Deregulated apoptosis in poor-prognosis CLL

CLL is a heterogeneous disease with marked variability in its clinical course. With the aim of identifying genes potentially related to disease progression, Fält et al., (2005) performed gene expression profiling on CLL patients with non-aggressive disease or with progressive disease requiring therapy. The Affymetrix GeneChip U95Av2 technique was used in 11 samples obtained from CLL patients with stable and 10 patients with clinically progressive disease. To discriminate samples from progressive and stable disease, a group of genes was chosen as markers; two genes in particular, *PPP2R5C* and *RBL2*, were included among the best discriminators as both were expressed at lower levels in progressive than in stable CLL. These genes are known to be key regulators of both the cell cycle and the mitochondria/cytochrome c apoptotic pathway. This procedure allowed samples with progressive and stable disease to be identified with 70-90% accuracy.

Stratowa et al., (2001) studied 54 peripheral blood lymphocyte samples obtained from patients with CLL to determine the expression levels of 1024 genes on a cDNA microarray and to correlate them with patient survival. Overall survival (OS) of CLL patients displaying low expression of genes coding for IL-1β, IL-8 and L-selectin was shorter than for patients with high expression of these genes. However, high expression of *TCL1* was connected with decreased patient survival. These findings suggest that CLL prognosis may be connected with a defect in lymphocyte trafficking, causing accumulation of leukemic B cells in the blood.

Edelmann et al., (2008) used a microarray-based GEP (Affymetrix U95A) to study how the stroma modulates the survival of CLL cells in *in vitro* co-culture model employing the murine fibroblast cell line M2-10B4. CLL cells cultured in direct contact with the stromal layer (STR) showed significantly better survival than cells cultured in transwell (TW) inserts above the M2-10B4 cells. STR induced a more marked up-regulation of the PI3K/NF-κB/Akt signaling pathway genes (*INPP4A, NFKB2, REL* and *MAPKAPK2*) than TW conditions and mediated a pro-angiogenetic switch in the CLL cells by up-regulating *VEGF* and *OPN* and down-regulating the anti-angiogenetic molecule *TSP-1*. The findings also suggest that *TSP-1* expression in CLL cells may be related to both disease stage and CLL subtype as defined by *ZAP70* and *CD38* expression. OPN protein secretion may be correlated to disease progression in CLL.

GEP used to predict the prognosis in CLL is presented in Table 1 and Table 2.

2.3 Contribution of GEP microarray study to pharmacogenomics

Drug resistance remains a major problem of CLL treatment. Owing to their high adaptability to therapeutic conditions, malignant tumour cells frequently develop escape mechanisms in response to cytostatic drugs. It is very difficult to predict a tumour's reaction to drugs because it can deploy multiple cellular mechanisms such as enhanced DNA repair, elevated levels of drug transporters, over-expression of detoxifying enzymes or apoptosis inhibition, which are often involved in the development of drug resistance. To monitor the multiple alterations by which CLL may become drug-insensitive, highly parallel analyses such as the DNA microarray technique are required. This technique affords new ways of predicting resistance and sensitivity to therapy (Dietel & Sers, 2006).

2.3.1 *In vitro* experiments

There is now well documented that some genes induce apoptosis, whereas the others can inhibit this phenomenon (Table 3). It is also known that drugs used for therapy regimens can change GEP and modify apoptosis. However, the knowledge concerning the drug influence on GEP is still insufficient and demands further studies.

The study by Vallat et al., (2003) combined two series of microarray analyses (Hu-FL GeneChips, Affymetrix, 7,070 genes) with four sensitive and three resistant CLL samples and compared their gene expression patterns before and after *in vitro* irradiation-induced apoptosis. Sixteen differentially expressed genes (≥2-fold, specifically in resistant cells) were disclosed by data analysis. After the validation of the selected genes by quantitative RT-PCR on seven microarray samples, their altered expression level was confirmed on a further 15 CLL samples not previously included in the microarray analysis. Eleven patients with

	Alterations in gene expression	Gene description
Good-prognosis CLL		*Cell cycle and transcription genes*
	RAF1 ⇑	V-raf-1 murine leukemia viral oncogene homolog 1
	PAX5 ⇑	Paired box gene 5
	TCF1 ⇑	Transcription factor 1
	CD44 ⇑	CD44 antigen
	SF1 (ZNF162) ⇑	Splicing factor 1 (zinc finger protein 162)
	S100A12 ⇑	S100 calcium binding protein A12
	NUP214 ⇑	Nucleoporin 214 kD
	DAF ⇑	CD55 molecule, decay accelerating factor for complement
	GLVR1 ⇑	Solute carrier family 20 (phosphate transporter) member 1 (Glv-r)
	MKK6 ⇑	Mitogen-activated protein kinase kinase 6 (MKK6, MAPKK6, MEK6)
	AF4 ⇑	Pre-B-cell monocytic leukemia partner 1; (AF4, AFF1, MLLT2)
	CX3CR1 ⇑	Chemokine (C-X3-C motif) receptor 1 (CCRL1, GPR13)
	NAF ⇑	T cell chemotactic factor (NAF, IL-8)
	HEX ⇑	Hematopoietically expressed homeobox (HEX, HHEX)
		Cell cycle and cell growth
	MCM4 ⇑	Minichromosome maintenance complex component 4
	RAPGEF2 ⇑	Rap guanine nucleotide exchange factor (GEF) 2 (RAPGEF2)
	OGG1 ⇑	8-oxoguanine DNA glycosylase (OGG1, HMMH, HOGG1)
	ESCO1 ⇑	Establishment of cohesion 1 homolog 1 (ESCO1, CTF, ECO1)
	ESR1 ⇑	Estrogen receptor 1 (ESR1, ER α)
	ACTL6A ⇑	Actin-like 6A (ACTL6A, Arp4, BAF53A, INO80K, MGC5382)
	CENPJ ⇑	Centromere protein J (CENPJ, BM032, CPAP, LAP, LIP1)
	ATG5 ⇑	ATG5 autophagy related 5 homolog (APG5-LIKE, APG5L, ASP)
		Ions regulation
	MYLC2PL ⇑	Myosin, light chain 10, regulatory (MYL10, MYLC2PL, PLRLC)
	ADRB1 ⇑	Adrenergic, beta-1-, receptor (ADRB1, B1AR, BETA1AR, RHR)
	TRPV5 ⇑	Transient receptor potential cation channel, subfamily V, member 5
	TMCO3 ⇑	Transmembrane and coiled-coil domains 3 (TMCO3, C13orf11)
		Cell signalling
	INPP4A ⇑	Inositol polyphosphate-4-phosphatase, type I (TVAS1, INPP4A)
	NFKβ2 ⇑	Nuclear factor of kappa light polypeptide gene enhancer in B-cells 2
	REL ⇑	V-rel reticuloendotheliosis viral oncogene homolog
	MAPKAPK2 ⇑	Mitogen-activated protein kinase-activated protein kinase 2 (MK2)

Gene expression: upregulation ⇑

Table 1. GEP in CLL, which may predict a good prognosis. (Edelmann et al., 2008; Fält et al., 2005; Fernandez et al., 2008; Ferrer et al., 2004; Stratowa et al., 2001)

	Alterations in gene expression	Gene description
Genes underexpressed		***Cell adhesion and motility***
	RAPGEF1 ⇓	Rap guanine nucleotide exchange factor (GEF) 2
	FLNA ⇓	Alpha-filamin; endothelial actin-binding protein
	PRAM1 ⇓	PML-RARA regulated adaptor molecule 1
	CDC42EP4 ⇓	CDC42 effector protein (Rho GTPase binding) 4
	COL4A2 ⇓	Collagen alpha-2(IV) chain
	PLCB2 ⇓	Phospholipase C, beta 2
	IL1β ⇓	Interleukin 1 beta
	IL-8 ⇓	Interleukin 8 (T cell chemotactic factor)
	L-selectin ⇓	Leukocyte-endothelial cell adhesion molecule 1 (LECAM-1)
		Cell cycle and signal transduction
	PPP2R5C ⇓	Protein phosphatase 2, regulatory subunit B', gamma
	RBL2 ⇓	Retinoblastoma-like 2 (p130)
		Cell growth
	TSP-1 ⇓	Thrombospondin-1
Genes overexpressed		***Cell adhesion and motility***
	TCL-1 ⇑	T-cell leukemia/lymphoma 1A
		Cell cycle and signal transduction
	VH 3.21 ⇑	Immunoglobulin heavy variable 3-21
	ZAP70 ⇑	Tyrosine-protein kinase ZAP-70
		Cell growth
	OPN ⇑	Osteopontin
	VEGF ⇑	Vascular Endothelial Growth Factor

Gene expression: up ⇑ - and downregulation ⇓

Table 2. GEP in CLL, which may predict the poor prognosis. (Edelmann et al., 2008; Fält et al., 2005; Stratowa et al., 2001; Thorselius et al., 2006)

malignant B cells that were sensitive to *in vitro* radiation-induced apoptosis had never been treated, whereas eight of the 11 patients with resistant disease had previously been treated with fludarabine (FA), cyclophosphamide (C) or chlorambucil (CHB). In the 11 sensitive and 11 resistant CLL samples tested, genes were found to be specific for all the resistant samples; *TR3, HLA-DQA1, MTMR6, C-MYC, C-REL, C-IAP1, MAT2A* and *FMOD* were up-regulated, whereas *MIP1A/GOS19-1* homolog, *STAT1, BLK, HSP27* and *ECH1* were down-regulated. The result of this study was defining clinically relevant new molecular markers specific to resistant CLL subtypes.

Morales et al., (2005) investigated the regulation of apoptosis in B-CLL cells using cDNA microarrays (Human Apoptosis GEArray Q Series, Superarray) with 96 known genes. Data were obtained from and compared between two groups of CLL patients with either non-progressive, non-aggressive, previously untreated disease in which the leukemic cells were sensitive to *in vitro* FA-induced apoptosis, referred to as sensitive B-CLL (sB-CLL), or progressive, chemotherapy-refractory disease in which the leukemic cells were resistant to *in vitro* FA-induced apoptosis, referred to as resistant B-CLL (rB-CLL). By performing a supervised clustering of genes that most clearly discriminated rB-CLL from sB-CLL, a small group of genes was identified. *BFL1* was the most strongly discriminating gene, with higher expression in rB-CLL. This finding suggests that *BFL1* may be an important regulator of CLL apoptosis, which could contribute to disease progression and resistance to chemotherapy, and could be a potential future therapeutic target.

Direct physical interaction of stromal cells with CLL cells and overexpression of *RAD51* and *LIG4* (DNA ligase IV) in the leukemic cells have been found. These genes code for DNA repair enzymes in mammalian cells (Edelmann et al., 2008). Given that *RAD51* expression in CLL was previously reported to correlate with resistance to CHB. These findings may provide a molecular-level explanation of the capacity of stromal cells to protect CLL cells from drug-induced apoptosis (Christodoulopoulos et al., 1999).

Segel et al., (2003) have used a cDNA microarray containing approximately 40,000 human gene sequences to obtain GEP for untreated and tetradecanoyl phorbol acetate (TPA)-treated B-CLL cells. Three genes, *EGR1, DUSP2* and *CD69*, showed a 2-fold or greater increase in mRNA transcription in two studies. Several genes (*PKC, N-MYC, JUN D* and *BCL2*), previously reported to be overexpressed in CLL lymphocytes, were also overexpressed in these studies but were not altered by TPA treatment. These findings suggest that the products of these three genes may be central to early steps in the TPA-induced evolution of B-CLL cells to a plasma-cell phenotype. A variety of stimulators such as TPA, bryostatin, IL-2 and others can induce CLL lymphocytes to mature *in vitro* to an immunoglobulin-producing and -secreting phenotype. Such treatment corrects some metabolic defects such as impairment of the L-system amino acid transport, but not others such as diminished membrane gamma-glutamyl transpeptidase (GGTP) activity.

GEP allows the study of a large number of genes and analysis of global pathways rather than single targets. Stamatopoulos et al., (2009) revealed the influence of valproic acid (VPA) on molecular changes in two key pathways in cancer: apoptosis and proliferation. The study was conducted on purified B cells obtained from 14 CLL patients. Microarray analysis was performed with an Affymetrix GeneChip Human Genome U133 Plus 2.0 array. Several genes (i.e. *CD5, BCL2, CD23, LCK, PIM1*) described as overexpressed in CLL by Wang et al., (2004) were downregulated by VPA in this study, whereas genes described by Wang et al., (2004) as underexpressed in CLL (i.e. *BCLA1, C-MYC, DUSP2* and *PEA15*) were upregulated by VPA. The authors suppose that these results indicate that VPA could restore a more 'normal' epigenetic code and, in this way, could allow normal cellular processes that were silenced after malignant transformation. No differences among the GEP of ZAP^+ and ZAP^- patients (poor and good prognosis, respectively) were found, indicating that VPA was acting independently of disease aggressiveness. It had also been observed that VPA acted on an important number of genes involved in apoptosis: *BCL2, XIAP, FLIP, BCL-xL, AVEN* and *cIAP*, which as a result, were significantly downregulated, whereas *CASP 2, 3, 6, 8, 9,* and *BAX, BAK, APAF1* and *P53* were all significantly upregulated. The ratio of anti- and proapoptotic genes determines the tendency towards cell death or cell survival. Moreover, a large number of cell-cycle genes were upregulated, not only *CDK1, 2, 4,* and *6, cyclin B1, B2, D1, D2, E1* and *E2,* but also inhibitors of cell cycle, such as *P15, 16, 18, 19* and *21.* The deregulated and simultaneous expression of all these genes is probably one of the reasons for proliferation inhibition (Stamatopoulos et al., 2009).

In our department, we identified differentially expressed genes in lymphocytes obtained from CLL patients and incubated with FA or cladribine (2-chlorodeoxyadenosine; 2-CdA) (Table 4). Among 93 studied apoptotic genes by means of 384 TaqMan Low Density Array (Applied Biosystems) most of them were downregulated, whereas such a few of them were upregulated: *BAD, TNFRSF21, DAPK1* – in 2-CdA cultured group and *CARD6* and *CARD9* in FA cultured group. We have also noticed 4 genes (*BAK1, BAX, FAS* and *PUMA*) with about a 20- or more –fold decrease in gene expression with respect to control samples. Interestingly, in the above-mentioned genes we have found great differences in fold change value between FA and 2-CdA. The expression of two of them, *BAX* and *PUMA,* were considerably decreased when lymphocytes were incubated with FA. It may be hypothesized that the high ratio between anti- and proapoptotic gene expression might account for the failure to achieve complete response after purine nucleoside analogues (PNAs) therapy. Additionally, 2-CdA has inhibited to a lower extent the expression of *PUMA* and *BID* as compared to FA (Franiak-Pietryga I, Korycka-Wolowiec A, unpublished data), which might confirm the results reported by Robak et al., (2009) that 2-CdA, but not FA, is the most effective drug against *P53*-defective cells. At this stage of our knowledge, probably it is too far-fetched to make a suggestion that FA mostly triggers apoptosis in intrinsic pathways to caspase activation, while 2-CdA induces apoptosis via death receptor activation (extrinsic pathway) and by stress-inducing stimuli (intrinsic pathway). To confirm this hypothesis, further experiments are to be conducted in our department. Besides the *in vitro* experiments also *in vivo* studies play an important role in the increase of our knowledge on gene expression profiling.

2.3.2 *In vivo* studies

The study of CLL by Plate et al., (2000) was directed at understanding the signals that maintain viability *in vivo* and are lost when the leukemic cells are removed from the body, such that they immediately begin to undergo apoptosis *ex vivo*. Differences in gene expression between freshly isolated B-CLL cells and those maintained *in vitro* with and without FA were measured using the ATLAS apoptosis cDNA microarray (Clontech, Palo Alto, CA). Many genes, especially *cyclin D1*, were under-expressed after culturing. The anti-apoptotic genes *BAG1* and *AKT2* were over-expressed. The greatest positive effect of FA was the up-regulation of *JNK1*.

Rosenwald et al., (2004) profiled gene expression in CLL leukemic samples obtained before and during FA administration using Lymphochip DNA arrays prepared from 17,856 cDNA clones. The procedure selected 27 microarray elements, 18 of which represented named genes while the other 9 represented novel genes of unknown function. In seven CLL samples, a consistent gene expression (GE) signature of *in vivo* FA exposure was identified. Many of the FA signature genes were known *P53* target genes and genes involved in DNA repair (*P21, MDM2, DDB2, TNFRSF10B, PCNA* and *PPMID*). Because *in vivo* treatment with FA induces a *P53*-dependent GE response, it has the potential to select *P53* mutant CLL cells, which are more drug-resistant and are associated with an aggressive clinical course. Therefore, treatment of CLL patients with FA has the potential to select for outgrowth of *P53* mutant subclones that would be cross-resistant to several other chemotherapeutic agents. Moreover, the gene expression response to γ radiation was highly similar to the response to FA.

The purine metabolism of B-CLL lymphocytes was studied by Marinello et al., (2006). Gene expression analysis was performed on samples obtained from 2 B-CLL patients. Data analysis revealed 17 genes whose expression varied at least 2-fold. Some purine metabolism genes expressed differently from controls were identified. Among the de novo enzymes, the *Gars-Airs-Gart* complex was over-expressed and *IMPDH1* and *APRT* seemed under-expressed. An imbalance in the expression of the adenosine-related protein gene was also observed, with over-expression of *CD26, CD38* and *mtAK3,* while *ADORA 1* and *cAK1* were under-expressed (Table 5). Simultaneous gene profiling of apoptosis-related factors and purine metabolism enzymes is of particular interest for drugs such as FA and 2-CdA, which are commonly used in CLL treatment. Three years later the above-mentioned data was confirmed on samples obtained from 5 B-CLL patients on a chip prepared with 57 genes. To the group of genes described previously some of new ones were added, including apoptosis-related proteins. *CASP6, CASP8* and *BCL2L1* (*BCL-xL*) were under-expressed, whereas *IL-4, IL-18* were over-expressed. In contrast, less significant changes were observed in the expression of some other anti- or proapoptotic factors like *BAX* and *BCL10*, respectively.

To identify novel genes involved in the molecular pathogenesis of CLL, Proto-Siqueira et al., (2008) performed a serial analysis of gene expression (SAGE) in CLL cells and compared it with healthy B cells (nCD19+). A gene ontology analysis revealed that *TOSO,* which plays a functional role upstream of the *FAS* extrinsic apoptosis pathway, was over-expressed in CLL cells. A positive correlation was observed between *TOSO* and *BCL2,* but not between *TOSO* and *FLIP*. The over-expression of *TOSO* and *BCL2* might be responsible for *BAX* inhibition, which leads to the suppression of apoptosis and might be associated with poor prognosis in CLL. It is also known that bortezomib blocks *BAX* degradation in malignant B cells. *TOSO* might therefore be considered a possible target for small molecule therapy in combination with newer pro-apoptotic drugs such as bortezomib and lumiliximab.

Giannopoulos et al., (2009) provided novel biological insights into the molecular effects of thalidomide and suggested the existence of a signature predictive of thalidomide response in CLL. GEP data on day 0 and 7, based on a paired supervised analysis, revealed a thalidomide-induced signature comprising 123 differentially expressed genes. Upon thalidomide monotherapy, an upregulation of genes, known to be involved in mediating thalidomide response, was observed. Such genes as *FAS* and *CDKN1A,* as well as novel candidate genes, such as *STAT1* and *IKZF1* were reported. Gene expression differences in responders as compared to nonresponders after thalidomide monotherapy on day 7 were determined. Responders showed lower expression of gene coding pro-survival cytokine such as *IL-8* and lower level of *TGFB1,* whereas genes involved in apoptosis, i.e. *CASP1,* were more highly expressed than in nonresponders. Higher expression of *ZAP70,* as well as anti-apoptotic genes such as *TRAF1,* and genes involved in angiogenesis, (eg. *ECGF1)* was observed in nonresponders group. Thalidomide responders showed also lower *JUN* and *CASP9* expression levels associated with deregulated insulin and *RAS* signalling pathways. In CLL being induced by *NFKB* activation, *IL-8* may function as an autocrine growth and apoptosis resistance factor promoting cell survival.

Our data depicts changes in apoptotic GEP in CLL patients treated with cladribine, cyclophosphamide and rituximab (CCR). The measurements were conducted by means of 384 TaqMan Low Density Arrays (Applied Biosystems). Data analysis pointed 20 out of 93 examined apoptotic genes, whose expression has significantly changed. Changes in GEP are mostly related to the intrinsic apoptotic pathway. The most significant differences in gene expression before, as opposed to after, treatment are demonstrated by antiapoptotic genes such as *BCL2, BCL2L1, BIRC1, BIRC5* and *BIRC8,* whose expression is considerably decreased. Of the proapoptotic genes, *NOXA, CASP10, ESRRBL1* and *NFKBIZ* are particularly distinguished, because they are significantly overexpressed (Table 4). Additionally, genes specifically clustered in terms of GEP, which was different in particular genes depending *IGHV* mutational status (Franiak-Pietryga et al., 2010).

	Gene expression	**Gene description**	**Response to drugs and other chemical substances**
Genes overexpressed	***BAG1***	BCL2-associated athanogene	Positive effect to FA
	AKT2	Protein kinase Akt-2; promoter of cell survival	Positive effect to FA
	BCL2	B cell lymphoma 2 associated oncogene	Positive effect to TPA
	JNK1	Mitogen-activated protein kinase 8; stress-activated protein kinase; *MAPK8*	Positive effect to FA
	TR3	TR3 orphan receptor; early response protein NAK1	Resistance to FA, C, CHB
	MTMR6	Myotubularin related protein 6	Resistance to FA, C, CHB
	C-MYC	Transcription factor, puf, and kinase	Resistance to FA, C, CHB; Positive effect to VPA
	C-REL	Proto-oncogene c-Rel	Resistance to FA, C, CHB
	C-IAP1	Apoptosis inhibitor 1; *BIRC2*	Resistance to FA, C, CHB
	N-MYC	V-myc myelocytomatosis viral related oncogene	Positive effect to TPA
	JUND	Transcription factor jun-D	Positive effect to TPA
	P21	Cyclin-dependent kinase inhibitor 1A, *CDKN1A*	FA signature genes involved in DNA repair
	MDM2	P53 binding protein homolog	FA signature genes involved in DNA repair
	TNFRSF10B	Tumor necrosis factor receptor superfamily, member 10b, apoptosis inducing protein	FA signature genes involved in DNA repair
	BFL1	BCL2-related protein A1, *BCL2A1*	Resistance to F, Positive effect to VPA
	BAX	BCL2 associated protein, apoptotic death-initiating protein	FA, 2-CdA
	BCL10	CARD-containing apoptotic signaling protein	FA, 2-CdA
	TOSO	Fas apoptotic inhibitory molecule 3; *FAIM3*	Bortezomib, Lumiliximab
	DUSP2	Dual specificity phosphatase 2	Positive effect to TPA, VPA

Genes underexpressed	*FAS*	TNF receptor superfamily, member 6; *TNFRSF6*	Positive effect to Thalidomide Resistance to FA, C, CHB
	CASP6	Caspase 6, enzyme of apoptotic pathway	FA, 2-CdA
	CASP8	Caspase 8, enzyme of apoptotic pathway	FA, 2-CdA
	BAX	BCL2 associated protein, apoptotic death-initiating protein	Bortezomib, Lumiliximab
	BCL-xL	Anti-apoptotic BCL2-like 1; *BCL2L1*	Positive effect to FA
	BCL2	B cell lymphoma 2 associated oncogene	Positive effect to TPA

C - cyclophosphamide, 2-CdA - cladribine, CHB - chlorambucil, FA - fludarabine,
TPA - tetradecanoyl phorbol acetate, VPA - valproic acid

Table 3. Expression of apoptotic genes under the influence of drugs and other chemical substances. (Giannopoulos et al., 2009; Marinello et al., 2006; Morales et al., 2005; Plate et al., 2000; Proto-Siqueira et al., 2008; Rosenwald et al., 2004; Segel et al., 2003; Stamatopoulos et al., 2009; Vallat et al., 2003).

	Gen expression	**Gen description**	**Response to drug**
Proapoptotic genes	***BAD*** ⇑	BCL2-associated agonist of cell death	2-CdA
	TNFRSF21 ⇑	Tumor necrosis factor receptor superfamily, member 21	2-CdA
	DAPK1 ⇑	Death associated protein kinase 1	2-CdA
	CARD6 ⇑	Caspase recruitment domain family member 6	FA
	CARD9 ⇑	Caspase recruitment domain family member 9	FA
	BAK1 ⇓	BCL2-antagonist/killer1; *BAK1*	2-CdA, FA
	BAX ⇓	BCL2-associated X protein, isoform delta	2-CdA, FA
	PUMA ⇓	BCL2 binding component 3; p53 up-regulated modulator of apoptosis; *BBC3*	2-CdA, FA
	FAS ⇓	TNF receptor superfamily, member 6; *TNFRSF6*	2-CdA, FA, CCR
	NOXA ⇑	Phorbol-12-myristate-13-acetate-induced protein 1; *PMAIP1*	CCR
	CASP10 ⇑	Caspase 10, apoptosis-related cysteine peptidase	CCR
	ESRRBL1 ⇑	Intraflagellar transport 57 homolog-IFT57; *HIP1*	CCR
	NFKBIZ ⇑	Nuclear factor of kappa light polypeptide gene enhancer in B-cells inhibitor, zeta; *IKBZ*	CCR
Antiapoptotic genes	***BCL2*** ⇓	B-cell leukemia/lymphoma 2	CCR
	BCL2L1 ⇓	BCL2 like isoform 1	CCR
	BIRC1 ⇓	Baculoviral IAP repeat-containing 1	CCR
	BIRC5 ⇓	Baculoviral IAP repeat-containing 5	CCR
	BIRC8 ⇓	Baculoviral IAP repeat-containing 8	CCR

Gene expression: up ⇑ - and downregulation ⇓

2-CdA - cladribine, CCR - cladribine, cyclophosphamide and rituximab; FA - fludarabine

Table 4. Genes involved in apoptosis (Franiak-Pietryga et al., 2010; Franiak-Pietryga I, Korycka-Wolowiec A, unpublished data)

GEP may have a predictive value for the effectiveness of anti-cancer therapy. Although numerous experiments remain to be performed, it might become possible to predict chemoresistance and to avoid ineffective drugs. The possibility of pretherapeutic discrimination between responders and non-responders will further stimulate the development of an individualised therapeutic strategy using a personalised combination of drugs (Dietel & Sers, 2006). A list of the genes and their response to therapy and drug resistance is presented in Table 5.

	Gene	Description	Response to drugs
Genes overexpressed	***HLA-DQA1***	HLA class II histocompatibility antigen, DQ alpha 1 chain	Resistance to FA, C, CHB
	MAT2A	Methionine adenosyltransferase 2	Resistance to FA, C, CHB
	FMOD	Fibromodulin	Resistance to FA, C, CHB
	EGR1	Early growth response protein 1	Positive effect to TPA
	CD69	Early lymphocyte activation antigen	Positive effect to TPA
	PKC	Protein kinase C	Positive effect to TPA
	DPB2	DNA polymerase epsilon	FA signature genes involved in DNA repair
	PCNA	Proliferating cell nuclear antigen	FA signature genes involved in DNA repair
	ADORA3	Adenosine A3 receptor	FA, 2-CdA
	Gars-Airs-Gar complex	Phosphoribosylglycinamide synthetasephosphoribosylaminoimidazole synthetase-phosphoribosylglycinamide formyltransferase	FA, 2-CdA
	mtAK3	Adenylate kinase 3 (mitochondrial)	FA, 2-CdA
	NMN	Myodenylate deaminase	FA, 2-CdA
	CD26	Adenosine deaminase complexing protein	FA, 2-CdA
	CD38	Cyclic ADP-ribose hydrolase	FA, 2-CdA
	IL-18	Interleukin 18; interferon-gamma-inducing factor	FA, 2-CdA
	IL-4	Interleukin-4; lymphocyte stimulatory factor 1	FA, 2-CdA
	RAD51	DNA repair protein	Resistance to CHB
	BFL1	BCL2-related protein A1, *BCL2A1*	Positive effect to VPA
	C-MYC	Transcription factor, puf, and kinase	Positive effect to VPA
	DUSP2	Serine/threonine specific protein phosphatase	Positive effect to VPA
	PEA15	Homolog of mouse MAT-1 oncogene	Positive effect to VPA

Genes underexpressed	***STAT1***	Signal transducer and activator of transcription 1	Positive effect to Thalidomide Resistance to FA, C, CHB
	BLK	B lymphoid tyrosine kinase	Positive effect to Thalidomide Resistance to FA, C, CHB
	HSP27	Heat shock protein beta-2	Positive effect to Thalidomide Resistance to FA, C, CHB
	ECH1	Enoyl CoA hydratase 1, peroxisomal	Positive effect to Thalidomide Resistance to FA, C, CHB
	P21	CDKN1A, cyclin-dependent kinase inhibitor 1A	Positive effect to Thalidomide Resistance to FA, C, CHB
	APRT	Adenine phosphoribosyltransferase	FA, 2-CdA
	IMPDH1	IMP dehydrogenase 1	FA, 2-CdA
	ADORA1	Adenosine A1 receptor	FA, 2-CdA
	cAK1	Cytosolic adenylate kinase 1	FA, 2-CdA
	GRK6	G-prot-coupled receptor kinase 6	FA, 2-CdA
	CD73	5'-nucleotidase, ecto	Bortezomib, Lumiliximab Positive effect to FA
	CD5	Lymphocyte antigen T1/Leu-1	Positive effect to VPA
	BCL2	B cell lymphoma 2 associated oncogene	Positive effect to VPA
	CD23	FCER2, Fc fragment of IgE, low affinity II, receptor for CD23	Positive effect to VPA
	PIM1	Proto-oncogene serine/threonine-protein kinase PIM-1	Positive effect to VPA

C - cyclophosphamide, 2-CdA - cladribine, CHB - chlorambucil, FA - fludarabine,
TPA - tetradecanoyl phorbol acetate, VPA - valproic acid

Table 5. The influence of GEP on response to therapy or drug resistance (Edelmann et al., 2008; Giannopoulos et al., 2009; Marinello et al., 2006; Plate et al., 2000; Proto-Siqueira et al., 2008; Rosenwald et al., 2004; Segel et al., 2003; Stamatopoulos et al., 2009; Vallat et al., 2003).

3. Genotyping

3.1 Introduction

Owing to a greater availability of the human genome sequence, the focus of research has now been shifted to identifying sequence polymorphisms. It is of utmost importance to understand how biological functions may be affected by these variations and be associated with heritable phenotypes.

A single nucleotide polymorphism (SNP) array is a type of DNA microarray that is used to detect polymorphisms within a population. SNPs are the most frequent type of variation in the genome. It is estimated that about 10 million SNPs have been identified in humans, an average of one SNP every 400–1000 base pairs (Botstein & Risch, 2003). Currently, about 5.6 million have been typed (dbSNP Build ID: 126), about half of which are estimated to have a minor allele frequency over 10% (Kruglyak & Nickerson, 2001). As SNPs are highly conserved throughout evolution and within a population, a map of SNPs serves as an excellent genotypic marker for research. SNPs from the whole genome form a *genetic fingerprint.* Although SNPs are spaced randomly throughout the genome and could therefore lie in coding sequences, only a small fraction has functional significance (i.e. are non-silent), such as those found in the transcribed or regulatory regions of genes (Mohr et al., 2002). SNPs on a small chromosomal segment tend to be transmitted as a block, forming a haplotype. This correlation between alleles at nearby sites is known as linkage disequilibrium (LD) and enables genotypes at a large number of SNP loci to be predicted from known genotypes at a smaller number of representative SNPs, called 'tag SNPs' or 'haplotype tag SNPs' (Gabriel et al., 2002; Dutt & Beroukhim, 2007). This reduction in the complexity of genetic variation among individuals enables an overall genotype to be determined much more efficiently and economically; roughly 500,000 tag SNPs are sufficient to genotype an individual with European ancestry (Dutt & Beroukhim, 2007; Nicolas et al., 2006).

The mechanisms of an SNP array and the DNA microarray are identical; the convergence of DNA hybridization, fluorescence microscopy and solid surface DNA capture. In order to study the genetic vulnerability of a germline to complex diseases, oligonucleotide arrays have been developed to interrogate such large numbers of SNP markers in multiple databases (Dutt & Beroukhim, 2007; Gunderson et al., 2005).

3.2 Genome-wide association studies

CLL and other B-cell lymphoproliferative disorders (LPDs) show clear evidence of familial aggregation, but the inherited basis is still largely unknown. To identify a susceptibility gene for CLL, Sellick et al., (2005) conducted a genome-wide linkage analysis of 115 families, using a high-density SNP array (GeneChip Mapping 10Kv1 Xba, Affymetrix) containing 11,560 markers. Multipoint linkage analyses were undertaken using both nonparametric (model-free) and parametric (model-based) methods. It confirmed that high LD between SNP markers could lead to inflated nonparametric linkage (NLP) and LOD scores (Dawn Tare & Barrett, 2005). After the high-LD SNPs were removed, a maximum NPL of 3.14 ($p<0.0008$) on chromosome (11)(p11) was obtained. The highest multipoint heterogeneity LOD (HLOD) score under both dominant (HLOD 1.95) and recessive (HLOD 2.78) models was yielded by the same genomic position. Moreover, four other chromosomal positions (5)(q22-23), (6)(p22),

(10)(q25) and (14)(q32) displayed HLOD scores >1.15 (p<0.01). None of those regions coincided with areas of common chromosomal abnormalities frequently observed for CLL. These results support an inherited predisposition to CLL and related B-cell LPDs.

Pfeifer at al., (2007) explored high-density 10k and 50k Affymetrix SNP arrays to assess genetic aberrations in the tumour B-cells of patients with CLL. Among the prognostically important aberrations, del(13)(q14) was present in 51%, trisomy 12 (+12) in 13%, del(11)(q22) in 13% and del(17)(p13) in about 6% of cases. A prominent clustering of breakpoints on both sides of the genes *MIRN15A/MIRN16-1* indicated the presence of recombination hot spots in the 13q14 region. Patients with a mono-allelic del(13)(q14) had slower lymphocyte growth kinetics than patients with bi-allelic deletions. In four CLL cases with unmutated *HV* genes, a common minimal 3.5-Mb gain of 2p16 spanning the *REL* and *BCL11A* oncogenes was identified, implicating these genes in the pathogenesis of CLL.

New risk variants for CLL were identified by Crowther-Swanepoel et al., (2010). A genome-wide association (GWA) study of 299,983 tagging SNPs (by means of HumanCNV370-Duo BeadChips, Illumina) was conducted with validation in four additional series totalling 2,503 cases and 5,789 controls. In 2008, the authors reported the results of a GWA study of CLL based on an analysis of 299,983 tagging SNPs in 505 cases and 1, 438 controls and through fast track analysis of SNPs, identified risk loci at 2q13, 2q37.1, 6p25.3, 11q24.1, 15q23 and 19q13.32 (Di Bernardo et al., 2008). The authors identified 4 new risk loci for CLL at 8q24.21 (rs2456449, *TCF4*), 2q37.3 (rs757978, *FARP2*), 15q21.3 (rs7169431, *NEDD4, RFX7*) and 16q24.1 (rs305061, *IRF8*). The evidence for risk was found for two more loci: 15q25.2 (rs783540, *CPEB1*) and 18q21.1 (rs1036935, *CXXC1, MBD1*). *TCF4* binds to an enhancer for *MYC*, providing a mechanistic basis for this 8q24.21 association. It had also been shown that variation in *IRF4* influences CLL risk. There is a possibility that the effect of the other 8q24.21 cancer risk loci is by *MYC*, which is a direct target of *IRF4* in activated B-cells and this observation needs further study.

FARP2 is a gene connected with signalling downstream of G protein-coupled receptors. rs757978 is involved in the substitution of threonine for isoleucine at amino acid 260 (T260I), whereas rs305061 maps within a 30-kb region of LD at 16q24.1 locus and localises 19kb telomeric to *IRF8*, which regulates α and β-interferon response. There is still no evidence for a direct role of *NEDD4* in CLL, but it is a credible candidate gene because it has a role in regulating viral latency and pathogenesis of EBV. Particularly, *NEDD4* regulates EBV-LMP2A, which mimics signalling induced by the B-cell receptor, altering B-cell development. *CPEB1* plays a role in regulating cyclin B1 during embryonic cell division and differentiation. *CXXC1* and *MBD1* are involved in gene regulation. *MBD1* expression in EBV-transformed lymphocytes correlated with risk genotype. Although *MBD1* has no documented role in CLL, it can affect CLL development through translational control of *MYC*. No connection between 17p deletion status and genotype was observed. Although there was evidence that the rs305061 risk genotype was associated with worse overall survival, *IGHV*-mutation status was highly correlated with rs305061, but risk genotype correlating with unmutated-CLL (Crowther-Swanepoel et al., 2010; Di Bernardo et al., 2008).

To identify genetic variants associated with outcome of CLL, Sellick et al., (2008) genotyped 977 non-synonymous SNPs (nsSNPs) in 755 genes relevant to cancer biology in 425 patients participating in a trial comparing the efficacies of FA and CHB ± C in first-line treatment. A total of 78 SNPs (51 dominantly acting and 27 recessively acting) were associated with progression-free survival (PFS), nine of them also affecting overall survival (OS) at the 5% level. These included SNPs mapping to the immunoregulatory genes *IL16* P434S, *IL19* S213F, *LILRA4* P27L, *KLRC4* S29I and *CD5* V471A, as well as the DNA response genes *POLB* P242R and *TOPBP1* S730L, which were all independently prognostic of *IGHV* mutational status. A total of five SNPs associated with PFS were common to patients treated with CHB or FA (*DST* L22S, *LILRA4* P27L, *SEC23B* H489Q, *XRCC2* R188H and *ZAK* S531L); three SNPs were common to patients treated with either CHB or FA with C (*APBB3* C236R, *ENPPS* I171V, and *C21orf57* S2L); and four were common to patients treated with either FA alone or FA with C (*DDX27* G206V, *DPYD* S534N, *WNT16* G72R and *DHX16* D566G). The variants have proved to be invaluable prognostic markers of patient outcome (Table 6).

Gene	Description	Chemotherapy	Response to treatment
DST L22S	Dystonin	CHB or FA	PFS
LILRA4 P27L	Leukocyte immunoglobulin-like receptor, subfamily A (with TM domain), member 4		PFS
SEC23B H489Q	SEC23-related protein B		PFS, OS
XRCC2 R188H	DNA repair protein XRCC2; RAD51-like		PFS
ZAK S531L	MLK-like mitogen-activated protein triple kinase		PFS
APBB3 C236R	Amyloid beta A4 precursor protein-binding family B member 3	CHB or FC	PFS
ENPPS I171V	Ectonucleotide pyrophosphatase/phosphodiesterase 1		PFS
C21orf57 S2L	Chromosome 21 open reading frame 57		PFS
DDX27 G206V	DEAD box protein 27	FA or FC	PFS
DPYD S534N	Dihydropyrimidine dehydrogenase		PFS
WNT16 G72R	Wingless-type MMTV integration site family, member 16		PFS
DHX16 D566G	DEAH (Asp-Glu-Ala-His) box polypeptide 16		PFS

FA – fludarabine, FC – fludarabine with cyclophosphamide, CHB – chlorambucil;
PFS – progression-free survival, OS – overall survival

Table 6. Relationship between SNPs and drug response (Sellic et al., 2008)

3.3 Copy number variation analyses

Gunnarsson et al., (2008) compared platform dynamics, an in-depth analysis of copy-number alterations (CNAs) using four high-resolution microarray platforms: BAC arrays (32K), oligonucleotide arrays (185K, Agilent) and two SNP arrays (250K, Affymetrix and 317K, Illumina). Ten CLL samples were analysed. The evaluation of baseline variation and copy-number ratio response showed that the Agilent platform performed best and confirmed the robustness of BAC arrays. These platforms demonstrated more platform-specific CNAs. The SNP arrays showed more technical diversity, although the high density of elements compensated for this. Affymetrix detected more CNAs than Illumina, but the latter showed a lower noise level and a higher detection rate in the LOH analysis. Application of high-resolution microarrays will enhance the possibility of detecting new recurrent microevents in CLL leading to identification of new important subgroups, refining the prognostic hierarchy established by FISH. The whole-genome screening with SNP arrays (Affymetrix GeneChip Mapping 250K Nsp1) was conducted and a high frequency of known recurrent alterations in 203 newly diagnosed CLL patients was revealed (Gunnarsson et al., 2010). Moreover, the genome-wide analysis allowed detection of a novel combination of gain of 2p and del(11q), and additional large and small CNAs, which are important for the evaluation of overall complexity in CLL patients. The authors identified genomic complexity as a poor prognostic marker in the survival analysis. However, they noted that this characteristic was strongly linked to established poor-risk molecular markers. The small alterations were mostly non-overlapping. It seems unlikely that there are unknown recurrent CNAs > 200 kbp involved in the CLL pathophysiology detectable in this setting (Gunnarsson et al., 2010). Similar results have been presented by Kujawski et al., (2008), who reported a correlation between genomic complexity and a significantly shorter time to first and second treatment and presented the number of CNAs as an independent prognosis factor.

The discovery of microRNA and its biological functions is a significant step towards the understanding of the molecular bases of human physiology and pathology. MicroRNAs constitute a class of short, non-coding RNA molecules involved in the regulation of a number of important biological process including cell proliferation, differentiation and apoptosis by down-regulation of gene expression during the translation phase. On the basis of these findings, CLL is a genetic disease in which the main alterations occur in microRNAs (miRNAs). Down-regulation of *MIR15A* and *MIR16* as a part of del(13)(q14) has been suggested as good prognostic factors. Both miRNAs negatively regulate *BCL2* at a post-transcriptional level. In CLL cases with unmutated *IGHV* or high level of expression *ZAP70* the overexpression of *TCL1* was observed. This is due to low-level expression of *MIR29* and *MIR181*, which directly targets this oncogene. The overexpression of *TCL1* is correlated with del(11)(q22) and with the aggressive CLL. These miRNAs might be used to target *BCL2* or *TCL1* for therapy of the disease (Calin et al., 2007; Cimmino et al., 2005).

Ouillette et al., (2008) analysed 171 CLL cases for LOH and subchromosomal copy loss on chromosome 13 in DNA from FACS-sorted $CD19^+$ cells by means of the Affymetrix *Xba*I 50k SNP array platform. Detailed analysis suggests the existence of distinct subtypes. Categorisation is based on del(13)(q14) lesions with Rb loss as type II [40% of del(13)(q14) cases] and consequently without such a loss as type I [60% of del(13)(q14) cases]. Rb is a decisive regulator of cell cycle progression and genomic stability. The loss of one or two alleles could differentially affect the biology of CLL cases Hernando et al., 2004. In the type I 198 genes were analysed. In this group reduced expression of *FLJ11712, KCNRG, RFP2, RFP2OS* and *DLEU1* was identified. Many other genes have emerged as candidate differentially expressed genes by means of qPCR: *LATS2, DFNA5, PHLPP, LPIN1, SERPINE2, ARHGAP20, CYTB5, SLA2,* and *AQP3. LATS2* RNA levels were lower in CLL cases with del(13)(q14) type I as opposed to type II cases or all other CLL cases without del(13)(q14). *LATS2* is involved in cell cycle progression control. It is possible that Rb and *LATS2* may be regulators [in non-del(13)(q14) cases] in different processes of CLL subsets (Ouillette et al., 2008). Further subdivision of del(13)(q14) type I cases into type Ia and type Ib is suggested by the occurrence of deletions that appear of relatively uniform length [del(13)(q14) type Ia] and that displays centromeric breaks within the vicinity of the *MIR15A/MIR16* cluster. Bi-allelic del(13)(q14) type Ia lesions were associated with significant reductions in *MIR15A/MIR16* expression levels. As opposed to Calin et al. (2007), this observation reveals that *BCL2* levels were not correlated with *MIR15A/MIR16* levels. In important recent discovery is that about 50% of all CLL cases with del(13)(q14) do not express the *PHLPP* gene. *PHLPP* dephosphorylates activated *AKT* and low or absent *PHLPP* expression may allow for sustained *AKT* signalling after proper cell surface stimuli (Ouilette et al., 2008).

Multiple, discrete, genomic alterations in the 13q region, including *MIR15A/MIR16, Rb* and others were also observed by Grubor et al., (2009). It might suggest greater complexity of lesions in the 13q region than already known. Moreover, they focused on intraclonal heterogeneity within CLL patients and they searched for genomic differences between CD38$^+$ and CD38$^-$ populations in the same patient. The study was conducted by means of a high-resolution CGH technique called representational oligonucleotide microarray analysis (ROMA). This method is very sensitive to examining the clonal heterogeneity of CLL within the same patient from mixed subpopulations. Copy number differences, in separated CD38$^+$ and CD38$^-$ fractions, were detected in 3 of 4 samples at various loci throughout the genome, some of clinical relevance (ie. *ATM* and *TP53*). With the exception of the del(6)(q21), reported major cytogenetic imbalances have been observed previously. The majority of lesions (315/419) were deletions and not amplifications, which is typical of CLL. Two novel regions were observed: del(8)(p21.2-p12) and del(2)(q37.1), including genes *TRIM35* and *SP100/110/140*, respectively. The apparent on-going evolution of CLL clones in a patient may improve the understanding of the disease and the ability to identify patients at risk. The above-demonstrated capabilities offer opportunities for patient treatment individualisation and the identification of new therapeutic agents.

Lehmann et al., (2008) performed molecular allelokaryotyping on 56 samples of early stage CLL using the 50k XbaI GeneChip from Affymetrix (50,000 SNP probes). Excluding the four common abnormalities [+12, del(17)(p13), del(11)(q22) and del(13)(q14)], SNP-chip analysis identified a total of 45 copy number changes in 25 CLL samples (45%). Four samples had del(6)(q21) that involved *AIM1*. UPD was detected in four samples, two of them involved the whole of chromosome 13, resulting in homozygous deletion of *MIR15A/MIR16-1*. The data suggests that genetic abnormalities including gain, loss and UPD of genetic materials frequently occur at an early stage of CLL. In addition to well-documented common genetic abnormalities, deletions of 5q, 6q and Xp were observed to be frequent in early-stage CLL. *AIM1* was examined as a target of this deletion. In the study, expression levels of *ZAP70* and the mutational status of *IGHV* were analysed. It was demonstrated for the first time that *ZAP70* expression was correlated with del(11)(q22) in early-stage CLL. It was also observed that non-hypermutation of *IGHV* was correlated with +12, del(11)(q22) and del(13)(q14) in early-stage CLL.

4. Conclusion

Microarray technology provides comprehensive data on the expression patterns of thousands of genes in parallel, which positions this method in the centre of optimisation of diagnosis and the classification of leukemias. GEP may lead to the detection of new biologically defined and clinically relevant subtypes of chronic lymphocytic leukemia as a basis for specific therapeutic decision. If such testing is to be used as a routine method for diagnostic purposes in parallel with current standard methods, it is crucial to include GEP in future routine diagnostic applications and in clinical trials. With promising initial results, genome-wide association studies using SNPs are becoming increasingly well established as tools for discovering disease genes. SNP array is an important application in determining disease susceptibility, and consequently in pharmacogenomics, by measuring the specific effectiveness of a form of drug therapy for the patient. As each individual has many SNPs that together create a unique DNA sequence. SNPs may be performed to map disease loci, and hence determine individual-specific disease susceptibility genes. As a result, drugs can be personally designed to act efficiently on a group of individuals who share a common allele, or even a single individual.

5. Acknowledgements

This work was supported by grant No. PBZ/MNiSW/07/2006/28 from the Ministry of Science and Higher Education, Poland to I. F-P and partially by statutory means No. 503/3-015-02/503-01 of the Department of Pharmaceutical Biochemistry, Medical University of Lodz, Poland.

6. References

Alizadeh, A.A.; Eisen, M.; Davis, R.E.; et al. (2000). The lymphochip: a specialized cDNA microarray for the genomic-scale analysis of gene expression in normal and malignant lymphocytes. Proceedings of Cold Spring Harbor Symposia on Quantitative Biology; n.d.

Alizadeh, A.A. & Staudt, L.M. (2000). Genomic-scale gene expression profiling of normal and malignant immune cells. *Current Opinion in Immunology*, Vol.12, No.2, (April 2000), pp. 219-225, ISSN 0952-7915

Botstein, D. & Risch, N. (2003). Discovering genotypes underlying human phenotypes: past successes for mendelian disease, future approaches for complex disease. *Nature Genetics*, Vol.33, Suppl, (March 2003), pp. 228-237, ISSN 1061-4036

Caligaris-Cappio, F. & Hamblin, T.J. (1999). B-cell chronic lymphocytic leukemia: a bird of a different feather. *Journal of Clinical Oncology*, Vol.17, No.1, (Junuary 1999), pp. 399-408, ISSN 0732-183X

Calin, G.A.; Pekarsky, Y. & Croce, C.M. (2007). The role of microRNA and other non-coding RNA in the pathogenesis of chronic lymphocytic leukemia. *Best Practice & Research. Clinical Haematology*, Vol.20, No.3, (September 2007), pp. 425-437, ISSN 1521-6926

Christodoulopoulos, G.; Malapetsa, A.; Schipper, H.; Golub; E.; Radding, C. & Panasci L.C. (1999). Chlorambucil induction of HsRad51 in B-cell chronic lymphocytic leukemia. *Clinical Cancer Research*, Vol.5, No.8, (August 1999), pp. 2178-2184, ISSN 1076-0432

Cimmino, A.; Calin, G.A.; Fabbri, M; et al. (2005). Mir-15 and mir-16 induce apoptosis by targeting BCL2. *Proceedings of the National Academy of Sciences of the United States of America*, Vol.102, No.39, (September 2005), pp. 13944-13949, ISSN 0027-8424

Crowther-Swanepoel, D.; Broderick, P.; Chiara Di Bernardo, M.; et al. (2010). Common variants at 2q37.3, 8q24.21, 15q21.3 and 16q24.1 influence chronic lymphocytic leukemia risk. *Nature Genetics*, Vol.42, No.2, (January 2010), pp. 132-136, ISSN 1061-4036

Damle, R.N.; Wasil, T.; Fais, F.; et al. (1999). Ig V gene mutation status and CD38 expression as novel prognostic indicators in chronic lymphocytic leukemia. *Blood*, Vol.94, No.6, (September 1999), pp.1840-1847, ISSN 0006-4971

Dawn Tearre, M. & Barrett, J.H. (2005). Genetic linkage studies. *Lancet*, Vol.366, No.9490, (September 2005), pp. 1036-1044, ISSN 0140-6736

Di Bernardo, M.C.; Crowther-Swanepoel, D.; Broderick; P.; et al. (2008). A genome-wide association study identifies six susceptibility loci for chronic lymphocytic leukemia. *Nature Genetics*, Vol.40, No.10, (August 2008), pp. 1204-1210, ISSN 1061-4036

Dietel, M. & Sers, C. (2006). Personalized medicine and development of targeted therapies: the upcoming challenge for diagnostic molecular pathology. A review. *Virchows Archiv: An International Journal of Pathology*, Vol.448, No.6, (April 2006), pp. 744-755, ISSN 0945-6317

Döhner, H.; Stilgenbauer, S.; Benner, A.; et al. (2000). Genomic aberrations and survival in chronic lymphocytic leukemia. *New England Journal of Medicine*, Vol.343, No.26, (December 2000), pp. 1910-1916, ISSN 0028-4793

Dutt, A. & Beroukhim, R. (2007). Single nucleotide polymorphism array analysis of cancer. *Current Opinion in Oncology*, Vol.19, No.1, (January 2007), pp. 43-49, ISSN 1040-8746

Edelmann, J.; Klein-Hitpass, L.; Carpinteiro, A.; et al. (2008). Bone marrow fibroblasts induce expression of PI3K/NF-κB pathway genes and a pro-angiogenic phenotype in CLL cells. *Leukemia Research*, Vol.32, No.10, (April 2008), pp. 1565-1572, ISSN 0145-2126

Fält, S.; Merup, M.; Gahrton, G.; Lambert, B.; Wennborg, A. (2005). Identification of progression markers in B-CLL by gene expression profiling. *Experimental Hematology*, Vol.33, No.8, (August 2005), pp. 883-893, ISSN 0301-472X

Fernandez, V.; Jares, P.; Salaverria, I.; et al. (2008). Gene expression profile and genomic changes in disease progression of early-stage chronic lymphocytic leukemia. *Haematologica*, Vol.93, No.1, (January 2008), pp. 132-136, ISSN 0390-6078

Ferrer, A.; Ollila, J.; Tobin, G.; et al. (2004). Different gene expression in the immunoglobulin-mutated and immunoglobulin-unmutated forms of chronic lymphocytic leukemia. *Cancer Genetics and Cytogenetics*, Vol.153, No.1, (August 2004), pp. 69-72, ISSN 0165-4608

Franiak-Pietryga, I.; Sałagacka, A.; Maciejewski, H.; et al. (2010). Changes in apoptotic gene expression profile in CLL patients treated with cladribine, cyclophosphamide and rituximab (CCR), *Proceedings of the ASH 2010 52nd Annual Meeting and Exposition*, pp1025-1026, ISSN 0006-4971, Orlando, Florida, USA, December 4-7, 2010

Gabriel, S.B.; Schaffner, S.F.; Nguyen, H.; et al. (2002). The structure of haplotype blocks in the human genome. *Science*, Vol.296, No.5576, (May 2002), pp. 2225-2229, ISSN 0036-8075

Giannopoulos, K.; Dmoszynska, A.; Kowal, M.; et al. (2009). Thalidomide exerts distinct molecular antileukemic effects and combined thalidomide/fludarabine therapy is clinically effective in high-risk chronic lymphocytic leukemia. *Leukemia*, Vol.23, No.10, (May 2009), pp. 1771-1778, ISSN 0887-6924

Grubor, V.; Krasnitz, A.; Troge, J.E.; Meth, J.L.; et al. (2009). Novel genomic alterations and clonal evolution in chronic lymphocytic leukemia revealed by representational oligonucleotide microarray analysis (ROMA). *Blood*, Vol.113, No.6, (October 2008), pp. 1294-1303, ISSN 0666-4971

Gunderson, K.L.; Steemers, F.J.; Lee, G.; Mendoza, L.G. & Chee, M.S. (2005). A genome-wide scalable SNP genotyping assay using microarray technology. *Nature Genetics*, Vol.37, No.5, (April 2005), pp. 549-554, ISSN 1061-4036

Gunnarsson, R.; Isaksson, A.; Mansouri, M.; et al. (2010). Large but not small copy-number alterations correlate to high-risk genomic aberrations and survival in chronic lymphocytic leukemia: a high-resolution genomic screening of newly diagnosed patients. *Leukemia*, Vol.24, No.1, (September 2009), pp. 211-215, ISSN 0887-6924

Gunnarsson, R.; Staaf, J.; Jansson, M.; et al. (2008). Screening for copy-number alterations anl loss of heterozygosity in chronic lymphocytic leukemia - A comparative study of four differently designed, high resolution microarray platforms. *Genes, Chromosomes & Cancer*, Vol.47, No.8, (August 2008), pp. 697-711, ISSN 1045-2257

Hamblin, T.J.; Davis, Z.; Gardiner, A.; Oscier, D.G. & Stevenson, F.K. (1999). Unmutated IgV(H) genes are associated with a more aggressive form of chronic lymphocytic leukemia. *Blood*, Vol.94, No.6, (September 1999), pp. 1848-1854, ISSN 0006-4971

Hernando, E.; Nahle, Z.; Juan, G.; et al. (2004). Rb inactivation promotes genomic instability by uncoupling cell cycle progression from mitotic control. *Nature*, Vol.430, No.7001, (August 2004), pp. 797-802, ISSN 0028-0836

Klein, U.; Tu, Y.; Stolovitzky, G.A.; et al. (2001). Gene expression profiling of B cell chronic lymphocytic leukemia reveals a homogeneous phenotype related to memory B cells. *The Journal of Experimental Medicine*, Vol.194, No.11, (December 2001), pp. 1625-1638, ISSN 0022-1007

Klein, U. & Dalla-Favera, R. (2010). New insights into the pathogenesis of chronic lymphocytic leukemia. *Seminars in Cancer Biology*, Vol.20, No.6, (December 2010), pp. 377-383, ISSN 1044-579X

Krober, A.; Seiler, T.; Benner, A.; et al. (2002). V(H) mutation status, CD 38 expression level, genomic aberrations, and survival in chronic lymphocytic leukemia. *Blood*, Vol.100, No.4, (August 2002), pp. 1410-1416, ISSN 0006-4971

Kruglyak, L. & Nickerson, D.A. (2001). Variation is the spice of life. *Nature Genetics*, Vol.27, No.3, (March 2001), pp. 234-236, ISSN 1061-4036

Kujawski, L.; Ouillette, P.; Erba, H.; et al. (2008). Genomic complexity identifies patients with aggressive chronic lymphocytic leukemia. *Blood*, Vol.112, No.5, (April 2008), pp. 1993-2003, ISSN 0006-4971

Lehmann, S.; Ogawa, S.; Raynaud, S.D.; et al. (2008). Molecular allelokaryotyping of early stage, untreated chronic lymphocytic leukemia. *Cancer*, Vol.112, No.6, (March 2008), pp. 1296-1305, ISSN 0008-543X

Marinello, E.; Carlucci, F.; Rosi, F.; Floccari, F.; Raspadori, D. & Tabucchi, A. (2006). Purine metabolism in B-cell lymphocytic leukemia: a microarray approach. *Nucleosides, Nucleotides, and Nucleic Acids*, Vol.25, No.9-11, (n.d.), pp. 1277-1281, ISSN 1525-7770

Mohr, S.; Leikauf, G.D.; Keith, G. & Rihn, B.H. (2002). Microarrays as cancer keys: an array of possibilities. *Journal of Clinical Oncology*, Vol.20, No.14, (July 2002), pp. 3165-3175, ISSN 0732-183X

Morales, A.A.; Olsson, A.; Celsing, F.; Österborg, A.; Jondal, M. & Osorio, L.M. (2005). High expression of bfl-1 contributes to the apoptosis resistant phenotype in B-cell chronic lymphocytic leukemia. *International Journal of Cancer*, Vol.113, No.5, (February 2005), pp. 730-737, ISSN 0020-7136

Munk Pedersen, I. & Reed, J. (2004). Microenvironmental interactions and survival of CLL B-cells. *Leukemia &Lymphoma*, Vol.45, No.12, (December 2004), pp. 2365-2372, ISSN 1042-8194

Nicolas, P.; Sun, F. & Li, L.M. (2006). A model-based approach to selection of tag SNPs. *BMC Bioinformatics*, Vol.7, (June 2006), p. 303, ISSN 1471-2105

Orchard, J.A.; Ibbotson, R.E.; Davis, Z.; et al. (2004). ZAP-70 expression and prognosis in chronic lymphocytic leukaemia. *Lancet*, Vol.363, No.9403, (January 2004), pp. 105-111, ISSN 0140-6736

Ouilette, P.; Erba, H.; Kujawski, L.; Kaminski, M.; Shedden, K. & Malek, S.N. (2008). Integrated genomic profiling of chronic lymphocytic leukemia identifies subtypes of deletion 13q14. *Cancer Research*, Vol.68, No.4, (February 2008), pp. 1012-1021, ISSN 0008-5472

Pfeifer, D.; Pantic, M.; Skatulla, I.; et al. (2007). Genome-wide analysis of DNA copy number changes and LOH in CLL using high-density SNP arrays. *Blood*, Vol.109, No.3, (October 2006), pp. 1202-1210, ISSN 0006-4971

Plate, J.; Petersen, K.S.; Buckingham, L.; Shahidi, H. & Schofield, C.M. (2000). Gene expression in chronic lymphocytic leukemia B cells and changes during induction of apoptosis. *Experimental Hematology*, Vol.28, No.11, (November 2000), pp. 1214-1224, ISSN 0301-472X

Proto-Siqueira, R.; Panepucci, R.; Careta, F.P.; et al. (2008). SAGE analysis demonstrates increased expression of TOSO contributing to Fas-mediated resistance in CLL. *Blood*, Vol.112, No.2, (April 2008), pp. 394-397, ISSN 0006-4971

Reya, T.; O'Riordan, M.; Okamura, R.; et al. (2000). Wnt signaling regulates B lymphocyte proliferation through a LEF-1 dependent mechanism. *Immunity*, Vol.13, No.1, (n.d.), pp. 15-24, ISSN 1074-7613

Robak, T.; Blonski, J.Z.; Wawrzyniak, E.; et al. (2009). Activity of cladribine combined with cyclophosphamide in frontline therapy for chronic lymphocytic leukemia with 17p13.1/*TP53* deletion. *Cancer*, Vol.115, No.1, (January 2009), pp. 94-100, ISSN 0008-543X

Rosenwald, A.; Alizadeh, A.A.; Widhopf, G.; et al. (2001). Relation of gene expression phenotype to immunoglobulin mutation genotype in B cell chronic lymphocytic leukemia. *The Journal of Experimental Medicine*, Vol.194, No.11, (December 2001), pp. 1639-1647, ISSN 0022-1007

Rosenwald, A.; Chuang, E.Y.; Davis, R.E.; et al. (2004). Fludarabine treatment of patients with chronic lymphocytic leukemia induces a p53-dependent gene expression response. *Blood*, Vol.104, No.5, (May 2004), pp. 1428-1434, ISSN 0006-4971

Schena, M.; Shalon, D.; Davis, R.W. & Brown, P.O. (1995). Quantitative monitoring of gene expression patterns with a complementary DNA microarray. *Science*, Vol.270, No.5235, (October 1995), pp. 467-470, ISSN 0036-8075

Schroeder, H.W. Jr & Dighiero, G. (1994). The pathogenesis of chronic lymphocytic leukemia: analysis of the antibody repertoire. *Immunology Today*, Vol.15, No.6, (Juni 1994), pp. 228-294, ISSN 0167-5699

Segel, G.B.; Woodlock, T.J.; Xu, J.; et al. (2003). Early gene activation in chronic leukemic B-lymphocytes induced toward a plasma cell phenotype. *Blood Cells, Molecules & Diseases*, Vol.30, No.3, (May-June 2003), pp. 277-287, ISSN 1079-9796

Sellic, G.S.; Wade, R.; Richards, S.; Oscier, D.G.; Catovsky, D. & Houlston, R.S. (2008). Scan of 977 nonsynonymous SNPs in CLL4 trial patients for the identification of genetic variants influencing prognosis. *Blood*, Vol.111, No.3, (November 2007), pp. 1625-1633, ISSN 0006-4971

Sellick, G.S.; Webb, E.L.; Allinson, R.; et al. (2005). A high-density SNP genomwide linkage scan for chronic lymphocytic leukemia-susceptibility loci. *American Journal of Human Genetics*, Vol.77, No.3, (August 2005), pp. 420-429, ISSN 0002-9297

Stamatopoulos, B.; Meuleman, N.; De Bruyn, C.; Mineur, P.; Martiat, P.; Bron, D. & Lagneaux, L. (2009). Antileukemic activity of valproic acid in chronic lymphocytic leukemia B cells defined by microarray analysis. *Leukemia*, Vol.23, No.12, (August 2009), pp. 2281-2289, ISSN 0887-6924

Stratowa, C.; Löffler, G.; Lichter, P.; et al. (2001). cDNA microarray gene expression analysis of B-cell chronic lymphocytic leukemia proposes potential new prognostic markers involved in lymphocyte trafficking. *International Journal of Cancer*, Vol.91, No.4, (February 2001), pp. 474-480, ISSN 0020-7136

Vallat, L.; Magdelenat, H.; Merle-Beral, H.; et al. (2003). The resistance of B-CLL cells to DNA damage-induced apoptosis defined by DNA microarrays. *Blood*, Vol.101, No.11, (February 2003), pp. 4598-4606, ISSN 0006-4971

Wang, J.; Coombes, K.R.; Highsmith, W.E.; Keating, M.J. & Abruzzo, L.V. (2004). Differences in gene expression between B-cell chronic lymphocytic leukemia and normal B cells: a meta-analysis of three microarray studies. *Bioinformatics*, Vol.20, No.17, (July 2004), pp. 3166-3178, ISSN 1367-4803

Zent, C.S.; Zhan, F.; Schichman, S.A.; et al. (2003). The distinct gene expression profiles of chronic lymphocytic leukemia and multiple myeloma suggest different anti-apoptotic mechanisms but predict only some differences in phenotype. *Leukemia Research*, Vol.27, No.9, (September 2003), pp. 765-774, ISSN 0145-2126

6

Contribution of microRNAs to CLL Biology and Their Potential as New Biomarkers

Maria Rosa Garcia-Silva[1], Maria Catalina Güida[1] and Alfonso Cayota[1,2]
[1]*Institut Pasteur de Montevideo,*
[2]*Faculty of Medicine, Montevideo,*
Uruguay

1. Introduction

After the complete description of the human genome (approximately $3x10^9$ bases) the best estimates of protein-coding genes account for about 30,000 to 40,000 genes representing approximately 1% of the genome. A significantly remainder fraction of the genome is transcribed into RNAs that do not code for proteins which are classified as non-coding RNAs (ncRNAs) (Wright et al., 2001). These ncRNAs were unnoticed in the genome until recent improvements in high-throughput technology for gene expression assays led to the discovery that most human transcriptional units are ncRNAs. These ncRNAs have been segregated into two main classes; long and small non-coding RNAs. Over the last almost two decades, the family of small ncRNAs (i.e. microRNAs, siRNAs and piRNAs) has grown in number and relevance and emerged as new key regulators of gene expression. These small ncRNAs, which are ~19–32 nucleotides (nt) in length, act as sequence-specific triggers for mRNA degradation, translation repression, heterochromatin formation and genome stability affecting biological functions either by posttranscriptional silencing or stimulating transcript degradation. The most well known small ncRNAs are the microRNAs (miRNAs). To date, more than 1500 human miRNAs genes have been annotated. They are organized as mono- or policystronic transcriptional units in the genome located either in intergenic regions or within introns and exons of non-coding as well as coding transcription units (miRBase, release 18: November 2011).

1.1 Biogenesis and function of microRNAs

The defining features of these small silencing RNAs are, in addition to their short size, their association with members of the Argonaute family of proteins, which guide them to their regulatory targets. Biogenesis and effector functions of miRNAs require several complex steps (Figure 1). Most miRNAs are transcribed by the RNA Polymerase II as long primary transcripts (pri-miRNAs) with a 5′m7G cap and a 3′ poly-A tail. In humans, they are subsequently cleaved in the nucleus by an RNase III endonuclease, Drosha, assisted by a dsRNA-binding protein (DGCR8) to produce a stem-loop precursor of ≈ 70 nt in length (pre-miRNA). Pre-miRNAs are translocated to the cytoplasm by the Exportin-5/Ran complex and further processed by the cytoplasmic RNase III, Dicer, yielding ≈ 22-nt duplexes. Several dsRNA-binding accessory proteins assist human Dicer enabling both RNA unwinding and loading onto effector complexes containing members of the Argonaute family of proteins as key components (Chu & Rana, 2007). This complex (miRNA-induced silencing complex or miRISC) is loaded with the mature miRNA while the complementary "passenger" strand is degraded.

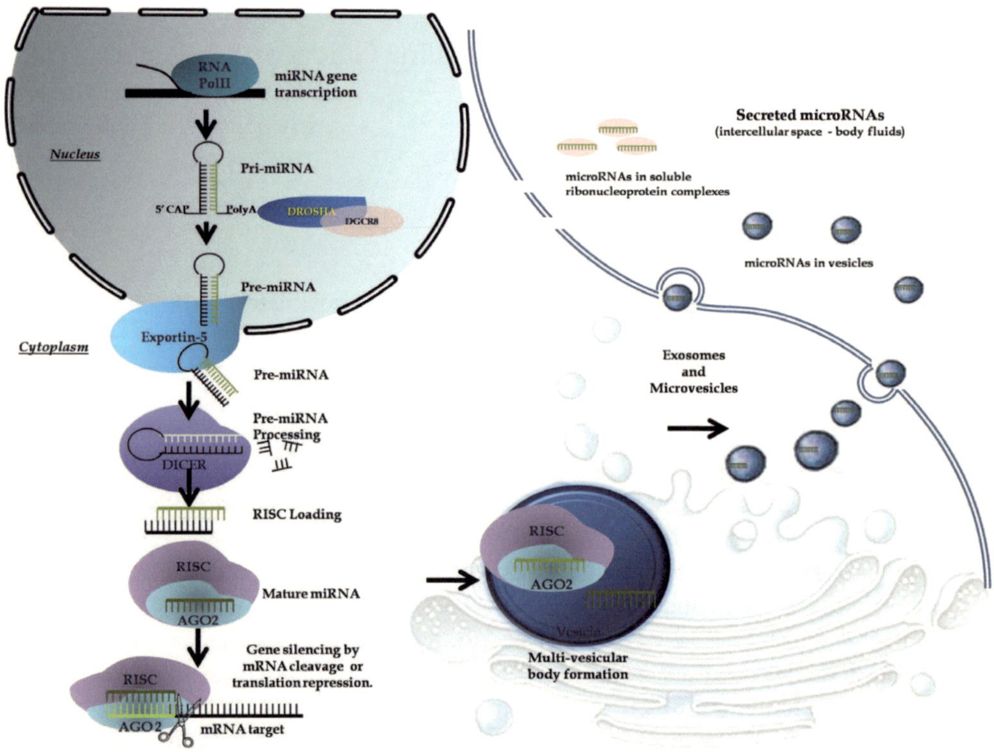

Fig. 1. miRNA biogenesis and effector pathways.

MicroRNAs are initially transcribed by RNA polymerase II as a primary (pri)-miRNA in the nucleus. Binding of the pri-miRNA to DGCR8 and Drosha results in the processing of the pri-miRNA to a 70 nt precursor miRNA (pre-miRNA). This complex is then transported to the cytoplasm by a complex consisting mainly of exportin-5. In the cytoplasm, a pre-miRNA processing complex containing a RNase III endonuclease (Dicer) at its core is formed cleaving the pre-miRNA to a double stranded of ≈22 nt miRNA molecule. The miRNA is then separated into two single-stranded molecules; the antisense strand is incorporated in the RNA-induced silencing complex (RISC) through its interaction with Argonaute (AGO) proteins while the other strand is degraded. The mature miRNA is then transported to either the 3′ or 5′ untranslated region of the target mRNA (UTR) for mRNA degradation of inhibition of translation. As a parallel pathway, the loaded RISC is linked to the Multi-vesicular bodies (MVB) and could be secreted to the extracellular medium an endocytosed by other cells. A significant fraction of miRNAs are secreted as ribonucleoprotein complexes.

This loaded complex is the effector responsible for the gene silencing of the mRNA target. Post-transcriptional gene silencing mediated by miRNAs involves their binding by partial or full complementarity to specific regions or binding sites on untranslated regions (UTRs) of target mRNAs. The commonly accepted mechanism of miRNA targeting in animals involves an interaction between the 5'-end of the miRNA called the "seed region" (about 7 nts) and the 3' untranslated region (3'-UTR) of the mRNA. This binding induces either translation inhibition or cleavage of target mRNAs.

1.2 Expression patterns of microRNAs

Numerous miRNAs exhibit characteristic expression patterns that could serve as a fingerprint of a particular tissue, cell type, biological state, etc. Some miRNAs are differentially expressed in developmental stages, like the first family members, lin-4 and let-7 in *C. elegans*. For this reason, they were called at the beginnings stRNA (small temporal RNA) because they are expressed in specific temporal phases of development and regulate the correct developmental timing. In mammalian cells, a miRNA expression pattern can usually be related to its possible role. Analogous to mRNA expression, miRNA expression is determined by intrinsic cellular factors as well as diverse environmental variables. The study and characterization of miRNAs was delayed several years due to their small size. However, the recent development of small RNA-adapted cloning, hybridization technologies and sequencing protocols allowed the use of high-throughput sequencing, microarrays and real time PCRs to characterize small RNAs in various genomics studies. Taken as a whole these technical improvements are expected to greatly extend the collection of miRNAs in a variety of biological systems.

1.3 MicroRNAs as key regulators of gene expression

It has become clear that miRNAs confer a novel layer of post-transcriptional regulation through fine-tuning gene expression, which is widely used in plants and animals. They are estimated to comprise 1%-5% of animal genes making them one of the most abundant classes of gene expression regulators. An increasing body of experimental data and bioinformatics prediction of miRNA targets revealed that miRNAs are expected to regulate more than 30% of protein coding genes (Croce, 2009). Most genes involved in basic processes common to all cells are under selective pressure to avoid miRNA-mediated regulation ("antitargets"). In contrast, many genes involved in developmental processes, cell proliferation, apoptosis, metabolism, cell differentiation, and morphogenesis ("targets") are enriched in miRNA binding sites by changes in 3′ UTR (and more recent discovered also in 5′ UTR) length and density during evolution (Farazi et al., 2011). These data induced many authors to speculate about a putative role of miRNAs in cancer and other human pathologies.

1.4 MicroRNAs as new actors in cancer biology

Nowadays, it is widely accepted that miRNAs could promote or suppress malignant processes in a similar manner to classical oncogenes and tumor suppressors. In the first case, miRNAs targeting mRNAs encoding for proteins that promote tumor initiation and progression are classified as tumor suppressor miRNAs. Thus, the loss of function of a tumor suppressor miRNA by genomic deletion, mutation, epigenetic silencing, and/or miRNA processing alterations ultimately leads to an inappropriate increase in levels of the respective mRNA target, which in turns initiate or contribute to the malignant transformation. On the other hand miRNAs are classified as oncogenes when their target mRNAs code for tumor suppressor proteins. Overexpression or amplification of these miRNAs is followed by down-modulation of the target tumor suppressor protein, which ultimately initiates or contributes to the malignant transformation (Rovira et al., 2010).

The levels of miRNAs usually are precisely controlled in the cells to guarantee a correct cell life cycle, function and differentiation. It was commonly observed that aberrant expression of miRNAs was associated to malignant transformation. The first description of a miRNA associated to cancer was reported in CLL by Calin et al (Calin et al., 2002). It is known that the most frequent chromosomal alteration, identified in more than 50% of patients suffering from B-cell Chronic Lymphocytic Leukemia, is a deletion of chromosome 13q14 that associated with longer survival. Deletions at 11q and 17p are also typical, although much less frequent, and correlate with up-regulation of the zeta-chain–associated protein kinase 70kDa (ZAP70) and a shorter overall survival. These findings led to extensive efforts to define a putative tumor suppressor gene or genes at the 13q14 locus. No plausible protein-encoding candidate was identified into this region. A perceptive change in the strategy for possible regulatory elements along this region unearthed the existence of two novel miRNAs; miR-15a and miR-16-1 (Calin et al., 2002). This was the first indication that miRNAs could function as tumor suppressors showing frequent deletions or down-modulation of miR-15a/16-1 in patients suffering from CLL, and the first link between miRNAs and cancer. A second report from this lab showed that about 50 % of annotated human miRNAs are located in "fragile sites" of the genome frequently associated with cancer (Calin et al., 2004b). Further studies found that these related miRNAs have as target the mRNA encoding the antiapoptotic protein B-cell CLL/lymphoma 2 (BCL2), the up-regulation of which is critical for CLL cell survival (Cimmino et al., 2005). Importantly, the direct interaction of *miR-15*/*miR-16* with *BCL2* transcripts delayed protein translation, induced apoptosis, and reinforced the role of miRNAs as part of a new class of tumor suppressor genes.

2. MicroRNAs reported in the initiation and progresion of CLL

The implication of miR-15a/16-1 in CLL patients described by Calin et al. and other fascinating results, led to Corney et al. (Corney et al., 2007) to explore the potential influence of the well known tumor protein p53 (TP53) on miRNA regulation. This work revealed that TP53 directly activates the expression of the *miR-34b*/*miR-34c* cluster situated at 11q, which is proximal to the region deleted in patients with CLL who have poor outcomes. Along with the noticeable location of the *TP53* gene at 17p, these findings were suggestive of a higher-order genetic connection in CLL pathogenesis.

These findings led to a rapidly expanding series of investigations linking miRNAs to CLL. As a result, miRNAs are currently under evaluation as novel putative diagnostic and prognostic biomarkers as well as potential therapeutic targets in CLL. Consequently, differential miRNA signatures distinguishing between tumor and normal tissues were reported in leukemia and solid tumors. Several recent reports suggested a miRNA signature associated with diagnosis, prognosis and progression of CLL.

As mentioned above, Calin et al. conducted a miRNA expression profiling on a well-annotated cohort of 94 CLL patients and identified a panel of 13 miRNAs that correlated with ZAP-70 expression and I_gV_H mutational status (Calin et al., 2005). In addition, a subgroup of nine miRNAs (*181b, 155, 146, 24-2, 23b, 23a, 222, 221,* and *29c*) differentiated patients with a short interval to therapy from patients with a longer interval to therapy. These authors also identified germ line or somatic mutations in miRNA genes in 15% of CLL patients studied. miRNA expression in B cells from a cohort of 50 CLL patients identified 7 upregulated miRNAs and 19 downregulated miRNAs (Calin et al., 2005). Similar to this previous study, the authors identified the upregulation of *miR-155* and downregulation of *miR-181a/b.* Although several studies have demonstrated a correlation between chromosomal alterations and miRNA deregulation, these studies failed to demonstrate such a connection, so the questions in this topic remain to be answered. Gain of methylation was present in pri-miRNAs for several deregulated miRNAs, including *miR-139* and *miR-582.* Thus, this suggests that epigenetic regulation is likely to have a role in altered miRNA expression in CLL (Nana-Sinkam & Croce, 2010).

Interestingly, it was recently reported (Fabbri et al., 2011) that the recurring deletion hot spots at 13q, 11q, and 17p actually represent nodes of a complex regulatory network in CLL that integrates the miR-15a/miR-16-1 and miR-34b/miR-34c clusters with the tumor suppressor p53. These studies have lighted a comprehensive hypothesis of CLL pathogenesis that makes a relationship between clinical heterogeneity, complex cytogenetic patterns and prognostic markers. The critical interactions of anti-apoptotic factors such as BCL2, the p53 tumor suppressor, and the ZAP-70 tyrosine kinase, all governed by miRNAs that derive from the long arms of chromosomes 13 and 11, may therefore be involved in managing the variety of indolent or aggressive phenotypes experienced by patients with CLL.

Different studies were performed to identify miRNAs profiles defining leukemic cells involved in CLL. Using different experimental approaches (i.e. qRT-PCR, cloning and microarrays of defined miRNAs) several groups reported at least 25 miRNAs that were differentially expressed in CLL cells versus normal cells. These miRNAs included miR-16-1, miR-26a, miR-206, and miR-223 (Calin et al., 2004a), miR-155, miR-21, miR-150, miR-92 and miR-222 (Fulci et al., 2007) and miR-181, miR-30d, let-7a and three newly reported miRNAs (miR-1201, miR-1202 and miR-1203) characteristics of the CLL cells (Marton et al., 2008).

Several reports identified miRNA signatures that could act as surrogate prognostic biomarkers in CLL, typically by correlating expression levels of these miRNAs with previously established prognostic markers such as IgV_H mutation status or ZAP-70 expression (Calin et al., 2005). This signature included miR-15a, miR-195, miR-221, miR-23b, miR-155, miR-223, miR29a-2, miR-24-1, miR-29b-2, miR-146, miR-16-1, miR-16-2, and miR-29c. Some authors have also developed a quantitative RT-PCR score combining miR-29c, miR-223, ZAP-70 and lipoprotein lipase (Stamatopoulos et al., 2009). Over-expression of miR-21 and low miR-181b expression has been reported as unfavorable prognostic factors independent of other clinical-pathologic factors (Rossi et al., 2010).

The rapid development of miRNA research in the past few years suggests that the roles of many more miRNAs in CLL have yet to be discovered. For instance, for some researchers, the miR-17-92 cluster is a group of miRNAs that have been studied in a wide variety of cancers ((Ward et al., 2011)). This miR-17-92 cluster consists of seven miRNAs: miR-17-5p, miR-17-3p, miR-18, miR-19a, miR-20, miR-19b-1 and miR-92-1 transcribed from the MIR17 Host Gene (MIR17HG) at locus 13q31.3, and members of this cluster are thought to co-express with the proto-oncogenic transcription factor MYC (He et al., 2005). Several profiling studies show that expression of members of the miR-17-92 cluster is altered to some degree in CLL (Calin et al., 2004a; Fulci et al., 2007). Thus, advances in miRNA biology will likely have an increasing influence in the diagnosis, prognosis and treatment of human cancers, including CLL. In addition, it is discussed below the discovery of the oncogenic and tumor-suppressive properties of various miRNAs that come up with the possibility of miRNA therapy for cancer in the near future.

2.1 The miR-15a/16-1

The association of miR-15a/16-1 in the pathogenesis of CLL was not only the first implication of miRNAs in this disease, but also in cancer. The authors of this finding were Calin et al. who determined that miR-15a/16-1 were located in 13q14.3, and were either deleted or down-regulated in 68% of patients with CLL (Calin et al., 2002).

As this chromosomal region is also deleted in other types of cancer (mantle cell lymphoma, multiple myeloma, DLBCL, mature T-cell lymphoma, and solid tumors) conducted several authors to search for the presence of tumor suppressor genes in this region. A region of more than 1.0 Mb was sequenced, but none of the protein genes identified were found implicated in the initiation or progression of CLL (Calin et al., 2005). That fact, give rise to some hypothesis that finally conducted authors to search for miRNAs candidates, unknown genes, or possibly, extremely small genes perhaps not detected by classic cloning methods that might reside in this region and be the real target of genomic alteration (Aqeilan et al., 2010). On this way, a minimal deleted region (MDR) that contains two tightly linked miRNAs, miR-15a and mirR-16-1 was identified (Calin et al., 2002; Lagos-Quintana et al., 2001; Migliazza et al., 2000) (Figure 2). Recent studies demonstrated that other genes located in the same region (deleted in leukemia gene, DLEU 2 and 7), may also function as tumor suppressors (Palamarchuk et al., 2010).

In addition to chromosomal abnormalities, other mechanisms as mutation, loss of heterozygosis, epigenetic deregulation and defects in the miRNA biogenesis machinery, could also contribute to deregulation of miRNA expression (Deng et al., 2008). In this respect, Calin et al. demonstrated that mutations in miR-16-1 could be responsible for the altered expression observed in CLL patients compared with subjects without cancer (Aqeilan et al., 2010).

Using bionformatic tools Cimmino et al. (Cimmino et al., 2005) found that miR-15a and miR-16- sequences share complementary homology with BCL2 (B-cell CLL/lymphoma 2) mRNA sequence. Bcl2 is an anti-apoptotic protein that is highly expressed in CLL as in other types of human cancer, including leukemias, lymphomas, and carcinomas (Sanchez-Beato et al., 2003)

As the BLC2 gene is overexpressed and that deletions or down-regulation of the miR-15a and miR-16-1 cluster have been reported to occur in the same proportion in CLL samples, it was proposed that miR-15a and miR-16-1 produce their anti-tumorigenic effect by targeting the BCL2 gene (Aqeilan et al., 2010; Cimmino et al., 2005). Its function has also been assayed *in vitro* and *in vivo*. In immunocompromised nude mice, ectopic expression of miR-15a/16-1 was found to cause dramatic suppression of tumorigenicity of MEG-01 leukemic cells exhibiting a loss of endogenous expression of miR-15a/ 16-1 (Calin et al., 2008) On the other hand, and besides the results obtained by Cimmino et al, other authors found no correlation between BCL2 and mir15a and miR-16-1 in cancer (Fulci et al., 2007; Hanlon et al., 2009; Klein et al., 2010; Linsley et al., 2007). Klein et al. (Klein & Dalla-Favera, 2010) confirmed the observation that the miR-15a/miR-16-1 locus controls B cell expansion by modulating proliferation, rather than influencing survival via regulation of BCL2 *in vivo*.

Nowadays, different methodological approaches revealed that CCND1 (encoding cyclin D1) and WNT3A mRNAs which promote several prostate tumorigenic features, could also be directly affected by miR-15a/16-1 (Bonci et al., 2008), like other cancer genes such as MCL1, ETS1 and PDCD6IP that directly or indirectly affect cell cycle and apoptosis.

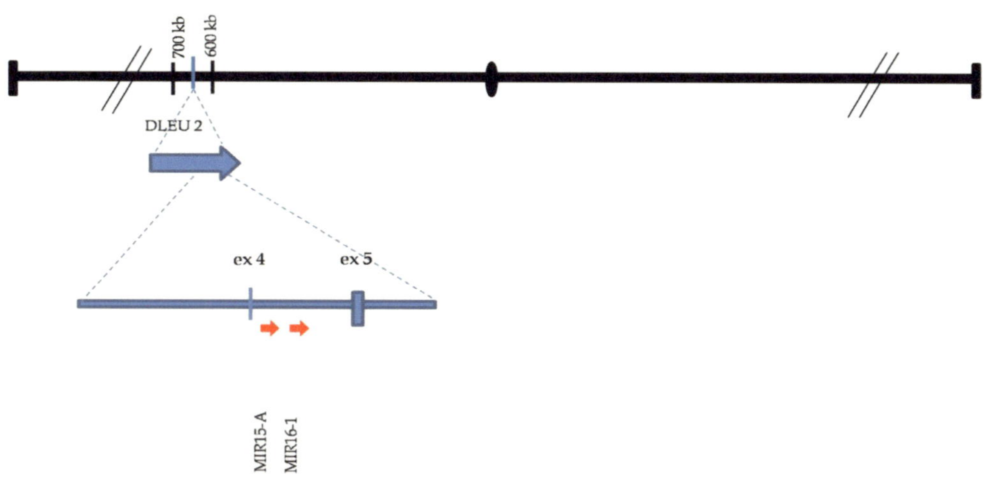

Fig. 2. Localization of miR15/16 cluster on human chromosome 13.

The 13q14 tumor suppressor locus deleted in CLL contain DLEU 2 gene where MIR15a/MIR16/b is located inside, between exon 4 and 5.

2.2 The miR-34 family

The miR-34 family has been implicated in several solid and hematological malignancies. The three members of the miR-34 family are encoded by two different genes: miR-34a is encoded by its own transcript, whereas miR-34b and miR-34c share a common primary transcript (Auer et al., 2007; Cole et al., 2008).

Deregulation of the miR-34a and miR-34b/c expression by chromosomal deletion and/or epigenectic inactivation, presumably occurs during tumorigenesis (Hermeking, 2010).

In the case of miR-34a, chromosomal deletion of the region in which it resides (locus 1p36) and epigenetic inactivation were identified in tumors. Moreover the epigenetic inactivation of miR-34a was identified in cell lines derived from some of the most common tumors and in primary melanoma. In addition, CpG methylation of miR-34b/c was also found in colorectal cancer, in oral squamous cell carcinoma and in malignant melanoma.

In the case of CLL, the variability of the mir-34a expression observed in patients is not precisely associated to the just mentioned process. It was demonstrated that members of the miR-34 family are direct p53 targets. MiR-34 genes are up-regulated by the tumor-suppressor protein p53, and their overexpression in turn causes senescence, apoptosis, or cell cycle arrest by regulating proteins such as BCL2, Cyclin D1, Cyclin E2, CDK4, and c-MYC Sirt-1, depending on the cell type (Corney et al., 2007; Ward et al., 2011). Further analysis effectively determined that miR-34a expression partially correlated with p53 status and patients with p53 mutations or deletions of 17p13.1, in general had lower miR-34a expression (Figure 3). However, in some patients decreased miR-34a was seen without p53 aberrations. These patients are homozygous for the single nucleotide polymorphism 309 (SNP309) in the intronic promoter of MDM2, a negative regulator of p53 (Asslaber et al., 2010). The down-regulation of miR-34 b/c is also related to a p53 inactivation and to one of the most characteristic chromosomal deletion in CLL: 11q23.1, where the miR-34 b/c cluster is located.

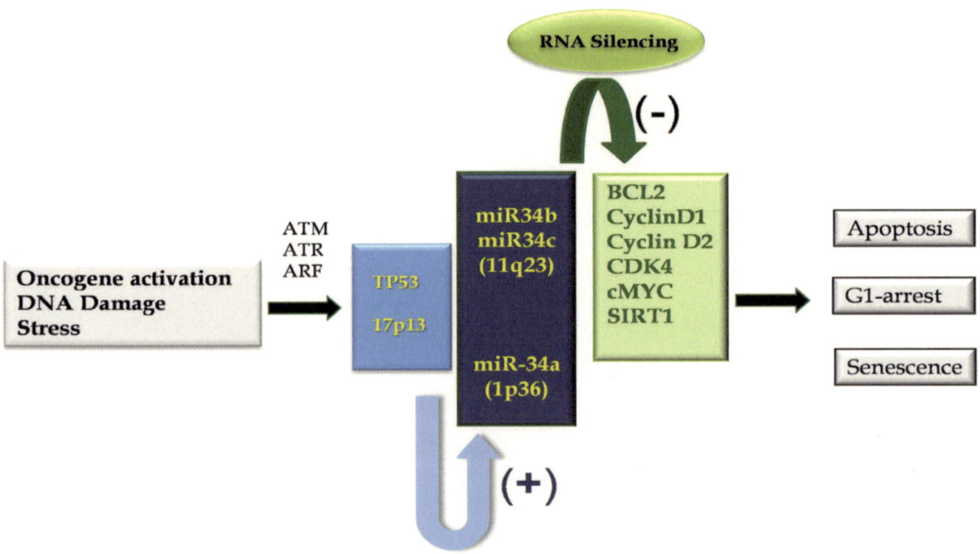

Fig. 3. MicroRNA-34 family regulation and targets involved in CLL. microRNA 34b (*miR-34b*)/microRNA 34c (*miR-34c*) cluster and miR-34a are regulated by tumor suppressor protein p53. After DNA damage or cellular stress, p53 is activated through ATM, ARF or ATR pathways and transactivates target genes including the miR-34 family members. The mature transcripts of the activated miR-34a/b/c induce either translation inhibition or cleavage of the indicated RNA targets.

2.3 The miR-29 and miR-181 in CLL

The members of miR-29 family are arranged in two different loci; the miR-29b-1/miR-29a located at 7q32 and the miR-29b-2/miR-29c at 1q32.

Downregulation of miR-29 members have been reported in various human cancers including aggressive chronic lymphocytic leukemia (Garzon et al., 2009). They were demonstrated to have a tumor suppressor activity by targeting several oncogenes as the T-cell leukemia/ lymphoma 1 (TCL1), the BCL2 family member MCL1, the cyclin-dependent kinase CDK6, and the transcriptional repressor Yy1 (Mott et al., 2007; Pekarsky et al., 2006; Zhao et al. 2010).).

Fabbri et al, showed that members of the miR-29 family target also the *de novo* DNA methyltransferases (DNMTs) and can reactivate tumor suppressor genes (Fabbri et al., 2007). Thus, loss of miR-29 family members could cause epigenetic changes associated with CLL and other cancer types.

Besides of the antitumoral activity of miR-29 overexpression by inhibition of cell proliferation, it was also observed that miR-29 up-regulation could also initiate acute and chronic leukemias in animal models. Santanam and co-workers (Santanam et al., 2010) developed a transgenic mice overexpressing mir-29 in mouse B cells. They reported that miR-29 is overexpressed in indolent CLL compared with normal B cells. In contrast, miR29 was down-regulated in aggressive CLL.

In addition, it was demonstrated that miR-29 inversely correlated with levels of TCL-1 in CLL patients. TCL-1 is a coactivator of AKT, an oncogene that inhibits apoptotic patways and has a critical role in the regulation of many relevant cell processes including cell proliferation and cell death (Santanam et al., 2010; Vasilatou et al., 2010). Taken together, these data led authors to hypothesize that TCL1 is mostly not expressed in indolent CLL and probably does not play an important role in this disease stage. Indeed, miR-29 overexpression is not sufficient to initiate aggressive CLL. In contrast, up-regulation of TCL1 is a critical event in the pathogenesis of the aggressive form of CLL and because miR-29 is down-regulated in aggressive CLL (compared with the indolent form), it contributes to the development of an aggressive phenotype (Santanam et al., 2010). As mir-29b, mir-181b acts as tumor-suppresor in aggressive CLL by targeting also the TCL-1 oncogene, there is an inverse correlation between TCL1 and miR-181 expression at different stages of B-cell development (Pekarsky et al., 2006).

The high expression of these miRNAs is associated with expression of unmutated IgV_H and high expression of ZAP-70, indicating an aggressive CLL phenotype (Vasilatou et al., 2010).

2.4 Other miRNAs potentially implicated in CLL pathogenesis

As was previously described in this chapter, several miRNAs have been reported to be differently expressed in B cells from CLL compared to normal B-cells.

The miR-155, for example, was reported overexpressed in solid tumors, including lung, colon, and breast cancer as well as in both acute myeloid leukemia and CLL (Garzon et al., 2009). Frenquelli et al. (Frenquelli et al., 2010) recently showed an inverse relationship between miR-221/222 and p27 expression and validated p27 as a functional target for miR-221/222 in CLL. Fulci and co-workers (Fulci et al., 2007) found an overexpression of miR-150, miR-223, miR-29b, and miR-29c in CLL patients with a mutated IgV_H phenotype compared to the patients with unmutated IgV_H phenotypes.

3. MicroRNA signatures and prognostic miRNAs in CLL

In addition to the well known molecular factors (mutational status of IgV_H, expression levels of ZAP-70 or β2-microglobulin and expression of CD38+) and chromosomal abnormalities (11q, 13q, 17p deletions) associated to the clinical course of CLL, the molecular basis for these correlations was largely unknown. However, several studies identified miRNAs that could act as prognostic indicators in CLL, typically by correlating expression levels of these miRNAs with previously mentioned established prognostic indicators (Ward et al., 2011).

One of the first works that described this relationship was published by Calin et al. in 2005. They described a signature of 13 miRNAs (miR- 15a, miR-195, miR-221, miR-23b, miR-155, miR-223, miR29a-2, miR- 24-1, miR-29b-2, miR-146, miR-16-1, miR-16-2, and miR-29c) differentially expressed between unmutated IgV_H/ ZAP70+ and mutated IgV_H/ZAP70 CLL patients. Further studies, using different molecular techniques, also confirmed the mentioned correlation (Fulci et al., 2007; Marton et al., 2008; Rossi et al., 2010; Stamatopoulos et al., 2009). They reveled also the implication of miR-150 and miR-181 as prognostic factors.

It was recently reported that the deregulation of miR-181b expression can be monitored throughout the course of the disease, which correlate with the overexpression of 4 genes with great significance in CLL biology and other cancers (i.e. MCL1, TCL1, BCL2 and AID (Visone et al., 2009).

An interesting link between the classical prognostic molecular and chromosomal markers of CLL and two groups of defined miRNAs have been recently described by Fabri et al. (Fabbri et al., 2011). They found that miR-15a/miR-16-1 cluster is associated with reduced expression levels of TP53, miR-34a, miR-34b, and miR-34c and increased protein levels of ZAP70. Low expression levels of ZAP70 have been found to be positively correlated with survival in patients with the indolent course of CLL carrying 13q deletions, and it was associated with increased TP53 levels and transactivation of miR-34b/ miR-34c. In this way, the authors found a microRNA/TP53 feedback circuitry associated with the pathogenesis and prognosis of CLL and revealed a new pathogenic model for human CLL.

As mentioned above, miR-29 expression correlated with the clinical course of CLL. Low expression of miR-29c was associated to patients who had a poor prognosis and shorter treatment-free survival as well as reduced overall survival (Calin & Croce, 2009).

Thus, advances in the identification of miRNAs as CLL biomarkers, as well as the mode of regulation of gene expression and the pathway in which they are involved, should provide a useful prognostic tool for patient stratification and more appropriated treatments.

3.1 Circulating miRNAs as novel biomarkers in CLL

Nowadays, after the identification of extracellular circulating microRNAs in plasma microvesicles or ribonucleoprotein complexes (Cortez et al., 2011; Valadi et al., 2007), they have become an attractive source of new nucleic acid-based biomarkers. Today miRNAs are considered powerful markers for early detection, prognosis, response, and recurrence surveillance of different cancers because they are widely involved in oncogenesis (Taylor & Gercel-Taylor, 2008). The diagnostic and prognostic potential of miRNAs as cancer biomarkers relies mainly on their high stability and resistance to storage handling. It has been consistently shown that serum miRNAs remain stable after being subjected to severe conditions that would normally degrade most RNAs. This stability can be partially explained by the discovery of lipoprotein complexes, including small membrane vesicles of endocytic origin called exosomes or microvesicles (30-1000 nm in diameter), containing miRNAs, mRNAs and proteins. Exosomes can be formed through inward budding of endosomal membranes, giving rise to intracellular multi vesicular bodies (MVBs) that later fuse with the plasma membrane, releasing the exosomes to the exterior (Figure 1). In contrast, microvesicles are originated by outward budding from the plasma membrane. The utility of miRNAs as diagnostic markers will be increased because samples of human plasma and serum can be obtained in a less invasive manner than can tissues.

Exosomes containing miRNAs were found in blood (Hunter et al., 2008), but also in other types of body fluids such as saliva and urine (Michael et al.). Importantly, exosomes represent a newly discovered mechanism by which donor cells can communicate and influence the gene expression of recipient cells. These findings were first demonstrated by the same study that discovered miRNAs in exosomes, in which mouse mast cell exosomes were added to human mast cells, leading to a subsequent detection of mouse proteins in the human cells (Valadi et al., 2007).

Tumor-specific miRNAs were first discovered in the serum of patients with diffuse large B cell lymphoma where high levels of miR-21 correlated with improved relapse-free survival (Lawrie et al., 2009). In an elegant experiment in a xenograft mouse prostate cancer model, the presence of circulating tumor-derived miR-629 and miR-660 was confirmed in blood with 100% sensitivity and specificity (Mitchell et al., 2008). In addition to showing that both serum and plasma samples are adequate for measuring specific miRNA levels, the investigators reported that by measuring serum levels of miR-141, they were able to distinguish patients with prostate cancer from healthy subjects. Since then, over 100 studies have assessed the potential use of serum or plasma miRNAs as biomarkers in different types of cancer (Cortez et al., 2011). In a comprehensive study, miRNA-expression profiles were identified in the sera of patients with lung or colorectal cancer, or diabetes by extracting miRNA from the serum (Chen et al., 2008). Although a unique expression profile of serum miRNAs was identified for each cancer type, an overlap was found in the profiles of specimens from all diseases analyzed in the study, including diabetes. In addition, this study also showed that miRNA-expression profiles differed between the serum and blood cells of lung cancer patients, while similar miRNA-expression profiles were seen in the serum and blood cells of healthy controls. These findings suggest that tumor-specific miRNAs in serum are derived not only from circulating blood cells but also cancer cells. An actualized compendium of relevant circulating miRNAs with potential as biomarkers for cancer was recently reviewed by Cortez et al. (Cortez et al., 2011).

Because most current approaches to cancer screening are invasive and unable to detect early-stage disease, it is important to determine when tumor-related circulating miRNAs can be detected in the bloodstream during disease development between other important factors. In this respect, it was recently reported that miRNAs can be also sensitive biomarkers for CLL, because certain extracellular miRNAs are present in CLL patient plasma at levels significantly different from healthy controls and from patients affected by other hematologic malignancies (Klein et al., 2010). Moreover, in this study the authors also determined that level of circulating miR-20a correlates reliably with diagnosis-to treatment time and miR-483-5p elevated almost six fold in plasma of CLL patients is predicted to target the mediators of IL-15 that induces CLL proliferation and drives CLL cell migration and infiltration. Although most of the miRNA–mRNA interactions are yet to be fully validated, the roles of these plasma miRNAs in CLL present intriguing biological questions with medically significant implications (Moussay et al., 2011; Ward et al., 2011).

4. MiRNAs as predictors of CLL responses to therapy

4.1 Chemotherapy resistance

In spite of the existence of effective treatments for patients suffering CLL, present therapeutic regimens are not totally effective and additional therapies are required.

Recently fludarabine-refractory CLL was linked to patients with p53 deletion and low miR-34a expression. It was previously mentioned that miR-34a is positively regulated by p53. Low miR-34a expression levels were statistically significantly associated with impaired DNA damage response, p53 mutations, and fludarabine-refractory CLL either with or without p53 deletion (Calin & Croce, 2009).

In addition, patients with resistant disease exhibited increased miR-181a and decreased miR-29a expression as consequence of their regulation by the myelocytomatosis viral oncogene homolog (MYC), which is increased in patients with fludarabine-resistant disease (Moussay et al., 2010).

These are the first identified miRNAs associated in the complex network of molecules associated to drug resistance and sensitivity in patients with CLL.

4.2 Therapy

According to the novel miRNAs described as biomarkers of prognosis and treatment in CLL, one of the most expecting use of them is the possible utility in the therapy of CLL.

The advantage to use these molecules for therapy, compared to other RNA inhibition strategies, relies on the fact that they are not only tiny and simple, but also they can target more than one mRNA relevant for the pathway of the disease (Calin & Croce, 2009).

Different chemical modification as are 2'-O-methylphosphorothioate oligonucleotides, locked nucleic acid and miRNA sponge are currently being used to improve the blocking capacity and half-life of miRNA. In addition Liposome–oligonucleotide Complexes, among other strategies are been improved for the delivery, specificity and reduction of toxicity of miRNAs.

As for miR-122, which seems to be effective for the treatment hepatitis C in ongoing clinical trials (Lanford et al.), the potential use of miRNAs in CLL treatment has only recently been envisioned and were only used *in vitro*.

5. Concluding remarks

In this chapter, we have analyzed the potential contribution of microRNAs as novel players and biomarkers in CLL pathogenesis.

The role of miRNAs as key regulatory molecules that control a wide variety of fundamental cellular processes, such as proliferation, death, differentiation, motility, invasiveness, etc., is increasingly recognized in almost all fields of biological and biomedical sciences. Over the last years, microRNAs have emerged as new actors in cancer biology as well as new diagnostic biomarkers and therapeutic targets in human cancer. This review attempts to briefly outline our current knowledge on the abnormalities of miRNAs found to be associated with CLL pathogenesis and possible mechanisms underlying the roles of miRNAs in CLL initiation and progression and to provide a perspective insight in using miRNAs as new CLL biomarkers. Nowadays, microRNAs are proposed as new sensitive, non-invasive and inexpensive biomarkers in CLL for early stage detection, predict outcome, monitor treatment and screen for disease recurrence. Understanding the significance of microRNAs in the pathogenesis of CLL represents an important dimension in miRNA research as it may lead to the development of miRNA-based novel therapeutic strategies or diagnostic/prognostic biomarkers. Additionally, microRNAs should also afford new avenues for exploring innovative pathways in CLL pathogenesis.

6. References

Aqeilan, R.I., Calin, G.A., and Croce, C.M. (2010). miR-15a and miR-16-1 in cancer: discovery, function and future perspectives. Cell death and differentiation *17*, 215-220.

Asslaber, D., Pinon, J.D., Seyfried, I., Desch, P., Stocher, M., Tinhofer, I., Egle, A., Merkel, O., and Greil, R. (2010). microRNA-34a expression correlates with MDM2 SNP309 polymorphism and treatment-free survival in chronic lymphocytic leukemia. Blood *115*, 4191-4197.

Auer, R.L., Riaz, S., and Cotter, F.E. (2007). The 13q and 11q B-cell chronic lymphocytic leukaemia-associated regions derive from a common ancestral region in the zebrafish. British journal of haematology *137*, 443-453.

Bonci, D., Coppola, V., Musumeci, M., Addario, A., Giuffrida, R., Memeo, L., D'Urso, L., Pagliuca, A., Biffoni, M., Labbaye, C., *et al.* (2008). The miR-15a-miR-16-1 cluster controls prostate cancer by targeting multiple oncogenic activities. Nature medicine *14*, 1271-1277.

Calin, G.A., Cimmino, A., Fabbri, M., Ferracin, M., Wojcik, S.E., Shimizu, M., Taccioli, C., Zanesi, N., Garzon, R., Aqeilan, R.I., *et al.* (2008). MiR-15a and miR-16-1 cluster functions in human leukemia. Proceedings of the National Academy of Sciences of the United States of America *105*, 5166-5171.

Calin, G.A., and Croce, C.M. (2009). Chronic lymphocytic leukemia: interplay between noncoding RNAs and protein-coding genes. Blood *114*, 4761-4770.

Calin, G.A., Dumitru, C.D., Shimizu, M., Bichi, R., Zupo, S., Noch, E., Aldler, H., Rattan, S., Keating, M., Rai, K., *et al.* (2002). Frequent deletions and down-regulation of micro-RNA genes miR15 and miR16 at 13q14 in chronic lymphocytic leukemia. Proceedings of the National Academy of Sciences of the United States of America *99*, 15524-15529.

Calin, G.A., Ferracin, M., Cimmino, A., Di Leva, G., Shimizu, M., Wojcik, S.E., Iorio, M.V., Visone, R., Sever, N.I., Fabbri, M., *et al.* (2005). A MicroRNA signature associated with prognosis and progression in chronic lymphocytic leukemia. The New England journal of medicine *353*, 1793-1801.

Calin, G.A., Liu, C.G., Sevignani, C., Ferracin, M., Felli, N., Dumitru, C.D., Shimizu, M., Cimmino, A., Zupo, S., Dono, M., *et al.* (2004a). MicroRNA profiling reveals distinct signatures in B cell chronic lymphocytic leukemias. Proceedings of the National Academy of Sciences of the United States of America *101*, 11755-11760.

Calin, G.A., Sevignani, C., Dumitru, C.D., Hyslop, T., Noch, E., Yendamuri, S., Shimizu, M., Rattan, S., Bullrich, F., Negrini, M., *et al.* (2004b). Human microRNA genes are frequently located at fragile sites and genomic regions involved in cancers. Proceedings of the National Academy of Sciences of the United States of America *101*, 2999-3004.

Cimmino, A., Calin, G.A., Fabbri, M., Iorio, M.V., Ferracin, M., Shimizu, M., Wojcik, S.E., Aqeilan, R.I., Zupo, S., Dono, M., *et al.* (2005). miR-15 and miR-16 induce apoptosis by targeting BCL2. Proceedings of the National Academy of Sciences of the United States of America *102*, 13944-13949.

Cole, K.A., Attiyeh, E.F., Mosse, Y.P., Laquaglia, M.J., Diskin, S.J., Brodeur, G.M., and Maris, J.M. (2008). A functional screen identifies miR-34a as a candidate neuroblastoma tumor suppressor gene. Mol Cancer Res *6*, 735-742.

Corney, D.C., Flesken-Nikitin, A., Godwin, A.K., Wang, W., and Nikitin, A.Y. (2007). MicroRNA-34b and MicroRNA-34c are targets of p53 and cooperate in control of cell proliferation and adhesion-independent growth. Cancer research *67*, 8433-8438.

Cortez, M.A., Bueso-Ramos, C., Ferdin, J., Lopez-Berestein, G., Sood, A.K., and Calin, G.A. (2011). MicroRNAs in body fluids--the mix of hormones and biomarkers. Nat Rev Clin Oncol *8*, 467-477.

Croce, C.M. (2009). Causes and consequences of microRNA dysregulation in cancer. Nature reviews *10*, 704-714.

Chen, X., Ba, Y., Ma, L., Cai, X., Yin, Y., Wang, K., Guo, J., Zhang, Y., Chen, J., Guo, X., *et al.* (2008). Characterization of microRNAs in serum: a novel class of biomarkers for diagnosis of cancer and other diseases. Cell Res *18*, 997-1006.

Chu, C.Y., and Rana, T.M. (2007). Small RNAs: regulators and guardians of the genome. Journal of cellular physiology *213*, 412-419.

Deng, S., Calin, G.A., Croce, C.M., Coukos, G., and Zhang, L. (2008). Mechanisms of microRNA deregulation in human cancer. Cell cycle (Georgetown, Tex *7*, 2643-2646.

Fabbri, M., Bottoni, A., Shimizu, M., Spizzo, R., Nicoloso, M.S., Rossi, S., Barbarotto, E., Cimmino, A., Adair, B., Wojcik, S.E., *et al.* (2011). Association of a microRNA/TP53 feedback circuitry with pathogenesis and outcome of B-cell chronic lymphocytic leukemia. Jama *305*, 59-67.

Fabbri, M., Garzon, R., Cimmino, A., Liu, Z., Zanesi, N., Callegari, E., Liu, S., Alder, H., Costinean, S., Fernandez-Cymering, C., *et al.* (2007). MicroRNA-29 family reverts aberrant methylation in lung cancer by targeting DNA methyltransferases 3A and 3B. Proceedings of the National Academy of Sciences of the United States of America *104*, 15805-15810.

Farazi, T.A., Spitzer, J.I., Morozov, P., and Tuschl, T. (2011). miRNAs in human cancer. The Journal of pathology *223*, 102-115.

Frenquelli, M., Muzio, M., Scielzo, C., Fazi, C., Scarfo, L., Rossi, C., Ferrari, G., Ghia, P., and Caligaris-Cappio, F. (2010). MicroRNA and proliferation control in chronic lymphocytic leukemia: functional relationship between miR-221/222 cluster and p27. Blood *115*, 3949-3959.

Fulci, V., Chiaretti, S., Goldoni, M., Azzalin, G., Carucci, N., Tavolaro, S., Castellano, L., Magrelli, A., Citarella, F., Messina, M., *et al.* (2007). Quantitative technologies establish a novel microRNA profile of chronic lymphocytic leukemia. Blood *109*, 4944-4951.

Garzon, R., Calin, G.A., and Croce, C.M. (2009). MicroRNAs in Cancer. Annual review of medicine *60*, 167-179.

Hanlon, K., Rudin, C.E., and Harries, L.W. (2009). Investigating the targets of MIR-15a and MIR-16-1 in patients with chronic lymphocytic leukemia (CLL). PloS one *4*, e7169.

He, L., Thomson, J.M., Hemann, M.T., Hernando-Monge, E., Mu, D., Goodson, S., Powers, S., Cordon-Cardo, C., Lowe, S.W., Hannon, G.J., *et al.* (2005). A microRNA polycistron as a potential human oncogene. Nature *435*, 828-833.

Hermeking, H. (2010). The miR-34 family in cancer and apoptosis. Cell death and differentiation *17*, 193-199.

Hunter, M.P., Ismail, N., Zhang, X., Aguda, B.D., Lee, E.J., Yu, L., Xiao, T., Schafer, J., Lee, M.L., Schmittgen, T.D., *et al.* (2008). Detection of microRNA expression in human peripheral blood microvesicles. PloS one *3*, e3694.

Klein, U., and Dalla-Favera, R. (2010). New insights into the pathogenesis of chronic lymphocytic leukemia. Seminars in cancer biology *20*, 377-383.

Klein, U., Lia, M., Crespo, M., Siegel, R., Shen, Q., Mo, T., Ambesi-Impiombato, A., Califano, A., Migliazza, A., Bhagat, G., *et al.* (2010). The DLEU2/miR-15a/16-1 cluster controls B cell proliferation and its deletion leads to chronic lymphocytic leukemia. Cancer cell *17*, 28-40.

Lagos-Quintana, M., Rauhut, R., Lendeckel, W., and Tuschl, T. (2001). Identification of novel genes coding for small expressed RNAs. Science (New York, NY *294*, 853-858.

Lanford, R.E., Hildebrandt-Eriksen, E.S., Petri, A., Persson, R., Lindow, M., Munk, M.E., Kauppinen, S., and Orum, H. Therapeutic silencing of microRNA-122 in primates with chronic hepatitis C virus infection. Science (New York, NY *327*, 198-201.

Lawrie, C.H., Ballabio, E., Dyar, O.J., Jones, M., Ventura, R., Chi, J., Tramonti, D., Gooding, S., Boultwood, J., Wainscoat, J.S., *et al.* (2009). MicroRNA expression in chronic lymphocytic leukaemia. British journal of haematology *147*, 398-402.

Linsley, P.S., Schelter, J., Burchard, J., Kibukawa, M., Martin, M.M., Bartz, S.R., Johnson, J.M., Cummins, J.M., Raymond, C.K., Dai, H., *et al.* (2007). Transcripts targeted by the microRNA-16 family cooperatively regulate cell cycle progression. Molecular and cellular biology *27*, 2240-2252.

Marton, S., Garcia, M.R., Robello, C., Persson, H., Trajtenberg, F., Pritsch, O., Rovira, C., Naya, H., Dighiero, G., and Cayota, A. (2008). Small RNAs analysis in CLL reveals a deregulation of miRNA expression and novel miRNA candidates of putative relevance in CLL pathogenesis. Leukemia *22*, 330-338.

Michael, A., Bajracharya, S.D., Yuen, P.S., Zhou, H., Star, R.A., Illei, G.G., and Alevizos, I. Exosomes from human saliva as a source of microRNA biomarkers. Oral diseases *16*, 34-38.

Migliazza, A., Cayanis, E., Bosch-Albareda, F., Komatsu, H., Martinotti, S., Toniato, E., Kalachikov, S., Bonaldo, M.F., Jelene, P., Ye, X., *et al.* (2000). Molecular pathogenesis of B-cell chronic lymphocytic leukemia: analysis of 13q14 chromosomal deletions. Current topics in microbiology and immunology *252*, 275-284.

Mitchell, P.S., Parkin, R.K., Kroh, E.M., Fritz, B.R., Wyman, S.K., Pogosova-Agadjanyan, E.L., Peterson, A., Noteboom, J., O'Briant, K.C., Allen, A., *et al.* (2008). Circulating microRNAs as stable blood-based markers for cancer detection. Proceedings of the National Academy of Sciences of the United States of America *105*, 10513-10518.

Mott, J.L., Kobayashi, S., Bronk, S.F., and Gores, G.J. (2007). mir-29 regulates Mcl-1 protein expression and apoptosis. Oncogene *26*, 6133-6140.

Moussay, E., Palissot, V., Vallar, L., Poirel, H.A., Wenner, T., El Khoury, V., Aouali, N., Van Moer, K., Leners, B., Bernardin, F., *et al.* (2010). Determination of genes and microRNAs involved in the resistance to fludarabine in vivo in chronic lymphocytic leukemia. Molecular cancer *9*, 115.

Moussay, E., Wang, K., Cho, J.H., van Moer, K., Pierson, S., Paggetti, J., Nazarov, P.V., Palissot, V., Hood, L.E., Berchem, G., *et al.* (2011). MicroRNA as biomarkers and regulators in B-cell chronic lymphocytic leukemia. Proceedings of the National Academy of Sciences of the United States of America *108*, 6573-6578.

Nana-Sinkam, S.P., and Croce, C.M. (2010). MicroRNA in chronic lymphocytic leukemia: transitioning from laboratory-based investigation to clinical application. Cancer genetics and cytogenetics *203*, 127-133.

Palamarchuk, A., Efanov, A., Nazaryan, N., Santanam, U., Alder, H., Rassenti, L., Kipps, T., Croce, C.M., and Pekarsky, Y. (2010). 13q14 deletions in CLL involve cooperating tumor suppressors. Blood *115*, 3916-3922.

Pekarsky, Y., Santanam, U., Cimmino, A., Palamarchuk, A., Efanov, A., Maximov, V., Volinia, S., Alder, H., Liu, C.G., Rassenti, L., *et al.* (2006). Tcl1 expression in chronic lymphocytic leukemia is regulated by miR-29 and miR-181. Cancer research *66*, 11590-11593.

Rossi, S., Shimizu, M., Barbarotto, E., Nicoloso, M.S., Dimitri, F., Sampath, D., Fabbri, M., Lerner, S., Barron, L.L., Rassenti, L.Z., *et al.* (2010). microRNA fingerprinting of CLL patients with chromosome 17p deletion identify a miR-21 score that stratifies early survival. Blood *116*, 945-952.

Rovira, C., Guida, M.C., and Cayota, A. (2010). MicroRNAs and other small silencing RNAs in cancer. IUBMB life *62*, 859-868.

Sanchez-Beato, M., Sanchez-Aguilera, A., and Piris, M.A. (2003). Cell cycle deregulation in B-cell lymphomas. Blood *101*, 1220-1235.

Santanam, U., Zanesi, N., Efanov, A., Costinean, S., Palamarchuk, A., Hagan, J.P., Volinia, S., Alder, H., Rassenti, L., Kipps, T., *et al.* (2010). Chronic lymphocytic leukemia modeled in mouse by targeted miR-29 expression. Proceedings of the National Academy of Sciences of the United States of America *107*, 12210-12215.

Stamatopoulos, B., Meuleman, N., Haibe-Kains, B., Saussoy, P., Van Den Neste, E., Michaux, L., Heimann, P., Martiat, P., Bron, D., and Lagneaux, L. (2009). microRNA-29c and microRNA-223 down-regulation has in vivo significance in chronic lymphocytic leukemia and improves disease risk stratification. Blood *113*, 5237-5245.

Taylor, D.D., and Gercel-Taylor, C. (2008). MicroRNA signatures of tumor-derived exosomes as diagnostic biomarkers of ovarian cancer. Gynecologic oncology *110*, 13-21.

Valadi, H., Ekstrom, K., Bossios, A., Sjostrand, M., Lee, J.J., and Lotvall, J.O. (2007). Exosome-mediated transfer of mRNAs and microRNAs is a novel mechanism of genetic exchange between cells. Nature cell biology *9*, 654-659.

Vasilatou, D., Papageorgiou, S., Pappa, V., Papageorgiou, E., and Dervenoulas, J. (2010). The role of microRNAs in normal and malignant hematopoiesis. European journal of haematology *84*, 1-16.

Visone, R., Rassenti, L.Z., Veronese, A., Taccioli, C., Costinean, S., Aguda, B.D., Volinia, S., Ferracin, M., Palatini, J., Balatti, V., *et al.* (2009). Karyotype-specific microRNA signature in chronic lymphocytic leukemia. Blood *114*, 3872-3879.

Ward, B.P., Tsongalis, G.J., and Kaur, P. (2011). MicroRNAs in chronic lymphocytic leukemia. Experimental and molecular pathology *90*, 173-178.

Wright, F.A., Lemon, W.J., Zhao, W.D., Sears, R., Zhuo, D., Wang, J.P., Yang, H.Y., Baer, T., Stredney, D., Spitzner, J., *et al.* (2001). A draft annotation and overview of the human genome. Genome biology *2*, RESEARCH0025.

Zhao, J.J., Lin, J., Lwin, T., Yang, H., Guo, J., Kong, W., Dessureault, S., Moscinski, L.C., Rezania, D., Dalton, W.S., *et al.* (2010) microRNA expression profile and identification of miR-29 as a prognostic marker and pathogenetic factor by targeting CDK6 in mantle cell lymphoma. Blood *115*, 2630-2639.

7

The Biological Relevance of ZAP-70 in CLL

Valerie Pede, Ans Rombout, Bruno Verhasselt and Jan Philippé
Ghent University
Belgium

1. Introduction

Initially, CLL was considered as a homogeneous disease caused by the accumulation of functionally incompetent B lymphocytes carrying no mutations in the immunoglobulin heavy chain variable (IgV_H) genes. However, further studies by Schroeder and Dighiero suggested that IgV_H genes may be mutated in CLL (Schroeder & Dighiero 1994). This report changed the general view of CLL and gained even more significance when the mutational status of the IgV_H genes was linked to the prognosis of the patients in two independent studies (Damle et al. 1999, Hamblin et al. 1999). These studies showed for the first time that patients with CLL cells expressing unmutated IgV_H genes presented with a more aggressive disease and shorter survival than those with cells carrying mutated IgV_H genes. Determination of the mutational status of the IgV_H genes in CLL patients became of great interest, but even today remains difficult to carry out in most medical centers since the technique is laborious, expensive and time-consuming. Therefore many efforts have been made to identify possible surrogate markers with the same prognostic value as the mutation status. In 2001, two independent groups published their studies in which they compared the gene expression profiles for IgV_H mutated versus unmutated CLL cells. Because, the description of the two groups of CLL with markedly different prognosis prompted the idea that CLL consisted of two different entities originating from either naive or memory cells, it was unexpected that only a few differentially expressed genes were found (Rosenwald et al. 2001, Klein et al. 2001). Among them, ZAP-70 appeared to be one of the most significant (Rosenwald et al. 2001). Subsequently, the correlation of ZAP-70 expression with the mutational status of the IgV_H genes was assessed in larger series of CLL patients, where ZAP-70 was mostly found expressed in unmutated CLL (reviewed in (Van Bockstaele et al. 2009)). Further clinical studies revealed that ZAP-70 was also an independent prognostic marker (Bosch et al. 2006). There were several attempts to standardize the determination of ZAP-70 expression by flow cytometry (Crespo et al. 2003, Wang et al. 2011, Van Bockstaele et al. 2006). Although, a successful standardized procedure was put forward by the European Research Initiative on CLL (ERIC), the determination and interpretation of ZAP-70 remains difficult (Letestu et al. 2006) and optimalization is still ongoing.

2. Structure of ZAP-70

The zeta-chain associated protein kinase with a molecular weight of 70 kDa, ZAP-70, is a member of the Syk family kinases predominantly involved in T cell receptor (TCR) signaling initiation and subsequent T cell activation (Chan et al. 1992). The ZAP-70 gene is located on chromosome 2q11.2 and is composed of 14 exons encoding a protein tyrosine kinase (PTK) made out of 619 amino acids building three functional domains; two Src homology 2 (SH_2) domains arranged in tandem at the amino-terminus and a tyrosine kinase domain at the carboxy-terminus (Figure 1) (Au-Yeung et al. 2009).

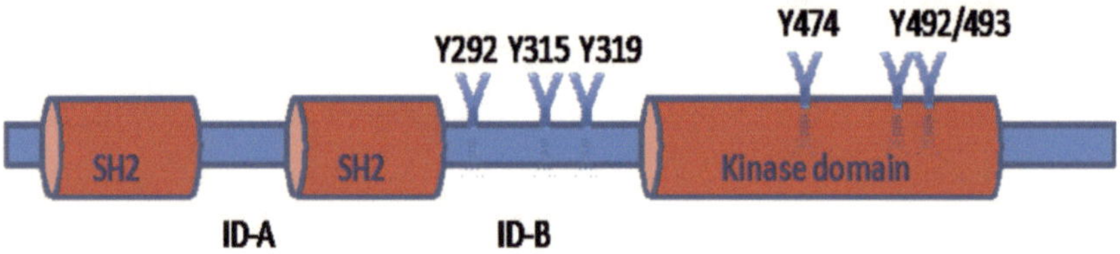

ID-A: interdomain A; ID-B: interdomain B; Y: Tyrosine residue

Fig. 1. Zeta-chain-associated protein kinase 70 (ZAP-70) protein structure.

The two SH_2 domains are separated by a linker region known as interdomain A (ID-A) and a linker region known as interdomain B (ID-B) connecting the SH2 domains to the kinase domain. SH2 domains are involved in the recruitment of ZAP-70 to phosphorylated immunoreceptor tyrosine-based activation motifs (ITAMs) on the CD3 ζ chain homodimers and both SH2 domains are responsible for ZAP-70 dependent signal transduction. The kinase domain of ZAP-70 contains two tyrosine residues, Tyr492 and Tyr493, which are phosphorylated by the Src tyrosine kinase, Lck, or autophosphorylated by ZAP-70 itself, after TCR engagement. Mutation of Tyr493 impairs ZAP-70 kinase activity, revealing a positive regulatory role of this residue, while mutation of Tyr492 increases kinase activity, indicating its inhibitory role (Wange et al. 1995). The tyrosine 474 of ZAP-70 is required for association with the Src Homology 2 domain Containing (Shc) adaptor protein and coupling of the activated TCR to the Ras/Raf/Erk pathways. Although the catalytic activity of ZAP-70 represents its major function, it is likely that interactions of ZAP-70 with other proteins contribute to its role in signal transduction. Interdomain B contains three tyrosines, Tyr292, Tyr315 and Tyr319, also representing important phosphorylation targets (Au-Yeung et al. 2009). These three tyrosines are phosphorylated by one of the Src family kinases, i.e. Lck or Fyn after TCR stimulation in T cells. Each of these binding sites, once phosphorylated, may bind to a different signaling molecule, conferring a role of ZAP-70 in the recruitment of additional signaling molecules to the antigen receptor complex. Tyr292 is able to bind the E3 ligase c-Cbl, which might be important for the turnover of the signaling complex (Rao et al. 2002). This implies a negative regulatory role for this tyrosine that however was recently shown to function also as a binding site for the p85 regulatory subunit of PI3K, indicating that it may also play a positive role in signal transduction. The two other tyrosines, Tyr315 and Tyr319 are positive regulators of ZAP-70 activity. Their phosphorylation is important for ZAP-70 activity, because it appears to prevent ZAP-70 from returning to an auto-inhibited conformation (Au-Yeung et al. 2009). Phosphorylated Tyr315 is a binding site for the SH2 domain of Vav-1. This plays a key role in activation of the Rho family of GTPases involved in cytoskeleton remodeling after receptor stimulation (Wu et al. 1997, Sanchez-Aguilera et al. 2010). Tyr319 is a binding site for the C terminal SH2 domain of phospholipase C γ (PLCγ), and phosphorylation of Tyr319 is required for PLCγ phosphorylation and subsequent activation of downstream signals, such as calcium mobilization or Il-2 production (Williams et al. 1999).

3. Expression of ZAP-70

3.1 Expression of ZAP-70 in T and B cells

For a long time ZAP-70 expression was considered to be restricted to T and NK cells, until it was found to be expressed as well in leukemic cells of CLL patients. Later studies have revealed ZAP-70 expression in a subset of normal tonsillar and splenic B cells (Cutrona et al. 2006, Nolz et al. 2005) and in bone marrow pro-B cells (Crespo et al. 2006, Guillaume et al. 2005). Besides the occurrence of ZAP-70 in a subset of CLL patients it was also found in a number of other human B cell tumors like some cases of mantle cell lymphoma, splenic marginal zone lymphoma, B-ALL and Burkitt lymphoma (Crespo et al. 2006, Guillaume et al. 2005, Admirand et al. 2004, Chiaretti et al. 2006, Scielzo et al. 2006, Sup et al. 2004, Orchard et al. 2005). A correlation was described between maturation of tumor cells and expression of ZAP-70, ZAP-70 being more expressed in the more mature cases with IgM, higher CD20 expression and pre-B rather than pro-B phenotype (Chiaretti et al. 2006) .

3.2 Regulation of ZAP-70 expression in CLL cells

In 2005, Corcoran et al. showed that there was an association between the methylation status of the ZAP-70 gene and expression status of ZAP-70 protein (Corcoran et al. 2005). It is well established that abnormal methylation is frequent in malignancy. Hypermethylation of CpG islands within gene promoters results in gene silencing, while hypomethylaion may cause genomic instability or the upregulation of gene expression (Herman & Baylin 2003). Specifically, they found that the majority of cases expressing ZAP-70 protein lacked methylation in the intron 1-exon 2 boundery region of the ZAP-70 gene. This region was found unmethylated in circulating ZAP-70 expressing T cells, but methylated in ZAP-70 negative normal B cells. These data give a possible explanation for ZAP-70 overexpression in a subset of CLL patients. But the absence of an association between ZAP-70 expression and methylation status indicates that other factors must play a role.

ZAP-70 expression in B cells may also be regulated by the heat shock protein (Hsp)90. Hsp90 is a molecular chaperone that catalyses the conformational maturation of a large number of signaling proteins in cancer that are collectively described as 'clients'. In advanced tumours, it exists in an activated form complexed with other molecular chaperones, whereas in normal tissue it is present in a latent, uncomplexed state (Kamal et al. 2003). Using inhibitors, Castro et al. have demonstrated that ZAP-70 is an Hsp90 client protein in tumour cells, but not in T cells (Castro et al. 2005).

4. ZAP-70 in lymphocyte receptor signaling

4.1 ZAP-70 in T cell signaling

Ligation of the TCR triggers a cascade of intracellular signals that culminate in cytokine gene expression, proliferation, and the execution of T cell effector functions. After engagement of the TCR with a peptide bound to a major histocompatibility complex molecule, a signaling cascade is activated by the sequential activation of two families of PTKs. First of all, members of the Src family, Lck and FynT, initiate this process by phosphorylating tyrosine residues at the ITAMs of the CD3 ζ subunits. Once the ITAMs in the receptor cytoplasmic tails have been phosphorylated, they can recruit the next player in the signaling cascade, ZAP-70, belonging to the second family of the PTKs, the Syk family. ZAP-70 binds to the double phosphorylated ITAMs via its SH_2 domains with high affinity. Recruitment of ZAP-70 to the ITAMs leads to ZAP-70 itself becoming phosphorylated. The subsequent activation of bound ZAP-70 by phosphorylation leads to three important signaling pathways. ZAP-70 phosphorylates the adaptor proteins linker for activation of T cells (LAT) and SH2-domain-containing leukocyte protein (SLP)-76, which in turn leads to the activation of PLCγ and the Rho-GTPase Ras. PLCγ cleaves phosphatidylinositol biphosphate (PIP_2) to yield diacylglycerol (DAG) and inositol triphosphate (IP_3). IP_3 increases intracellular Ca^{2+} concentration, activating the phosphatase calcineurin, and subsequently calcineurin activates a transcription factor, nuclear factor of activated T cells (NFAT). DAG and the increase in Ca^{2+} concentration activate protein kinase C (PKC). PKC will in turn activate the transcription factor, nuclear factor κappaB (NFκB). Another pathway involves the Rho-GTPase Ras, which activates a mitogen-activated protein (MAP) kinase cascade. This Ras-induced kinase cascade induces and activates Fos, a component of the activator protein (AP)-1 transcription factor. The three transcription factors NFκB, NFAT and AP-1 act to induce specific gene transcription, leading to cell proliferation and differentiation (Figure 2).

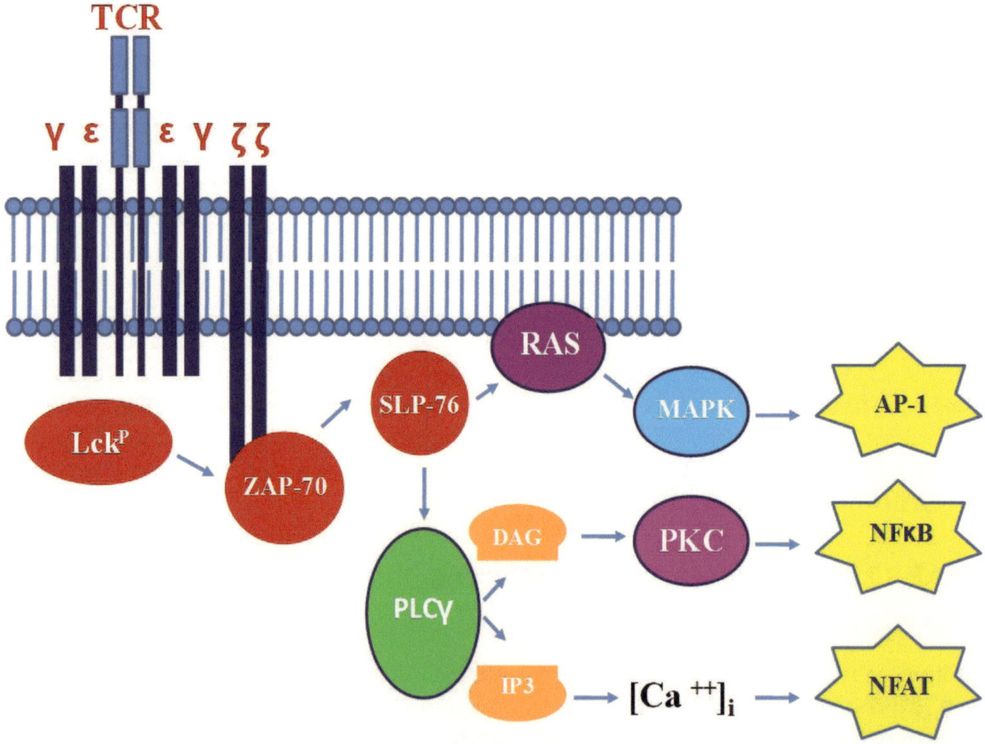

Schematic presentation of the intracellular signaling pathways initiated by the T cell receptor complex (TCR) leading to activation of three important transcription factors.

Fig. 2. ZAP-70 in T cell signaling

In addition to its importance in T cell signaling through the TCR, ZAP-70 has also been shown to be required for effective signaling by the chemokine CXCL12 (Ticchioni et al. 2002). CXCL12 is an important chemoattractant for T cells, driving them from the blood to tissue sites where they are likely to encounter antigens. Binding of CXCL12 to its ligand CXCR4 results in phosphorylation of ZAP-70, which is required for activation of downstream proteins, such as ERK and Vav-1, leading to T cell migration.

4.2 ZAP-70 in CLL B cell signaling

4.2.1 Normal B cell signaling

Signaling in normal B cells occurs after crosslinking of the surface immunoglobulin molecules (Igα and Igβ) with an antigen. On clustering of the receptors, the receptor-associated Src-family protein tyrosine kinases Blk, FynB and Lyn are activated. These activated kinases phosphorylate the ITAMs in the receptor complex, which bind and activate the cytosolic protein kinase Syk. Subsequently, Syk phosphorylates other targets, inlucing the adaptor protein BLNK, which help to recruit Tec kinases that in turn phosphorylate and activate the enzyme PLCγ. Similar to T cell signaling, PLCγ together with Ras, leads to activation of the three main signaling pathways to the nucleus: activation of NFκB, NFAT and AP-1, initiating new gene transcription that results in the differentiation, proliferation and effector actions of B cells (Figure 3).

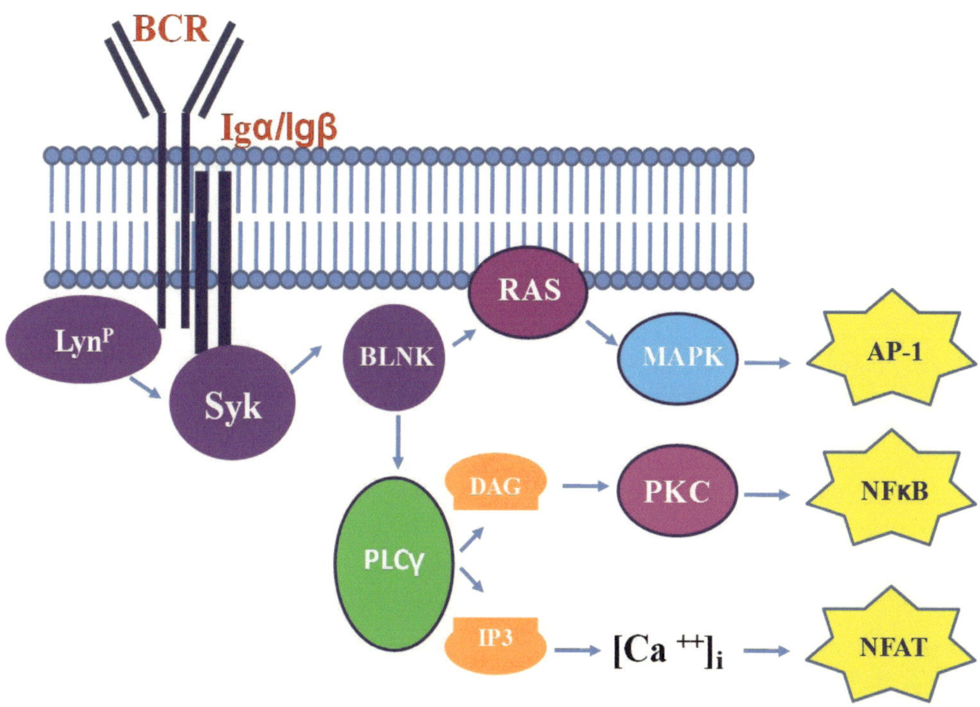

Schematic presentation of the intracellular signaling pathways initiated by cross-linking of B cell receptors (BCR) by an antigen, leading to activation of three important transcription factors.

Fig. 3. B cell signaling

4.2.2 Interplay between ZAP-70, Syk and CLL B cells

The role of ZAP-70 in proximal signaling after TCR activation and its homology with Syk, suggest that ZAP-70 may augment signaling through the BCR, thus, providing a biological explanation for the more aggressive clinical outcome of the ZAP-70 positive subgroup of patients (Chen et al. 2002). Nevertheless, the molecular mechanisms underlying the role of ZAP-70 in BCR signaling remain largely unknown. In Figure 4 the interactions between ZAP-70, Syk and BCR signaling is shown.

Studies, performed in the eighties and nineties had indicated that CLL cells varied in their capacity to respond to IgM ligation (Hivroz et al. 1986, Karray et al. 1987). In general, CLL cells were less able to respond to BCR stimulation than normal B cells (Lankester et al. 1995). Furtermore, several investigators found that, upon IgM crosslinking, CLL cells with unmutated Ig genes showed significantly increased levels of tyrosine-phosphorylated proteins, including Syk, compared to CLL cells that expressed mutated Ig receptors (Lanham et al. 2003, Chen et al. 2002). Remarkably, this was not related to differences in the levels of Syk protein found (Semichon et al. 1997).

In 2002, Chen et al. linked this phenomenon to the expression of ZAP-70. They found a greater increase in Syk tyrosine phosphorylation in cells expressing ZAP-70 compared to CLL cells lacking the protein. Consistent with this notion, they found that, besides Syk, also ZAP-70 itself undergoes tyrosine phosphorylation and complexes with the proteins of the BCR complex. At that time, two possible explanations were put forward. ZAP-70 might function to enhance BCR signaling by phosphorylation of specific motifs in CLL cells and thereby lower the threshold for Syk phosphorylation. Alternatively, expression of ZAP-70 in CLL cells might enhance the stability of phosphorylated Syk, allowing accumulation of the functional form of Syk in CLL cells.

In a subsequent study, the same group (Chen et al. 2005) examined samples that expressed unmutated IgV_H genes without ZAP-70 or samples carrying mutated IgV_H genes with ZAP-70, allowing them to examine the relative importance of ZAP-70 versus the IgV_H mutational status in influencing the relative intensity of IgM signaling. A greater Ca^{2+} influx was seen in samples expressing ZAP-70 independently of the mutational status. Therefore, it was concluded that the induced increase in phosphorylated forms of Syk, BLNK or PLCγ and Ca^{2+} influx after IgM ligation appeared more closely associated with the expression of ZAP-70, rather than with the expression of unmutated IgV_H. However, it could not be excluded that secondary factors other than ZAP-70 might also have been associated with the mutational status of the leukemic cells. To challenge this hypothesis it was required to transduce the CLL cells. Transduction studies revealed that expression of ZAP-70 in initially ZAP-70-negative CLL cells was sufficient to enhance IgM signaling.

4.2.3 ZAP-70 tyrosine phosphorylation

Gobessi et al. explored in 2007 the phosphorylation of ZAP-70 in CLL cells (Gobessi et al. 2007). ZAP-70 was found to be inefficiently activated in CLL and relatively weakly activated compared to Syk. Phosphorylation of Tyr319 and Tyr493 could not be detected. Phosphorylation of these tyrosines are required for the catalytic activation of ZAP-70 (Figure 1). Phosphorylation of the corresponding tyrosines in Syk was readily detectable with the same phospho-specific antibodies (Gobessi et al. 2007). ZAP-70 contains additional sites of tyrosine phosphorylation (Figure 1) not involved in the regulation of its catalytic activity, but regulating the recruitment of downstream signaling molecules and adaptor proteins. With the use of specific antibodies against Tyr292 constitutive phosphorylation of Tyr292 in CLL B cells was demonstrated. Although, BCR stimulation did not induce a significant change in the level of Tyr292 phosphorylation, suggesting that the interactions mediated by this tyrosine do not require additional phosphorylation. Instead, after IgM ligation an association between c-Cbl and PI3K and ZAP-70 (Gobessi et al. 2007) was observed. Additionally, an association between ZAP-70 and Shc, which requires phosphorylation at Tyr474, was detected. The same authors, in agreement with Chen et al. (2005), reported a stronger and prolonged BCR-induced phosphorylation of Syk, ERK and Akt in ZAP-70 transfected CLL cells.

4.2.4 Molecular interactions of ZAP-70 in CLL and downstream effects

To our knowledge, how ZAP-70 enhances BCR signaling in CLL cells is not known. It is conceivable that the capacity of ZAP-70 to enhance BCR signaling is not dependent upon its kinase activity. Two findings support this hypothesis. First, although Syk and ZAP-70 play similar roles in receptor signaling, Syk has approximately a 100-fold greater kinase activity in vitro than does ZAP-70 (Latour et al. 1996). Second, the kinase specific tyrosines are not phosphorylated in CLL cells (Gobessi et al. 2007). To address this, Chen et al. (Chen et al. 2007) transduced ZAP-70 negative cells with an adenovirus containing a ZAP-70 lacking kinase activity. In these cells, similar responses were observed after IgM stimulation compared to CLL cells naturally expressing ZAP-70 or cells being transduced with the wild-type ZAP-70. This unequivocally shows that ZAP-70 doesn't enhance BCR signaling by means of its intrinsic kinase activity.

Subsequently, Chen et al. as well as Gobessi et al. considered the hypothesis that ZAP-70 instead may enhance BCR signaling indirectly by enhancing the stability of activated Syk following ligation of the BCR. It is known that activated ZAP-70 and Syk are targets of the E3 ubiquitin ligase, c-Cbl, which in turn directs polyubiquitination and proteosomal degradation of the activated PTK (Fournel et al. 1996, Lupher et al. 1998, Rao et al. 2002). Possibly, the activated ZAP-70 may compete with activated Syk for binding to c-Cbl and thereby prolong the half-life of activated Syk. However, transduction of CLL cells with an adenovirus encoding a mutant form of ZAP-70 carrying a mutation at position 292, which abrogates the ability of the mutant form to interact with c-Cbl, also enhanced BCR signaling of ZAP-70 negative CLL cells. So, binding of C-cbl to Tyr292 (Gobessi et al. 2007) is unlikely to account for the capacity of ZAP-70 to enhance BCR signaling in CLL B cells.

Another explanation, proposed by both groups, is that ZAP-70 functions as an adaptor protein that facilitates the recruitment of other signaling molecules to the activated BCR. The associations with PI3K and Shc after IgM stimulation are noteworthy in this respect because these proteins are involved in the activation of Akt and ERK, respectively (Gobessi et al. 2007). In addition to this, examination of additional constructs encoding mutant forms of ZAP-70 that lacked a functional SH2 domain revealed that both SH2 domains are required for enhanced IgM signaling. This suggests that docking at the ITAM may be necessary for ZAP-70 to have an effect on CLL Ig receptor signaling (Chen et al. 2007).

The finding that ZAP-70 may enhance IgM signaling by functioning as an adaptor protein is further confirmed by zum Buschenfelde et al. (2010). The interaction of Ig receptors with their ligands has been shown to occur within an organized contact zone known as the immune synapse. Formation of the immune synapse is accompanied by a remodeling of specialized membrane microdomains enriched in sphingolipids and cholesterol known as lipid rafts (Viola & Gupta 2007). In T cells, ZAP-70 is known to be required for clustering signaling molecules into lipid rafts (Blanchard et al. 2002). This group investigated the distribution of ZAP-70 and signaling molecules like PKC-βII in lipid raft domains before and after BCR stimulation . They found that ZAP-70 was constitutively expressed in the raft domains. Accordingly, these cells constitutively expressed PKC-βII in lipid rafts, whereas the expression of PKC-βII was negligible in raft fractions of ZAP-70 negative patients, although total amounts of PKC-βII was expressed in the same amounts in whole-cell lysates in both groups. Signaling through the BCR recruited accessory ZAP-70 and PKC-βII into lipid raft domains (zum Buschenfelde et al. 2010). These experiments demonstrate that ZAP-70 may function as an adaptor protein in specific lipid raft domains, and therefore recruits specific signaling molecules towards the immune synapse.

Although reduced BCR internalization by ZAP-70 is never established in CLL cells, it could be a fourth explanation for increasing the magnitude and duration of BCR signaling. Transfection of ZAP-70 in BJAB B cells downmodulates BCR internalization (Gobessi et al. 2007) explaining how ZAP-70 could contribute to the stronger signaling observed in CLL B cells.

As described above, an important mediator of BCR signaling is NFκB, encoded by a family of transcription factors which are key regulators of differentiation and survival in B cells. In humans they include five members: c-Rel, Rel B, p50, p52 and p65 or Rel A. These factors form homo- or heterodimers, which in the resting state are retained in the cytoplasm by binding to the inhibitory IκB proteins. Upon different stimuli, including ligation of BCR, the IκB proteins are phosphorylated by IκB kinases (IKK) and degraded by the proteasome. Consequently, the NFκB dimers become free to translocate to the nucleus and activate the transcription of their target genes. These include antiapoptotic genes (Bcl-2, Mcl-1, Survivin), inflammatory genes (COX-2, MMP-9, VEGF) and genes encoding adhesion molecules, chemokines (IL-1β, IL-6, IL-8) and cell cycle regulatory proteins (Cyclin D1, c-Myc) (Hayden & Ghosh 2008). More generally, NFκB has been implicated in tumorigenesis and survival of a growing list of leukemias and lymphomas (Karin & Lin 2002).

CLL cells have been reported to exhibit high constitutive NFκB activation compared with normal B lymphocytes (Cuni et al. 2004, Furman et al. 2000, Tracey et al. 2005). Although the exact factors responsible for the constitutive expression of NFκB are not fully resolved, many factors, including Akt activation, BCR signaling, CD40 ligation, IL-4 and B cell activating factor (BAFF), have been shown to increase NFκB activity and enhance CLL survival, with members of the Bcl-2 family being principal transcriptional targets (Petlickovski et al. 2005). Hewamana (2008) found an association between ZAP-70 expression and the ability of CLL cells to activate NFκB (Hewamana et al. 2008). Furthermore, they found that the magnitude of the change in NFκB after stimulation with anti-IgM is associated with the suppression of in vitro apoptosis. Lopez-Guerra et al. (2009) tested a specific IκB kinase inhibitor, BMS-435541, and found that CLL cells expressing ZAP-

70 are more sensitive to this IKK inhibitor compared to CLL cells without ZAP-70. This supports the hypothesis that there is a functional link between ZAP-70 and NFκB. On the other hand, these results also imply that the therapeutic combination of NFκB inhibitors with other chemotherapeutic drugs, represents a novel strategy especially for the group with high ZAP-70, known to be more resistant to agents currently in use (Lopez-Guerra et al. 2009).

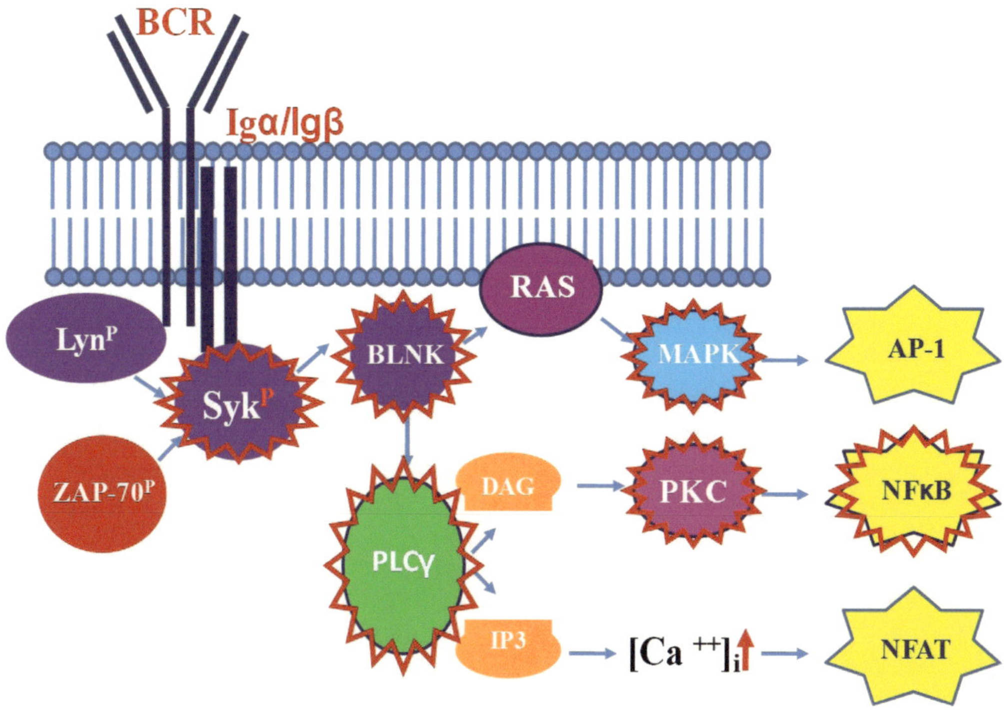

Schematic presentation of the interaction of ZAP-70 into the intracellular signaling pathways occurring in a CLL cell after stimulation of the B cell receptor. Syk, BLNK, PLCγ, MAPK, PKC and NFκB (enclosed by a red line) are potentially stimulated by ZAP-70. Also the phosphorylation of Syk (red P) and calcium influx (red arrow) may be augmented by ZAP-70.

Fig. 4. ZAP-70 in CLL signaling in poor prognosis CLL

5. Interaction of ZAP-70 with the leukemic microenvironment

In contrast with their long-living capacities in the human body, CLL cells tend to undergo rapid apoptotic cell death when incubated in vitro. This has raised the hypothesis of pro-survival environmental factors existing *in vivo*, supporting the CLL cells in their survival and growth (Ghia et al. 2002).

The peripheral blood of CLL patients contains an accumulation of mature B cells that have escaped programmed cell death and have undergone cell cycle arrest in the G0/G1 phase lacking metabolic activity. However, when in *in vivo* experiments patients drank deuterated water (^2H_2O) cell generation rates were in the range between 0,1 to 1,75 % of the entire CLL clone per day (Messmer et al. 2005). Considering a CLL clone to contain 10^{12}-10^{14} cells, an extensive number of 10^9 to 10^{12} cells are produced each day. This implies that, although there is a virtual absence of proliferative cells in peripheral blood, ill-defined areas of proliferation are existing in the bone marrow and affected lymph nodes (Herishanu et al. 2011). Indeed, interactions with stromal cells, or nurse-like cells, or interactions between CD38 and its ligand CD31 rescue CLL cells from apoptosis in vitro and probably do the same in vivo (Chiorazzi et al. 2005), and furthermore enhance proliferation of the cells. Below, several interactions between CLL cells and by-stander cells will be discussed, especially those findings that correlate with the more aggressive nature of the ZAP-70 positive disease.

5.1 CD38 and ZAP-70

CD38 is a transmembrane glycoprotein that mediates cell-cell interactions (Deaglio et al. 1998). CD38 expression is significantly associated with unmutated IgVH genes in CLL, also with ZAP-70 and subsequently with a more aggressive disease (Damle et al. 1999).

In CLL, chemokines are reported to contribute significantly to the delivery of growth signals to the malignant CLL cells expressing functional receptors. Knowing that ZAP-70 is an essential element in the signaling cascade initiated via CXCR4 in T cells and knowing that the combination of CD38 and ZAP-70 defines a subgroup of patients with the highest migratory potential towards the ligand for CXCR4, SDF1α, it is tempting to speculate that the CD38-ZAP-70 axis synergizes with the SDF1α-CXCR4 pathway (Deaglio et al. 2007).

SDF1α has previously been shown to exert both a chemotactic effect and a prosurvival effect on CLL cells, being a crucial mechanism through which stromal cells or nurse like cells support CLL cells in vitro (Burger et al. 1999, Burger et al. 2000). The finding that CLL cells proliferate at sites where stromal cells are present suggest that SDF1α is an important factor in CLL pathogenesis. Moreover, several groups confirmed an increased level of CXCR4 on the surface of CLL cells when compared with normal B cells (Richardson et al. 2006, Mohle et al. 1999, Burger et al. 1999). Treatment of CLL cells with SDF1α resulted in a rapid and sustained ERK activation profile only in the ZAP-70 positive subgroup. Furthermore, treatment with SDF1α in vitro of ZAP-70 positive but not in ZAP-70 negative cells, resulted in a longer survival. Sustained ERK activation can lead to the initiation of transcription of genes involved in both proliferation and survival (Burger et al. 2000, Xia et al. 1995, Murphy et al. 2002). This could be the explanation for both survival and proliferative advantages seen in ZAP-70 positive cells. These results indicate that ZAP-70 positive cells are more responsive to signals derived from their surrounding environment.

5.2 CCR7 and ZAP-70

Several groups found that CCR7 is upregulated on the surface of circulating peripheral blood CLL cells when compared with healthy control peripheral blood B cells (Richardson et al. 2006, Till et al. 2002, Lopez-Giral et al. 2004, Ghobrial et al. 2004). Moreover, Richardson et al. (2006) demonstrates that CCR7 levels are increased in ZAP-70 positive CLL cells when compared with ZAP-70 negative CLL cells. This upregulation in CCR7 confers an increased ability to respond to its ligands, CCL19 and CCL21. Both chemokines are important in both T and B lymphocyte trafficking (Figure 5). Prior studies in B cells (Reif et al. 2002) have shown that antigen engagement upregulates expression of CCR7 and can facilitate the movement of these cells into the lymph nodes and localization to the B/T cells

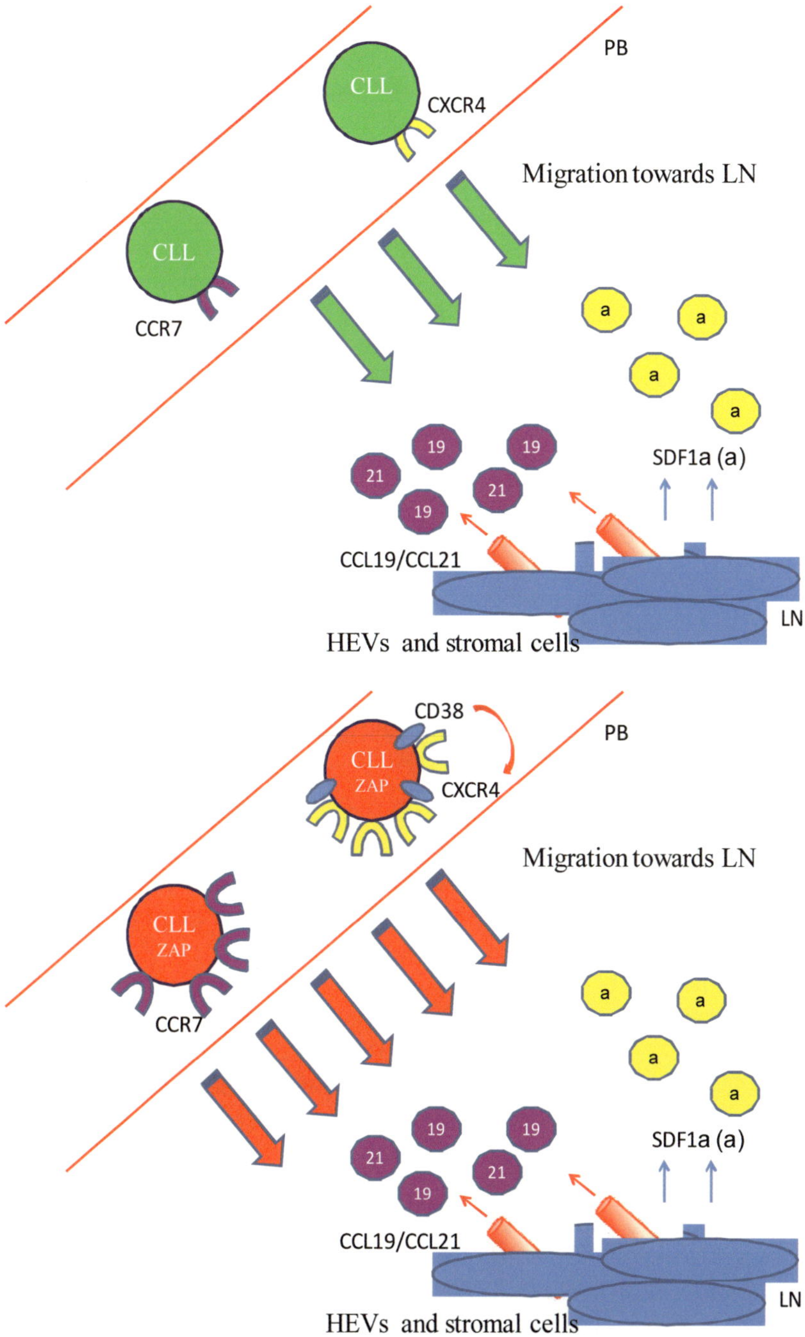

LN: lymph nodes; HEV: high endothelial venules
Upper: CLL ZAP⁻ cells;
Lower: CLL ZAP⁺ cells: In ZAP-70 positive cells, increased levels of CCR7 and the interplay between ZAP-70, CD38 and CXCR4 facilitate movement and migratory potential towards lymph nodes.

Fig. 5. Migration of CLL cells towards the lymph nodes

boundary. Since increased CCR7 expression has been documented following antigen contact, this could be reflecting either an increased level of antigen contact, which is likely to be the case for both ZAP-70 positive and ZAP-70 negative CLL B cells, as both cell types have been shown to resemble activated B cells (Damle et al. 2002, Herishanu et al. 2011), or an increased ability to respond to antigen contact. Herishanu et al. (2011) further described the increased proliferative signature of the CLL cells residing in the lymph nodes and bone marrow, due to a more intensive BCR triggering. ZAP-70 helps in a more sustained activation state after BCR triggering. The finding that CCR7 levels are lower in lymph node CLL cells than in peripheral blood CLL cells is suggestive of it being involved in migration to the lymph nodes (Till et al. 2002, Lopez-Giral et al. 2004, Ghobrial et al. 2004).

6. Summary

It remains largely unkown why ZAP-70 is or is not expressed in CLL. Hsp90 may be important in this respect. Although the precise molecular mechanism of the role of ZAP-70 in CLL B cells is not yet fully resolved, many hypotheses have been put forward suggesting multiple functions. Strikingly, it is improbable that ZAP-70 exerts its role by its kinase activity. ZAP-70 in CLL may be stabilizing SYK, creating more sustained phosphorylation and in association increasing the proliferative capacity. Moreover, ZAP-70 functions as an adaptor protein that facilitates the recruitment of other signaling molecules to the activated BCR. Also the internalization of the BCR after stimulation may be reduced due to intervention of ZAP-70. An important mechanism explaining prolonged survival of CLL cells has been attributed to its interaction with the microenvironment. In this interaction, ZAP-70 may also be of relevance.

7. References

Admirand, J. H., G. Z. Rassidakis, L. V. Abruzzo, J. R. Valbuena, D. Jones & L. J. Medeiros (2004) Immunohistochemical detection of ZAP-70 in 341 cases of non-Hodgkin and Hodgkin lymphoma. *Mod Pathol,* 17, 954-61.

Au-Yeung, B. B., S. Deindl, L. Y. Hsu, E. H. Palacios, S. E. Levin, J. Kuriyan & A. Weiss (2009) The structure, regulation, and function of ZAP-70. *Immunological reviews,* 228, 41-57.

Blanchard, N., V. Di Bartolo & C. Hivroz (2002) In the immune synapse, ZAP-70 controls T cell polarization and recruitment of signaling proteins but not formation of the synaptic pattern. *Immunity,* 17, 389-99.

Bosch, F., A. Muntanola, E. Gine, A. Carrio, N. Villamor, C. Moreno, M. Crespo & E. Montserrat (2006) Clinical implications of ZAP-70 expressionin chronic lymphocytic leukemia. *Cytometry B Clin Cytom,* 70, 214-7.

Burger, J. A., M. Burger & T. J. Kipps (1999) Chronic lymphocytic leukemia B cells express functional CXCR4 chemokine receptors that mediate spontaneous migration beneath bone marrow stromal cells. *Blood,* 94, 3658-67.

Burger, J. A., N. Tsukada, M. Burger, N. J. Zvaifler, M. Dell'Aquila & T. J. Kipps (2000) Blood-derived nurse-like cells protect chronic lymphocytic leukemia B cells from spontaneous apoptosis through stromal cell-derived factor-1. *Blood,* 96, 2655-63.

Castro, J. E., C. E. Prada, O. Loria, A. Kamal, L. Chen, F. J. Burrows & T. J. Kipps (2005) ZAP-70 is a novel conditional heat shock protein 90 (Hsp90) client: inhibition of Hsp90 leads to ZAP-70 degradation, apoptosis, and impaired signaling in chronic lymphocytic leukemia. *Blood,* 106, 2506-12.

Chan, A. C., M. Iwashima, C. W. Turck & A. Weiss (1992) ZAP-70: a 70 kd protein-tyrosine kinase that associates with the TCR zeta chain. *Cell,* 71, 649-62.

Chen, L., J. Apgar, L. Huynh, F. Dicker, T. Giago-McGahan, L. Rassenti, A. Weiss & T. J. Kipps (2005) ZAP-70 directly enhances IgM signaling in chronic lymphocytic leukemia. *Blood,* 105, 2036-41.

Chen, L., L. Huynh, J. Apgar, L. Tang, L. Rassenti, A. Weiss & T. J. Kipps (2007) ZAP-70 enhances IgM signaling independent of its kinase activity in chronic lymphocytic leukemia. *Blood.*

Chen, L., G. Widhopf, L. Huynh, L. Rassenti, K. R. Rai, A. Weiss & T. J. Kipps (2002) Expression of ZAP-70 is associated with increased B-cell receptor signaling in chronic lymphocytic leukemia. *Blood,* 100, 4609-14.

Chiaretti, S., A. Guarini, M. S. De Propris, S. Tavolaro, S. Intoppa, A. Vitale, S. Iacobelli, L. Elia, C. Ariola, J. Ritz & R. Foa (2006) ZAP-70 expression in acute lymphoblastic leukemia: association with the E2A/PBX1 rearrangement and the pre-B stage of differentiation and prognostic implications. *Blood,* 107, 197-204.

Chiorazzi, N., K. R. Rai & M. Ferrarini (2005) Chronic lymphocytic leukemia. *N Engl J Med,* 352, 804-15.

Corcoran, M., A. Parker, J. Orchard, Z. Davis, M. Wirtz, O. J. Schmitz & D. Oscier (2005) ZAP-70 methylation status is associated with ZAP-70 expression status in chronic lymphocytic leukemia. *Haematologica,* 90, 1078-88.

Crespo, M., F. Bosch, N. Villamor, B. Bellosillo, D. Colomer, M. Rozman, S. Marce, A. Lopez-Guillermo, E. Campo & E. Montserrat (2003) ZAP-70 expression as a surrogate for immunoglobulin-variable-region mutations in chronic lymphocytic leukemia. *N Engl J Med,* 348, 1764-75.

Crespo, M., N. Villamor, E. Gine, A. Muntanola, D. Colomer, T. Marafioti, M. Jones, M. Camos, E. Campo, E. Montserrat & F. Bosch (2006) ZAP-70 expression in normal pro/pre B cells, mature B cells, and in B-cell acute lymphoblastic leukemia. *Clin Cancer Res,* 12, 726-34.

Cuni, S., P. Perez-Aciego, G. Perez-Chacon, J. A. Vargas, A. Sanchez, F. M. Martin-Saavedra, S. Ballester, J. Garcia-Marco, J. Jorda & A. Durantez (2004) A sustained activation of PI3K/NF-kappa B pathway is critical for the survival of chronic lymphocytic leukemia B cells. *Leukemia,* 18, 1391-1400.

Cutrona, G., M. Colombo, S. Matis, D. Reverberi, M. Dono, V. Tarantino, N. Chiorazzi & M. Ferrarini (2006) B lymphocytes in humans express ZAP-70 when activated in vivo. *Eur J Immunol,* 36, 558-69.

Damle, R. N., F. Ghiotto, A. Valetto, E. Albesiano, F. Fais, X. J. Yan, C. P. Sison, S. L. Allen, J. Kolitz, P. Schulman, V. P. Vinciguerra, P. Budde, J. Frey, K. R. Rai, M. Ferrarini & N. Chiorazzi (2002) B-cell chronic lymphocytic leukemia cells express a surface membrane phenotype of activated, antigen-experienced B lymphocytes. *Blood,* 99, 4087-93.

Damle, R. N., T. Wasil, F. Fais, F. Ghiotto, A. Valetto, S. L. Allen, A. Buchbinder, D. Budman, K. Dittmar, J. Kolitz, S. M. Lichtman, P. Schulman, V. P. Vinciguerra, K. R. Rai, M. Ferrarini & N. Chiorazzi (1999) Ig V gene mutation status and CD38 expression as novel prognostic indicators in chronic lymphocytic leukemia. *Blood,* 94, 1840-7.

Deaglio, S., M. Morra, R. Mallone, C. M. Ausiello, E. Prager, G. Garbarino, U. Dianzani, H. Stockinger & F. Malavasi (1998) Human CD38 (ADP-ribosyl cyclase) is a counter-receptor of CD31, an Ig superfamily member. *Journal of Immunology,* 160, 395-402.

Deaglio, S., T. Vaisitti, S. Aydin, L. Bergui, G. D'Arena, L. Bonello, P. Omede, M. Scatolini, O. Jaksic, G. Chiorino, D. Efremov & F. Malavasi (2007) CD38 and ZAP-70 are functionally linked and mark CLL cells with high migratory potential. *Blood,* 110, 4012-21.

Fournel, M., D. Davidson, R. Weil & A. Veillette (1996) Association of tyrosine protein kinase Zap-70 with the protooncogene product p120c-cbl in T lymphocytes. *The Journal of experimental medicine,* 183, 301-6.

Furman, R. R., Z. Asgary, J. O. Mascarenhas, H. C. Liou & E. J. Schattner (2000) Modulation of NF-kappa B activity and apoptosis in chronic lymphocytic leukemia B cells. *Journal of Immunology,* 164, 2200-2206.

Ghia, P., L. Granziero, M. Chilosi & F. Caligaris-Cappio (2002) Chronic B cell malignancies and bone marrow microenvironment. *Semin Cancer Biol,* 12, 149-55.

Ghobrial, I. M., N. D. Bone, M. J. Stenson, A. Novak, K. E. Hedin, N. E. Kay & S. M. Ansell (2004) Expression of the chemokine receptors CXCR4 and CCR7 and disease progression in B-cell chronic lymphocytic leukemia/ small lymphocytic lymphoma. *Mayo Clinic proceedings. Mayo Clinic,* 79, 318-25.

Gobessi, S., L. Laurenti, P. G. Longo, S. Sica, G. Leone & D. G. Efremov (2007) ZAP-70 enhances B-cell-receptor signaling despite absent or inefficient tyrosine kinase activation in chronic lymphocytic leukemia and lymphoma B cells. *Blood,* 109, 2032-9.

Guillaume, N., C. Alleaume, D. Munfus, J. C. Capiod, G. Touati, B. Pautard, B. Desablens, J. J. Lefrere, F. Gouilleux, K. Lassoued & V. Gouilleux-Gruart (2005) ZAP-70 tyrosine kinase is constitutively expressed and phosphorylated in B-lineage acute lymphoblastic leukemia cells. *Haematologica,* 90, 899-905.

Hamblin, T. J., Z. Davis, A. Gardiner, D. G. Oscier & F. K. Stevenson (1999) Unmutated Ig V(H) genes are associated with a more aggressive form of chronic lymphocytic leukemia. *Blood,* 94, 1848-54.

Hayden, M. S. & S. Ghosh (2008) Shared principles in NF-kappaB signaling. *Cell,* 132, 344-62.

Herishanu, Y., P. Perez-Galan, D. Liu, A. Biancotto, S. Pittaluga, B. Vire, F. Gibellini, N. Njuguna, E. Lee, L. Stennett, N. Raghavachari, P. Liu, J. P. McCoy, M. Raffeld, M. Stetler-Stevenson, C. Yuan, R. Sherry, D. C. Arthur, I. Maric, T. White, G. E. Marti, P. Munson, W. H. Wilson & A. Wiestner (2011) The lymph node microenvironment promotes B-cell receptor signaling, NF-kappaB activation, and tumor proliferation in chronic lymphocytic leukemia. *Blood,* 117, 563-74.

Herman, J. G. & S. B. Baylin (2003) Gene silencing in cancer in association with promoter hypermethylation. *The New England journal of medicine,* 349, 2042-54.

Hewamana, S., S. Alghazal, T. T. Lin, M. Clement, C. Jenkins, M. L. Guzman, C. T. Jordan, S. Neelakantan, P. A. Crooks, A. K. Burnett, G. Pratt, C. Fegan, C. Rowntree, P. Brennan & C. Pepper (2008) The NF-kappa B subunit Rel A is associated with in vitro survival and clinical disease progression in chronic lymphocytic leukemia and represents a promising therapeutic target. *Blood,* 111, 4681-4689.

Hivroz, C., C. Grillot-Courvalin, J. C. Brouet & M. Seligmann (1986) Heterogeneity of responsiveness of chronic lymphocytic leukemic B cells to B cell growth factor or interleukin 2. *European journal of immunology,* 16, 1001-4.

Kamal, A., L. Thao, J. Sensintaffar, L. Zhang, M. F. Boehm, L. C. Fritz & F. J. Burrows (2003) A high-affinity conformation of Hsp90 confers tumour selectivity on Hsp90 inhibitors. *Nature,* 425, 407-10.

Karin, M. & A. Lin (2002) NF-kappaB at the crossroads of life and death. *Nature immunology,* 3, 221-7.

Karray, S., H. Merle-Beral, A. Vazquez, J. P. Gerard, P. Debre & P. Galanaud (1987) Functional heterogeneity of B-CLL lymphocytes: dissociated responsiveness to growth factors and distinct requirements for a first activation signal. *Blood,* 70, 1105-10.

Klein, U., Y. Tu, G. A. Stolovitzky, M. Mattioli, G. Cattoretti, H. Husson, A. Freedman, G. Inghirami, L. Cro, L. Baldini, A. Neri, A. Califano & R. Dalla-Favera (2001) Gene expression profiling of B cell chronic lymphocytic leukemia reveals a homogeneous phenotype related to memory B cells. *J Exp Med,* 194, 1625-38.

Lanham, S., T. Hamblin, D. Oscier, R. Ibbotson, F. Stevenson & G. Packham (2003) Differential signaling via surface IgM is associated with V-H gene mutational status and CD38 expression in chronic lymphocytic leukemia. *Blood,* 101, 1087-1093.

Lankester, A. C., G. M. van Schijndel, C. E. van der Schoot, M. H. van Oers, C. J. van Noesel & R. A. van Lier (1995) Antigen receptor nonresponsiveness in chronic lymphocytic leukemia B cells. *Blood,* 86, 1090-7.

Latour, S., L. M. Chow & A. Veillette (1996) Differential intrinsic enzymatic activity of Syk and Zap-70 protein-tyrosine kinases. *The Journal of biological chemistry,* 271, 22782-90.

Letestu, R., A. Rawstron, P. Ghia, N. Villamor, N. Boeckx, S. Boettcher, A. M. Buhl, J. Duerig, R. Ibbotson, A. Kroeber, A. Langerak, M. Le Garff-Tavernier, I. Mockridge, A. Morilla, R. Padmore, L. Rassenti, M. Ritgen, M. Shehata, P. Smolewski, P. Staib, M. Ticchioni, C. Walker & F. Ajchenbaum-Cymbalista (2006) Evaluation of ZAP-70 expression by flow cytometry in chronic lymphocytic leukemia: A multicentric international harmonization process. *Cytometry. Part B, Clinical cytometry,* 70, 309-14.

Lopez-Giral, S., N. E. Quintana, M. Cabrerizo, M. Alfonso-Perez, M. Sala-Valdes, V. G. De Soria, J. M. Fernandez-Ranada, E. Fernandez-Ruiz & C. Munoz (2004) Chemokine receptors that mediate B cell homing to secondary lymphoid tissues are highly expressed in B cell chronic lymphocytic leukemia and non-Hodgkin lymphomas with widespread nodular dissemination. *Journal of leukocyte biology,* 76, 462-71.

Lopez-Guerra, M., G. Roue, P. Perez-Galan, R. Alonso, N. Villamor, E. Montserrat, E. Campo & D. Colomer (2009) p65 activity and ZAP-70 status predict the sensitivity of chronic lymphocytic leukemia cells to the selective IkappaB kinase inhibitor BMS-345541. *Clinical cancer research : an official journal of the American Association for Cancer Research,* 15, 2767-76.

Lupher, M. L., Jr., N. Rao, N. L. Lill, C. E. Andoniou, S. Miyake, E. A. Clark, B. Druker & H. Band (1998) Cbl-mediated negative regulation of the Syk tyrosine kinase. A critical role for Cbl phosphotyrosine-binding domain binding to Syk phosphotyrosine 323. *The Journal of biological chemistry,* 273, 35273-81.

Messmer, B. T., D. Messmer, S. L. Allen, J. E. Kolitz, P. Kudalkar, D. Cesar, E. J. Murphy, P. Koduru, M. Ferrarini, S. Zupo, G. Cutrona, R. N. Damle, T. Wasil, K. R. Rai, M. K. Hellerstein & N. Chiorazzi (2005) In vivo measurements document the dynamic cellular kinetics of chronic lymphocytic leukemia B cells. *The Journal of Clinical Investigation,* 115, 755-764.

Mohle, R., C. Failenschmid, F. Bautz & L. Kanz (1999) Overexpression of the chemokine receptor CXCR4 in B cell chronic lymphocytic leukemia is associated with increased functional response to stromal cell-derived factor-1 (SDF-1). *Leukemia : official journal of the Leukemia Society of America, Leukemia Research Fund, U.K,* 13, 1954-9.

Murphy, L. O., S. Smith, R. H. Chen, D. C. Fingar & J. Blenis (2002) Molecular interpretation of ERK signal duration by immediate early gene products. *Nature cell biology,* 4, 556-64.

Nolz, J. C., R. C. Tschumper, B. T. Pittner, J. R. Darce, N. E. Kay & D. F. Jelinek (2005) ZAP-70 is expressed by a subset of normal human B-lymphocytes displaying an activated phenotype. *Leukemia,* 19, 1018-24.

Orchard, J., R. Ibbotson, G. Best, A. Parker & D. Oscier (2005) ZAP-70 in B cell malignancies. *Leuk Lymphoma,* 46, 1689-98.

Petlickovski, A., L. Laurenti, X. P. Li, S. Marietti, P. Chiusolo, S. Sica, G. Leone & D. G. Efremov (2005) Sustained signaling through the B-cell receptor induces Mcl-1 and promotes survival of chronic lymphocytic leukemia B cells. *Blood,* 105, 4820-4827.

Rao, N., I. Dodge & H. Band (2002) The Cbl family of ubiquitin ligases: critical negative regulators of tyrosine kinase signaling in the immune system. *Journal of leukocyte biology,* 71, 753-63.

Reif, K., E. H. Ekland, L. Ohl, H. Nakano, M. Lipp, R. Forster & J. G. Cyster (2002) Balanced responsiveness to chemoattractants from adjacent zones determines B-cell position. *Nature,* 416, 94-9.

Richardson, S. J., C. Matthews, M. A. Catherwood, H. D. Alexander, B. S. Carey, J. Farrugia, A. Gardiner, S. Mould, D. Oscier, J. A. Copplestone & A. G. Prentice (2006) ZAP-70 expression is associated with enhanced ability to respond to migratory and survival signals in B-cell chronic lymphocytic leukemia (B-CLL). *Blood,* 107, 3584-92.

Rosenwald, A., A. A. Alizadeh, G. Widhopf, R. Simon, R. E. Davis, X. Yu, L. Yang, O. K. Pickeral, L. Z. Rassenti, J. Powell, D. Botstein, J. C. Byrd, M. R. Grever, B. D. Cheson, N. Chiorazzi, W. H. Wilson, T. J. Kipps, P. O. Brown & L. M. Staudt (2001) Relation of gene expression phenotype to immunoglobulin mutation genotype in B cell chronic lymphocytic leukemia. *J Exp Med,* 194, 1639-47.

Sanchez-Aguilera, A., I. Rattmann, D. Z. Drew, L. U. Muller, V. Summey, D. M. Lucas, J. C. Byrd, C. M. Croce, Y. Gu, J. A. Cancelas, P. Johnston, T. Moritz & D. A. Williams (2010) Involvement of RhoH GTPase in the development of B-cell chronic lymphocytic leukemia. *Leukemia : official journal of the Leukemia Society of America, Leukemia Research Fund, U.K*, 24, 97-104.

Schroeder, H. W., Jr. & G. Dighiero (1994) The pathogenesis of chronic lymphocytic leukemia: analysis of the antibody repertoire. *Immunol Today*, 15, 288-94.

Scielzo, C., A. Camporeale, M. Geuna, M. Alessio, A. Poggi, M. R. Zocchi, M. Chilosi, F. Caligaris-Cappio & P. Ghia (2006) ZAP-70 is expressed by normal and malignant human B-cell subsets of different maturational stage. *Leukemia*, 20, 689-95.

Semichon, M., H. Merle-Beral, V. Lang & G. Bismuth (1997) Normal Syk protein level but abnormal tyrosine phosphorylation in B-CLL cells. *Leukemia : official journal of the Leukemia Society of America, Leukemia Research Fund, U.K*, 11, 1921-8.

Sup, S. J., R. Domiati-Saad, T. W. Kelley, R. Steinle, X. Zhao & E. D. Hsi (2004) ZAP-70 expression in B-cell hematologic malignancy is not limited to CLL/SLL. *Am J Clin Pathol*, 122, 582-7.

Ticchioni, M., C. Charvet, N. Noraz, L. Lamy, M. Steinberg, A. Bernard & M. Deckert (2002) Signaling through ZAP-70 is required for CXCL12-mediated T-cell transendothelial migration. *Blood*, 99, 3111-8.

Till, K. J., K. Lin, M. Zuzel & J. C. Cawley (2002) The chemokine receptor CCR7 and alpha4 integrin are important for migration of chronic lymphocytic leukemia cells into lymph nodes. *Blood*, 99, 2977-84.

Tracey, L., A. Perez-Rosado, M. J. Artiga, F. I. Camacho, A. Rodriguez, N. Martinez, E. Ruiz-Ballesteros, M. Mollejo, B. Martinez, M. Cuadros, J. F. Garcia, M. Lawler & M. A. Piris (2005) Expression of the NF-kappaB targets BCL2 and BIRC5/Survivin characterizes small B-cell and aggressive B-cell lymphomas, respectively. *The Journal of pathology*, 206, 123-34.

Van Bockstaele, F., A. Janssens, A. Piette, F. Callewaert, V. Pede, F. Offner, B. Verhasselt & J. Philippe (2006) Kolmogorov-Smirnov statistical test for analysis of ZAP-70 expression in B-CLL, compared with quantitative PCR and IgV(H) mutation status. *Cytometry B Clin Cytom*, 70, 302-8.

Van Bockstaele, F., B. Verhasselt & J. Philippe (2009) Prognostic markers in chronic lymphocytic leukemia: A comprehensive review. *Blood Reviews*, 23, 25-47.

Viola, A. & N. Gupta (2007) Tether and trap: regulation of membrane-raft dynamics by actin-binding proteins. *Nature reviews. Immunology*, 7, 889-96.

Wang, Y. H., L. Fan, W. Xu & J. Y. Li (2011) Detection methods of ZAP-70 in chronic lymphocytic leukemia. *Clinical and experimental medicine*.

Wange, R. L., R. Guitian, N. Isakov, J. D. Watts, R. Aebersold & L. E. Samelson (1995) Activating and inhibitory mutations in adjacent tyrosines in the kinase domain of ZAP-70. *The Journal of biological chemistry*, 270, 18730-3.

Williams, B. L., B. J. Irvin, S. L. Sutor, C. C. Chini, E. Yacyshyn, J. Bubeck Wardenburg, M. Dalton, A. C. Chan & R. T. Abraham (1999) Phosphorylation of Tyr319 in ZAP-70 is required for T-cell antigen receptor-dependent phospholipase C-gamma1 and Ras activation. *The EMBO journal*, 18, 1832-44.

Wu, J., Q. Zhao, T. Kurosaki & A. Weiss (1997) The Vav binding site (Y315) in ZAP-70 is critical for antigen receptor-mediated signal transduction. *The Journal of experimental medicine,* 185, 1877-82.

Xia, Z., M. Dickens, J. Raingeaud, R. J. Davis & M. E. Greenberg (1995) Opposing effects of ERK and JNK-p38 MAP kinases on apoptosis. *Science,* 270, 1326-31.

zum Buschenfelde, C. M., M. Wagner, G. Lutzny, M. Oelsner, Y. Feuerstacke, T. Decker, C. Bogner, C. Peschel & I. Ringshausen (2010) Recruitment of PKC-betaII to lipid rafts mediates apoptosis-resistance in chronic lymphocytic leukemia expressing ZAP-70. *Leukemia : official journal of the Leukemia Society of America, Leukemia Research Fund, U.K,* 24, 141-52.

8

Pathophysiology of Protein Kinase C Isozymes in Chronic Lymphocytic Leukaemia

John C. Allen and Joseph R. Slupsky
Department of Molecular and Clinical Cancer Medicine,
University of Liverpool, Liverpool,
United Kingdom

1. Introduction

This chapter will review the roles of protein kinase C (PKC) isozymes in chronic lymphocytic leukaemia (CLL) cells. PKC family proteins are central to many signalling pathways within cells, and some have been implicated in the oncogenesis of numerous cancers (Benimetskaya, *et al.*, 2001;Keenan, *et al.*, 1999;O'Brian, 1998). In CLL, inhibitors of PKC signalling have been shown to have cytotoxic effects on the malignant cells, and the α, β and δ isoforms of PKC have been shown to have pathophysiological roles (Holler, *et al.*, 2009;Nakagawa, *et al.*, 2006;Ringshausen, *et al.*, 2002). The aim of this chapter is to discuss whether PKC can be considered a drug target in the treatment of this disease. We will examine how inhibitors of PKCs have been used in past preclinical studies of CLL, and will discuss the roles of various PKC isozymes (namely PKCβII, PKCα, PKCδ and PKCε) in the pathology of CLL. This chapter will end with the proposal that inhibition of PKC may be useful in combination therapy through a potential role in regulating Mcl-1 expression.

2. PKC in CLL

Survival and expansion of the malignant clone in CLL involves a myriad of intrinsic and extrinsic signals and most, if not all of these signals will involve the kinase function of PKC. For example, chronic antigen stimulation of the B-cell receptor (BCR) is thought to play a key role in CLL cell survival (Chiorazzi, *et al.*, 2005), and the β isoform of PKC (PKCβ) is known to play an important role in BCR signalling (Kang, *et al.*, 2001;Saijo, *et al.*, 2002). In this context, specific targeting of PKCβ in CLL cells may either enhance or inhibit the pro-survival signals that BCR engagement provides.

A role for PKC function in CLL cell survival was first suggested in experiments using PKC agonists such as the phorbol ester 12-*0* tetradecanoylphorbol 13-acetate (TPA) and bryostatin (al-Katib, *et al.*, 1993;Drexler, *et al.*, 1989;Forbes, *et al.*, 1992;Totterman, *et al.*, 1980). These compounds are natural product analogues of diacylglycerol, which is the ligand of PKC within cells, and act to stimulate kinase activity of PKC. Initial observations showed that treatment of CLL cells with either TPA or bryostatin-1 resulted in the induction of differentiation and inhibition of spontaneous apoptosis (al-Katib, *et al.*, 1993;Barragan, *et al.*, 2002;Drexler, *et al.*, 1989;Forbes, *et al.*, 1992;Totterman, *et al.*, 1980;Varterasian, *et al.*, 2000). Exploration of the mechanism through which TPA and bryostatin induced CLL cell differentiation showed that this was likely due to PKC-mediated activation of the ERK pathway (Figure 1A). These early experiments prompted a phase I (Varterasian, *et al.*, 1998) and phase II (Varterasian, *et al.*, 2000) clinical trial of bryostatin in CLL. The findings of these studies showed that bryostatin could induce *in vivo* differentiation of the malignant cells in CLL patients (Varterasian, *et al.*, 2000). Combination of bryostatin with 2-chlorodeoxyadenosine showed promise in treating CLL in both an animal model of CLL (Mohammad, *et al.*, 1998) as well as a case report of a single patient (Ahmad, *et al.*, 2000), however, the use of bryostatin as a therapeutic agent has not been followed up. This could be because other studies have shown that TPA and bryostatin provide protection against dexamethasone- and fludarabine-induced apoptosis of CLL cells (Bellosillo, *et al.*, 1997;Kitada, *et al.*, 1999). Investigation of the mechanism through which this protection is provided showed that these compounds stimulate upregulation of the anti-apoptotic proteins Mcl-1 and XIAP (Thomas, *et al.*, 2004) (Figure 1A).

A second approach to address the role of PKC in CLL cell survival has used inhibitors of this enzyme. Thus, compounds such as UCN01 (Byrd, *et al.*, 2001;Kitada, *et al.*, 2000), PKC412 (Ganeshaguru, *et al.*, 2002), LY379196 (Abrams, *et al.*, 2007) and Bisindolymaleimide (Barragan, *et al.*, 2002;Snowden, *et al.*, 2003) have all been shown to potently induce apoptosis of CLL cells *in vitro*. Interestingly, treatment of CLL cells with UCN01 or Bisindolylmaleimide reduces the expression of Mcl-1 and XIAP (Kitada, *et al.*, 2000;Snowden, *et al.*, 2003), thereby making treated cells more susceptible to apoptosis (Figure 1B). This observation, when taken together with others showing that activation of PKC results in an upregulation of Mcl-1 and XIAP, strongly suggest that PKC is an important mediator of CLL cell survival signals.

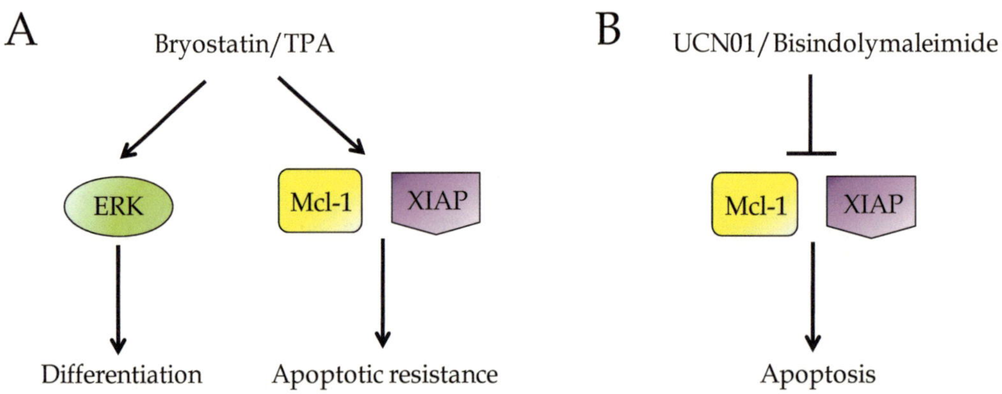

Fig. 1. Effects of PKC agonists and antagonists on CLL cells. (A) PKC agonists such as TPA and bryostatin induce ERK-mediated differentiation in CLL cells, and inhibit spontaneous apoptosis by stimulating the expression of Mcl-1 and XIAP. (B) PKC antagonists such as UCN01 or Bisindolymaleimide reduce the expression of Mcl-1 and XIAP in CLL cells thereby increasing the potential of CLL cells to undergo apoptosis.

2.1 PKC structure and function

PKCs are a family of serine/threonine kinases that share extensive structural homologies between different isotypes. Despite this homology, PKCs regulate different cellular functions in a variety of cell types, including proliferation, differentiation, apoptosis and cell survival (Tan & Parker, 2003). PKCs are divided into three subfamilies based on their regulatory domain composition, which determines what co-factors help induce their activation. Classical PKCs (PKC α, βI, βII, and γ) require the presence of DAG and calcium for activation, while novel PKCs (PKC δ, ε, η, θ) require only the presence of DAG. In contrast, atypical PKCs (PKC ζ, λ/ι) are both calcium and diacylglycerol-independent (Mellor & Parker, 1998).

The structure of all PKC family members is comprised of a C-terminal kinase domain linked by a flexible hinge segment to an N-terminal regulatory domain (Parker & Murray-Rust, 2004) (Figure 2). The kinase domain of PKC is highly conserved among isoforms and shows homology to the AGC superfamily of serine/threonine protein kinases. This domain contains the ATP- and substrate-binding sites, and also serves as a phosphorylation-dependent docking site for the regulatory molecules that interact with PKC (Newton, 2010).

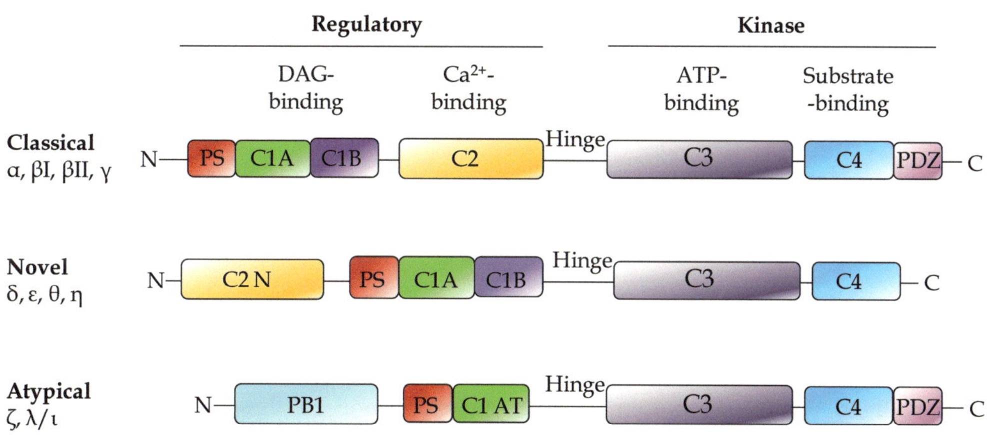

Fig. 2. Schematic representation of PKC isoform structure. The regulatory domain of PKC isoforms contain the regions necessary for membrane association and activation of the kinase. The C1 domain binds DAG/phorbol esters, and also contains a pseudosubstrate (PS) sequence at its N-terminus. The PS binds to the substrate-binding site within the catalytic domain to hold PKC in an inactive state. Atypical PKCs have a unique C1 region (C1 AT) as well as a Phox and Bem1 (PB1) region which are likely responsible for protein interaction resulting in kinase activation. The C2 domain regulates Ca^{2+}-mediated phospholipid binding in classical PKCs. Novel PKCs have a C2-like domain that does not bind Ca^{2+} (C2 N). The catalytic domain of all PKCs is conserved and contains the regions necessary for ATP-binding (the C3 domain) and for binding to substrate (the C4 domain). A PDZ region is also present in some PKC isoforms, and is responsible for protein-protein interactions following kinase activation.

The regulatory domain of PKC is divided into two regions. At the N-terminus there is a pseudosubstrate (PS) sequence that is responsible for binding the catalytic domain and maintaining the enzyme in an inactive conformation when it is in the cytoplasm (House & Kemp, 1987). This domain of PKC also contains the regions responsible for membrane targeting. Thus, classical PKCs contain motifs, termed C1 domains, that are able to bind DAG as well as phorbol esters (Newton, 1995a). Classical PKCs also have motifs, termed C2 domains, that are responsible for binding membrane phospholipids such as phosphatidylserine (PtS) and phosphatidylinositol-4-5-biphosphate (PIP_2) in a Ca^{2+}-dependent manner (Newton, 1995a). Novel and atypical PKC isoforms have a different regulatory domain structure. Novel PKCs contain tandem C1 domains that bind DAG with an affinity that is high enough to induce translocation to the membrane (Giorgione, *et al.*, 2006), and use a C2-like domain to bind phospholipids in a Ca^{2+}-independent manner (Newton, 1995a). In contrast, atypical PKCs lack a C2 domain in any format, and contain an impaired C1 domain that does not bind diacylglycerol (Newton, 1995a). Instead, atypical PKC isoforms depend largely upon protein-protein interactions for activation. For this purpose, these isoforms contain an N-terminal PB1 domain and a C-terminal PDZ ligand binding domain.

The flexible hinge region of PKCs is important in as much as it allows the close apposition of the regulatory and catalytic domains when PKC is in an inactive state. When PKC becomes activated, the hinge region allows the protein to unfold to the extent needed for the catalytic domain to interact with substrates and regulatory proteins.

2.2 PKC regulation

PKC is regulated by four key mechanisms: phosphorylation, co-factor binding, protein-protein interactions and regulated degradation. All help regulate the subcellular localisation, structure, and function of the enzyme.

2.2.1 Processing of PKC

Newly synthesised PKC is associated with membrane fractions where it is processed by a series of tightly coupled phosphorylations on serine and/or threonine residues in the catalytic domain (Newton, 2010) (Figure 3). These phosphorylations are essential before PKC can become activated, and the series in which they take place is analogous to other AGC protein kinases such as Akt. The binding of the chaperone protein heat shock protein 90 (HSP90) was identified as an initial step in the maturation of both classical and novel PKC isoforms (Gould, *et al.*, 2009). It binds to the catalytic domain of PKC and primes the enzyme for phosphorylation within the activation loop of the catalytic domain (Figure 3A). Failure of PKC to bind HSP90 results in inhibited phosphorylation at this site, misfolding of the entire protein and its consequent degradation (Balendran, *et al.*, 2000;Gould, *et al.*, 2009). Phosphorylation of the activation loop of PKC is catalyzed by 3-phosphoinositide-dependent kinase (PDK)-1, which binds to the exposed C-terminus of newly synthesised PKC that is in complex with HSP90 (Chou, *et al.*, 1998;Dutil, *et al.*, 1998;Dutil & Newton, 2000) (Figure 3A). This is followed by phosphorylation of the turn motif by the mTORC2 complex (Ikenoue, *et al.*, 2008) (Figure 3B). Phosphorylation of the turn motif stabilises the active conformation of PKC prior to autophosphorylation of the hydrophobic motif and generation of catalytically competent PKC (Behn-Krappa & Newton, 1999). Whether this latter step results from autophosphorylation is controversial because phosphorylation of the hydrophobic motif does not take place in mTORC2 deficient cells (Newton, 2010). However, because phosphorylation of the turn motif must take place before phosphorylation of the hydrophobic motif, it is likely to be very difficult to fully define the kinase(s) responsible. It is important to note here that phosphorylation of the activation loop, turn and hydrophobic motifs within PKC only results in an enzyme that is fully matured and catalytically competent, it should not be mistaken for active PKC as these sites will be phosphorylated on inactive PKC located within the cytoplasm of cells.

2.2.2 Mechanism(s) of activation

Fully matured PKC is predominantly localised to the cytosol, where it is likely maintained in specific microenvironments by interacting with regulatory proteins (Schechtman & Mochly-Rosen, 2001). Here, the enzyme is held in an inactive conformation by the N-terminal PS binding to the substrate-binding site of the catalytic domain (House & Kemp, 1987). Processes that result in a structural change in the protein so that the N-terminus of PKC is no longer in close proximity to the C-terminus result in activation of the enzyme. Typically, activation of classical isoforms of PKC occurs following the induction of PIP_2 hydrolysis within certain pathways of intracellular signalling. This generates Ca^{2+} and DAG, two second messengers crucial for the activation of classical PKCs (Beaven, 1996;Nishizuka, 1988). Ca^{2+} binds to the C2 domain of classical PKCs causing their translocation to the plasma membrane where they bind phospholipids such as PtS and PIP_2 (Cho, 2001;Newton, 1995b) (Figure 3C). Once at the membrane the C1 domain of PKC binds to membrane-bound DAG, an interaction aided by the binding of PtS (Bolsover, *et al.*, 2003;Cho, 2001). The engagement of both the C1 and C2 domains then causes a structural change in PKC that induces the release of the PS from the substrate-binding site of the catalytic domain, freeing PKC to catalyze the phosphorylation of downstream substrates (Newton, 1995a). The greater affinity of the C1 domain of novel PKC isoforms for DAG (Giorgione, *et al.*, 2006) allows the recruitment of these isoforms to membranes without the need for Ca^{2+}. Once at the membrane, novel PKC isozymes, like classical ones, unfold the regulatory domains from the catalytic domains and kinase activities ensue.

However, there are additional mechanisms of activation involving post-translational modification. Tyrosine kinases such as $pp60^{src}$ are able to bind some PKC isoforms, such as PKCδ, and catalyze their tyrosine phosphorylation (Joseloff, *et al.*, 2002;Kronfeld, *et al.*, 2000;Yuan, *et al.*, 1998). Phosphorylated tyrosine residues within PKCδ then act as docking sites for SH2 domain-containing proteins, which can further regulate the function of this PKC isoform (Leitges, *et al.*, 2002). The specific tyrosine residue where phosphorylation occurs dictates the response induced by PKCδ. The location of this phosphorylation and resultant cellular response is largely dependent upon the inciting stimulus and cell type. For example, the use of a mutant form of PKCδ containing several tyrosine residue mutations found that phosphorylation of Y^{64} and Y^{187} were important sites for regulating etoposide-induced apoptosis in C6 glioma cells (Blass, *et al.*, 2002). In contrast, viral infection of PC12 cells induced the phosphorylation of Y^{52}, Y^{64} and Y^{155} in PKCδ and these sites proved essential in mediating the antiapoptotic effects of this PKC isoform (Wert & Palfrey, 2000).

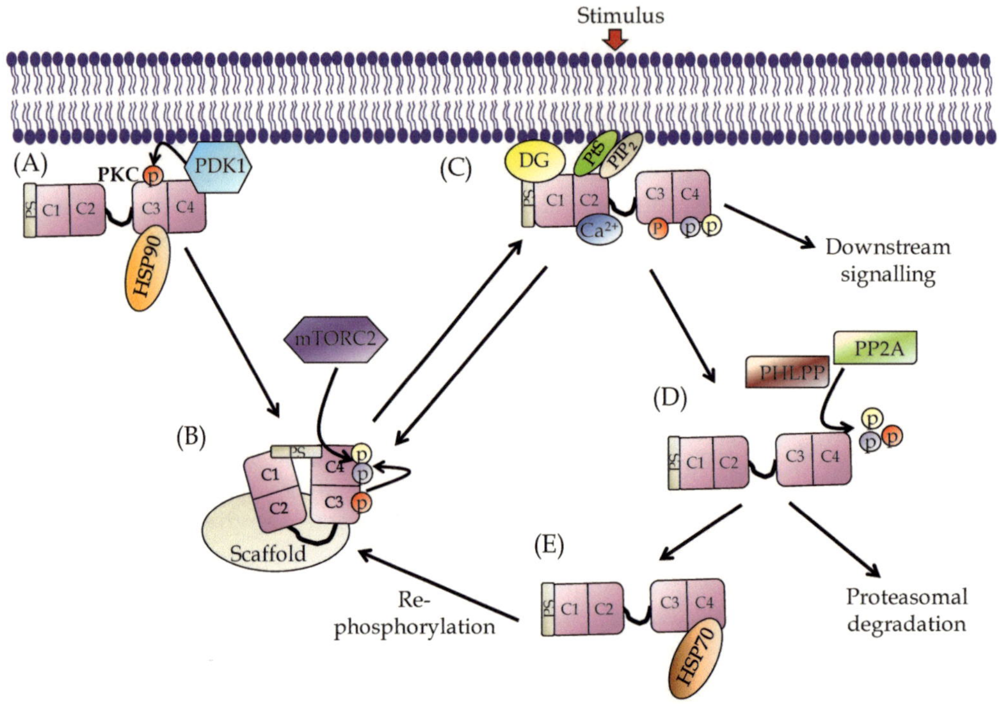

Fig. 3. PKC regulation (adapted from Newton, *et al.*, 2010). (A) HSP90 binds the kinase domain of newly synthesised PKC within the C3 region and primes it for phosphorylation of the activation motif by PDK-1. (B) mTORC2 and/or autophosphorylation is then responsible for phosphorylating the turn and then hydrophobic motifs within the C4 region of the catalytic domain. This results in fully-matured PKC which is then maintained in different cytosolic locations by interacting with scaffold proteins, and in an inactive state through interaction of the pseudosubstrate (PS) in the C1 region of the regulatory domain with the substrate binding site (C4) in the catalytic domain. (**C**) Specific stimuli induce the production of PIP_2, DAG and Ca^{2+}. This causes the recruitment of PKC to the membrane where the C1 domain binds DAG and the C2 domain binds phospholipids such as PIP_2 and phosphotidylserine (PtS) in a Ca^{2+}-dependant way. Membrane association of PKC releases the PS from the substrate-binding site to allow the protein to assume an active conformation and induce downstream signalling. (**D**) Active PKC is prone to dephosphorylation by phosphatases. PHLPP (PH domain leucine-rich repeat protein phosphatase) dephosphorylates the hydrophobic motif, while the activation and turn motifs are likely dephosphorylated by PP2A. (**E**) Dephosphorylated PKC is then either degraded, or HSP70 can bind the unphosphorylated turn motif and allow rephosphorylation of PKC to occur.

Other examples of post-translational modification include the oxidation of cysteines within the C1 domain. This causes a conformational change similar to that induced by lipid binding to result in increased PKC activity (Knapp & Klann, 2000). This phenomenon has been observed for PKCα, -βII, -γ and ε isoforms following exposure to superoxide anions (Knapp & Klann, 2000). Finally, nitrosylation of tyrosine residues can also activate certain PKC isozymes. Tyrosine nitrosylation occurs in the presence of peroxynitrite and can affect PKCε activation (Balafanova, *et al.*, 2002). Pathologically, this is important for constitutive activation of ERK pathway signalling in hairy cell leukaemia cells (Slupsky, *et al.*, 2007).

Another mechanism of PKC activation is through the generation of an autonomous kinase by caspase-cleavage of the hinge domain. This form of the enzyme lacks the regulatory PS and is therefore maintained in an active conformation. This mechanism is best exemplified by PKCδ, which can be cleaved by caspases following the onset of apoptosis. Such cleavage causes the now autonomous catalytic domain of PKCδ to translocate to the nucleus where it catalyzes histone phosphorylation and chromosomal decondensation to aid in the production of DNA ladders that are characteristic of apoptotic cell death (Brodie & Blumberg, 2003;Kikkawa, *et al.*, 2002).

2.2.3 Co-factor binding

The activity of all PKC isoforms is tightly coordinated by interacting with different scaffold proteins. These interactions help localise the enzyme to different microenvironments where they are in proximity to particular lipid regulators, key proteins and substrates. The C2 (Brandman, *et al.*, 2007) , PB1 (Hirano, *et al.*, 2004;Moscat & Diaz-Meco, 2000) and PDZ (Staudinger, *et al.*, 1997) binding domains of PKCs are specifically engineered for this purpose, and define the individual functions of each isozyme. Examples of such proteins include receptors for activated C kinase (RACKs). RACK1 and RACK2 can competitively bind PKC isozymes, trapping them in active conformations by relieving autoinhibition by the N-terminus (Ron & Mochly-Rosen, 1995). Such interactions have the potential of localising active PKC in areas where sustained ligand activation is not possible. PKC can also interact with the cytoskeleton, either directly through protein-protein interaction or by binding to cytoskeleton-associated proteins (Larsson, 2006). Like PKCs interaction with RACK proteins, these interactions can replace the need for lipid second messengers and induce an active PKC conformation.

Co-factor binding to PKC can also prevent activation of this enzyme. For example, the overexpression of 14-3-3 in jurkat cells inhibits phorbol ester-induced PKCθ translocation from the cytosol to the membrane (Meller, *et al.*, 1996). Taking this into consideration it is important to note that there are different scaffold proteins for all conformations of PKC, all helping to regulate PKC from the moment it is synthesised and activated, until when it is deactivated and degraded.

2.2.4 Downregulation and degradation

Despite having a long half-life in the absence of stimulation, sustained activation of PKC, such as that achieved when cells are treated with phorbol esters, results in its rapid degradation (Hansra, *et al.*, 1999;Huang, *et al.*, 1989;Szallasi, *et al.*, 1994). Active PKC adopts a membrane-bound open conformation that is vulnerable to dephosphorylation by phosphatases (Dutil, *et al.*, 1994). PH domain leucine-rich repeat protein phosphatases (PHLPP) are able to dephosphorylate the hydrophobic motif of novel and classical PKC isoforms when they are in this open membrane-bound conformation (Figure 3D). This dephosphorylation causes these PKC isozymes to shunt to a detergent-insoluble cell fraction where they are then further dephosphorylated on the turn motif, possibly by PP2A, before being degraded (Brognard & Newton, 2008;Gao, *et al.*, 2008). However, in some instances HSP70 can rescue PKC from this mechanism of degradation. Like HSP90, HSP70 can bind to the dephosphorylated turn motif of PKC and stabilise its conformation, and, in turn, promote its rephosphorylation and catalytic competence (Gao & Newton, 2002) (Figure 3E). This may be important because HSP70 is upregulated in cells undergoing stress, such as in response to chemotherapeutic agents (Jensen, *et al.*, 2009).

2.3 The role of different PKC isoforms in CLL

To gain a greater insight into the function of PKC in CLL pathobiology it is first important to determine the expression profile of this enzyme in CLL cells and to define the specific role each isoform plays in CLL signalling. Together, these findings may help design more customised clinical therapies targeting specific PKC isoforms.

2.3.1 Expression profile

Work in our lab discovered that CLL cells express PKCβI, -βII, -α, -δ, –ε, -ζ and PKC λ/ι (Abrams, *et al.*, 2007;Alkan, *et al.*, 2005). Furthermore, upon comparing the expression levels of these isoforms to the levels expressed in normal B cells, we discovered that CLL cells express less PKCβI and PKCα, and more PKCδ. However, what clearly distinguished CLL cells from normal B cells and other B-lymphoid malignancies was an overexpression of PKCβII equating to 0.53% ± 0.25% of total cellular protein (Abrams, *et al.*, 2007).

2.3.2 PKCβ

The PRKCB gene is transcribed as a single mRNA that is then alternatively spliced to produce PKCβI and PKCβII (Ono, *et al.*, 1986). In CLL cells, PKCβII is the predominant isoform and its elevated expression is thought to be due to increased transcription of the PKC gene by autocrine VEGF stimulation (Abrams, *et al.*, 2010). Furthermore, PKCβII is constitutively active in CLL cells and contributes to cell survival by protecting the cells from pro-apoptotic BCR signalling (Abrams, *et al.*, 2007). The importance of PKCβ in CLL development and propagation was more recently shown in a study using a CLL mouse model where the T-cell leukaemia (TCL1) protein is specifically overexpressed in B cells (Holler, *et al.*, 2009). This particular mouse model of CLL develops an aggressive disease that is similar to the aggressive form of CLL in humans (Yan, *et al.*, 2006). Thus, when this TCL1 transgenic mouse model of CLL was crossed with mice in which PKCβ was disrupted it was found that the CLL-like disease did not develop (Holler, *et al.*, 2009) (Figure 4A). Interestingly, in this same study the TCL1 transgenic PKCβ(+/-) heterozygous mice developed the CLL like disease with a slower kinetic than did TCL1 transgenic PKCβ wild type mice. Taken together, these data indicate that not only is PKCβ expression important for the development of CLL, but the level of expression plays a key role too. This same study also showed that the specific PKCβ inhibitor enzastaurin induced apoptosis of human CLL cells *in vitro*, suggesting that PKCβ was important in maintaining CLL cell survival.

Signals through the BCR are important for CLL cell survival and PKCβII activity inversely correlates with CLL cell response to BCR engagement (Abrams, *et al.*, 2007). An important substrate of PKCβ in B cells is Bruton's tyrosine kinase (Btk). Phosphorylation of Btk on serine 180 results in its removal from the cell membrane and downregulation of its contribution to BCR signal transduction (Kang, *et al.*, 2001) (Figure 4B). During BCR signalling PKCβ is downstream of Btk activation, therefore, PKCβ acts in a feedback fashion to provide inhibition of this signalling. In CLL cells, PKCβII activity provides inhibition of BCR-induced intracellular calcium release and other downstream signals. We believe that this effect is largely pro-survival because strong, pro-apoptotic BCR signals would be largely suppressed in these cells. However, in CLL cells with high levels of PKCβII activity the pro-survival effects of BCR signalling are lost. Experiments comparing cell survival and Mcl-1 protein levels have shown that both these parameters are increased in response to BCR signalling in CLL cells with low levels of PKCβII activity, whereas there was little effect on these parameters when CLL cells with high levels of PKCβII activity were stimulated by BCR engagement. The regulation of PKCβ activity in CLL cells is likely to involve factors such as VEGF and bFGF, which have been shown to increase PKCβ activity and downregulate BCR signalling (Abrams, *et al.*, 2010).

In addition to its role in downregulating BCR signalling in CLL cells, PKCβII has also been shown to augment anti-apoptotic BCR signalling pathways in CLL cells (Barragan, *et al.*, 2006;zum Buschenfelde, *et al.*, 2010). The expression of ZAP70 in CLL cells is associated with poor disease prognosis and it is thought to enhance BCR signal transduction by acting as a platform to recruit downstream signalling proteins (Chen, *et al.*, 2005). In CLL cells, ZAP70 was recently demonstrated to enhance the BCR signal by recruiting PKCβII into lipid raft domains (zum Buschenfelde, *et al.*, 2010). Here, PKCβII becomes active and is shuttled to the mitochondrial membrane where it is able to phosphorylate anti-apoptotic Bcl-2 and pro-apoptotic Bim_{EL} (Figure 4B). This process provides important pro-survival signals because phosphorylation of Bcl-2 increases its ability to sequester Bim_{EL} and promote cell survival, whilst the phosphorylation of Bim_{EL} results in its proteasomal degradation and protection from its pro-apoptotic effects (zum Buschenfelde, *et al.*, 2010). Another example of how PKCβII mediates BCR-induced survival signals in CLL cells is by activating Akt, a kinase that provides an important source of survival signals to CLL cells (Barragan, *et al.*, 2006;Longo, *et al.*, 2008) (Figure 4B).

Finally, one study has shown that PKCβII may provide pro-survival signals in B cells by inducing the activation of Akt following stimulation by B cell-activating factor (BAFF) (Patke, *et al.*, 2006). This may be important for the pathophysiology of CLL cells because both BAFF and Akt are important sources of pro-survival signals for CLL cells (Barragan, *et al.*, 2006;Nishio, *et al.*, 2005). In B cells, PKCβII also transmits BCR signals to the NFκB pathway by phosphorylating CARMA1, which, together with MALT1, Bcl10 and TAK1 acts to stimulate I-κB kinase activity and NFκB pathway activation (Shinohara, *et al.*, 2005, 2007). Again, this may be pathophysiologically important in CLL because constitutive activation of the NFκB pathway is a feature of the malignant cells of this disease (Hewamana, *et al.*, 2008). Support for this idea comes from studies of diffuse large B cell lymphoma. PKCβ has been shown to be a therapeutic target in the malignant cells of this disease that bear the activated B cell phenotype because of the role it plays in activating the NFκB pathway through the CARMA1/MALT1/Bcl10 complex (Naylor, *et al.*, 2011). Taken together, these studies provide strong support for PKCβII in maintaining CLL cell survival by decreasing pro-apoptotic signals and increasing anti-apoptotic signals.

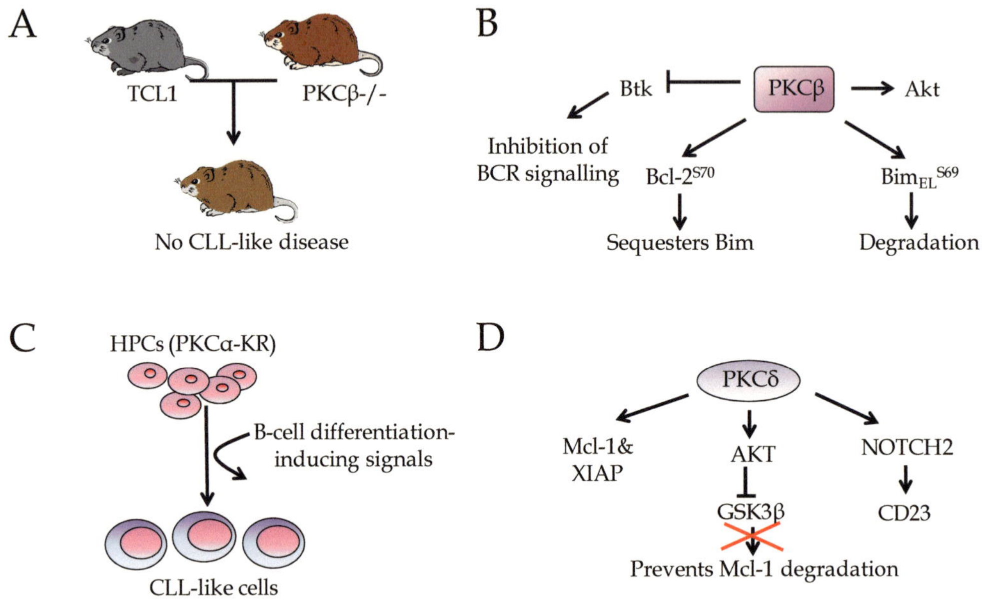

Fig. 4. PKC isoforms in CLL. (A) The T-cell leukaemia-1 (TCL1) mouse overexpresses TCL1 protein and develops an aggressive disease similar to aggressive CLL. TCL1 mice that do not express PKCβ (PKCβ-/-) do not develop the CLL-like disease. (B) PKCβII signalling. CLL cells express elevated levels of PKCβII, likely due to VEGF stimulation. High PKCβII-expressing CLL cases inhibit BCR-signalling by phosphorylating Btk on S^{180} which prevents its activation. Additionally, PKCβII augments antiapoptotic signalling by inducing S^{69} phosphorylation of Bim_{EL} and S^{70} phosphorylation of Bcl-2. Phosphorylation on these residues results in Bim_{EL} proteasomal degradation, and sequestration of Bim_{EL} by Bcl-2, respectively. PKCβII can also activate Akt which is an important mediator of CLL-cell survival. (**C**) Tumour suppressive effects of PKCα in CLL. When fetal-derived hematopoietic progenitor cells (HPCs) overexpressing a dominant negative form of PKCα (PKCα-KR) are induced to differentiate into B lineage cells, a population of CLL-like malignant cells is generated. (**D**) PKCδ signalling. PKCδ is constitutively active in CLL cells via a PI3Kδ-sensitive mechanism. Active PKCδ induces Akt phosphorylation which can then phosphorylate GSK3β. Hyperphosphorylated GSK3β is inactive, preventing it from phosphorylating Mcl-1 and inducing its proteasomal degradation. PKCδ may also induce the transcription of Mcl-1 and XIAP. More recent work has shown that PKCδ can induce the expression of CD23 by activating NOTCH2.

2.3.3 PKCα

Expression and function of PKCα is associated with both tumour promoting and tumour suppressing effects. For example, high levels of PKCα expression are associated with breast, prostrate, gastric and brain cancers (Griner & Kazanietz, 2007;Michie & Nakagawa, 2005) whilst low levels of PKCα expression are associated with cancers of epithelium, pancreas, colon and CLL (Abrams, *et al.*, 2007;Alvaro, *et al.*, 1997;Detjen, *et al.*, 2000;Neill, *et al.*, 2003). In its tumour promoting role PKCα is typically associated with anti-apoptotic signalling achieved through the ability of this kinase to phosphorylate Bcl-2 at the mitochondrial membrane and increase its ability to sequester Bim (Jiffar, *et al.*, 2004;Ruvolo, *et al.*, 1998). The tumour suppressive functions of PKCα are unclear. It has been shown that PKCα knockout mice spontaneously develop intestinal lesions with greater frequency than wild type littermate controls, and that the mitotic index of the malignant cells derived from the PKCα knockout mice is greater than that of malignant cells derived from wild type mice (Oster & Leitges, 2006). However, the mechanism through which this happens remains undefined.

With respect to CLL, a very interesting study by Nakagawa *et al* (Nakagawa, *et al.*, 2006) has suggested that PKCα may have important tumour suppressive effects in this disease (Figure 4C). Using a system whereby fetal liver-derived hematopoietic progenitor cells (HPCs) are induced to differentiate into B lineage cells, this group show that stable overexpression of a dominant negative PKCα (PKCα-KR) leads to the generation of a population of malignant cells bearing a CLL phenotype ($CD19^{hi}$, $CD23^{+}$, $CD5^{+}$, $sIgM^{lo}$) (Figure 4C). This population of malignant cells, like human CLL cells, are arrested in G_0/G_1 phase of the cell cycle and have enhanced expression of Bcl-2 (Hanada, *et al.*, 1993;Kitada, *et al.*, 1998;Mariano, *et al.*, 1992). However, when these cells are injected into SCID mice they have an enhanced proliferative capacity over mock-transfected and non-transfected control populations. This effect was specific for PKCα-KR because expression of other kinase dead PKC isoforms within the same system did not produce cells bearing the same phenotype (Michie & Nakagawa, 2006).

This system as a model for CLL is interesting for the reason that the malignant cells it generates have a high resemblance to the human CLL phenotype, as well as to CLL-like cells in mouse models of the disease (Holler, *et al.*, 2009;Nakagawa, *et al.*, 2006). This is important because in virtually all mouse models of CLL there is expansion of the B1 population of cells prior to development of disease (Hamano, *et al.*, 1998), and B1 cells in the mouse mainly derive from progenitor cells within the fetal liver (Dorshkind & Montecino-Rodriguez, 2007). Importantly, where the B1 population is absent, such as in PKCβ knockout mice, CLL does not develop in mouse models of this disease (Holler, *et al.*, 2009). Thus, by subverting the function of PKCα, this group has created a system whereby malignant expansion of B1 cells is promoted at the haematopoietic stage. Although this system may not represent the actual mechanism of CLL pathogenesis, it does reveal some important aspects within this mechanism. Since this system is easily manipulated at a genetic level, further study will provide important information on the tumour suppressive function of PKCα not only in CLL cells, but in other cancers as well.

2.3.4 PKCδ

In normal B cells PKCδ plays a key role in mediating signals for cell survival in response to BAFF (Mecklenbrauker, *et al.*, 2004). BAFF signalling is important for maintaining B cell survival in the periphery, particularly with respect to B cells that have become tolerant to autoantigens (Ota, *et al.*, 2010). Thus, mice in which BAFF is overexpressed develop autoimmune diseases such as systemic lupus erythematosis because autoreactive B cells are able to escape tolerance (Stohl, *et al.*, 2005). A similar situation is observed in mice where PKCδ expression is disrupted (Mecklenbrauker, *et al.*, 2004), indicating a pro-apoptotic role for this PKC isozyme within a process that maintains survival of tolerant B cells. The relationship of PKCδ to BAFF is illustrated by experiments showing that this cytokine prevents nuclear localization of this PKC isoform. The absence of BAFF-stimulated signals results in nuclear localisation of PKCδ where it contributes to phosphorylation of histone H2B at serine 14 and initiation of apoptosis (Mecklenbrauker, *et al.*, 2004). Whether BAFF-mediated signalling stimulates pro-survival functions of PKCδ or merely prevents nuclear localisation is not clear at the present time, however, the pro-survival signalling capabilities of PKCδ, particularly those potentially induced by BAFF, may be highly relevant for CLL cells.

A potential role of PKCδ in maintaining CLL cell survival was first proposed in a paper by Ringshausen *et al.* (Ringshausen, *et al.*, 2002, 2006). This paper demonstrated that PKCδ was constitutively active in a phosphatidylinositol 3 kinase (PI3K)-dependent manner in CLL cells, and that inhibition of this isozyme with rottlerin induced apoptosis of treated cells by reducing the expression of Mcl-1 and XIAP (Ringshausen, *et al.*, 2002, 2006) (Figure 4D). However, with respect to this latter aspect there are some controversies regarding the use of rottlerin. Rottlerin is described as a specific inhibitor of PKCδ, but its pro-apoptotic activity is associated with PKC-independent effects (Villalba, *et al.*, 1999), particularly with respect to the uncoupling and depolarization of mitochondrial membranes (Soltoff, 2007). This uncoupling in cells leads to a reduction in ATP levels and consequent activation of 5'-AMP-activated protein kinase (AMPK), with the end result resembling that produced by direct inhibition of PKCδ. Therefore, results using this inhibitor lack specificity and must be approached with caution. Nevertheless, there is evidence linking PI3K activity to PKCδ in B cells. BAFF signalling in B cells is impaired by the absence of the p110δ isoform of PI3K (Henley, *et al.*, 2008), and inhibition of PI3Kδ with a compound known as CAL101 has shown clinical efficacy both *in vitro* and *in vivo* in CLL cells (Herman, *et al.*, 2010, 2011;Hoellenriegel, *et al.*, 2011). Moreover, other recent findings have shown that PKCδ regulates CLL cell survival by activating the Akt pathway and stabilising the expression of Mcl-1 (Baudot, *et al.*, 2009) (Figure 4D). These findings provide confirmation that PKCδ may play an anti-apoptotic role in CLL cells.

Our own work has discovered that PKC may be important for the survival of CLL cells through its ability to phosphorylate STAT3 on serine 727, and cause increased transcription of the gene for Mcl-1 (Allen, *et al.*, 2011) (Figure 4D). We found that treatment of CLL cells with Bis-1, a specific inhibitor of the novel isoforms PKCδ and PKCε, inhibited the phosphorylation of $STAT3^{S727}$ and decreased the expression of Mcl-1. Conversely, treatment with bryostatin, to activate classical and novel PKC isoforms, induced $STAT3^{S727}$ phosphorylation and increased Mcl-1 expression in CLL cells. Of course, the identity of the PKC isoform phosphorylating STAT3 in CLL cells remains to be characterised by more specific investigations, such as siRNA-mediated knock down of specific PKC isoform expression. Indeed, investigation of the mechanism of Syk-mediated CLL cell survival used siRNA to knock down PKCδ expression and showed a concomitant downregulation of Mcl-1 expression (Baudot, *et al.*, 2009). This study does not address whether PKCδ can phosphorylate STAT3 in CLL cells, but studies using other cell types have shown that PKCδ and PKCε can perform this function (Aziz, *et al.*, 2010;Gartsbein, *et al.*, 2006). Thus, there is ample support for our findings that these PKC isoforms may promote CLL cell survival by activating STAT3-mediated Mcl-1 transcription. Such a mechanism may be useful therapeutically. High expression levels of Mcl-1 correlate with more aggressive and poor prognosis disease in CLL by providing the malignant cells with protection against chemotherapy (Pepper, *et al.*, 2008). Inhibiting PKC may reduce Mcl-1 expression in CLL cells, thereby lowering the apoptosis threshold and making them more susceptible to other chemotherapeutic agents.

Another way in which PKCδ may contribute to CLL cell pathophysiology is through NOTCH2. One study has used RNAi to knock down PKCδ expression in CLL cells and found that this procedure antagonises PMA-induced NOTCH2 activation (Hubmann, *et al.*, 2010). This result is important because one characteristic of CLL cells is high expression of CD23, and NOTCH2 is known to regulate CD23 expression in these cells (Hubmann, *et al.*, 2002). Taken together, these results suggest that PKCδ and NOTCH2 are critically involved in maintaining the malignant phenotype of CLL cells.

2.3.5 Other PKC isoforms

The function of the remaining PKC isoforms in CLL cells remains poorly defined. However, their role in other cell types is well documented and may provide clues as to what function they have in CLL cells. Intriguingly, PKCε is known to phosphorylate and activate signalling proteins such as Akt (Matsumoto, *et al.*, 2001), PKD (Waldron & Rozengurt, 2003) and STAT3 (Aziz, *et al.*, 2010), pathways which all provide an important source of anti-apoptotic signals to CLL cells. Furthermore, in hairy cell leukaemia, PKCε is activated by nitration of a tyrosine residue causing it to co-localise with ERK1/2 at the mitochondrial membrane and induce activation of the MAPK pathway (Slupsky, *et al.*, 2007). Given that ERK1/2 has been shown to phosphorylate and stabilise the expression of Mcl-1 (Domina, *et al.*, 2004), its activation in CLL cells may provide additional anti-apoptotic signals to CLL cells. Moreover, knockout mouse models have highlighted the importance of the atypical PKCζ in B-cell survival and proliferation by regulating the activation of ERK and NFκB signalling pathways (Martin, *et al.*, 2002).

The above findings are important because Akt, NFκB and STAT3 signalling pathways are known to be constitutively active in CLL cells, and because these pathways are essential in maintaining CLL cell viability (Allen, *et al.*, 2011;de Frias, *et al.*, 2009;Hazan-Halevy, *et al.*, 2010;Hewamana, *et al.*, 2008;Zhuang, *et al.*, 2010). The level of NFκB activation is regarded as an essential component of CLL survival because it correlates with *in vitro* survival of CLL cells as well as with clinical disease progression (Hewamana, *et al.*, 2008). Furthermore, our own work has demonstrated that STAT3 mediates CLL cell survival by inducing Mcl-1 transcription (Allen, *et al.*, 2011), and more recent studies have shown that both pathways can work in concert to induce the expression of anti-apoptotic proteins (Liu, *et al.*, 2011). Collectively, these findings highlight that PKC has the potential to activate numerous anti-apoptotic pathways and that further work is now critical to help understand the specific role these isoforms play in CLL cell signalling.

2.4 CLL cell microenvironment and PKC

It is clear that PKC-mediated signalling pathways seem to provide important survival signals to CLL cells *in vitro*, but how close do these conditions mimic those of *in vivo*? The CLL microenvironment is a milieu rich in signals generated by the interaction of the malignant cells with IL-6 (Moreno, *et al.*, 2001), IL-4 (Dancescu, *et al.*, 1992) , SDF-1 (Burger, *et al.*, 2000), BAFF and April (Endo, *et al.*, 2007). These cytokines have all been shown to have anti-apoptotic effects on CLL cells. Moreover, the interaction of CLL cells with bone marrow stromal cells (Lagneaux, *et al.*, 1998;Panayiotidis, *et al.*, 1996), follicular dendritic cells (Pedersen, *et al.*, 2002), endothelial cells (Moreno, *et al.*, 2001), nurse-like cells (Burger, *et al.*, 2000) and CD40L-expressing cells (Hallaert, *et al.*, 2008) results in an increase apoptotic threshold. This may be due to the induction of anti-apoptotic genes by these interactions; a comparison of the apoptosis regulatory genes and proteins in neoplastic B cells derived from CLL lymph node proliferation centres and peripheral blood found that lymph node-derived cells had increased expression of anti-apoptotic Mcl-1, Bcl-XL and A1/Bfl-1 (Smit, *et al.*, 2007). Moreover, co-culture of CLL cells on CD40L-expressing fibroblasts strongly induces the expression of these anti-apoptotic proteins, and this culminates in drug resistance (Hallaert, *et al.*, 2008). PKC activation is likely to play a role in all of the microenvironmental interactions CLL cells are likely to encounter in an *in vivo* setting. However, whether inhibition of PKC lowers the threshold of apoptosis in CLL cells within their microenvironment is unknown and requires proper assessment before PKC inhibition becomes a therapeutic target in the treatment of this disease. Recent studies have begun to address this area and have demonstrated the importance of PKC in the survival of CLL cells that have been co-cultured with accessory cells (Martins, *et al.*, 2011).

3. Conclusion

There are convincing demonstrations that PKC-mediated signalling is an important contributor to the development and propagation of the malignant clone in CLL. Inhibition of PKC, therefore, poses an attractive therapeutic approach for the treatment of this debilitating disease, particularly when we consider the roles of the individual PKC isozymes in CLL pathobiology. Within this review we have addressed the potential functions of PKCβ, α, δ and, to a lesser extent, PKCε and PKCζ. There is clear contribution of PKCβ to the pathogenesis of CLL, because disruption of PKCβ expression blocks the development of the CLL-like disease in TCL1-transgenic mice. This same type of experiment now needs to be done for the other PKC isoforms. Thus, disruption of PKCα may accelerate disease progression in TCL1 mice because of the tumour suppressive action of this PKC isoform. The effect of PKCδ disruption is harder to predict. On one hand, disruption of PKCδ should accelerate disease development because the pro-apoptotic effects of this isoform would be lost. However, this prediction does not take into account the pro-survival functions of PKCδ in CLL cells, particularly its potential role in regulating STAT3 phosphorylation and Mcl-1 protein expression. Finally, targeted disruption of PKC isoforms would potentially yield useful information on the role these isoforms play in CLL cell–microenvironment interactions.

Within this review we have not addressed opposing functions of different PKC isoforms. For example, PKCα and PKCδ can act antagonistically to regulate cellular proliferation and apoptosis in glioma cells (Mandil, *et al.*, 2001). It is conceivable that more general inhibitors of PKC, through their ability to inhibit tumour suppressive or pro-apoptotic functions of PKC, may have an adverse effect by actually promoting CLL cell survival and proliferation. Nevertheless, PKC inhibitors such as N-benzoyl-staurosporine (PKC412) have already been tested in clinical trials, and were found to be effective at inducing CLL cell apoptosis in patients that were refractory to fludarabine and chlorambucil (Ganeshaguru, *et al.*, 2002). Furthermore, a more recent drug called sotrastaurin (AEB071) has been introduced as an immunosuppressant following organ transplant, and for the treatment of psoriasis. Early clinical trials suggest sotrastaurin has no clinically relevant side effects and has the potential to become a long term treatment option (Skvara, *et al.*, 2008). Another study has suggested that AEB071 may even be useful in the treatment of diffuse large B-cell lymphoma (DLCBL) through inhibition of BCR-mediated NFκB pathway activation (Naylor, *et al.*, 2011). Thus, given the potential role of PKC in regulating CLL cell survival and disease pathogenesis and that side effects associated with the use of some inhibitors can be adequately managed within a clinical setting, PKC inhibitors may have therapeutic application in the treatment of CLL.

4. Acknowledgement

JCA and JRS thank Leukaemia and Lymphoma Research U.K. for their support in publishing this article.

5. References

Abrams, S.T., Lakum, T., Lin, K., Jones, G.M., Treweeke, A.T., Farahani, M., Hughes, M., Zuzel, M. & Slupsky, J.R. (2007). B-cell receptor signaling in chronic lymphocytic leukemia cells is regulated by overexpressed active protein kinase CβII. *Blood*, Vol.109, No.3, (Feb 2007), pp. 1193-1201, ISSN 0006-4971

Abrams, S.T., Brown, B.R., Zuzel, M. & Slupsky, J.R. (2010). Vascular endothelial growth factor stimulates protein kinase CβII expression in chronic lymphocytic leukemia cells. *Blood*, Vol.115, No.22, (Jun 2010), pp. 4447-4454, ISSN 0006-4971

Ahmad, I., Al-Katib, A.M., Beck, F.W. & Mohammad, R.M. (2000). Sequential treatment of a resistant chronic lymphocytic leukemia patient with bryostatin 1 followed by 2-chlorodeoxyadenosine: case report. *Clinical Cancer Research*, Vol.6, No.4, (Apr 2000), pp. 1328-1332, ISSN 1078-0432

al-Katib, A., Mohammad, R.M., Dan, M., Hussein, M.E., Akhtar, A., Pettit, G.R. & Sensenbrenner, L.L. (1993). Bryostatin 1-induced hairy cell features on chronic lymphocytic leukemia cells in vitro. *Experimental Hematology*, Vol.21, No.1, (Jan 1993), pp. 61-65, ISSN 0301-472X

Alkan, S., Huang, Q., Ergin, M., Denning, M.F., Nand, S., Maududi, T., Paner, G.P., Ozpuyan, F. & Izban, K.F. (2005). Survival role of protein kinase C (PKC) in chronic lymphocytic leukemia and determination of isoform expression pattern and genes altered by PKC inhibition. *American Journal of Hematology*, Vol.79, No.2, (Jun 2005), pp. 97-106, ISSN 0361-8609

Allen, J.C., Talab, F., Zuzel, M., Lin, K. & Slupsky, J.R. (2011). c-Abl regulates Mcl-1 gene expression in chronic lymphocytic leukemia cells. *Blood*, Vol.117, No.8, (Feb 2011), pp. 2414-2422, ISSN 0006-4971

Alvaro, V., Prevostel, C., Joubert, D., Slosberg, E. & Weinstein, B.I. (1997). Ectopic expression of a mutant form of PKCα originally found in human tumors: aberrant subcellular translocation and effects on growth control. *Oncogene*, Vol.14, No.6, (Feb 1997), pp. 677-685, ISSN 0950-9232

Aziz, M.H., Hafeez, B.B., Sand, J.M., Pierce, D.B., Aziz, S.W., Dreckschmidt, N.E. & Verma, A.K. (2010). Protein kinase Cε mediates Stat3 Ser^{727} phosphorylation, Stat3-regulated gene expression, and cell invasion in various human cancer cell lines through integration with MAPK cascade (RAF-1, MEK1/2, and ERK1/2). *Oncogene*, Vol.29, No.21, (May 2010), pp. 3100-3109, ISSN 0950-9232

Balafanova, Z., Bolli, R., Zhang, J., Zheng, Y., Pass, J.M., Bhatnagar, A., Tang, X.L., Wang, O., Cardwell, E. & Ping, P. (2002). Nitric oxide (NO) induces nitration of protein kinase Cε (PKCε), facilitating PKCε translocation via enhanced PKCε -RACK2 interactions: a novel mechanism of no-triggered activation of PKCε. *The Journal of Biological Chemistry*, Vol.277, No.17, (Apr 2002), pp. 15021-15027, ISSN 0021-9258

Balendran, A., Hare, G.R., Kieloch, A., Williams, M.R. & Alessi, D.R. (2000). Further evidence that 3-phosphoinositide-dependent protein kinase-1 (PDK1) is required for the stability and phosphorylation of protein kinase C (PKC) isoforms. *FEBS Letters*, Vol.484, No.3, (Nov 2000), pp. 217-223, ISSN 0014-5793

Barragan, M., Bellosillo, B., Campas, C., Colomer, D., Pons, G. & Gil, J. (2002). Involvement of protein kinase C and phosphatidylinositol 3-kinase pathways in the survival of B-cell chronic lymphocytic leukemia cells. *Blood*, Vol.99, No.8, (Apr 2002), pp. 2969-2976, ISSN 0006-4971

Barragan, M., de Frias, M., Iglesias-Serret, D., Campas, C., Castano, E., Santidrian, A.F., Coll-Mulet, L., Cosialls, A.M., Domingo, A., Pons, G. & Gil, J. (2006). Regulation of Akt/PKB by phosphatidylinositol 3-kinase-dependent and -independent pathways in B-cell chronic lymphocytic leukemia cells: role of protein kinase Cβ. *Journal of Leukocyte Biology*, Vol.80, No.6, (Dec 2006), pp. 1473-1479, ISSN 0741-5400

Baudot, A.D., Jeandel, P.Y., Mouska, X., Maurer, U., Tartare-Deckert, S., Raynaud, S.D., Cassuto, J.P., Ticchioni, M. & Deckert, M. (2009). The tyrosine kinase Syk regulates the survival of chronic lymphocytic leukemia B cells through PKCδ and proteasome-dependent regulation of Mcl-1 expression. *Oncogene*, Vol.28, No.37, (Sep 2009), pp. 3261-3273, ISSN 0950-9232

Beaven, M.A. (1996). Calcium signalling: sphingosine kinase versus phospholipase C? *Current Biology*, Vol.6, No.7, (Jul 1996), pp. 798-801, ISSN 0960-9822

Behn-Krappa, A. & Newton, A.C. (1999). The hydrophobic phosphorylation motif of conventional protein kinase C is regulated by autophosphorylation. *Current Biology*, Vol.9, No.14, (Jul 1999), pp. 728-737, ISSN 0960-9822

Bellosillo, B., Dalmau, M., Colomer, D. & Gil, J. (1997). Involvement of CED-3/ICE proteases in the apoptosis of B-chronic lymphocytic leukemia cells. *Blood*, Vol.89, No.9, (May 1997), pp. 3378-3384, ISSN 0006-4971

Benimetskaya, L., Miller, P., Benimetsky, S., Maciaszek, A., Guga, P., Beaucage, S.L., Wilk, A., Grajkowski, A., Halperin, A.L. & Stein, C.A. (2001). Inhibition of potentially anti-apoptotic proteins by antisense protein kinase C-α (Isis 3521) and antisense bcl-2 (G3139) phosphorothioate oligodeoxynucleotides: relationship to the decreased viability of T24 bladder and PC3 prostate cancer cells. *Molecular Pharmacology*, Vol.60, No.6, (Dec 2001), pp. 1296-1307, ISSN 0026-895X

Blass, M., Kronfeld, I., Kazimirsky, G., Blumberg, P.M. & Brodie, C. (2002). Tyrosine phosphorylation of protein kinase Cδ is essential for its apoptotic effect in response to etoposide. *Molecular Cell Biology*, Vol.22, No.1, (Jan), pp. 182-195, ISSN 0270-7306

Bolsover, S.R., Gomez-Fernandez, J.C. & Corbalan-Garcia, S. (2003). Role of the Ca^{2+}/phosphatidylserine binding region of the C2 domain in the translocation of protein kinase Cα to the plasma membrane. *Journal of Biological Chemistry*, Vol.278, No.12, (Mar 2003), pp. 10282-10290, ISSN 0021-9258

Brandman, R., Disatnik, M.H., Churchill, E. & Mochly-Rosen, D. (2007). Peptides derived from the C2 domain of protein kinase C ε (ε PKC) modulate ε PKC activity and identify potential protein-protein interaction surfaces. *Journal of Biological Chemistry*, Vol.282, No.6, (Feb 2007), pp. 4113-4123, ISSN 0021-9258

Brodie, C. & Blumberg, P.M. (2003). Regulation of cell apoptosis by protein kinase c δ. *Apoptosis*, Vol.8, No.1, (Jan 2003), pp. 19-27, ISSN 1360-8185

Brognard, J. & Newton, A.C. (2008). PHLiPPing the switch on Akt and protein kinase C signaling. *Trends in Endocrinology and Metabolism*, Vol.19, No.6, (Aug 2008), pp. 223-230, ISSN 1043-2760

Burger, J.A., Tsukada, N., Burger, M., Zvaifler, N.J., Dell'Aquila, M. & Kipps, T.J. (2000). Blood-derived nurse-like cells protect chronic lymphocytic leukemia B cells from spontaneous apoptosis through stromal cell-derived factor-1. *Blood*, Vol.96, No.8, (Oct 2000), pp. 2655-2663, ISSN 0006-4971

Byrd, J.C., Shinn, C., Willis, C.R., Flinn, I.W., Lehman, T., Sausville, E., Lucas, D. & Grever, M.R. (2001). UCN-01 induces cytotoxicity toward human CLL cells through a p53-independent mechanism. *Experimental Hematology*, Vol.29, No.6, (Jun 2001), pp. 703-708, ISSN 0301-472X

Chen, L., Apgar, J., Huynh, L., Dicker, F., Giago-McGahan, T., Rassenti, L., Weiss, A. & Kipps, T.J. (2005). ZAP-70 directly enhances IgM signaling in chronic lymphocytic leukemia. *Blood*, Vol.105, No.5, (Mar 2005), pp. 2036-2041, ISSN 0006-4971

Chiorazzi, N., Rai, K.R. & Ferrarini, M. (2005). Chronic lymphocytic leukemia. The *New England Journal of Medicine*, Vol.352, No.8, (Feb 2005), pp. 804-815, ISSN 0028-4793

Cho, W. (2001). Membrane targeting by C1 and C2 domains. *Journal of Biological Chemistry*, Vol.276, No.35, (Aug 2001), pp. 32407-32410, ISSN 0021-9258

Chou, M.M., Hou, W., Johnson, J., Graham, L.K., Lee, M.H., Chen, C.S., Newton, A.C., Schaffhausen, B.S. & Toker, A. (1998). Regulation of protein kinase C ζ by PI 3-kinase and PDK-1. *Current Biology*, Vol.8, No.19, (Sep 1998), pp. 1069-1077, ISSN 0960-9822

Dancescu, M., Rubio-Trujillo, M., Biron, G., Bron, D., Delespesse, G. & Sarfati, M. (1992). Interleukin 4 protects chronic lymphocytic leukemic B cells from death by apoptosis and upregulates Bcl-2 expression. *The Journal of Experimental Medicine*, Vol.176, No.5, (Nov 1992), pp. 1319-1326, ISSN 0022-1007

de Frias, M., Iglesias-Serret, D., Cosialls, A.M., Coll-Mulet, L., Santidrian, A.F., Gonzalez-Girones, D.M., de la Banda, E., Pons, G. & Gil, J. (2009). Akt inhibitors induce apoptosis in chronic lymphocytic leukemia cells. *Haematologica*, Vol.94, No.12, (Dec 2009), pp. 1698-1707, ISSN 0390-6078

Detjen, K.M., Brembeck, F.H., Welzel, M., Kaiser, A., Haller, H., Wiedenmann, B. & Rosewicz, S. (2000). Activation of protein kinase Cα inhibits growth of pancreatic cancer cells via p21(cip)-mediated G(1) arrest. *Journal of Cell Science*, Vol.113 (Pt 17), (Sep 2000), pp. 3025-3035, ISSN 0021-9533

Domina, A.M., Vrana, J.A., Gregory, M.A., Hann, S.R. & Craig, R.W. (2004). MCL1 is phosphorylated in the PEST region and stabilized upon ERK activation in viable cells, and at additional sites with cytotoxic okadaic acid or taxol. *Oncogene*, Vol.23, No.31, (Jul 2004), pp. 5301-5315, ISSN 0950-9232

Dorshkind, K. & Montecino-Rodriguez, E. (2007). Fetal B-cell lymphopoiesis and the emergence of B-1-cell potential. *Nature reviews. Immunology*, Vol.7, No.3, (Mar 2007), pp. 213-219, ISSN 1474-1733

Drexler, H.G., Gignac, S.M., Jones, R.A., Scott, C.S., Pettit, G.R. & Hoffbrand, A.V. (1989). Bryostatin 1 induces differentiation of B-chronic lymphocytic leukemia cells. *Blood*, Vol.74, No.5, (Oct 1989), pp. 1747-1757, ISSN 0006-4971

Dutil, E.M., Keranen, L.M., DePaoli-Roach, A.A. & Newton, A.C. (1994). In vivo regulation of protein kinase C by trans-phosphorylation followed by autophosphorylation. *Journal of Biological Chemistry*, Vol.269, No.47, (Nov 1994), pp. 29359-29362, ISSN 0021-9258

Dutil, E.M., Toker, A. & Newton, A.C. (1998). Regulation of conventional protein kinase C isozymes by phosphoinositide-dependent kinase 1 (PDK-1). *Current Biology*, Vol.8, No.25, (Dec 1998), pp. 1366-1375, ISSN 0960-9822

Dutil, E.M. & Newton, A.C. (2000). Dual role of pseudosubstrate in the coordinated regulation of protein kinase C by phosphorylation and diacylglycerol. *Journal of Biological Chemistry*, Vol.275, No.14, (Apr 2000), pp. 10697-10701, ISSN 0021-9258

Endo, T., Nishio, M., Enzler, T., Cottam, H.B., Fukuda, T., James, D.F., Karin, M. & Kipps, T.J. (2007). BAFF and APRIL support chronic lymphocytic leukemia B-cell survival through activation of the canonical NF-κB pathway. *Blood*, Vol.109, No.2, (Jan 2007), pp. 703-710, ISSN 0006-4971

Forbes, I.J., Zalewski, P.D., Giannakis, C. & Cowled, P.A. (1992). Induction of apoptosis in chronic lymphocytic leukemia cells and its prevention by phorbol ester. *Experimental Cell Research*, Vol.198, No.2, (Feb 1992), pp. 367-372, ISSN 0014-4827

Ganeshaguru, K., Wickremasinghe, R.G., Jones, D.T., Gordon, M., Hart, S.M., Virchis, A.E., Prentice, H.G., Hoffbrand, A.V., Man, A., Champain, K., Csermak, K. & Mehta, A.B. (2002). Actions of the selective protein kinase C inhibitor PKC412 on B-chronic lymphocytic leukemia cells in vitro. *Haematologica*, Vol.87, No.2, (Feb 2002), pp. 167-176, ISSN 0390-6078

Gao, T. & Newton, A.C. (2002). The turn motif is a phosphorylation switch that regulates the binding of Hsp70 to protein kinase C. *Journal of Biological Chemistry*, Vol.277, No.35, (Aug 2002), pp. 31585-31592, ISSN 0021-9258

Gao, T., Brognard, J. & Newton, A.C. (2008). The phosphatase PHLPP controls the cellular levels of protein kinase C. *Journal of Biological Chemistry*, Vol.283, No.10, (Mar 2008), pp. 6300-6311, ISSN 0021-9258

Gartsbein, M., Alt, A., Hashimoto, K., Nakajima, K., Kuroki, T. & Tennenbaum, T. (2006). The role of protein kinase C δ activation and STAT3 Ser^{727} phosphorylation in insulin-induced keratinocyte proliferation. *Journal of Cell Science* Vol.119, No.Pt 3, (Feb 2006), pp. 470-481, ISSN 0021-9533

Giorgione, J.R., Lin, J.H., McCammon, J.A. & Newton, A.C. (2006). Increased membrane affinity of the C1 domain of protein kinase Cδ compensates for the lack of involvement of its C2 domain in membrane recruitment. *Journal of Biological Chemistry*, Vol.281, No.3, (Jan 2006), pp. 1660-1669, ISSN 0021-9258

Gould, C.M., Kannan, N., Taylor, S.S. & Newton, A.C. (2009). The chaperones Hsp90 and Cdc37 mediate the maturation and stabilization of protein kinase C through a conserved PXXP motif in the C-terminal tail. *Journal of Biological Chemistry*, Vol.284, No.8, (Feb 2009), pp. 4921-4935, ISSN 0021-9258

Griner, E.M. & Kazanietz, M.G. (2007). Protein kinase C and other diacylglycerol effectors in cancer. *Nat Rev Cancer*, Vol.7, No.4, (Apr 2007), pp. 281-294, ISSN 1474-175X

Hallaert, D.Y., Jaspers, A., van Noesel, C.J., van Oers, M.H., Kater, A.P. & Eldering, E. (2008). c-Abl kinase inhibitors overcome CD40-mediated drug resistance in CLL: implications for therapeutic targeting of chemoresistant niches. *Blood*, Vol.112, No.13, (Dec 2008), pp. 5141-5149, ISSN 0006-4971

Hamano, Y., Hirose, S., Ida, A., Abe, M., Zhang, D., Kodera, S., Jiang, Y., Shirai, J., Miura, Y., Nishimura, H. & Shirai, T. (1998). Susceptibility alleles for aberrant B-1 cell proliferation involved in spontaneously occurring B-cell chronic lymphocytic leukemia in a model of New Zealand white mice. *Blood*, Vol.92, No.10, (Nov 1998), pp. 3772-3779, ISSN 0006-4971

Hanada, M., Delia, D., Aiello, A., Stadtmauer, E. & Reed, J.C. (1993). bcl-2 gene hypomethylation and high-level expression in B-cell chronic lymphocytic leukemia. *Blood*, Vol.82, No.6, (Sep 1993), pp. 1820-1828, ISSN 0006-4971

Hansra, G., Garcia-Paramio, P., Prevostel, C., Whelan, R.D., Bornancin, F. & Parker, P.J. (1999). Multisite dephosphorylation and desensitization of conventional protein kinase C isotypes. *The Biochemical Journal*, Vol.342 (Pt 2), (Sep 1999), pp. 337-344, ISSN 0264-6021

Hazan-Halevy, I., Harris, D., Liu, Z., Liu, J., Li, P., Chen, X., Shanker, S., Ferrajoli, A., Keating, M.J. & Estrov, Z. (2010). STAT3 is constitutively phosphorylated on serine 727 residues, binds DNA, and activates transcription in CLL cells. *Blood*, Vol.115, No.14, (Apr 2010), pp. 2852-2863, ISSN 0006-4971

Henley, T., Kovesdi, D. & Turner, M. (2008). B-cell responses to B-cell activation factor of the TNF family (BAFF) are impaired in the absence of PI3K δ. *European Journal of Immunology* Vol.38, No.12, (Dec 2008), pp. 3543-3548, ISSN 0014-2980

Herman, S.E., Lapalombella, R., Gordon, A.L., Ramanunni, A., Blum, K.A., Jones, J., Zhang, X., Lannutti, B.J., Puri, K.D., Muthusamy, N., Byrd, J.C. & Johnson, A.J. (2011). The role of phosphatidylinositol 3-kinase-δ in the immunomodulatory effects of lenalidomide in chronic lymphocytic leukemia.. *Blood*, Vol.117, No.16, (Apr 2011), pp. 4323-4327, ISSN 0006-4971

Herman, S.E., Gordon, A.L., Wagner, A.J., Heerema, N.A., Zhao, W., Flynn, J.M., Jones, J., Andritsos, L., Puri, K.D., Lannutti, B.J., Giese, N.A., Zhang, X., Wei, L., Byrd, J.C. & Johnson, A.J. (2010). Phosphatidylinositol 3-kinase-δ inhibitor CAL-101 shows promising preclinical activity in chronic lymphocytic leukemia by antagonizing intrinsic and extrinsic cellular survival signals. *Blood*, Vol.116, No.12, (Sep 2010), pp. 2078-2088, ISSN 0006-4971

Hewamana, S., Alghazal, S., Lin, T.T., Clement, M., Jenkins, C., Guzman, M.L., Jordan, C.T., Neelakantan, S., Crooks, P.A., Burnett, A.K., Pratt, G., Fegan, C., Rowntree, C., Brennan, P. & Pepper, C. (2008). The NF-κB subunit Rel A is associated with in vitro survival and clinical disease progression in chronic lymphocytic leukemia and represents a promising therapeutic target. *Blood*, Vol.111, No.9, (May 2008), pp. 4681-4689, ISSN 0006-4971

Hirano, Y., Yoshinaga, S., Ogura, K., Yokochi, M., Noda, Y., Sumimoto, H. & Inagaki, F. (2004). Solution structure of atypical protein kinase C PB1 domain and its mode of interaction with ZIP/p62 and MEK5. *Journal of Biological Chemistry*, Vol.279, No.30, (Jul 2004), pp. 31883-31890, ISSN 0021-9258

Hoellenriegel, J., Meadows, S.A., Sivina, M., Wierda, W.G., Kantarjian, H., Keating, M.J., Giese, N., O'Brien, S., Yu, A., Miller, L.L., Lannutti, B.J. & Burger, J.A. (2011). The phosphoinositide 3'-kinase δ inhibitor, CAL-101, inhibits B-cell receptor signaling and chemokine networks in chronic lymphocytic leukemia. *Blood*, (Jul 2011), pp. ISSN 0006-4971

Holler, C., Pinon, J.D., Denk, U., Heyder, C., Hofbauer, S., Greil, R. & Egle, A. (2009). PKCβ is essential for the development of chronic lymphocytic leukemia in the TCL1 transgenic mouse model: validation of PKCβ as a therapeutic target in chronic lymphocytic leukemia. *Blood*, Vol.113, No.12, (Mar 2009), pp. 2791-2794, ISSN 0006-4971

House, C. & Kemp, B.E. (1987). Protein kinase C contains a pseudosubstrate prototope in its regulatory domain. *Science*, Vol.238, No.4834, (Dec 1987), pp. 1726-1728, ISSN 0036-8075

Huang, F.L., Yoshida, Y., Cunha-Melo, J.R., Beaven, M.A. & Huang, K.P. (1989). Differential down-regulation of protein kinase C isozymes. *Journal of Biological Chemistry*, Vol.264, No.7, (Mar 1989), pp. 4238-4243, ISSN 0021-9258

Hubmann, R., Schwarzmeier, J.D., Shehata, M., Hilgarth, M., Duechler, M., Dettke, M. & Berger, R. (2002). Notch2 is involved in the overexpression of CD23 in B-cell chronic lymphocytic leukemia. *Blood*, Vol.99, No.10, (May 2002), pp. 3742-3747, ISSN 0006-4971

Hubmann, R., Duchler, M., Schnabl, S., Hilgarth, M., Demirtas, D., Mitteregger, D., Holbl, A., Vanura, K., Le, T., Look, T., Schwarzmeier, J.D., Valent, P., Jager, U. & Shehata, M. (2010). NOTCH2 links protein kinase C δ to the expression of CD23 in chronic lymphocytic leukaemia (CLL) cells. *British Journal of Haematology*, Vol.148, No.6, (Mar 2010), pp. 868-878, ISSN 0007-1048

Ikenoue, T., Inoki, K., Yang, Q., Zhou, X. & Guan, K.L. (2008). Essential function of TORC2 in PKC and Akt turn motif phosphorylation, maturation and signalling. *The EMBO Journal*, Vol.27, No.14, (Jul 2008), pp. 1919-1931, ISSN 0261-4189

Jensen, H., Andresen, L., Hansen, K.A. & Skov, S. (2009). Cell-surface expression of Hsp70 on hematopoietic cancer cells after inhibition of HDAC activity. *Journal of Leukocyte Biology* Vol.86, No.4, (Oct 2009), pp. 923-932, ISSN 0741-5400

Jiffar, T., Kurinna, S., Suck, G., Carlson-Bremer, D., Ricciardi, M.R., Konopleva, M., Andreeff, M. & Ruvolo, P.P. (2004). PKC α mediates chemoresistance in acute lymphoblastic leukemia through effects on Bcl2 phosphorylation. *Leukemia*, Vol.18, No.3, (Mar 2004), pp. 505-512, ISSN 0887-6924

Joseloff, E., Cataisson, C., Aamodt, H., Ocheni, H., Blumberg, P., Kraker, A.J. & Yuspa, S.H. (2002). Src family kinases phosphorylate protein kinase C δ on tyrosine residues and modify the neoplastic phenotype of skin keratinocytes. *Journal of Biological Chemistry*, Vol.277, No.14, (Apr 2002), pp. 12318-12323, ISSN 0021-9258

Kang, S.W., Wahl, M.I., Chu, J., Kitaura, J., Kawakami, Y., Kato, R.M., Tabuchi, R., Tarakhovsky, A., Kawakami, T., Turck, C.W., Witte, O.N. & Rawlings, D.J. (2001). PKCβ modulates antigen receptor signaling via regulation of Btk membrane localization. *The EMBO Journal*, Vol.20, No.20, (Oct 2001), pp. 5692-5702, ISSN 0261-4189

Keenan, C., Thompson, S., Knox, K. & Pears, C. (1999). Protein kinase C-α is essential for Ramos-BL B cell survival. *Cellular Immunology*, Vol.196, No.2, (Sep 1999), pp. 104-109, ISSN 0008-8749

Kikkawa, U., Matsuzaki, H. & Yamamoto, T. (2002). Protein kinase C δ (PKC δ): activation mechanisms and functions. *Journal of Biochemistry*, Vol.132, No.6, (Dec 2002), pp. 831-839, ISSN 0021-924X

Kitada, S., Andersen, J., Akar, S., Zapata, J.M., Takayama, S., Krajewski, S., Wang, H.G., Zhang, X., Bullrich, F., Croce, C.M., Rai, K., Hines, J. & Reed, J.C. (1998). Expression of apoptosis-regulating proteins in chronic lymphocytic leukemia: correlations with In vitro and In vivo chemoresponses. *Blood*, Vol.91, No.9, (May 1998), pp. 3379-3389, ISSN 0006-4971

Kitada, S., Zapata, J.M., Andreeff, M. & Reed, J.C. (1999). Bryostatin and CD40-ligand enhance apoptosis resistance and induce expression of cell survival genes in B-cell chronic lymphocytic leukaemia. *British Journal of Haematology*, Vol.106, No.4, (Sep 1999), pp. 995-1004, ISSN 0007-1048

Kitada, S., Zapata, J.M., Andreeff, M. & Reed, J.C. (2000). Protein kinase inhibitors flavopiridol and 7-hydroxy-staurosporine down-regulate antiapoptosis proteins in B-cell chronic lymphocytic leukemia. *Blood*, Vol.96, No.2, (Jul 2000), pp. 393-397, ISSN 0006-4971

Knapp, L.T. & Klann, E. (2000). Superoxide-induced stimulation of protein kinase C via thiol modification and modulation of zinc content. *Journal of Biological Chemistry*, Vol.275, No.31, (Aug 2000), pp. 24136-24145, ISSN 0021-9258

Kronfeld, I., Kazimirsky, G., Lorenzo, P.S., Garfield, S.H., Blumberg, P.M. & Brodie, C. (2000). Phosphorylation of protein kinase Cδ on distinct tyrosine residues regulates specific cellular functions. *Journal of Biological Chemistry*, Vol.275, No.45, (Nov 2000), pp. 35491-35498, ISSN 0021-9258

Lagneaux, L., Delforge, A., Bron, D., De Bruyn, C. & Stryckmans, P. (1998). Chronic lymphocytic leukemic B cells but not normal B cells are rescued from apoptosis by contact with normal bone marrow stromal cells. *Blood*, Vol.91, No.7, (Apr 1998), pp. 2387-2396, ISSN 0006-4971

Larsson, C. (2006). Protein kinase C and the regulation of the actin cytoskeleton. *Cell Signal*, Vol.18, No.3, (Mar 2006), pp. 276-284, ISSN 0898-6568

Leitges, M., Gimborn, K., Elis, W., Kalesnikoff, J., Hughes, M.R., Krystal, G. & Huber, M. (2002). Protein kinase C-δ is a negative regulator of antigen-induced mast cell degranulation. *Molecular and Cellular Biology*, Vol.22, No.12, (Jun 2002), pp. 3970-3980, ISSN 0270-7306

Liu, Z., Hazan-Halevy, I., Harris, D.M., Li, P., Ferrajoli, A., Faderl, S., Keating, M.J. & Estrov, Z. (2011). STAT-3 activates NF-κB in chronic lymphocytic leukemia cells. *Mol Cancer Research*, Vol.9, No.4, (Apr 2011), pp. 507-515, ISSN 1541-7786

Longo, P.G., Laurenti, L., Gobessi, S., Sica, S., Leone, G. & Efremov, D.G. (2008). The Akt/Mcl-1 pathway plays a prominent role in mediating antiapoptotic signals downstream of the B-cell receptor in chronic lymphocytic leukemia B cells. *Blood*, Vol.111, No.2, (Jan 2008), pp. 846-855, ISSN 0006-4971

Mandil, R., Ashkenazi, E., Blass, M., Kronfeld, I., Kazimirsky, G., Rosenthal, G., Umansky, F., Lorenzo, P.S., Blumberg, P.M. & Brodie, C. (2001). Protein kinase Cα and protein kinase Cδ play opposite roles in the proliferation and apoptosis of glioma cells. *Cancer Research*, Vol.61, No.11, (Jun 2001), pp. 4612-4619, ISSN 0008-5472

Mariano, M.T., Moretti, L., Donelli, A., Grantini, M., Montagnani, G., Di Prisco, A.U., Torelli, G., Torelli, U. & Narni, F. (1992). bcl-2 gene expression in hematopoietic cell differentiation. *Blood*, Vol.80, No.3, (Aug 1992), pp. 768-775, ISSN 0006-4971

Martin, P., Duran, A., Minguet, S., Gaspar, M.L., Diaz-Meco, M.T., Rennert, P., Leitges, M. & Moscat, J. (2002). Role of ζ PKC in B-cell signaling and function. *The EMBO Journal*, Vol.21, No.15, (Aug 2002), pp. 4049-4057, ISSN 0261-4189

Martins, L.R., Lucio, P., Silva, M.C., Gameiro, P., Silva, M.G. & Barata, J.T. (2011). On CK2 regulation of chronic lymphocytic leukemia cell viability. *Molecular and Cellular Biochemistry*, (Jul 2001), pp. ISSN 0300-8177

Matsumoto, M., Ogawa, W., Hino, Y., Furukawa, K., Ono, Y., Takahashi, M., Ohba, M., Kuroki, T. & Kasuga, M. (2001). Inhibition of insulin-induced activation of Akt by a kinase-deficient mutant of the epsilon isozyme of protein kinase C. *Journal of Biological Chemistry*, Vol.276, No.17, (Apr 2001), pp. 14400-14406, ISSN 0021-9258

Mecklenbrauker, I., Kalled, S.L., Leitges, M., Mackay, F. & Tarakhovsky, A. (2004). Regulation of B-cell survival by BAFF-dependent PKCδ-mediated nuclear signalling. *Nature*, Vol.431, No.7007, (Sep 2004), pp. 456-461, ISSN 0028-0836

Meller, N., Liu, Y.C., Collins, T.L., Bonnefoy-Berard, N., Baier, G., Isakov, N. & Altman, A. (1996). Direct interaction between protein kinase C θ (PKC θ) and 14-3-3 τ in T cells: 14-3-3 overexpression results in inhibition of PKC θ translocation and function. *Molecular and Cellular Biology*, Vol.16, No.10, (Oct 1996), pp. 5782-5791, ISSN 0270-7306

Mellor, H. & Parker, P.J. (1998). The extended protein kinase C superfamily. *The Biochemical Journal*, Vol.332 (Pt 2), (Jun 1998), pp. 281-292, ISSN 0264-6021

Michie, A.M. & Nakagawa, R. (2005). The link between PKCα regulation and cellular transformation. Immunology Letters, Vol.96, No.2, (Jan 2005), pp. 155-162, ISSN 0165-2478

Michie, A.M. & Nakagawa, R. (2006). Elucidating the role of protein kinase C in chronic lymphocytic leukaemia. *Hematolgical Oncology*, Vol.24, No.3, (Sep 2006), pp. 134-138, ISSN 0278-0232

Mohammad, R.M., Katato, K., Almatchy, V.P., Wall, N., Liu, K.Z., Schultz, C.P., Mantsch, H.H., Varterasian, M. & al-Katib, A.M. (1998). Sequential treatment of human chronic lymphocytic leukemia with bryostatin 1 followed by 2-chlorodeoxyadenosine: preclinical studies. *Clinical Cancer Research*, Vol.4, No.2, (Feb 1998), pp. 445-453, ISSN 1078-0432

Moreno, A., Villar, M.L., Camara, C., Luque, R., Cespon, C., Gonzalez-Porque, P., Roy, G., Lopez-Jimenez, J., Bootello, A. & Santiago, E.R. (2001). Interleukin-6 dimers produced by endothelial cells inhibit apoptosis of B-chronic lymphocytic leukemia cells. *Blood*, Vol.97, No.1, (Jan 2001), pp. 242-249, ISSN 0006-4971

Moscat, J. & Diaz-Meco, M.T. (2000). The atypical protein kinase Cs. Functional specificity mediated by specific protein adapters. *EMBO Reports* Vol.1, No.5, (Nov 2000), pp. 399-403, ISSN 1469-221X

Nakagawa, R., Soh, J.W. & Michie, A.M. (2006). Subversion of protein kinase C α signaling in hematopoietic progenitor cells results in the generation of a B-cell chronic lymphocytic leukemia-like population in vivo. *Cancer Research*, Vol.66, No.1, (Jan 2006), pp. 527-534, ISSN 0008-5472

Naylor, T.L., Tang, H., Ratsch, B.A., Enns, A., Loo, A., Chen, L., Lenz, P., Waters, N.J., Schuler, W., Dorken, B., Yao, Y.M., Warmuth, M., Lenz, G. & Stegmeier, F. (2011). Protein kinase C inhibitor sotrastaurin selectively inhibits the growth of CD79 mutant diffuse large B-cell lymphomas. *Cancer Research*, Vol.71, No.7, (Apr 2011), pp. 2643-2653, ISSN 0008-5472

Neill, G.W., Ghali, L.R., Green, J.L., Ikram, M.S., Philpott, M.P. & Quinn, A.G. (2003). Loss of protein kinase Cα expression may enhance the tumorigenic potential of Gli1 in basal cell carcinoma. *Cancer Research*, Vol.63, No.15, (Aug 2003), pp. 4692-4697, ISSN 0008-5472

Newton, A.C. (1995a). Protein kinase C: structure, function, and regulation. *Journal of Biological Chemistry*, Vol.270, No.48, (Dec 1995), pp. 28495-28498, ISSN 0021-9258

Newton, A.C. (1995b). Protein kinase C. Seeing two domains. *Current Biology*, Vol.5, No.9, (Sep 1995), pp. 973-976, ISSN 0960-9822

Newton, A.C. (2010). Protein kinase C: poised to signal. *American Journal of Physiology. Endocrinology and Metabolism* Vol.298, No.3, (Mar 2010), pp. E395-402, ISSN 0193-1849

Nishio, M., Endo, T., Tsukada, N., Ohata, J., Kitada, S., Reed, J.C., Zvaifler, N.J. & Kipps, T.J. (2005). Nurselike cells express BAFF and APRIL, which can promote survival of chronic lymphocytic leukemia cells via a paracrine pathway distinct from that of SDF-1α. *Blood*, Vol.106, No.3, (Aug 2005), pp. 1012-1020, ISSN 0006-4971

Nishizuka, Y. (1988). The molecular heterogeneity of protein kinase C and its implications for cellular regulation. *Nature*, Vol.334, No.6184, (Aug 1998), pp. 661-665, ISSN 0028-0836

O'Brian, C.A. (1998). Protein kinase C-α: a novel target for the therapy of androgen-independent prostate cancer? (Review-hypothesis). *Oncology Reports*, Vol.5, No.2, (Mar-Apr 1998), pp. 305-309, ISSN 1021-335X

Ono, Y., Kurokawa, T., Fujii, T., Kawahara, K., Igarashi, K., Kikkawa, U., Ogita, K. & Nishizuka, Y. (1986). Two types of complementary DNAs of rat brain protein kinase C. Heterogeneity determined by alternative splicing. *FEBS Letters*, Vol.206, No.2, (Oct 1986), pp. 347-352, ISSN 0014-5793

Oster, H. & Leitges, M. (2006). Protein kinase C α but not PKCζ suppresses intestinal tumor formation in $Apc^{Min/+}$ mice. *Cancer Research*, Vol.66, No.14, (Jul 2006), pp. 6955-6963, ISSN 0008-5472

Ota, M., Duong, B.H., Torkamani, A., Doyle, C.M., Gavin, A.L., Ota, T. & Nemazee, D. (2010). Regulation of the B cell receptor repertoire and self-reactivity by BAFF. Journal of Immunology, Vol.185, No.7, (Oct 2010), pp. 4128-4136, ISSN 0022-1767

Panayiotidis, P., Jones, D., Ganeshaguru, K., Foroni, L. & Hoffbrand, A.V. (1996). Human bone marrow stromal cells prevent apoptosis and support the survival of chronic lymphocytic leukaemia cells in vitro. *British Journal of Haematology*, Vol.92, No.1, (Jan 1996), pp. 97-103, ISSN 0007-1048

Parker, P.J. & Murray-Rust, J. (2004). PKC at a glance. *Journal of Cell Science* Vol.117, No.Pt 2, (Jan 2004), pp. 131-132, ISSN 0021-9533

Patke, A., Mecklenbrauker, I., Erdjument-Bromage, H., Tempst, P. & Tarakhovsky, A. (2006). BAFF controls B cell metabolic fitness through a PKC β- and Akt-dependent mechanism. *The Journal of Experimental Medicine*, Vol.203, No.11, (Oct 2006), pp. 2551-2562, ISSN 0022-1007

Pedersen, I.M., Kitada, S., Leoni, L.M., Zapata, J.M., Karras, J.G., Tsukada, N., Kipps, T.J., Choi, Y.S., Bennett, F. & Reed, J.C. (2002). Protection of CLL B cells by a follicular dendritic cell line is dependent on induction of Mcl-1. *Blood*, Vol.100, No.5, (Sep 2002), pp. 1795-1801, ISSN 0006-4971

Pepper, C., Lin, T.T., Pratt, G., Hewamana, S., Brennan, P., Hiller, L., Hills, R., Ward, R., Starczynski, J., Austen, B., Hooper, L., Stankovic, T. & Fegan, C. (2008). Mcl-1 expression has in vitro and in vivo significance in chronic lymphocytic leukemia and is associated with other poor prognostic markers. *Blood*, Vol.112, No.9, (Nov 2008), pp. 3807-3817, ISSN 0006-4971 (Linking)

Ringshausen, I., Schneller, F., Bogner, C., Hipp, S., Duyster, J., Peschel, C. & Decker, T. (2002). Constitutively activated phosphatidylinositol-3 kinase (PI-3K) is involved in the defect of apoptosis in B-CLL: association with protein kinase Cδ. *Blood*, Vol.100, No.10, (Nov 2002), pp. 3741-3748, ISSN 0006-4971

Ringshausen, I., Oelsner, M., Weick, K., Bogner, C., Peschel, C. & Decker, T. (2006). Mechanisms of apoptosis-induction by rottlerin: therapeutic implications for B-CLL. *Leukemia*, Vol.20, No.3, (Mar 2006), pp. 514-520, ISSN 0887-6924

Ron, D. & Mochly-Rosen, D. (1995). An autoregulatory region in protein kinase C: the pseudoanchoring site. *Proceedings of the National Academy of Sciences of the United States of America*, Vol.92, No.2, (Jan 1995), pp. 492-496, ISSN 0027-8424

Ruvolo, P.P., Deng, X., Carr, B.K. & May, W.S. (1998). A functional role for mitochondrial protein kinase Cα in Bcl2 phosphorylation and suppression of apoptosis. *Journal of Biological Chemistry*, Vol.273, No.39, (Sep 1998), pp. 25436-25442, ISSN 0021-9258 (Print)

Saijo, K., Mecklenbrauker, I., Santana, A., Leitger, M., Schmedt, C. & Tarakhovsky, A. (2002). Protein kinase C β controls nuclear factor κB activation in B cells through selective regulation of the IκB kinase α. *The Journal of Experimental Medicine*, Vol.195, No.12, (Jun 2002), pp. 1647-1652, ISSN 0022-1007

Schechtman, D. & Mochly-Rosen, D. (2001). Adaptor proteins in protein kinase C-mediated signal transduction. *Oncogene*, Vol.20, No.44, (Oct 2001), pp. 6339-6347, ISSN 0950-9232

Shinohara, H., Yasuda, T., Aiba, Y., Sanjo, H., Hamadate, M., Watarai, H., Sakurai, H. & Kurosaki, T. (2005). PKC β regulates BCR-mediated IKK activation by facilitating the interaction between TAK1 and CARMA1. *The Journal of Experimental Medicine*, Vol.202, No.10, (Nov 2005), pp. 1423-1431, ISSN 0022-1007

Shinohara, H., Maeda, S., Watarai, H. & Kurosaki, T. (2007). IκB kinase β-induced phosphorylation of CARMA1 contributes to CARMA1 Bcl10 MALT1 complex formation in B cells. *The Journal of Experimental Medicine*, Vol.204, No.13, (Dec 2007), pp. 3285-3293, ISSN 0022-1007

Skvara, H., Dawid, M., Kleyn, E., Wolff, B., Meingassner, J.G., Knight, H., Dumortier, T., Kopp, T., Fallahi, N., Stary, G., Burkhart, C., Grenet, O., Wagner, J., Hijazi, Y., Morris, R.E., McGeown, C., Rordorf, C., Griffiths, C.E., Stingl, G. & Jung, T. (2008). The PKC inhibitor AEB071 may be a therapeutic option for psoriasis. *The Journal of Clinical Investigation*, Vol.118, No.9, (Sep 2008), pp. 3151-3159, ISSN 0021-9738

Slupsky, J.R., Kamiguti, A.S., Harris, R.J., Cawley, J.C. & Zuzel, M. (2007). Central role of protein kinase Cε in constitutive activation of ERK1/2 and Rac1 in the malignant cells of hairy cell leukemia. *The American Journal of Pathology*, Vol.170, No.2, (Feb 2007), pp. 745-754, ISSN 0002-9440

Smit, L.A., Hallaert, D.Y., Spijker, R., de Goeij, B., Jaspers, A., Kater, A.P., van Oers, M.H., van Noesel, C.J. & Eldering, E. (2007). Differential Noxa/Mcl-1 balance in peripheral versus lymph node chronic lymphocytic leukemia cells correlates with survival capacity. *Blood*, Vol.109, No.4, (Feb 2007), pp. 1660-1668, ISSN 0006-4971

Snowden, R.T., Sun, X.M., Dyer, M.J. & Cohen, G.M. (2003). Bisindolylmaleimide IX is a potent inducer of apoptosis in chronic lymphocytic leukaemic cells and activates cleavage of Mcl-1. *Leukemia*, Vol.17, No.10, (Oct 2003), pp. 1981-1989, ISSN 0887-6924

Soltoff, S.P. (2007). Rottlerin: an inappropriate and ineffective inhibitor of PKCδ. *Trends Pharmacol Sci*, Vol.28, No.9, (Sep 2007), pp. 453-458, ISSN 0165-6147

Staudinger, J., Lu, J. & Olson, E.N. (1997). Specific interaction of the PDZ domain protein PICK1 with the COOH terminus of protein kinase C-α. *Journal of Biological Chemistry*, Vol.272, No.51, (Dec 1997), pp. 32019-32024, ISSN 0021-9258

Stohl, W., Xu, D., Kim, K.S., Koss, M.N., Jorgensen, T.N., Deocharan, B., Metzger, T.E., Bixler, S.A., Hong, Y.S., Ambrose, C.M., Mackay, F., Morel, L., Putterman, C., Kotzin, B.L. & Kalled, S.L. (2005). BAFF overexpression and accelerated glomerular disease in mice with an incomplete genetic predisposition to systemic lupus erythematosus. *Arthritis and rheumatism*, Vol.52, No.7, (Jul 2005), pp. 2080-2091, ISSN 0004-3591

Szallasi, Z., Smith, C.B., Pettit, G.R. & Blumberg, P.M. (1994). Differential regulation of protein kinase C isozymes by bryostatin 1 and phorbol 12-myristate 13-acetate in NIH 3T3 fibroblasts. *Journal of Biological Chemistry*, Vol.269, No.3, (Jan 1994), pp. 2118-2124, ISSN 0021-9258

Tan, S.L. & Parker, P.J. (2003). Emerging and diverse roles of protein kinase C in immune cell signalling. *The Biochemical Journal*, Vol.376, No.Pt 3, (Dec 2003), pp. 545-552, ISSN 0264-6021

Thomas, A., Pepper, C., Hoy, T. & Bentley, P. (2004). Bryostatin induces protein kinase C modulation, Mcl-1 up-regulation and phosphorylation of Bcl-2 resulting in cellular differentiation and resistance to drug-induced apoptosis in B-cell chronic lymphocytic leukemia cells. *Leukemia & Lymphoma*, Vol.45, No.5, (May 2004), pp. 997-1008, ISSN 1026-8022

Totterman, T.H., Nilsson, K. & Sundstrom, C. (1980). Phorbol ester-induced differentiation of chronic lymphocytic leukaemia cells. *Nature*, Vol.288, No.5787, (Nov 1980), pp. 176-178, ISSN 0028-0836

Varterasian, M.L., Mohammad, R.M., Eilender, D.S., Hulburd, K., Rodriguez, D.H., Pemberton, P.A., Pluda, J.M., Dan, M.D., Pettit, G.R., Chen, B.D. & Al-Katib, A.M. (1998). Phase I study of bryostatin 1 in patients with relapsed non-Hodgkin's lymphoma and chronic lymphocytic leukemia. *Journal of Clinical Oncology*, Vol.16, No.1, (Jan 1998), pp. 56-62, ISSN 0732-183X

Varterasian, M.L., Mohammad, R.M., Shurafa, M.S., Hulburd, K., Pemberton, P.A., Rodriguez, D.H., Spadoni, V., Eilender, D.S., Murgo, A., Wall, N., Dan, M. & Al-Katib, A.M. (2000). Phase II trial of bryostatin 1 in patients with relapsed low-grade non-Hodgkin's lymphoma and chronic lymphocytic leukemia. *Clinical Cancer Research*, Vol.6, No.3, (Mar 2000), pp. 825-828, ISSN 1078-0432

Villalba, M., Kasibhatla, S., Genestier, L., Mahboubi, A., Green, D.R. & Altman, A. (1999). Protein kinase cθ cooperates with calcineurin to induce Fas ligand expression during activation-induced T cell death. *Journal of Immunology*, Vol.163, No.11, (Dec 1999), pp. 5813-5819, ISSN 0022-1767

Waldron, R.T. & Rozengurt, E. (2003). Protein kinase C phosphorylates protein kinase D activation loop Ser744 and Ser748 and releases autoinhibition by the pleckstrin homology domain. *Journal of Biological Chemistry*, Vol.278, No.1, (Jan 2003), pp. 154-163, ISSN 0021-9258

Wert, M.M. & Palfrey, H.C. (2000). Divergence in the anti-apoptotic signalling pathways used by nerve growth factor and basic fibroblast growth factor (bFGF) in PC12 cells: rescue by bFGF involves protein kinase C δ. *The Biochemical Journal*, Vol.352 Pt 1, (Nov 2000), pp. 175-182, ISSN 0264-6021

Yan, X.J., Albesiano, E., Zanesi, N., Yancopoulos, S., Sawyer, A., Romano, E., Petlickovski, A., Efremov, D.G., Croce, C.M. & Chiorazzi, N. (2006). B cell receptors in TCL1 transgenic mice resemble those of aggressive, treatment-resistant human chronic lymphocytic leukemia. *Proceedings of the National Academy of Sciences of the United States of America* Vol.103, No.31, (Aug 2006), pp. 11713-11718, ISSN 0027-8424

Yuan, Z.M., Utsugisawa, T., Ishiko, T., Nakada, S., Huang, Y., Kharbanda, S., Weichselbaum, R. & Kufe, D. (1998). Activation of protein kinase C δ by the c-Abl tyrosine kinase in response to ionizing radiation. *Oncogene*, Vol.16, No.13, (Apr 1998), pp. 1643-1648, ISSN 0950-9232

Zhuang, J., Hawkins, S.F., Glenn, M.A., Lin, K., Johnson, G.G., Carter, A., Cawley, J.C. & Pettitt, A.R. (2010). Akt is activated in chronic lymphocytic leukemia cells and delivers a pro-survival signal: the therapeutic potential of Akt inhibition. *Haematologica*, Vol.95, No.1, (Jan 2010), pp. 110-118, ISSN 0390-6078

zum Buschenfelde, C.M., Wagner, M., Lutzny, G., Oelsner, M., Feuerstacke, Y., Decker, T., Bogner, C., Peschel, C. & Ringshausen, I. (2010). Recruitment of PKC-βII to lipid rafts mediates apoptosis-resistance in chronic lymphocytic leukemia expressing ZAP-70. *Leukemia*, Vol.24, No.1, (Jan 2010), pp. 141-152, ISSN 0887-6924

9

The Role of Polymorphisms in Co-Signalling Molecules' Genes in Susceptibility to B-Cell Chronic Lymphocytic Leukaemia

Lidia Karabon[1,2] and Irena Frydecka[1,2]
[1]*Institute of Immunology & Experimental Therapy, Polish Academy of Science, Wroclaw,*
[2]*Wroclaw Medical University, Wroclaw,*
Poland

1. Introduction

Chronic lymphocytic leukaemia (CLL) is associated with several humoural and cellular immune abnormalities (Scrivener *et al*, 2003; Stevenson & Caligaris-Cappio, 2004) that could lead to an inadequate anti-tumour response. The immune surveillance of tumour cells depends on the recognition of antigens presented in the context of human leukocyte receptor HLA class I molecules by cytotoxic T lymphocytes (CTLs), via their T-cell receptors (TCRs) (Rosenberg, 2001). However, antigen alone is insufficient to drive the activation of naïve T-cells (Lafferty *et al*, 1978), and the two-signal model of T-cell activation was proposed. According to this model, the effective activation of naïve T cells requires second, antigen independent, co-stimulatory signal provided by the interaction between a co-stimulatory receptor and its ligand on an antigen-presenting cell (Jenkins *et al*, 1990; Schwartz *et al*, 1989). The lack of co-stimulation results in T-cell tolerance and anergy. Over the past several years, a large number of molecules have been identified that function as second signals following TCR engagement, and many have been revealed to be negative co-stimulatory molecules, which dampen T-cell activation and regulate immune tolerance. Some have been shown to be upregulated in the tumour microenvironment and have become potential targets for augmenting anti-tumour immunity (Sharpe, 2009).

Polymorphisms in genes can influence the level of protein expression (Anjos *et al*, 2002; Kouki *et al*, 2000; Wang *et al*, 2002b; Oki *et al*, 2011). Therefore, genetic variation in genes encoding co-signalling molecules may also alter the antitumour response and influence cancer susceptibility, particularly susceptibility to CLL.

Here we focus on polymorphisms in genes encoding co-signalling molecules that belong to the best-characterized B7/CD28 family, which plays a crucial role in T-cell activation.

2. Co-signalling molecules – Overview

2.1 Cluster of differentiation 28 (CD28)

CD28 is the primary co-stimulatory molecule constitutively expressed on the majority of T cells (95% of $CD4^+$ T cells and approximately 50% of $CD8^+$ T cells). Upon interaction with its ligands CD80 (B7.1) and CD86 (B7.2), CD28 transduces a signal that enhances the activation and proliferation of T cells and IL-2 production (Frauwirth & Thompson, 2002; Carreno & Collins, 2002). In addition, a higher level of secretion of other cytokines such as IFN-γ, GM-CSF, IL-4, IL-8 and IL-13, can be observed after CD28 ligation. Moreover, CD28 signalling promotes cell survival via Bcl-x_L transcriptions and prevents anergy (Boise *et al*, 1995). It has been shown that mice deficient in CD28 or both of its ligands (B7.1 and B7.2) have severely impaired $CD4^+$ T cell proliferation (Shahinian *et al*, 1993; Borriello *et al*, 1997) and lymphokine secretion after stimulation with concanavalin A (Con A) or superantigen (Mittrucker *et al*, 1996). Furthermore, CD28-deficient mice exhibit lower levels of certain isotypes of immunoglobulins, and germinal centres are not formed in response to immunisation (Ferguson *et al*, 1996). The requirement for CD28 for the co-stimulation of $CD8^+$ T cells is more controversial; it was postulated that $CD8^+$ T cells are less CD28 dependent than $CD4^+$ cells (Green *et al*, 1995).

The *CD28* is located on the q33 region of chromosome 2. The gene encoding *CD28* consist of four exons, of which exon 1 encodes the leader peptide, exon 2 the ligand binding domain, exon 3 the transmembrane segment, and exon 4 the cytoplasmic tail. Within the gene encoding the CD28 molecule several polymorphic sites have been identified. Three of these sites are non-synonymous gene polymorphisms: the *CD28c.73G>A* (rs3181099) single nucleotide polymorphism (SNP) in exon 1, which leads to change from Gly 25 to Arg; the *CD28c.224G>A* (rs35290181) SNP in exon 2 which changes Ser 75 to Asn, and the *CD28c.272G>A* (rs75899942) SNP that is also in the second exon, which changes Gly91 to Asp. Moreover, 4 synonymous SNP were found, all in the third exon.

It has been reported that variations in non-coding regions can regulate gene expression by altering the motif of functional DNA binding sites, thereby affecting their affinity to transcription factors.

In the intronic region of *CD28* gene eleven SNPs have been described, but CD28c*.17+3T>C* (rs3116496) is the best studied in the context of susceptibility to autoimmune and neoplastic disease. This polymorphism is located near the splice receptor site and might influence the mRNA splicing efficiency and thus the expression of the CD28 molecule (Ahmed *et al*, 2001). Another widely investigated SNP in the *CD28* gene is *CD28 -372G>A* (rs35593994), which is situated in the promoter (Teutsch *et al*, 2004). The potential functional effect of this SNP remains to be elucidated, but a search for transcription factor binding sites suggested that the *CD28-372G>A* [A] allele differs from the *CD28-372G>A* [G] allele by the presence of a binding site for the CCAAT enhancer-binding protein and the lack of a binding site for growth factor independence 1 (Teutsch *et al*, 2004). Only one microsatellite polymorphism was described in the *CD28* gene and in comparison with many other microsatellites, it presented a low degree of polymorphism. The most common allele occurred at frequencies higher than 0.8, and the gene diversity is close to 0.3 (Pincerati *et al*, 2010).

2.2 Inducible co-stimulator (ICOS)

The second co-stimulatory molecule is ICOS, which appears on T lymphocytes rapidly upon activation (Hutloff *et al*, 1999) and on unpolarised as well as Th1, Th2, Th17, and Treg subpopulations of $CD4^+$ cells (McAdam *et al*, 2000; Tan *et al*, 2008; Nakae *et al*, 2007; Akiba *et al*, 2005; Burmeister *et al*, 2008). This co-stimulatory molecule binds the B7-related protein

B7RP-1 (Yoshinaga *et al*, 1999). Like CD28, ICOS provides a signal for T-cell activation and differentiation, and in one model, animals lacking this molecule had a reduced CD4$^+$ T-cell response (Dong *et al*, 2003).

While CD28 and ICOS have overlapping functions in early T-cell activation, ICOS augments the T-cell effector function, in particular the production of IL-4, IL-5, IL-10, IFN-α, and IFN- γ (Beier *et al*, 2000), but not IL-2 (Hutloff *et al*, 1999). In addition, ICOS is important for the generation of chemokine receptor 5 (CXCR5)$^+$ follicular helper T cells (T_{FH}), a unique T-cell subset that regulates germinal centre formation and humoural immunity (Nurieva *et al*, 2008).

ICOS knockout mice have reduced CD4$^+$ T-cell responses, an increased risk of experimental autoimmune encephalomyelitis (Dong *et al*, 2001), and defects in immunoglobulin class switching and germinal centre formation (McAdam *et al*, 2001).

In human, the homozygous loss of the *ICOS* gene is the cause of the ICOS deficiency (ICOSD) form of common variable immunodeficiency (CVID). ICOSD patients suffer from recurrent bacterial infections of the respiratory and digestive tracts, which are characteristic of humoural immunodeficiency, but do not have other complicating features, such as splenomegaly, autoimmune phenomena, or sarcoid-like granulomas, or clinical signs of overt T-cell immunodeficiency (Grimbacher *et al*, 2003). A severe disturbance of T cell-dependent B-cell maturation occurs in the secondary lymphoid tissue; B cells exhibit a naive IgD$^+$/IgM$^+$ phenotype, and the numbers of IgM memory and switched memory B cells are substantially reduced in individuals with ICOSD (Grimbacher *et al*, 2003).

The *ICOS* gene also located in the 2q33 region contains five exons. Exons 1-4 are parallel to those of *CD28*, while exon 5 encodes an additional fragment of the cytoplasmic tail. In the *ICOS* gene, two microsatellites in the fourth intron and 31 single-nucleotide polymorphisms (SNPs) (http://www.hapmap.org) have been found. None of the described *ICOS* SNPs leads to changes in the amino acid sequence, although a few have been demonstrated to be functional variants (Kaartinen *et al*, 2007; Haimila *et al*, 2009; Castelli *et al*, 2007; Shilling *et al*, 2005).

The *ICOSc.1624C>T* (rs10932037) polymorphism has been shown to influence the ICOS mRNA level (Kaartinen *et al*, 2007). The authors described that activated CD4$^+$ T cells from *ICOSc.1624C>T* [CC] homozygous people had higher actual levels of ICOS mRNA than cells from [TC] heterozygous people 1 h and 3 h after activation, following which this difference disappeared.

The *ICOSc.1624C>T (rs10932037)*, *ICOSc.1624C>T*(rs10932037), and *ICOSc.2373G>C* (rs10183087) SNPs, which are located in the 3' untranslated region (UTR) of the *ICOS* gene, influence the functions of the *ICOS* gene (Castelli *et al*, 2007). Three major haplotypes, which were associated with different levels of expression of ICOS in CD3$^+$ cells and IL-10 secretion have been identified. The AA genotype, characterised by presence of *ICOSc.1624C>T*[CC], *ICOSc.602A>*C[AA], and *ICOSc.2373G>*C[GG] was shown to be associated with the lowest percentage of CD3+ activated cells expressing ICOS and the highest levels of IL-10 secretion.

The *ICOSISV1+173T>*C (rs10932029) polymorphism, which is located close to the *CTLA-4* gene, has been reported to affect the expression of the CTLA-4 isoforms (Kaartinen *et al*, 2007; Brown *et al*, 2007).

Two microsatellite polymorphisms have been described in the fourth intron of the *ICOS* gene. The first is a GT repeats at position 1554, the location of an Sp1 binding site, and the second, a T repeats, is at a position near the splice donor site (Ihara *et al*, 2001).

2.3 Cytotoxic T lymphocyte- associated antigen-4 (CTLA-4)

CTLA-4 has been well established as negative regulator of T-cell function (Walunas *et al*, 1994; Walunas *et al*, 1996). CTLA-4 is rapidly expressed on T cells following activation and is highly up-regulated by CD28 engagement. CTLA-4 shares the B7 ligands with CD28.

CTLA-4 binding with its ligands antagonises early T-cell activation, leading to decreased IL-2 production, the inhibition of cell-cycle progression, decreased cyclin expression, and the modulation of TCR signalling (Luhder *et al*, 2000). CTLA-4-deficient mice develop a severe lymphoproliferative disease and die within 3-4 weeks (Tivol *et al*, 1995; Waterhouse *et al*, 1995). CTLA-4 is also important in the function of regulatory cells, which suppress effector T-cell activation and function (Tang *et al*, 2004; Tai *et al*, 2005).

Many mechanistic models have been postulated for the function of CTLA-4. These models include competition with the co-stimulatory CD28 molecule by more effectively binding their common ligands, the inhibition of downstream TCR signalling by the phosphates SH2 domain, the inhibition of lipid-raft and microcluster formation, and the negative regulation of the immune response by extrinsic components such as TGF-β and the tryptophan-degrading enzyme indoleamine 2,3-dioxygenase (IDO) (Rudd *et al*, 2009).

The *CTLA-4* gene is located between *CD28* and *ICOS* genes. It is similar to *CD28* gene and consists of four exons, of which exon 1 encodes the leader peptide, exon 2 the ligand binding domain, exon 3 the transmembrane segment, and exon 4 the cytoplasmic tail. The functional significance of the polymorphisms in the *CTLA-4* gene have been widely explored and described. The most studied is the *CTLA-4c.49A>G* (rs231775) transition. This non-synonymous SNP causes an amino acid change from threonine to alanine. It influences T-cell activation and could have a role in antitumour immunity. The presence of the [AA] genotype as opposed to the [GG] genotype has been shown to be associated with significantly lower levels of activation of T lymphocytes and lower proliferation. The protein product encoded by the *CTLA-4c.49A>G*[AA] genotype, CTLA-4^{17}Thr, had a higher capacity to bind B7.1 and a stronger inhibitory effect on T-cell activation compared with CTLA-4^{17}Ala (Sun *et al*, 2008). It was also postulated that the *CTLA-4c.49A>G* polymorphism in the leader sequence of the protein alters the inhibitory function of the molecule by influencing the rate of endocytosis or surface trafficking (Kouki *et al*, 2000) and the glycosylation of CTLA-4 (Anjos *et al*, 2002).

The *CTLA-4*g.319C>T (rs5742909) SNP located in the promoter region also has documented functional significance. The *CTLA-4*g.319C>T[T] allele has been associated with a higher promoter activity (Wang *et al*, 2002b), probably due to the creation of a lymphoid enhancer factor-1 (LEF1) binding site in the *CTLA-4* promoter (Chistiakov *et al*, 2006). This allele has also been associated with significantly increased mRNA and surface expression of CTLA-4 in stimulated and non-stimulated cells (Ligers *et al*, 2001; Anjos *et al*, 2002).

The *CTLA-4g.1661A>C* (rs4553808) SNP, also located in the promoter, appears to be involved in the transcription-associated binding activity of nuclear factor (NF-1) and C/EBPβ and might cause abnormal alternative spicing and affect the expression of CTLA-4 (Wang *et al*, 2008).

The *CTLA*-4g.*6230G>A (CT60) (rs3087243) polymorphism situated in the 3′ UTR was shown to be associated with variations in the mRNA level of soluble CTLA-4, an isoform lacking the transmembrane domain, that is generated by the alternative splicing of the primary transcript (Ueda *et al*, 2003). Our recent results indicate that the CT60 polymorphism together with the Jo31 SNP (*CTLA*-4g.10223G>T, rs11571302, also located in the 3′ region) is associated with the levels of membrane and cytoplasmic CTLA-4 in $CD4^+$ T lymphocytes from multiple sclerosis patients (Karabon *et al*, 2009) and with the altered levels of soluble CTLA-4 in the serum of Graves' disease patients (Daroszewski *et al*, 2009).

Another widely investigated genetic marker situated in the 3′ UTR region of *CTLA*-4 gene is a microsatellite polymorphism *CTLA*-4g.*642AT(8_33). The number of dinucleotide (AT) repeats at position 642 in the 3′UTR region has been shown to be associated with the stability of the mRNA transcripts (Wang *et al*, 2002a).

2.4 Programmed death-1 (PD-1)

Similar to CTLA-4, PD-1 has been described as a negative regulator of T- and B-cell function. PD-1 is an inducible molecule expressed on activated T- and B-cells (Greenwald *et al*, 2005). In reactive lymph nodes, PD-1 was mainly expressed in follicular T cells (Dorfman *et al*, 2006). PD-1 binding limits T-cell functions, including T-cell proliferation, apoptosis and interferon-γ production (Freeman *et al*, 2000).

Knockout PD-1 mice develop different autoimmune diseases depending on the genetic background: BALBc mice develop autoimmune cardiomyopathy (Nishimura *et al*, 2001); C57BL mice develop progressive arthritis and lupus-like glomerulonephritis (Nishimura *et al*, 1999); and NOD mice develop autoimmune diabetes (Wang *et al*, 2005). PD-1 also has a critical role in murine experimental encephalomyelitis (Salama *et al*, 2003).

PD-1 has two ligands, which belong to the B7 superfamily: PD-L1 (B7-H) and PD-L2 (B7-DC). The mRNA expression patterns of PD-L1 and PD-L2 are different. PD-L1 is broadly expressed in different human and mouse cells, such as leukocytes, non-haematopoietic cells and non-lymphoid tissue (Freeman *et al*, 2000), while PD-L2 is present exclusively on dendritic cells and monocytes (Latchman *et al*, 2001; Liang *et al*, 2006). The differential expression patterns of PD-L1/PD-L2 and CD80/CD86 are crucial differences between CTLA-4 and PD-1, and this fact raises the hypothesis that CTLA-4 has a key role in the early stages of tolerance induction, while PD-1 functions late for the maintenance of long-term tolerance. The expression of PD-1 ligands limits T-cell function within tissue-specific sites, while CTLA-4 limits T cells in lymphoid structures because CD80 and CD86 are expressed on antigen-presenting cells.

The *PD-1* gene is also located on the long arm of chromosome 2, but in the 37.3 region. Similar to the *ICOS* gene, it consists of 5 exons: exon 1 encodes leader peptide, exon 2 extracellular IgV-like domain, exon 3 the transmembrane domain, exon 4 and 5 the intracellular domain. So far, more than 30 SNPs have been identified in the *PD-1* gene. These polymorphisms have been investigated mainly in context of susceptibility to autoimmune disease, such as rheumatoid arthritis (RA) (Kong *et al*, 2005), type I diabetes (Flores *et al*, 2010), ankylosis spondylitis (AS) (Lee *et al*, 2006), and systemic lupus erytrhomatosus (SLE) (Velazquez-Cruz *et al*, 2007), but only a few studies have been devoted to determining the functional significance of these genetic variations. Among the *PD-1* gene polymorphisms, seven namely PD-1.1, PD-1.2, PD-1.3, PD-1.4, PD-1.5, PD-1.6 and PD-1.9, have been studied the most frequently. Two SNPs (PD-1.5 (*57785C>T* - rs2227981) and PD-1.9 *(7625C>T* - rs2227982)) occur in exon 5. The C>T transition in the PD-1.9 SNP causes a change in amino acid from valine to alanine, while PD1.5 is a synonymous coding variant.

PD-1.1 (*−538G>A* - rs58398280) is located in promoter region, PD-1.2 (*6438G>A* - rs34819229), PD1.3 (*7146G>A - rs11568821*), and PD1.4 (*7499G>A* - rs6705653)) are situated in introns 2, 4, and 4, respectively, while the PD1.6 (*8737G>A*) SNP is in the 3′ UTR (Ferreiros-Vidal *et al*, 2004).

The data describing the functional roles of the *PD-1* gene polymorphisms are limited. It has been shown that the PD-1.3 (7146G>A) polymorphism has functional significance, and the presence of PD-1.3. The [A] allele has been associated with a significantly lower expression of the PD-1 receptor in SLE patients, their relatives and healthy individuals (Kristjansdottir *et al*, 2010).

Patients homozygous for PD-1.3[AA], but not heterozygous for PD-1.3[AG], had reduced basal and induced PD-1 expression on activated $CD4^+$ T cells. In an autologous mixed lymphocyte reactions (AMLRs), activated $CD4^+$ cells from SLE patients had defective PD-1 induction, and this abnormality was more pronounced in homozygotes than heterozygotes. Moreover, the A allele conferred decreased transcriptional activity in transfected Jurkat cells (Bertsias *et al*, 2009).

The *7209C>T* SNP located in intron 4 of the *PD-1* gene was also found to be associated with protein expression. Using a luciferase reporter assay, it was shown that the *PD-1 7209C>T*[T] allele creates a negative *cis*-element for gene transcription (Zheng *et al*, 2010).

The promoter polymorphism *PD-1-606G>A* (rs360488323) alters the promoter activity. The significantly higher promoter activity was observed with the construct with the *PD-1-606G>A* [G] allele than with the *PD-1-606G>A* [A] allele *(*Ishizaki *et al, 2010).*

2.5 B and T lymphocyte attenuator (BTLA)

Although BTLA shares only 9-13% amino acid identity with CTLA-4 and PD-1, it is structurally similar to them. The presence of two ITIM motifs in its cytoplasmic region suggests, that it has an inhibitory function. In mice, it is expressed at a very low level on resting T cells, and it is induced during activation. Interestingly, after T-cell differentiation, only T helper type Th1, but not Th2, cells express BTLA, and its expression is independent of interleukin 12 (IL-12) or IFN-γ, suggesting a specific role for BTLA in Th-1 cells (Watanabe *et al*, 2003). However, BTLA transcripts have been detected in primary B cells and B-cell lines, which indicates its role in the regulation of the B-cell response. In comparison with other co-inhibitory molecules, BTLA is more widely expressed than CTLA-4, which is expressed only on T-cells, but has more limited expression than PD-1, which is expressed on T, B and myeloid cells.

Blocking BTLA prevents proliferation and cytokine production by T cells. BTLA-deficient mice exhibit a moderate increase in specific antibody responses and increased susceptibility to experimentally induced autoimmune encephalomyelitis (EAC) (Watanabe *et al*, 2003).

In humans, BTLA is highly expressed on $CD14^+$ monocytes and $CD19^+$ B cells, constituently on $CD4^+$ and $CD8^+$ lymphocytes and weakly on $CD56^+$ NK-cells. Among normal B cells, the highest level of BTLA-expression is found in naïve B cells. Of normal T cells, high levels of BTLA expression are found in T follicular helper (T_{FH}) cells (M'Hidi *et al*, 2009). When PBMCs were stimulated 2 days with LPS, the expression of BTLA on $CD14^+$ monocytes and $CD19^+$ B cells decreased to some extent, while the expression on the other cell types, $CD4^+$ and $CD8^+$ lymphocytes and $CD56^+$ NK cells, is upregulated.

BTLA binds the herpes virus entry mediator (HVEM). Interestingly HVEM is a member of the TNFR family, and its interaction with BTLA is the first demonstration of crosstalk between CD28 and the TNFR family. HVEM is expressed on resting T cells, B cells, macrophages and immature dendritic cells, and its expression is downregulated on activated T cells (Sedy *et al*, 2005; Gonzalez *et al*, 2005)

Unlike the other co-signalling molecules described, the *BTLA* gene is located on chromosome 3 in q13.2 region. However, like *ICOS* it has 5 exons (Garapati VP & Lefranc MP, 2007). Because *BTLA* was relatively recently described in the literature, there are only a few studies that address *BTLA* gene polymorphisms, and most have investigated its role in susceptibility to autoimmune diseases, such as RA (Lin *et al*, 2006; Oki *et al*, 2011), SLE and type 1 diabetes mellitus (Inuo *et al*, 2009). The non-synonymous *BTLAc.800G>A* SNP (rs9288952) which leads to a Pro 219 to Leu exchange, has been associated with susceptibility to RA (Lin *et al*, 2006).

Another study has described a functional polymorphism, *BTLAc.590A>C* (rs76844316) (Oki *et al*, 2011). This polymorphism is located in forth exon of the *BTLA* gene gene and leads to the exchange of asparagine to threonine in the intracellular domain. It was found that the C allele is associated with decreased inhibitory activity of BTLA in ConA- and anti-CD3-induced IL-2 production, although the surface expression level is similar in transfectants of both the A and C alleles. It was postulated that the change in amino acids interferes with BTLA signalling and downregulates the association of an unidentified kinase that phosphorylates BTLA or SHP1/SHP2 (Oki *et al*, 2011).

3. Polymorphisms in co-signalling genes and susceptibility to cancer

Because the significance of co-signalling molecules in the regulation of immune response has been clearly documented, polymorphisms in the genes encoding those molecules have been widely investigated, previously as susceptibility determinants for autoimmune disease and recently for cancer. Among others, *CTLA-4* gene polymorphisms have been investigated the most intensively. It was found that the *CTLA-4c.49A>G*[A] allele was associated with an increased risk of many types of cancers, including oesophageal cancer, gastric cardia cancer (Sun *et al*, 2008), non-Hodgkin's lymphoma (Piras *et al*, 2005), breast cancer (Ghaderi *et al*, 2004; Sun *et al*, 2008), renal cancer (Cozar *et al*, 2007) and lung cancer, esophagus and gastric cardia cancer (Sun *et al*, 2008). Wong *et al* (2006) reported that although the *CTLA-4c.49A>G*[AA] genotype did not increase the risk of oral squamous cell cancer, it correlated significantly with a younger age at onset and poorer survival. Notably, the *CTLA-4c.49A>G*[GG] genotype was found to be prevalent in mucosa-associated lymphoid tissue lymphoma (Cheng *et al*, 2006) and in multiple myeloma (Karabon *et al*, 2011c). There was no association between the *CTLA-4c.49A>G* SNP and colorectal cancer (Solerio *et al*, 2005; Hadinia *et al*, 2007), B-cell chronic lymphocytic leukaemia (Suwalska *et al*, 2008), cervical squamous cell carcinoma (Su *et al*, 2007), malignant melanoma (Bouwhuis *et al*, 2009), or non-malignant melanoma (Welsh *et al*, 2009).

The *CTLA-4*g.319C>T polymorphism was shown to be associated with female-related cancers such as sporadic breast cancer (Wong *et al*, 2006) cervical cancer (Su *et al*, 2007; Pawlak *et al*, 2010) and lung cancer in women (Karabon *et al.* 2011). However, this polymorphism was not associated with lung cancer (without stratification by gender) (Sun *et al*, 2008) or other cancers, such as colon cancer (Cozar *et al*, 2007), colorectal cancer (Dilmec *et al*, 2008) or multiple myeloma (Karabon *et al*, 2011c).

A limited number of studies have been devoted to the association between the CT60 and Jo31 SNPs and cancers. No association was found between CT60 and Jo31 and lung cancers (Karabon *et al*, 2011b; Sun *et al*, 2008), cervical squamous cell carcinoma (Su *et al*, 2007;Pawlak *et al*, 2010) or malignant melanoma (Bouwhuis *et al*, 2009). However, the CT60 [AA] homozygosity correlated with an increased risk of renal cell cancer and with tumour grade (Cozar *et al*, 2007), while the presence of the A allele is associated with increased susceptibility to non-melanoma skin cancer (Welsh *et al*, 2009). In contrast, the CT60[G] alleles were found to be prevalent in patients with sporadic breast cancer (Wong *et al*, 2006) and in multiple myeloma patients (Karabon *et al*, 2011c).

Only one study indicates a possible predisposing role for the *CTLA-4g.1661A>G* [G] allele in susceptibility to oral squamous cell carcinoma (OSCC) (Kammerer *et al*, 2010).

In summary, the latest meta-analysis, which summarised data from 48 studies, confirmed that the presence of the G allele in *CTLA-4c.49A>G* polymorphisms decreased the risk of cancer compared with that with the homozygous *CTLA-4c.49A>G*[AA] genotype. Interestingly, the *CTLA-4c.49A>G*[AG+GG] genotype was associated with a decreased risk of cancer in Asians, but not among Europeans, while the *CTLA-4*g.319C>T[T] allele was associated with an increased risk among Europeans but not Asians. The meta-analysis did not confirm the role of the CT60 SNP as a cancer risk factor (Zhang *et al*, 2011).

Polymorphisms in the *CD28* gene have not been as widely investigated. The *CD28*c.17+3T>C SNP was not associated in an indirect way with non-solid tumour cancer, while several conditioner associations were established. Our study revealed a lack of association between the *CD28*c.17+3T>C polymorphism and CSCC, while we found an association with well-differentiated tumours (Pawlak *et al*, 2010). No association with the *CD28*c.17+3T>C polymorphism was found in a previous study with cervical cancer, but Guzman showed an epistatic effect between *CD28* and *IFNG* genes in susceptibility to cervical cancer (Guzman *et al*, 2008). Recently a Chinese study and a Swedish study confirmed the *CD28*c.17+3T>C polymorphism as an independent risk factor for the development of that cancer (Ivansson *et al*, 2010;Chen *et al*, 2011).

The *CD28c.17+3T>C* SNP is not susceptibility locus for gastric mucosa-associated lymphoid tissue (MALT) lymphoma (Cheng *et al*, 2006), colorectal cancer (Dilmec *et al*, 2008) or, together with other tag polymorphisms in the *CD28* gene, malignant melanoma (Bouwhuis *et al*, 2009). Two polymorphic sites, rs3181100 and rs3181113, were shown to not be associated with OSCC (Kammerer *et al*, 2010).

ICOS gene polymorphisms have been widely examined for their potential role as susceptibility locus for melanoma (Bouwhuis *et al*, 2009), but none of the tested tag polymorphisms was associated with this disease. The *ICOSc.602A>C* and *ICOSc.1624C>T* polymorphisms are not related to the risk for MALT (Cheng *et al*, 2006). Similarly, the distribution of alleles and genotypes of *ICOSc.602A>C* and *ICOSc.1599C>T* polymorphisms were no different between OSCC patients and controls (Kammerer *et al*, 2010).

The *PD-1* gene polymorphism mentioned in the previous subsection (2.4) has been widely explored as a susceptibility locus for autoimmune diseases (Kong *et al*, 2005; Flores *et al*, 2010; Lee *et al*, 2006; Velazquez-Cruz *et al*, 2007). Only a few studies have been devoted to the relationship between *PD-1* polymorphisms and cancer. Recently, it has been shown that polymorphisms (PD-1.1, and PD-1.5) alone and as a part of haplotype confers susceptibility to breast cancer in Chinese population (Hua *et al*, 2011). In contrast, in an Iranian population, neither PD1.3 nor PD-1.5 was associated with the risk of breast cancer (Haghshenas *et al*, 2011).

Polymorphisms in the gene of another co-signalling molecule *BTLA* have been investigated mostly in context of autoimmunity. Only one Chinese study was performed to investigate the relationship between *BTLA* polymorphisms and breast cancer (Fu *et al*, 2010). A strong association was found between three polymorphisms, rs9288952, rs2705535 and rs1844089, and the risk of breast cancer. Moreover, associations were also found with tumour size, the oestrogen receptor, the progesterone receptor, C-erbB-2 and the P53 status.

The more important polymorphisms in *CD28, CTLA-4, ICOS, PD-1 and BTLA* genes and their associations with susceptibility to cancer are displaying on Figure 1.

4. Expression of co-signalling molecules in B-cell chronic lymphocytic leukaemia

One of the mechanisms by which neoplastic cells escape elimination by host cells is the downregulation of the co-stimulatory pathway. Actually, a decreased expression of co-stimulatory molecules and the overexpression of co-inhibitory molecules in peripheral blood (PB) T cells have been reported in patients with several neoplastic diseases.

The downregulated expression of the CD28 antigen on peripheral blood T lymphocytes was reported in patients with solid tumours such as: gastric carcinoma, cervical cancer and malignant melanoma (reviewed by (Bocko *et al*, 2002)), and in patients with multiple myeloma (Brown *et al*, 1998; Robillard *et al*, 1998) and hairy-cell leukaemia (van de Corp *et al*, 1999)

Considering the pivotal role of the co-signalling pathway in the antitumour response, several studies have been devoted to examining the expression level of co-signaling molecules in patients with CLL. The investigation by Rossi et al. (Rossi *et al*, 1996), which was confirmed by Van den Hove et al. (1997) showed significantly lower expression of CD28 on T-cell subsets of chronic lymphocytic leukaemia, and this lower expression was more pronounced in the $CD8^+$ subset than in the $CD4^+$ subset. Scrivener et al. (2003) reported a decreased proportion of $CD2^+/CD28^+$ cells in unstimulated and stimulated PB from CLL patients.

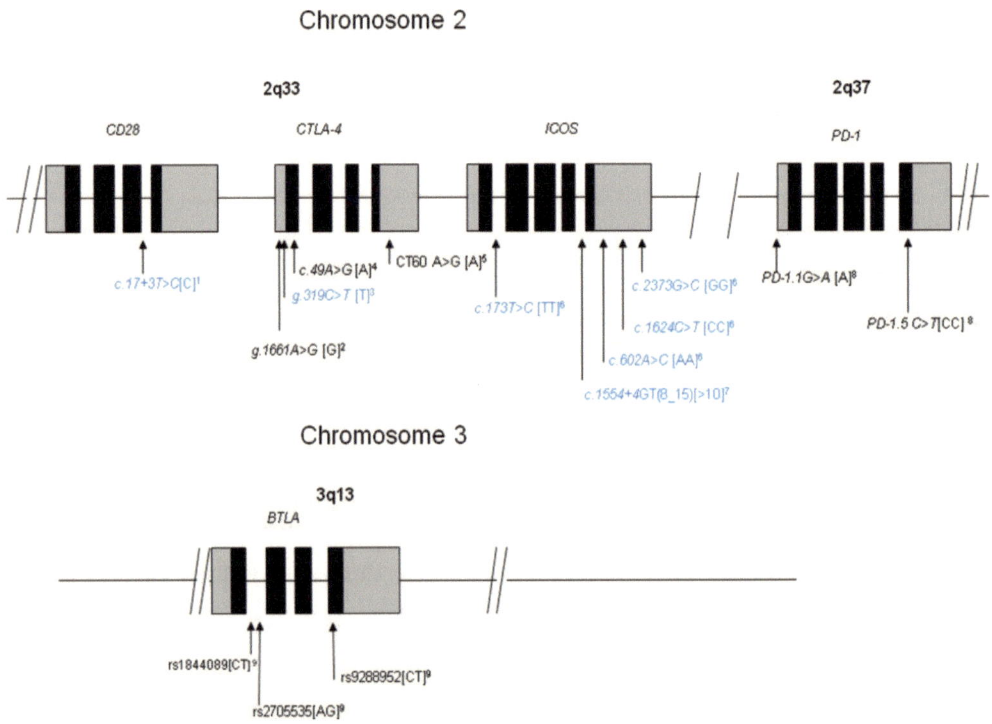

1. predisposing to cervical cancer (Ivansson *et al.* 2010, Chen *et al.* 2011) and CLL (Suwalska *et al.* 2008)
2. predisposing to oral squamous cell carcinoma (Kammerer *et al*, 2010)
3. predisposing to breast cancer (Wong *et al*, 2006), cervical cancer (Su *et al*, 2007;Pawlak *et al*, 2010), lung cancer in women (Karabon *et al.* 2011) and CLL (Suwalska *et al.* 2008); in general for cancer especially in European (Zhang *et al*, 2011)
4. predisposing to oesophageal cancer, gastric cardia cancer (Sun *et al*, 2008), non-Hodgkin's lymphoma (Piras *et al*, 2005), breast cancer (Ghaderi *et al*, 2004; Sun *et al*, 2008), renal cancer (Cozar *et al*, 2007), lung cancer, esophagus and gastric cardia cancer (Sun *et al*, 2008); in general for cancer especially in Asian (Zhang *et al*, 2011)
5. predisposing to renal cell cancer (Cozar *et al*, 2007), non-melanoma skin cancer (Welsh *et al*, 2009).
6. associated with lower rate of CLL progression (Karabon et al. 2011a)
7. predisposing to CLL (Suwalska *et al.* 2008)
8. predisposing to breast cancer (Hua *et al*, 2011)
9. predisposing to breast cancer (Fu *et al*, 2010)

Fig. 1. Structure of genes *CD28, CTLA-4, ICOS, PD-1* and *BTLA* and location of polymorphisms associated with susceptibility to cancer and in particular to CLL - (distances are not to scale). Genetic variants associated with cancer are marked in black, those associated with cancer and CLL in blue.

In contrast, increased CTLA-4 expression has been observed on peripheral blood T-cells in multiple myeloma (Brown *et al*, 1998; Mozaffari *et al*, 2004), Hodgkin's disease (Vandenborre *et al*, 1998; Kosmaczewska *et al*, 2002), non-Hodgkin's lymphoma (Vyth-Dreese *et al*, 1998), and neoplastic skin diseases (Alaibac *et al*, 2000).

Results from our lab indicated abnormal kinetics and levels of CD28 expression on T cells in CLL patients. The mean percentages of $CD4^+$ and $CD8^+$ cells expressing CD28 were significantly lower in CLL patients than in controls. Moreover, after anti-CD3 and rIL-2 stimulation, the mean percentages of those cells decreased rapidly, and the return to the basal level took longer than it did in healthy individuals (Frydecka *et al*, 2004)

In contrast to the results above, we observed a markedly increased expression of CTLA-4 on unstimulated $CD4^+$ and $CD8^+$ T cells in CLL patients than in controls. The pattern and kinetics of CTLA-4 expression on $CD4^+$ and $CD8^+$ cells in CLL patients after stimulation also differed from that observed in normal subjects. In CLL patient samples, the highest proportion of T cells co-expressing CTLA-4 was found after 24 h of culture as compared to 72 h in samples from normal individuals, and the basal levels were achieved after 5 days compared to 4 days in normal individual samples (Frydecka *et al*, 2004). The dysregulated expression of both the co-stimulatory CD28 and the inhibitory CTLA-4 molecules in peripheral blood T cells might contribute to the T cell-mediated anti-tumour responses in CLL.

Our group also observed a higher expression of both intracellular and surface CTLA-4 in malignant B cells from CLL patients compared with the normal population of $CD19^+/CD5^+$ cells, and the level of its expression in leukaemic cells positively correlated with the progression of the disease. The upregulated CTLA-4 expression in CLL cells was also previously described by (Pistillo *et al*, 2003) in 3 of 4 studied patients. Furthermore, we observed positive correlations between the frequency of $CD19^+/CD5^+/CTLA\text{-}4^+$ cells with the frequency of leukaemic B cells co-expressing the inhibitory protein p27KIP1 and the early G1 phase regulator cyclin D2. We also found a negative association between $CD19^+/CD5^+/CTLA\text{-}4^+$ lymphocytes and $CD19^+/CD5^+$ positive for cyclin D3, which is expressed in the late G1 phase of cell cycle progression. These findings led us to hypothesise that CTLA-4 might contribute to the arrest of leukaemic cells in the G0/G1 phase of the cell cycle (Kosmaczewska *et al*, 2005).

Similar to our results, it has been shown that both BTLA and PD-1 are strongly expressed on malignant B cells from chronic lymphocytic leukaemia/small lymphocytic leukaemia (CLL/SLL) compared with other small-cell lymphomas, such as follicular lymphoma, mantle cell lymphoma and marginal zone lymphoma (M'Hidi *et al*, 2009; Xerri *et al*, 2008). An explanation for why the expression of both BTLA and PD1 is increased in CLL/SLL was proposed by M'Hidi *et al.*, (2009). According to this hypothesis, CLL is considered a monoclonal expansion of antigen selected B lymphocytes with varying degrees of autospecificity. The upregulation of inhibitory receptors on CLL precursor cells may result from an attempt by the immune system to prevent autoimmune disorders. To this extent, the simultaneous expression of BTLA and HVEM in CLL cells suggests the triggering of an inefficient autocrine inhibitory loop. This hypothesis is strongly supported by the study of Costello *et al* (2003) who described the upregulated expression of HVEM in human B-cell malignancies.

5. Polymorphisms in co-signalling molecules' genes and susceptibility to B-cell chronic leukaemia

Despite the strong familial basis to CLL, with the risk in first-degree relatives being increased approximately sevenfold, the inherited genetic basis of the disease is yet largely unknown, and the major disease-causing locus has not been established. Therefore, a model of genetic predisposition based on the inheritance of multiple risk variants has been proposed (Houlston & Catovsky, 2008).

Our group focused on the co-signalling pathway, because the development of CLL could be regarded as a failure of immunological surveillance. Therefore genes involved in the regulation of the immunological response might be predisposing loci for disease development. We found that among the three polymorphisms studied in the *CTLA-4* gene (*CTLA-4c.49A>G, CTLA*-4g.319C>T and CT60) only one, *CTLA*-4g.319C>T, which is located in the promoter region, confers susceptibility to CLL. We have shown that the presence of the [T] allele or a [T]-positive phenotype increases the risk of the disease about twofold. Moreover, the [T]-positive phenotype correlates with the progression of disease (about 30% of patients with this phenotype increased their Rai stage during the 24 months follow-up compared with 12% of the [CC] patients) (Suwalska *et al*, 2008).

Interestingly, we observed that the intracellular distribution of CTLA-4 was markedly higher in CLL patients possessing *CTLA*-4g.*642AT(8_33) [AT_8] repeat allele compared to patients possessing longer alleles. That allele was shown by Wang et al., (2002) to be associated with higher mRNA transcription than longer alleles (Kosmaczewska *et al.* 2005).

Moreover, we found an association between the *CD28* gene polymorphism with the incidence of CLL. The presence of the *CD28c.17+3T>C* [C] allele and the [C] phenotype confers an approximately twofold increased risk of CLL in the Polish population. Additionally, the *CD28c.17+3T>C* polymorphism tended to associate with a higher frequency of Rai stage progression (Suwalska *et al*, 2008).

We also studied a polymorphism of the *ICOS* gene. We found a relationship between micro satellite gene *c.1544+4GT(8_15)* polymorphism and susceptibility to disease. The long alleles (>11 repeats) were associated with protection from disease, while short alleles (< 10) predispose to CLL (Suwalska *et al*, 2008). Further studies on functional the *ICOS SNP: ICOSISV1+173C>T[TT], ICOSc.602A>C, ICOSc.1624C>T,* and *ICOSc.2373G>C* showed that these SNPs do not modulate the risk of CLL in the Polish population. However, we noted that *ICOSISV1+173T>*C[TT] alone, *ICOSc.602A>*C[AA] alone, and together as part of the genotype AA defined by Casteli et al (2007), (*ISV1+173T>*C[TT], *ICOSc.602A>*C[AA], *ICOSc.1624C>T*[CC], and *ICOSc.2373G>*C[GG]) were associated with a lower rate of disease progression. Only about 20% of patients carrying the genotype *ICOSISV1+173T>C* [TT], *ICOSc.602A>*C[AA], *ICOSc.1624C>T*[CC], and *ICOSc.2373G>*C[GG] increased in the Rai stage during the 60 months of follow-up, compared to more than 40% of the patients possessing other genotypes (Karabon *et al*, 2011a).

Polymorphisms in the 2q33 region were also investigated by (Monne *et al*, 2004; Piras *et al*, 2005) in non- Hodgkin's lymphoma. In both studies the group of patients was very heterogenous and patients with small lymphocytic leukaemia/chronic lymphocytic leukaemia, marginal zone lymphoma, follicular lymphoma, mantle-cell lymphoma, large B-cell lymphoma and T-cell lymphoma were included in these studies. The results obtained by the Sardinian group differed from ours, wherein the *CTLA-4c.49A>G* and the microsatellite *CTLA-4g.**642AT(8_33) polymorphism alone and as a part of the *CTLA-4c.49A>G/CTLA-*4g.319C>T/*CTLA-4g.**642AT(8_33) haplotype were related to the risk of NHL. No independent association was found between *CD28* or *ICOS* gene polymorphisms and NHL in that study.

The explanation for the different results might be the fact that the patients and controls originated from a Sardinian population, which is genetically distinct from other European populations. Moreover, the Sardinian study was performed on a patient group comprising different subtypes of non-Hodgkin`s lymphoma, with only 29 (of a total of 100) patients with CLL/small lymphocytic lymphoma.

Recently, we have focused on *BTLA* gene polymorphisms. Our preliminary (not published) results indicate that the *BTLA+800A>G* (rs9288952) non-synonymous polymorphism is not associated with susceptibility to CLL in a Polish population.

To the best of our knowledge, there have been no studies on *PD-1* gene polymorphisms and CLL risk.

The described association between polymorphisms in *CD28, CTLA-4* and *ICOS* gene and their associations with susceptibility or course of CLL are displaying on Figure 1.

6. Conclusions

Considering the pivotal role of co-inhibitory molecules in tumourgenesis and, genetic predisposition to various rates of gene transcription, translation and amino acid sequence caused by polymorphisms, investigation for genetic markers predisposing to the development and influencing prognosis of cancer, in particular CLL is eligible and important.

7. References

Ahmed,S., Ihara,K., Kanemitsu,S., Nakashima,H., Otsuka,T., Tsuzaka,K., Takeuchi,T., & Hara,T. (2001) Association of CTLA-4 but not CD28 gene polymorphisms with systemic lupus erythematosus in the Japanese population. *Rheumatology.(Oxford)*, 40, 662-667.

Akiba,H., Takeda,K., Kojima,Y., Usui,Y., Harada,N., Yamazaki,T., Ma,J., Tezuka,K., Yagita,H., & Okumura,K. (2005) The role of ICOS in the CXCR5+ follicular B helper T cell maintenance in vivo. *J.Immunol.*, 175, 2340-2348.

Alaibac,M., Belloni,F.A., Poletti,A., Vandenberghe,P., Marino,F., Tarantello,M., & Peserico,A. (2000) In situ expression of the CTLA-4 receptor in T-cell-mediated inflammatory and neoplastic skin diseases. *Arch.Dermatol.Res.*, 292, 472-474.

Anjos,S., Nguyen,A., Ounissi-Benkalha,H., Tessier,M.C., & Polychronakos,C. (2002) A common autoimmunity predisposing signal peptide variant of the cytotoxic T-lymphocyte antigen 4 results in inefficient glycosylation of the susceptibility allele. *J.Biol.Chem.*, 277, 46478-46486.

Beier,K.C., Hutloff,A., Dittrich,A.M., Heuck,C., Rauch,A., Buchner,K., Ludewig,B., Ochs,H.D., Mages,H.W., & Kroczek,R.A. (2000) Induction, binding specificity and function of human ICOS. *Eur.J.Immunol.*, 30, 3707-3717.

Bertsias,G.K., Nakou,M., Choulaki,C., Raptopoulou,A., Papadimitraki,E., Goulielmos,G., Kritikos,H., Sidiropoulos,P., Tzardi,M., Kardassis,D., Mamalaki,C., & Boumpas,D.T. (2009) Genetic, immunologic, and immunohistochemical analysis of the programmed death 1/programmed death ligand 1 pathway in human systemic lupus erythematosus. *Arthritis Rheum.*, 60, 207-218.

Bocko,D., Kosmaczewska,A., Ciszak,L., Teodorowska,R., & Frydecka,I. (2002) CD28 costimulatory molecule--expression, structure and function. *Arch.Immunol.Ther.Exp.(Warsz.)*, 50, 169-177.

Boise,L.H., Minn,A.J., Noel,P.J., June,C.H., Accavitti,M.A., Lindsten,T., & Thompson,C.B. (1995) CD28 costimulation can promote T cell survival by enhancing the expression of Bcl-XL. *Immunity.*, 3, 87-98.

Borriello,F., Sethna,M.P., Boyd,S.D., Schweitzer,A.N., Tivol,E.A., Jacoby,D., Strom,T.B., Simpson,E.M., Freeman,G.J., & Sharpe,A.H. (1997) B7-1 and B7-2 have overlapping, critical roles in immunoglobulin class switching and germinal center formation. *Immunity.*, 6, 303-313.

Bouwhuis,M.G., Gast,A., Figl,A., Eggermont,A.M., Hemminki,K., Schadendorf,D., & Kumar,R. (2009) Polymorphisms in the CD28/CTLA4/ICOS genes: role in malignant melanoma susceptibility and prognosis? *Cancer Immunol.Immunother* 59,303-312.

Brown,E.E., Lan,Q., Zheng,T., Zhang,Y., Wang,S.S., Hoar-Zahm,S., Chanock,S.J., Rothman,N., & Baris,D. (2007) Common variants in genes that mediate immunity and risk of multiple myeloma. *Int.J.Cancer*, 120, 2715-2722.

Brown,R.D., Pope,B., Yuen,E., Gibson,J., & Joshua,D.E. (1998) The expression of T cell related costimulatory molecules in multiple myeloma. *Leuk.Lymphoma*, 31, 379-384.

Burmeister,Y., Lischke,T., Dahler,A.C., Mages,H.W., Lam,K.P., Coyle,A.J., Kroczek,R.A., & Hutloff,A. (2008) ICOS controls the pool size of effector-memory and regulatory T cells. *J.Immunol.*, 180, 774-782.

Carreno,B.M. & Collins,M. (2002) The B7 family of ligands and its receptors: new pathways for costimulation and inhibition of immune responses. *Annu.Rev.Immunol.*, 20, 29-53.

Castelli,L., Comi,C., Chiocchetti,A., Nicola,S., Mesturini,R., Giordano,M., D'Alfonso,S., Cerutti,E., Galimberti,D., Fenoglio,C., Tesser,F., Yagi,J., Rojo,J.M., Perla,F., Leone,M., Scarpini,E., Monaco,F., & Dianzani,U. (2007) ICOS gene haplotypes correlate with IL10 secretion and multiple sclerosis evolution. *J.Neuroimmunol.*, 186, 193-198.

Chen,X., Li,H., Qiao,Y., Yu,D., Guo,H., Tan,W., & Lin,D. (2011) Association of CD28 gene polymorphism with cervical cancer risk in a Chinese population. *Int.J.Immunogenet.*, 38, 51-54.

Cheng,T.Y., Lin,J.T., Chen,L.T., Shun,C.T., Wang,H.P., Lin,M.T., Wang,T.E., Cheng,A.L., & Wu,M.S. (2006) Association of T-cell regulatory gene polymorphisms with susceptibility to gastric mucosa-associated lymphoid tissue lymphoma. *J.Clin.Oncol.*, 24, 3483-3489.

Chistiakov,D.A., Savost'anov,K.V., Turakulov,R.I., Efremov,I.A., & Demurov,L.M. (2006) Genetic analysis and functional evaluation of the C/T(-318) and A/G(-1661) polymorphisms of the CTLA-4 gene in patients affected with Graves' disease. *Clin.Immunol.*, 118, 233-242.

Cozar,J.M., Romero,J.M., Aptsiauri,N., Vazquez,F., Vilchez,J.R., Tallada,M., Garrido,F., & Ruiz-Cabello,F. (2007) High incidence of CTLA-4 AA (CT60) polymorphism in renal cell cancer. *Hum.Immunol.*, 68, 698-704.

Daroszewski,J., Pawlak,E., Karabon,L., Frydecka,I., Jonkisz,A., Slowik,M., & Bolanowski,M. (2009) Soluble CTLA-4 receptor an immunological marker of Graves' disease and severity of ophthalmopathy is associated with CTLA-4 Jo31 and CT60 gene polymorphisms. *Eur.J.Endocrinol.*, 161, 787-793.

Dilmec,F., Ozgonul,A., Uzunkoy,A., & Akkafa,F. (2008) Investigation of CTLA-4 and CD28 gene polymorphisms in a group of Turkish patients with colorectal cancer. *Int.J.Immunogenet.*, 35, 317-321.

Dong,C., Juedes,A.E., Temann,U.A., Shresta,S., Allison,J.P., Ruddle,N.H., & Flavell,R.A. (2001) ICOS co-stimulatory receptor is essential for T-cell activation and function. *Nature*, 409, 97-101.

Dong,C., Nurieva,R.I., & Prasad,D.V. (2003) Immune regulation by novel costimulatory molecules. *Immunol.Res.*, 28, 39-48.

Dorfman,D.M., Brown,J.A., Shahsafaei,A., & Freeman,G.J. (2006) Programmed death-1 (PD-1) is a marker of germinal center-associated T cells and angioimmunoblastic T-cell lymphoma. *Am.J.Surg.Pathol.*, 30, 802-810.

Ferguson,S.E., Han,S., Kelsoe,G., & Thompson,C.B. (1996) CD28 is required for germinal center formation. *J.Immunol.*, 156, 4576-4581.

Ferreiros-Vidal,I., Gomez-Reino,J.J., Barros,F., Carracedo,A., Carreira,P., Gonzalez-Escribano,F., Liz,M., Martin,J., Ordi,J., Vicario,J.L., & Gonzalez,A. (2004) Association of PDCD1 with susceptibility to systemic lupus erythematosus: evidence of population-specific effects. *Arthritis Rheum.*, 50, 2590-2597.

Flores,S., Beems,M., Oyarzun,A., Carrasco,E., & Perez,F. (2010) [Programmed cell death 1 (PDCD1) gene polymorphisms and type 1 diabetes in Chilean children]. *Rev.Med.Chil.*, 138, 543-550.

Frauwirth,K.A. & Thompson,C.B. (2002) Activation and inhibition of lymphocytes by costimulation. *J.Clin.Invest*, 109, 295-299.

Freeman,G.J., Long,A.J., Iwai,Y., Bourque,K., Chernova,T., Nishimura,H., Fitz,L.J., Malenkovich,N., Okazaki,T., Byrne,M.C., Horton,H.F., Fouser,L., Carter,L., Ling,V., Bowman,M.R., Carreno,B.M., Collins,M., Wood,C.R., & Honjo,T. (2000) Engagement of the PD-1 immunoinhibitory receptor by a novel B7 family member leads to negative regulation of lymphocyte activation. *J.Exp.Med.*, 192, 1027-1034.

Frydecka,I., Kosmaczewska,A., Bocko,D., Ciszak,L., Wolowiec,D., Kuliczkowski,K., & Kochanowska,I. (2004) Alterations of the expression of T-cell-related costimulatory CD28 and downregulatory CD152 (CTLA-4) molecules in patients with B-cell chronic lymphocytic leukaemia. *Br.J.Cancer*, 90, 2042-2048.

Fu,Z., Li,D., Jiang,W., Wang,L., Zhang,J., Xu,F., Pang,D., & Li,D. (2010) Association of BTLA gene polymorphisms with the risk of malignant breast cancer in Chinese women of Heilongjiang Province. *Breast Cancer Res.Treat.*, 120, 195-202.

Garapati VP, Lefranc MP. (2007) IMGT Colliers de Perles and IgSF domain standardization for T cell costimulatory activatory (CD28, ICOS) and inhibitory (CTLA4, PDCD1 and BTLA) receptors. Dev Comp Immunol.,31,1050-72.

Ghaderi,A., Yeganeh,F., Kalantari,T., Talei,A.R., Pezeshki,A.M., Doroudchi,M., & Dehaghani,A.S. (2004) Cytotoxic T lymphocyte antigen-4 gene in breast cancer. *Breast Cancer Res.Treat.*, 86, 1-7.

Gonzalez,L.C., Loyet,K.M., Calemine-Fenaux,J., Chauhan,V., Wranik,B., Ouyang,W., & Eaton,D.L. (2005) A coreceptor interaction between the CD28 and TNF receptor family members B and T lymphocyte attenuator and herpesvirus entry mediator. *Proc.Natl.Acad.Sci.U.S.A*, 102, 1116-1121.

Green,J.M., Noel,P.J., Sperling,A.I., Walunas,T.L., Lenschow,D.J., Stack,R., Gray,G.S., Bluestone,J.A., & Thompson,C.B. (1995) T cell costimulation through the CD28 receptor. *Proc.Assoc.Am.Physicians*, 107, 41-46.

Greenwald,R.J., Freeman,G.J., & Sharpe,A.H. (2005) The B7 family revisited. *Annu.Rev.Immunol.*, 23, 515-548.

Grimbacher,B., Hutloff,A., Schlesier,M., Glocker,E., Warnatz,K., Drager,R., Eibel,H., Fischer,B., Schaffer,A.A., Mages,H.W., Kroczek,R.A., & Peter,H.H. (2003) Homozygous loss of ICOS is associated with adult-onset common variable immunodeficiency. *Nat.Immunol.*, 4, 261-268.

Guzman,V.B., Yambartsev,A., Goncalves-Primo,A., Silva,I.D., Carvalho,C.R., Ribalta,J.C., Goulart,L.R., Shulzhenko,N., Gerbase-Delima,M., & Morgun,A. (2008) New approach reveals CD28 and IFNG gene interaction in the susceptibility to cervical cancer. *Hum.Mol.Genet.*, 17, 1838-1844.

Hadinia,A., Hossieni,S.V., Erfani,N., Saberi-Firozi,M., Fattahi,M.J., & Ghaderi,A. (2007) CTLA-4 gene promoter and exon 1 polymorphisms in Iranian patients with gastric and colorectal cancers. *J.Gastroenterol.Hepatol.*, 22, 2283-2287.

Haghshenas,M.R., Naeimi,S., Talei,A., Ghaderi,A., & Erfani,N. (2011) Program death 1 (PD1) haplotyping in patients with breast carcinoma. *Mol.Biol.Rep.*, 38, 4205-4210.

Haimila,K., Turpeinen,H., Alakulppi,N.S., Kyllonen,L.E., Salmela,K.T., & Partanen,J. (2009) Association of genetic variation in inducible costimulator gene with outcome of kidney transplantation. *Transplantation*, 87, 393-396.

Houlston,R.S. & Catovsky,D. (2008) Familial chronic lymphocytic leukemia. *Curr.Hematol.Malig.Rep.*, 3, 221-225.

Hua,Z., Li,D., Xiang,G., Xu,F., Jie,G., Fu,Z., Jie,Z., Da,P., & Li,D. (2011) PD-1 polymorphisms are associated with sporadic breast cancer in Chinese Han population of Northeast China. *Breast Cancer Res.Treat.*, 129,195-201

Hutloff,A., Dittrich,A.M., Beier,K.C., Eljaschewitsch,B., Kraft,R., Anagnostopoulos,I., & Kroczek,R.A. (1999) ICOS is an inducible T-cell co-stimulator structurally and functionally related to CD28. *Nature*, 397, 263-266.

Ihara,K., Ahmed,S., Nakao,F., Kinukawa,N., Kuromaru,R., Matsuura,N., Iwata,I., Nagafuchi,S., Kohno,H., Miyako,K., & Hara,T. (2001) Association studies of CTLA-4, CD28, and ICOS gene polymorphisms with type 1 diabetes in the Japanese population. *Immunogenetics*, 53, 447-454.

Inuo,M., Ihara,K., Matsuo,T., Kohno,H., & Hara,T. (2009) Association study between B- and T-lymphocyte attenuator gene and type 1 diabetes mellitus or systemic lupus erythematosus in the Japanese population. *Int.J.Immunogenet.*, 36, 65-68.

Ishizaki,Y., Yukaya,N., Kusuhara,K., Kira,R., Torisu,H., Ihara,K., Sakai,Y., Sanefuji,M., Pipo-Deveza,J.R., Silao,C.L., Sanchez,B.C., Lukban,M.B., Salonga,A.M., & Hara,T. (2010) PD1 as a common candidate susceptibility gene of subacute sclerosing panencephalitis. *Hum.Genet.*, 127, 411-419.

Ivansson,E.L., Juko-Pecirep,I., & Gyllensten,U.B. (2010) Interaction of immunological genes on chromosome 2q33 and IFNG in susceptibility to cervical cancer. *Gynecol.Oncol.*, 116, 544-548.

Jenkins,M.K., Chen,C.A., Jung,G., Mueller,D.L., & Schwartz,R.H. (1990) Inhibition of antigen-specific proliferation of type 1 murine T cell clones after stimulation with immobilized anti-CD3 monoclonal antibody. *J.Immunol.*, 144, 16-22.

Kaartinen,T., Lappalainen,J., Haimila,K., Autero,M., & Partanen,J. (2007) Genetic variation in ICOS regulates mRNA levels of ICOS and splicing isoforms of CTLA4. *Mol.Immunol.*, 44, 1644-1651.

Kammerer,P.W., Toyoshima,T., Schoder,F., Kammerer,P., Kuhr,K., Brieger,J., & Al-Nawas,B. (2010) Association of T-cell regulatory gene polymorphisms with oral squamous cell carcinoma. *Oral Oncol.*, 46, 543-548.

Karabon,L., Jedynak,A., Tomkiewicz,A., Wolowiec,D., Kielbinski,M., Woszczyk,D., Kuliczkowski,K., & Frydecka,I. (2011a) ICOS gene polymorphisms in B-cell chronic lymphocytic leukemia in the Polish population. *Folia Histochem.Cytobiol.*, 49, 49-54.

Karabon,L., Kosmaczewska,A., Bilinska,M., Pawlak,E., Ciszak,L., Jedynak,A., Jonkisz,A., Noga,L., Pokryszko-Dragan,A., Koszewicz,M., & Frydecka,I. (2009) The CTLA-4 gene polymorphisms are associated with CTLA-4 protein expression levels in multiple sclerosis patients and with susceptibility to disease. *Immunology*, 128, e787-e796.

Karabon,L., Pawlak,E., Tomkiewicz,A., Jedynak,A., Passowicz-Muszynska,E., Zajda,K., Jonkisz,A., Jankowska,R., Krzakowski,M., & Frydecka,I. (2011b) CTLA-4, CD28, and ICOS gene polymorphism associations with non-small-cell lung cancer. *Hum.Immunol.*, 72, 947-954

Karabon,L., Pawlak-Adamska,E., Tomkiewicz,A., Jedynak,A., Kielbinski,M., Woszczyk,D., Potoczek,S., Jonkisz,A., Kuliczkowski,K., & Frydecka,I. (2011c) Variations in Suppressor Molecule CTLA-4 Gene Are Related to Susceptibility to Multiple Myeloma in a Polish Population. *Pathol.Oncol.Res.* 9. [Epub ahead of print]

Kong,E.K., Prokunina-Olsson,L., Wong,W.H., Lau,C.S., Chan,T.M., Alarcón-Riquelme M, & Lau,Y.L. (2005) A new haplotype of PDCD1 is associated with rheumatoid arthritis in Hong Kong Chinese. *Arthritis Rheum.*, 52, 1058-1062.

Kosmaczewska,A., Ciszak,L., Suwalska,K., Wolowiec,D., & Frydecka,I. (2005) CTLA-4 overexpression in CD19+/CD5+ cells correlates with the level of cell cycle regulators and disease progression in B-CLL patients. *Leukemia*, 19, 301-304.

Kosmaczewska,A., Frydecka,I., Bocko,D., Ciszak,L., & Teodorowska,R. (2002) Correlation of blood lymphocyte CTLA-4 (CD152) induction in Hodgkin's disease with proliferative activity, interleukin 2 and interferon-gamma production. *Br.J.Haematol.*, 118, 202-209.

Kouki,T., Sawai,Y., Gardine,C.A., Fisfalen,M.E., Alegre,M.L., & DeGroot,L.J. (2000) CTLA-4 gene polymorphism at position 49 in exon 1 reduces the inhibitory function of CTLA-4 and contributes to the pathogenesis of Graves' disease. *J.Immunol.*, 165, 6606-6611.

Kristjansdottir,H., Steinsson,K., Gunnarsson,I., Grondal,G., Erlendsson,K., & Alarcón-Riquelme M, (2010) Lower expression levels of the programmed death 1 receptor on CD4+CD25+ T cells and correlation with the PD-1.3A genotype in patients with systemic lupus erythematosus. *Arthritis Rheum.*, 62, 1702-1711.

Lafferty,K.J., Warren,H.S., Woolnough,J.A., & Talmage,D.W. (1978) Immunological induction of T lymphocytes: role of antigen and the lymphocyte costimulator. *Blood Cells*, 4, 395-406.

Latchman,Y., Wood,C.R., Chernova,T., Chaudhary,D., Borde,M., Chernova,I., Iwai,Y., Long,A.J., Brown,J.A., Nunes,R., Greenfield,E.A., Bourque,K., Boussiotis,V.A., Carter,L.L., Carreno,B.M., Malenkovich,N., Nishimura,H., Okazaki,T., Honjo,T., Sharpe,A.H., & Freeman,G.J. (2001) PD-L2 is a second ligand for PD-1 and inhibits T cell activation. *Nat.Immunol.*, 2, 261-268.

Lee,S.H., Lee,Y.A., Woo,D.H., Song,R., Park,E.K., Ryu,M.H., Kim,Y.H., Kim,K.S., Hong,S.J., Yoo,M.C., & Yang,H.I. (2006) Association of the programmed cell death 1 (PDCD1) gene polymorphism with ankylosing spondylitis in the Korean population. *Arthritis Res.Ther.*, 8, R163.

Liang,S.C., Greenwald,R.J., Latchman,Y.E., Rosas,L., Satoskar,A., Freeman,G.J., & Sharpe,A.H. (2006) PD-L1 and PD-L2 have distinct roles in regulating host immunity to cutaneous leishmaniasis. *Eur.J.Immunol.*, 36, 58-64.

Ligers,A., Teleshova,N., Masterman,T., Huang,W.X., & Hillert,J. (2001) CTLA-4 gene expression is influenced by promoter and exon 1 polymorphisms. *Genes Immun.*, 2, 145-152.

Lin,S.C., Kuo,C.C., & Chan,C.H. (2006) Association of a BTLA gene polymorphism with the risk of rheumatoid arthritis. *J.Biomed.Sci.*, 13, 853-860.

Luhder,F., Chambers,C., Allison,J.P., Benoist,C., & Mathis,D. (2000) Pinpointing when T cell costimulatory receptor CTLA-4 must be engaged to dampen diabetogenic T cells. *Proc.Natl.Acad.Sci.U.S.A*, 97, 12204-12209.

M'Hidi,H., Thibult,M.L., Chetaille,B., Rey,F., Bouadallah,R., Nicollas,R., Olive,D., & Xerri,L. (2009) High expression of the inhibitory receptor BTLA in T-follicular helper cells and in B-cell small lymphocytic lymphoma/chronic lymphocytic leukemia. *Am.J.Clin.Pathol.*, 132, 589-596.

McAdam,A.J., Chang,T.T., Lumelsky,A.E., Greenfield,E.A., Boussiotis,V.A., Duke-Cohan,J.S., Chernova,T., Malenkovich,N., Jabs,C., Kuchroo,V.K., Ling,V., Collins,M., Sharpe,A.H., & Freeman,G.J. (2000) Mouse inducible costimulatory molecule (ICOS) expression is enhanced by CD28 costimulation and regulates differentiation of CD4+ T cells. *J.Immunol.*, 165, 5035-5040.

McAdam,A.J., Greenwald,R.J., Levin,M.A., Chernova,T., Malenkovich,N., Ling,V., Freeman,G.J., & Sharpe,A.H. (2001) ICOS is critical for CD40-mediated antibody class switching. *Nature*, 409, 102-105.

Mittrucker,H.W., Shahinian,A., Bouchard,D., Kundig,T.M., & Mak,T.W. (1996) Induction of unresponsiveness and impaired T cell expansion by staphylococcal enterotoxin B in CD28-deficient mice. *J.Exp.Med.*, 183, 2481-2488.

Monne,M., Piras,G., Palmas,A., Arru,L., Murineddu,M., Latte,G., Noli,A., & Gabbas,A. (2004) Cytotoxic T-lymphocyte antigen-4 (CTLA-4) gene polymorphism and susceptibility to non-Hodgkin's lymphoma. *Am.J.Hematol.*, 76, 14-18.

Mozaffari,F., Hansson,L., Kiaii,S., Ju,X., Rossmann,E.D., Rabbani,H., Mellstedt,H., & Osterborg,A. (2004) Signalling molecules and cytokine production in T cells of multiple myeloma-increased abnormalities with advancing stage. *Br.J.Haematol.*, 124, 315-324.

Nakae,S., Iwakura,Y., Suto,H., & Galli,S.J. (2007) Phenotypic differences between Th1 and Th17 cells and negative regulation of Th1 cell differentiation by IL-17. *J.Leukoc.Biol.*, 81, 1258-1268.

Nishimura,H., Nose,M., Hiai,H., Minato,N., & Honjo,T. (1999) Development of lupus-like autoimmune diseases by disruption of the PD-1 gene encoding an ITIM motif-carrying immunoreceptor. *Immunity.*, 11, 141-151.

Nishimura,H., Okazaki,T., Tanaka,Y., Nakatani,K., Hara,M., Matsumori,A., Sasayama,S., Mizoguchi,A., Hiai,H., Minato,N., & Honjo,T. (2001) Autoimmune dilated cardiomyopathy in PD-1 receptor-deficient mice. *Science*, 291, 319-322.

Nurieva,R.I., Chung,Y., Hwang,D., Yang,X.O., Kang,H.S., Ma,L., Wang,Y.H., Watowich,S.S., Jetten,A.M., Tian,Q., & Dong,C. (2008) Generation of T follicular helper cells is mediated by interleukin-21 but independent of T helper 1, 2, or 17 cell lineages. *Immunity.*, 29, 138-149.

Oki,M., Watanabe,N., Owada,T., Oya,Y., Ikeda,K., Saito,Y., Matsumura,R., Seto,Y., Iwamoto,I., & Nakajima,H. (2011) A functional polymorphism in B and T lymphocyte attenuator is associated with susceptibility to rheumatoid arthritis. *Clin.Dev.Immunol.*, 2011, 305656.

Pawlak,E., Karabon,L., Wlodarska-Polinska,I., Jedynak,A., Jonkisz,A., Tomkiewicz,A., Kornafel,J., Stepien,M., Ignatowicz,A., Lebioda,A., Dobosz,T., & Frydecka,I. (2010) Influence of CTLA-4/CD28/ICOS gene polymorphisms on the susceptibility to cervical squamous cell carcinoma and stage of differentiation in the Polish population. *Hum.Immunol.*, 71, 195-200.

Pincerati,M.R., la-Costa,R., Pavoni,D.P., & Petzl-Erler,M.L. (2010) Genetic polymorphisms of the T-cell coreceptors CD28 and CTLA-4 in Afro- and Euro-Brazilians. *Int.J.Immunogenet.*, 37, 253-261.

Piras,G., Monne,M., Uras,A., Palmas,A., Murineddu,M., Arru,L., Bianchi,A., Calvisi,A., Curreli,L., Gaviano,E., Lai,P., Murgia,A., Latte,G.C., Noli,A., & Gabbas,A. (2005) Genetic analysis of the 2q33 region containing CD28-CTLA4-ICOS genes: association with non-Hodgkin's lymphoma. *Br.J.Haematol.*, 129, 784-790.

Pistillo,M.P., Tazzari,P.L., Palmisano,G.L., Pierri,I., Bolognesi,A., Ferlito,F., Capanni,P., Polito,L., Ratta,M., Pileri,S., Piccioli,M., Basso,G., Rissotto,L., Conte,R., Gobbi,M., Stirpe,F., & Ferrara,G.B. (2003) CTLA-4 is not restricted to the lymphoid cell lineage and can function as a target molecule for apoptosis induction of leukemic cells. *Blood*, 101, 202-209.

Robillard,N., Jego,G., Pellat-Deceunynck,C., Pineau,D., Puthier,D., Mellerin,M.P., Barille,S., Rapp,M.J., Harousseau,J.L., Amiot,M., & Bataille,R. (1998) CD28, a marker associated with tumoral expansion in multiple myeloma. *Clin.Cancer Res.*, 4, 1521-1526.

Rosenberg,S.A. (2001) Progress in the development of immunotherapy for the treatment of patients with cancer. *J.Intern.Med.*, 250, 462-475.

Rossi,E., Matutes,E., Morilla,R., Owusu-Ankomah,K., Heffernan,A.M., & Catovsky,D. (1996) Zeta chain and CD28 are poorly expressed on T lymphocytes from chronic lymphocytic leukemia. *Leukemia*, 10, 494-497.

Rudd,C.E., Taylor,A., & Schneider,H. (2009) CD28 and CTLA-4 coreceptor expression and signal transduction. *Immunol.Rev.*, 229, 12-26.

Salama,A.D., Chitnis,T., Imitola,J., Ansari,M.J., Akiba,H., Tushima,F., Azuma,M., Yagita,H., Sayegh,M.H., & Khoury,S.J. (2003) Critical role of the programmed death-1 (PD-1) pathway in regulation of experimental autoimmune encephalomyelitis. *J.Exp.Med.*, 198, 71-78.

Schwartz,R.H., Mueller,D.L., Jenkins,M.K., & Quill,H. (1989) T-cell clonal anergy. *Cold Spring Harb.Symp.Quant.Biol.*, 54 Pt 2, 605-610.

Scrivener,S., Goddard,R.V., Kaminski,E.R., & Prentice,A.G. (2003) Abnormal T-cell function in B-cell chronic lymphocytic leukaemia. *Leuk.Lymphoma*, 44, 383-389.

Sedy,J.R., Gavrieli,M., Potter,K.G., Hurchla,M.A., Lindsley,R.C., Hildner,K., Scheu,S., Pfeffer,K., Ware,C.F., Murphy,T.L., & Murphy,K.M. (2005) B and T lymphocyte attenuator regulates T cell activation through interaction with herpesvirus entry mediator. *Nat.Immunol.*, 6, 90-98.

Shahinian,A., Pfeffer,K., Lee,K.P., Kundig,T.M., Kishihara,K., Wakeham,A., Kawai,K., Ohashi,P.S., Thompson,C.B., & Mak,T.W. (1993) Differential T cell costimulatory requirements in CD28-deficient mice. *Science*, 261, 609-612.

Sharpe,A.H. (2009) Mechanisms of costimulation. *Immunol.Rev.*, 229, 5-11.

Shilling,R.A., Pinto,J.M., Decker,D.C., Schneider,D.H., Bandukwala,H.S., Schneider,J.R., Camoretti-Mercado,B., Ober,C., & Sperling,A.I. (2005) Cutting edge: polymorphisms in the ICOS promoter region are associated with allergic sensitization and Th2 cytokine production. *J.Immunol.*, 175, 2061-2065.

Solerio,E., Tappero,G., Iannace,L., Matullo,G., Ayoubi,M., Parziale,A., Cicilano,M., Sansoe,G., Framarin,L., Vineis,P., & Rosina,F. (2005) CTLA4 gene polymorphism in Italian patients with colorectal adenoma and cancer. *Dig.Liver Dis.*, 37, 170-175.

Stevenson,F.K. & Caligaris-Cappio,F. (2004) Chronic lymphocytic leukemia: revelations from the B-cell receptor. *Blood*, 103, 4389-4395.

Su,T.H., Chang,T.Y., Lee,Y.J., Chen,C.K., Liu,H.F., Chu,C.C., Lin,M., Wang,P.T., Huang,W.C., Chen,T.C., & Yang,Y.C. (2007) CTLA-4 gene and susceptibility to human papillomavirus-16-associated cervical squamous cell carcinoma in Taiwanese women. *Carcinogenesis*, 28, 1237-1240.

Sun,T., Zhou,Y., Yang,M., Hu,Z., Tan,W., Han,X., Shi,Y., Yao,J., Guo,Y., Yu,D., Tian,T., Zhou,X., Shen,H., & Lin,D. (2008) Functional genetic variations in cytotoxic T-lymphocyte antigen 4 and susceptibility to multiple types of cancer. *Cancer Res.*, 68, 7025-7034.

Suwalska,K., Pawlak,E., Karabon,L., Tomkiewicz,A., Dobosz,T., Urbaniak-Kujda,D., Kuliczkowski,K., Wolowiec,D., Jedynak,A., & Frydecka,I. (2008) Association studies of CTLA-4, CD28, and ICOS gene polymorphisms with B-cell chronic lymphocytic leukemia in the Polish population. *Hum.Immunol.*, 69, 193-201.

Tai,X., Cowan,M., Feigenbaum,L., & Singer,A. (2005) CD28 costimulation of developing thymocytes induces Foxp3 expression and regulatory T cell differentiation independently of interleukin 2. *Nat.Immunol.*, 6, 152-162.

Tan,A.H., Goh,S.Y., Wong,S.C., & Lam,K.P. (2008) T helper cell-specific regulation of inducible costimulator expression via distinct mechanisms mediated by T-bet and GATA-3. *J.Biol.Chem.*, 283, 128-136.

Tang,Q., Boden,E.K., Henriksen,K.J., Bour-Jordan,H., Bi,M., & Bluestone,J.A. (2004) Distinct roles of CTLA-4 and TGF-beta in CD4+CD25+ regulatory T cell function. *Eur.J.Immunol.*, 34, 2996-3005.

Teutsch,S.M., Booth,D.R., Bennetts,B.H., Heard,R.N., & Stewart,G.J. (2004) Association of common T cell activation gene polymorphisms with multiple sclerosis in Australian patients. *J.Neuroimmunol.*, 148, 218-230.

Tivol,E.A., Borriello,F., Schweitzer,A.N., Lynch,W.P., Bluestone,J.A., & Sharpe,A.H. (1995) Loss of CTLA-4 leads to massive lymphoproliferation and fatal multiorgan tissue destruction, revealing a critical negative regulatory role of CTLA-4. *Immunity.*, 3, 541-547.

Ueda,H., Howson,J.M., Esposito,L., Heward,J., Snook,H., Chamberlain,G., Rainbow,D.B., Hunter,K.M., Smith,A.N., Di,G.G., Herr,M.H., Dahlman,I., Payne,F., Smyth,D., Lowe,C., Twells,R.C., Howlett,S., Healy,B., Nutland,S., Rance,H.E., Everett,V., Smink,L.J., Lam,A.C., Cordell,H.J., Walker,N.M., Bordin,C., Hulme,J., Motzo,C., Cucca,F., Hess,J.F., Metzker,M.L., Rogers,J., Gregory,S., Allahabadia,A., Nithiyananthan,R., Tuomilehto-Wolf,E., Tuomilehto,J., Bingley,P., Gillespie,K.M., Undlien,D.E., Ronningen,K.S., Guja,C., Ionescu-Tirgoviste,C., Savage,D.A., Maxwell,A.P., Carson,D.J., Patterson,C.C., Franklyn,J.A., Clayton,D.G., Peterson,L.B., Wicker,L.S., Todd,J.A., & Gough,S.C. (2003) Association of the T-cell regulatory gene CTLA4 with susceptibility to autoimmune disease. *Nature*, 423, 506-511.

van de Corp, Falkenburg,J.H., Kester,M.G., Willemze,R., & Kluin-Nelemans,J.C. (1999) Impaired expression of CD28 on T cells in hairy cell leukemia. *Clin.Immunol.*, 93, 256-262.

Van den Hove,L.E., Van Gool,S.W., Vandenberghe,P., Bakkus,M., Thielemans,K., Boogaerts,M.A., & Ceuppens,J.L. (1997) CD40 triggering of chronic lymphocytic leukemia B cells results in efficient alloantigen presentation and cytotoxic T lymphocyte induction by up-regulation of CD80 and CD86 costimulatory molecules. *Leukemia*, 11, 572-580.

Vandenborre,K., Delabie,J., Boogaerts,M.A., De,V.R., Lorre,K., De Wolf-Peeters,C., & Vandenberghe,P. (1998) Human CTLA-4 is expressed in situ on T lymphocytes in germinal centers, in cutaneous graft-versus-host disease, and in Hodgkin's disease. *Am.J.Pathol.*, 152, 963-973.

Velazquez-Cruz,R., Orozco,L., Espinosa-Rosales,F., Carreno-Manjarrez,R., Solis-Vallejo,E., Lopez-Lara,N.D., Ruiz-Lopez,I.K., Rodriguez-Lozano,A.L., Estrada-Gil,J.K., Jimenez-Sanchez,G., & Baca,V. (2007) Association of PDCD1 polymorphisms with childhood-onset systemic lupus erythematosus. *Eur.J.Hum.Genet.*, 15, 336-341.

Vyth-Dreese,F.A., Boot,H., Dellemijn,T.A., Majoor,D.M., Oomen,L.C., Laman,J.D., Van,M.M., De Weger,R.A., & de,J.D. (1998) Localization in situ of costimulatory molecules and cytokines in B-cell non-Hodgkin's lymphoma. *Immunology*, 94, 580-586.

Walunas,T.L., Bakker,C.Y., & Bluestone,J.A. (1996) CTLA-4 ligation blocks CD28-dependent T cell activation. *J.Exp.Med.*, 183, 2541-2550.

Walunas,T.L., Lenschow,D.J., Bakker,C.Y., Linsley,P.S., Freeman,G.J., Green,J.M., Thompson,C.B., & Bluestone,J.A. (1994) CTLA-4 can function as a negative regulator of T cell activation. *Immunity.*, 1, 405-413.

Wang,J., Yoshida,T., Nakaki,F., Hiai,H., Okazaki,T., & Honjo,T. (2005) Establishment of NOD-Pdcd1-/- mice as an efficient animal model of type I diabetes. *Proc.Natl.Acad.Sci.U.S.A*, 102, 11823-11828.

Wang,X.B., Kakoulidou,M., Giscombe,R., Qiu,Q., Huang,D., Pirskanen,R., & Lefvert,A.K. (2002a) Abnormal expression of CTLA-4 by T cells from patients with myasthenia gravis: effect of an AT-rich gene sequence. *J.Neuroimmunol.*, 130, 224-232.

Wang,X.B., Pirskanen,R., Giscombe,R., & Lefvert,A.K. (2008) Two SNPs in the promoter region of the CTLA-4 gene affect binding of transcription factors and are associated with human myasthenia gravis. *J.Intern.Med.*, 263, 61-69.

Wang,X.B., Zhao,X., Giscombe,R., & Lefvert,A.K. (2002b) A CTLA-4 gene polymorphism at position -318 in the promoter region affects the expression of protein. *Genes Immun.*, 3, 233-234.

Watanabe,N., Gavrieli,M., Sedy,J.R., Yang,J., Fallarino,F., Loftin,S.K., Hurchla,M.A., Zimmerman,N., Sim,J., Zang,X., Murphy,T.L., Russell,J.H., Allison,J.P., & Murphy,K.M. (2003) BTLA is a lymphocyte inhibitory receptor with similarities to CTLA-4 and PD-1. *Nat.Immunol.*, 4, 670-679.

Waterhouse,P., Penninger,J.M., Timms,E., Wakeham,A., Shahinian,A., Lee,K.P., Thompson,C.B., Griesser,H., & Mak,T.W. (1995) Lymphoproliferative disorders with early lethality in mice deficient in Ctla-4. *Science*, 270, 985-988.

Welsh,M.M., Applebaum,K.M., Spencer,S.K., Perry,A.E., Karagas,M.R., & Nelson,H.H. (2009) CTLA4 variants, UV-induced tolerance, and risk of non-melanoma skin cancer. *Cancer Res.*, 69, 6158-6163.

Wong,Y.K., Chang,K.W., Cheng,C.Y., & Liu,C.J. (2006) Association of CTLA-4 gene polymorphism with oral squamous cell carcinoma. *J.Oral Pathol.Med.*, 35, 51-54.

Xerri,L., Chetaille,B., Serriari,N., Attias,C., Guillaume,Y., Arnoulet,C., & Olive,D. (2008) Programmed death 1 is a marker of angioimmunoblastic T-cell lymphoma and B-cell small lymphocytic lymphoma/chronic lymphocytic leukemia. *Hum.Pathol.*, 39, 1050-1058.

Yoshinaga,S.K., Whoriskey,J.S., Khare,S.D., Sarmiento,U., Guo,J., Horan,T., Shih,G., Zhang,M., Coccia,M.A., Kohno,T., Tafuri-Bladt,A., Brankow,D., Campbell,P., Chang,D., Chiu,L., Dai,T., Duncan,G., Elliott,G.S., Hui,A., McCabe,S.M., Scully,S., Shahinian,A., Shaklee,C.L., Van,G., Mak,T.W., & Senaldi,G. (1999) T-cell co-stimulation through B7RP-1 and ICOS. *Nature*, 402, 827-832.

Zhang,Y., Zhang,J., Deng,Y., Tian,C., Li,X., Huang,J., & Fan,H. (2011) Polymorphisms in the cytotoxic T-lymphocyte antigen 4 gene and cancer risk: A meta-analysis. *Cancer.*

Zheng,L., Li,D., Wang,F., Wu,H., Li,X., Fu,J., Chen,X., Wang,L., Liu,Y., & Wang,S. (2010) Association between hepatitis B viral burden in chronic infection and a functional single nucleotide polymorphism of the PDCD1 gene. *J.Clin.Immunol.*, 30, 855-860.

Part 3

CLL Animal Models

10

Mouse Models of Chronic Lymphocytic Leukemia

Gema Pérez-Chacón and Juan M. Zapata
Instituto de Investigaciones Biomédicas "Alberto Sols", CSIC/UAM, Madrid Spain

1. Introduction

Genetically modified mice mimicking the expression of candidate genes implicated in the etiology of disease are essential tools not only to demonstrate the role of these genes in disease, but also as preclinical platforms for testing new therapies. The absence of mouse models of CLL was a problem hindering CLL research for long time. This problem was exacerbated because the development of xenograft models of human CLL cells was also troublesome as a result of the non-proliferative nature of circulating CLL cells. However, this situation has turned around in the last few years, and several groups have generated a collection of genetically modified mice of CLL representing different subtypes of the disease. These mice not only have provided new insights into the genes and mechanisms involved in development and progression of CLL but also reflect the heterogeneity and complexity of this disease. In this chapter we will summarize the most defining characteristics of the available mouse models of CLL and how they relate to the different CLL subtypes seen in human patients.

2. Chronic lymphocytic leukemia

Chronic lymphocytic leukemia (CLL) remains as the most common leukemia in Western countries with an age-adjusted incidence rate of 4.2 per 100,000 individuals and an age-adjusted death rate of 1.5 per 100,000 individuals in the United States, according to the National Cancer Institute. CLL shows significant differences in incidence rates by race (Whites/Asians ratio of 4.8:1) and gender (male/female ratio of 2:1) (http://seer.cancer.gov/csr/1975_2008).

Several decades ago CLL was defined as an accumulative disease of immunologically incompetent lymphocytes (Dameshek, 1967). Nowadays, CLL is described as a disease characterized by the accumulation of slowly proliferating CD5+ CD23+ B lymphocytes with a surface membrane phenotype of activated B cells and a gene profile related to memory B cells (Damle et al., 2002; Klein et al., 2001). The origin of CLL B cells remains unknown, and evidence is accumulating suggesting that different B cell types may be the source of CLL (Chiorazzi & Ferrarini, 2011). It is however well established that CLL is a heterogeneous disease consisting of at least two separate entities, based on phenotypic and genetic features. Approximately 50% of CLL patients have transformed B cells with mutations in IgV_H genes

(Fais et al., 1998; Schroeder & Dighiero, 1994). The rest of the patients have unmutated IgV_H CLL clones, which correlates with poor prognosis (Damle et al., 1999; Hamblin et al., 1999). Exposure to antigens seems to play a role in both malignant transformation in CLL and in selection and expansion of more aggressive clones (Damle et al., 2002; Ghia et al., 2008; Klein et al., 2001). Mutational status of the expanded clones could be associated with the type of antigen inducing the immune response, that is, T-dependent stimulation in germinal center, in the case of mutated clones, or T-dependent out of germinal center or T-independent stimulation, in the case of unmutated clones (Chiorazzi & Ferrarini, 2003).

Several genetic alterations are found in CLL, including chromosome translocations and gene promoter unmethylation (Coll-Mulet and Gil, 2009; Klein & Dalla-Favera, 2010). Epigenetic changes affecting the expression and function of genes have also been described in CLL (Marton et al., 2008; Plass et al., 2007). The variability in the origin of the CLL is also reflected in its clinical progression with patients suffering a mild, indolent disease that do not need treatment, patients with aggressive disease, and patients that became resistant to current treatments. Therefore, the development of mouse models based on the different alterations observed in CLL patients that recapitulate distinctive aspects of specific CLL subtypes will help to better understand the molecular mechanisms of CLL transformation and disease progression.

2.1 NZB mice in the crossroad of autoimmunity and CLL

As indicated above, human CLL cells usually express CD5 on their surface. Naturally occurring CD5+ B cells expansions are observed in two strains of New Zealand mice. One of these strains is the New Zealand White (NZW) (Hamano et al., 1998), where these CD5+ B-1 cell expansions might progress to CLL-like disease in a fraction of elder mice. Three major susceptibility loci in chromosomes 17 and 13 have been implicated in this abnormal B-1 cell proliferation. The second strain is the New Zealand Black (NZB), where clonal expansions of immunosuppresive CD5+ B cells are found in spleens of aged mice. These expansions will progress to CLL in a majority of elder mice (Phillips et al., 1992; Raveche, 1990). These two mouse strains have provided the first link between CLL and autoimmunity. Indeed, the hybrid F1 offspring of NZBxNZW backcrosses spontaneously developed systemic lupus erithematosus (SLE)-like disease, with glomerulonephritis caused by IgM depositions and higher titers of anti-DNA and anti-erythrocytes antibodies compared to the parental strains (Okada et al., 1990; Tokado el al., 1991). In contrast, the NZBxNZW hybrids showed lower incidence of B cell malignancies compared to the pure NZB and NZW backgrounds (Scaglione et al., 2007). Further studies demonstrated that development of either autoimmunity or CLL-like disease was dependent on the MHC haplotypes of the parental NZB, NZW and their progeny. Thus, MHC heterozygosis predisposed to SLE-like disease while MHC homozygosis predisposed to CLL-like disease (reviewed in (Scaglione et al., 2007)).

Studies aimed to identify loci linked to the development of CLL in NZB mice were carried out by Raveche and coworkers (Raveche et al., 2007). These studies led to the identification of three loci on chromosomes 14, 18 and 19 implicated in CLL development. Interestingly, the locus on NZB chromosome 14 has synteny with human 13q14, which is deleted in almost 50% of patients with CLL (see below). This result further stresses the relevance of this locus in CLL development. Both the mouse locus on chromosome 14 and the human 13q14 region harbor the genes encoding miR15a and miR16-1, and both human CLL with

13q14 translocations and NZB mouse with CLL-like disease showed reduced expression of miR16 (Raveche et al., 2007). However, new studies indicate that other genes in human 13q14 besides *miR15a/16-1* might be also implicated in CLL development and progression (Klein et al., 2010).

Beyond the identification of the genetic alterations in the NZB and NZW mice responsible for disease, these mice provide a unique tool to understand how the lymph node microenvironment and cytokines might influence the development of either SLE or CLL. Several studies carried out in the NZB and NZW mice have shown that cytokines play distinct roles in SLE and CLL development. In this regard, Ramachandra and coworkers (Ramachandra et al., 1996) demonstrated that high interleukin (IL)-10 levels in NZB mice were correlated with B-1 cell transformation. In agreement with a role for IL-10 in CLL development in this mouse model, IL-10 depletion achieved either by targeting deletion of the *IL-10* gene (Czarneski et al., 2004) or by *in vivo* administration of antisense IL-10 (Parker et al., 2000; Peng et al., 1995) delayed, and even prevented, CLL development. IL-5 is another member of the IL family that seems to play an important role as a switch for SLE or CLL development. Several studies (Herron et al., 1988; Kanno et al., 1992; Umland et al., 1989) have shown that B-1 cells in (NZBxNZW)F1 mice are hyper-responsive to IL-5. Indeed, *in vitro* activation of (NZBxNZW)F1 B-1 cells with IL-5 results in B-1 cells differentiation to Mott cells (Jiang et al., 1997) and IgM overproduction (Herron et al., 1988; Kanno et al., 1992; Umland et al., 1989), strongly suggesting that IL-5 overproduction might exacerbate the disease. To prove the role of IL-5 in SLE, Wen and coworkers (Wen et al., 2004) generated (NZBxNZW)F1 congenic for an IL-5 transgene. Contrary to expectations, these mice showed a significant amelioration of SLE symptoms but increased incidence of B cell malignancy. Indeed, 40% of these mice exhibited an anomalous accumulation of B-1 cells that by month 20 met the criteria for CLL.

The relevance of the New Zealand mouse strains, and particularly the NZB strain, as a CLL model can be summarized in these characteristics: 1) it is a naturally occurring model of late onset CLL that resembles familiar CLL; 2) transformed B cells are $B220^{low}IgM^{high}CD5^{+}$, they express zeta-chain associated protein kinase (ZAP)-70 and have germline Ig sequence; 3) transformed cells show DNA repair defects and chromosomal instability; 4) the mice develop clinical features also observed in CLL patients, such as autoimmune hemolytic anemia; 5) it provides a unique model for studying the relation between CLL and autoimmunity; and 6) CLL developed by these mice could be transplanted into recipient mice, which makes it suitable for preclinical studies (Scaglione et al., 2007). The identification of the gene(s) accounting for CLL and/or SLE predisposition in these mouse strains and also of the extrinsic factors influencing whether CLL or SLE is developed would be a breakthrough in our understanding of the mechanisms governing autoimmunity and tumorigenesis.

2.2 The *IgH-Eμ-Tcl-1* transgenic mouse as a model of aggressive CLL

The proto-oncogene T cell leukemia (TCL)-1 family is composed by three isoforms: TCL-1, TCL-1B and Mature T cell Proliferation (MTCP)-1 (Teitell, 2005). All three members of the family lack any known enzymatic activity, but they interact with AKT and enhance its kinase activity (Pekarsky et al., 2000). Dysregulated expression of the TCL-1 family members as a result of chromosome rearrangements is common in a variety of T cell leukemias of the mature phenotype (Pekarsky et al., 2001) and has been also found in Epstein-Barr virus positive Burkitt lymphomas (Kiss et al., 2003). Virgilio and coworkers (Virgilio et al., 1998) generated transgenic mice with *tcl-1* under the control of the *lck* proximal promoter to enforce its expression in T cells. These mice developed T-cell leukemias, thus demonstrating that TCL-1 is a *bona fide* oncogene. Furthermore, transgenic mice with *mtcp-1* under the control of the T cell specific *CD2* promoter also developed T cell leukemia (Gritti et al., 1998).

Two other TCL-1 transgenic mouse models extended its transforming capacity to B cells. One of these transgenic mice had *tcl-1* gene under the control of *pEμ-B29* promoter, causing the development of Burkitt-like lymphoma and diffuse large B cell lymphoma (DLBCL) (Hoyer et al., 2002). The other model had *tcl-1* gene expression under the control of a V_H promoter and an *IgH-Eμ* enhancer whose activity targets expression of the transgene to immature and mature B cells. The *IgH-Eμ-Tcl-1* mice have demonstrated a role for TCL-1 in CLL/SLL development (Bichi et al., 2002). Indeed, these mice showed slightly enlarged spleens with marginal zone overgrowth, and they developed expanded $B220^{low}IgM^{+}CD5^{+}$ B cells populations in peripheral blood starting at 6 months of age. All mice around 13-18 months became visibly ill, presenting splenomegaly, hepatomegaly, and overt leukemia (180 x 10^6 cells/ml compared to 2.8 x 10^6 cells/ml in wild-type littermates). Expanded B cells show clonal *IgH* rearrangements and have low proliferative activity (Bichi et al., 2002). Studies on the B cell receptors in the *IgH-Eμ-Tcl-1* transgenic mice showed that they displayed minimal levels of somatic mutations and resemble those of aggressive, treatment-resistant human CLL (Yan et al., 2006).

The demonstration that TCL-1 had a role in CLL development in mice prompted the characterization of TCL-1 expression in CLL patients. Indeed, TCL-1 is expressed in the majority of CLL (90% by IHC) but shows a differential and regulated expression pattern among patients. Higher TCL-1 expression correlates with markers of the pre-germinal center subtype including unmutated V_H status, ZAP-70 expression and presence of 11q22-23 deletions. Interestingly, TCL-1 expression was absent in CLL proliferation centers (Herling et al., 2006). However, high TCL-1 expression strongly associated to aggressive disease features, such as higher white blood cell counts and shorter duplication time (Herling et al., 2009). In agreement with these data, two independent studies have shown that high TCL-1 expression correlates with worse disease outcome (Herling et al., 2009), while low TCL-1 expression showed a trend toward improved complete remission rate after treatment (Browning et al., 2007). In agreement with these data, Enzler and coworkers (Enzler et al., 2009) have found that CLL-like cells from the *IgH-Eμ-Tcl-1* transgenic mice have also high proliferation rates. However, these cells also have an increased death rate, which slows down disease progression.

AKT is a key component of the BCR signaling, and its activation promotes CLL cell survival following BCR engagement (Longo et al., 2008; Petlickovski et al., 2005). Herling and coworkers (Herling et al., 2009) have shown that high TCL-1 expression levels are found in patients with CLL cells with higher proliferation rates upon BCR engagement. These authors found that TCL-1 increases BCR-mediated CLL proliferation by favoring AKT recruitment to the activated BCR. Furthermore, decreasing TCL1A levels by small interfering RNA reduces AKT activation and sensitizes the fludarabine-resistant CLL cell line MEC-2 to fludarabine-triggered apoptosis (Hofbauer et al., 2010)

2.2.1 The *IgH-Eμ-Tcl-1* transgenic mouse model as a tool for the identification of genes involved in CLL progression

The *IgH-Eμ-Tcl-1* transgenic mice have proved to be an invaluable tool to demonstrate *in vivo* the involvement of different genes in the pathogenesis and progression of CLL. Among the genes studied so far are the BCR regulators *rhoH, pkcβ,* and *hs1,* the TLR regulators *id4* and *tir8,* and the TNFR family member *baff.*

RhoH is a GTPase-deficient member of the GTPase family that facilitates the recruitment of ZAP-70 to the immunological synapse. RhoH mRNA expression is slightly upregulated in CLL and positively correlates with ZAP-70 expression, a known prognostic marker in CLL (Sanchez-Aguilera et al., 2010). To show whether RhoH might have a role in CLL progression, *IgH-Eμ-Tcl-1*(Tg);*RhoH-/-* mice were generated. In the absence of RhoH expression, disease burden and accumulation of CLL cells in blood were delayed. Although *RhoH-/-* B cells showed no defects in BCR signaling, BCR-mediated AKT and ERK phosphorylation was reduced in the *IgH-Eμ-Tcl-1* (Tg);*RhoH -/-* leukemic cells, suggesting a cooperation between TCL-1 and RhoH in the control of BCR signaling (Sanchez-Aguilera et al., 2010).

A role for TCL-1 in BCR signaling and its relevance in CLL development and progression was further supported with findings showing that *IgH-Eμ-Tcl-1* transgenic mice in which protein kinase beta (*pkcβ*) gene was knocked down failed to develop CLL (Holler et al., 2009). This result is particularly relevant because PKCβ is an essential component of the BCR signaling complex (Shinohara & Kurosaki, 2009) and its expression and activity is upregulated in CLL cells (Abrams et al., 2007).

Downstream signaling of the BCR in CLL is dominated by the kinases lyn and syk, which transduce pro-survival signals after antigen-mediated BCR activation. Lyn was also identified as a major contributor to antigen-independent BCR signaling (Contri et al., 2005). Scielzo and coworkers (Scielzo et al., 2010) have studied the role in CLL of the hematopoietic cell-specific Lyn substrate (HS)-1, a poorly defined component of the Lyn signaling pathway. Their results suggest that this protein regulates cytoskeleton remodeling that controls lymphocyte trafficking and homing. Mice overexpressing TCL-1 (*IgH-Eμ-Tcl-1* tg) were crossed with *hs-1* deficient mice. These mice showed an earlier disease onset and a reduced survival compared to the TCL-1-tg mice with normal HS-1 expression levels. The authors concluded that HS-1 deficiency increases tissue invasion and infiltration capabilities of CLL cells.

The Inhibitor of DNA binding protein (ID)-4 is a member of the basic helix-loop-helix (bHLH) transcription factor family that lacks DNA binding activity but retains the ability to bind and inhibit the function of other bHLH proteins, thus conferring ID4 a tumor suppressor function (Norton et al., 1998). Chen and coworkers (Chen et al., 2010) have shown that ID4 expression is uniformly silenced in CLL cells. The crossing of *id4+/-* mice with *IgH-Eμ-Tcl-1* transgenic mice demonstrated that *ID4* haploinsufficiency was enough to shift CLL to a more aggressive phenotype, as measured by lymphocyte count and reduced survival. *Id4* hemizygosity in nontransformed TCL-1 positive B cells protected cells from dexamethasone-induced apoptosis and enhanced Toll like receptor (TLR)-9-mediated B cell proliferation, suggesting a role for ID4 in apoptosis protection and enhanced immune responses to T-independent antigens.

Indeed, a role for TLRs in development and progression of CLL has been long suspected (Reviewed in (Chiron et al., 2008; Muzio et al., 2009a)). Different TLR agonists, particularly those of TLR9, trigger proliferation of unmutated CLL cells, while frequently triggering apoptosis of V_H mutated CLL cells. Interestingly, these differences observed between patients in these two CLL subgroups did not correlate with TLR9 expression levels (Jahrsdorfer et al., 2005; Longo et al., 2007; Muzio et al., 2009b), but rather with prolonged activation of signaling pathways, including Akt, MAP kinase p38 and NFκB. Consistent with these data, *IgH-Eμ-Tcl-1* transgenic mice with targeted deletion of the gene encoding the inhibitory receptor *TIR8* (*IgH-Eμ-Tcl-1*(Tg);*tir8-/-*), that allows an unabated TLR-mediated stimulation, developed a more aggressive CLL. The CLL developed by these mice was characterized for the appearance of prolymphocytes, reproducing progression of human CLL to a terminal phase (Bertilaccio et al., 2011).

The role of BAFF in promoting CLL in the *IgH-Eμ-Tcl-1* transgenic mice will be discussed below.

2.3 Targeted deletion of *miR-29* in mice causes indolent CLL

MicroRNAs (miRs) are endogenous non-coding RNAs 19-25 nucleotides in size that play relevant roles in various cellular processes including DNA methylation, cellular growth, cell differentiation and apoptosis. They control the expression of specific genes by regulating the translation and degradation of target mRNAs (Fabbri et al., 2007). Recent studies revealed that nearly half of human miRs are located within fragile sites and genomic regions altered in various cancers and there is accumulating evidence of a role for several miRs in the etiology of CLL (Calin et al., 2004; Mraz et al., 2009).

Different lines of evidence suggested that *miR-29* should function as an anti-oncogene in CLL. First, the expression of the three miR-29 isoforms was downregulated in aggressive CLL *versus* indolent CLL (Calin et al., 2004). Second, *miR-29* was shown to target the expression of genes implicated in CLL progression and pharmacological resistance, such as *Tcl-1* (Pekarsky et al., 2006), *mcl-1* (Mott et al., 2007), and *cdk6* (Garzon et al., 2009).

Therefore, it came out as a surprise when Santanam and coworkers (Santanam et al., 2010) showed that mice with enforced expression of *miR-29* under the control of the V_H promoter and the *IgH-Eμ* enhancer developed B cell malignancies similar to CLL/SLL. Indeed, clonal expansions of CD19+IgM+CD5+ B-cells were found in spleens of a majority (85%) of 12-24 months old mice. However, only 20% of the mice developed frank leukemia and died of the disease. Similar to human patients with indolent CLL, *IgH-Eμ-miR-29* transgenic mice were immune incompetent, as demonstrated by their inability to mount humoral responses against T-dependent antigens, and also contained low levels of IgG in serum.

Additional studies on miR-29 expression levels in CLL cells from patients showed that although miR-29 expression was indeed downmodulated in aggressive versus indolent CLL, miR29 level in indolent CLL samples was 4-4.5 fold higher than in normal B cells (Pekarsky & Croce, 2010). As discussed by Pekarsky and Croce (Pekarsky & Croce, 2010) these results suggest that miR-29 overexpression might predispose to CLL, as demonstrated by the *miR-29* transgenic mice. However, miR-29 overexpression might preclude progression of the disease to more aggressive stages, maybe by targeting TCL-1, whose expression is associated with the most aggressive forms of CLL (see above). Other targets of miR-29 might also be implicated in CLL progression, such as MCL-1, CDK6 and peroxidasin (Pekarsky & Croce, 2010). New studies to identify the miR-29 targets that are implicated in development of indolent CLL seem to be warranted.

2.4 Mouse models of CLL with dysregulated TNFR family signaling

TNF-family cytokines and their receptors (TNFRs) regulate a plethora of cellular activities. In B cells a restricted group of TNFR family members are expressed, but they tightly regulate B cell fate by controlling B cell survival, proliferation and differentiation. Dysregulation of these pathways causes severe immune dysfunctions including autoimmune disorders (Mackay et al., 2003).

2.4.1 The *Traf2DN/Bcl-2* mouse model of CLL/SLL

TNF-Receptors Associated Factors (TRAFs) are the molecules that are first recruited to the activated TNFR, initially acting as docking molecules for kinases and other effector proteins. TRAFs control the subcellular relocalization of the receptor-ligand complex and modulate the extent of the response by controlling the degradation of key proteins in the pathway (Zapata et al., 2007). TRAF family members are characterized by a conserved N-terminal domain of 180 amino-acid fold coined the TRAF domain, consisting on a bundle of 8 anti-parallel β-strands that are preceded by an α-helical segment. A total of 6 members of the TRAF family participate in the regulation of as many as 20 TNFRs. Some members of the family are also involved in the regulation of different members of the Toll-like Receptor (TLR) and interleukin-1 receptor (IL-1R) family. Furthermore, TNFR-family members generally utilize more than one TRAF family member for signaling, seemingly activating similar pathways and even the same downstream effectors. Therefore, the levels of expression of the different TRAF-family members and downstream effectors will likely play an important role in the outcome of the response. However, there is accumulating evidence supporting specific and unique roles for each member of the TRAF family in cell signaling (Zapata et al., 2007).

The first evidence of a direct implication of TRAF dysregulation in tumorigenesis came from our laboratory (Zapata et al., 2004). We crossed transgenic mice expressing a TRAF2 mutant lacking the N-terminal 240 amino acids encompassing the RING and zinc finger domains (TRAF2DN) (Lee et al., 1997) with transgenic mice expressing human BCL-2 specifically in B lymphocytes (Katsumata et al., 1992). The *Bcl-2* transgene mimics the (14,18)(q32;21) translocation involving *Bcl-2* and *IgH* found in human follicular lymphomas. The TRAF2DN mutant is defective in the E3 ubiquitin ligase activity that resides in the RING finger domain, but it could interact with the receptors (Ha et al., 2009). Single transgenic mice overexpressing either BCL-2 or TRAF2DN developed polyclonal expansions of B cells that very rarely progressed to malignancy. These mice also had a normal lifespan. The *Traf2DN/Bcl-2* double transgenic mice were normal at birth. The analysis of B cell populations in younger mice demonstrated higher B cell counts and expansion of marginal zone B cells, closely resembling those observed in the single *Traf2DN*-tg mice. However, starting at 6 months of age, the *Traf2DN/Bcl-2* mice developed severe splenomegaly and lymphadenopathy, and most animals also developed leukemia (as many as 130 x 10^6 B cells/ml), pleural effusion, and, in some cases, ascites associated with monoclonal and oligoclonal B cell neoplasms. The expanded B cell population of *Traf2DN/Bcl-2* double-transgenic mice was primarily comprised of small/medium-size non-cycling $B220^{Medium}IgM^{high}CD5^{+}CD11b^{+}$ cells. Transformed B cells also had high expression levels of the adhesion molecules CD49d, CD29, CD54, and CD11a in the surface, compared to wild-type B cells. Histopathologic features were consistent with mouse small lymphocytic lymphoma (SLL) progressing to leukemia with many similarities to human chronic lymphocytic leukemia. By month 14, as many as 80% of the mice died from the disease (Kress et al., 2007; Zapata et al., 2004).

B cells from the *Traf2DN/Bcl-2* double-transgenic did not show any increase in proliferation in culture compared to B cells either from the *Traf2DN* or the *Bcl-2* single transgenic mice and wild-type littermates. However, consistent with the overexpression of BCL-2, *Traf2DN/Bcl-2* B cells were partially resistant to apoptosis induced by chemotherapeutic drugs, such as dexamethasone and fludarabine. Interestingly, TRAF2DN B cells were also partially resistant to apoptosis induced by these drugs, suggesting that functional inhibition of TRAF2 might provide survival advantage to B cells (Zapata et al., 2004).

BCL-2 overexpression is a hallmark of many lymphoid malignancies, including CLL. BCL-2 protects transformed cells from apoptosis favoring disease progression and contributing to drug resistance (Buggins and Pepper, 2010; Reed, 2008). However, the role in tumorigenesis of dysregulated TRAF2 pathways is less characterized (Zapata et al., 2007). We have continued our studies to assess the role of TRAF2DN in B cell transformation and have shown that expression of the *Traf2DN* transgene causes proteosome-dependent degradation of endogenous TRAF2 (manuscript in preparation). Therefore, the TRAF2DN mice are indeed TRAF2 deficient mice. TRAF2DN B cells have deficient JNK activation and constitutive activation of the non-canonical NFκB pathway (NFκB2) (manuscript in preparation). B cell-specific *Traf2*-defficient mice have been already described (Gardam et al., 2008; Grech et al., 2004). Similar to *Traf2DN* and *Traf2DN/Bcl-2* mice, the *TRAF2-/-* mice also have expansion of marginal zone B cells. Furthermore, B cells from these mice are also deficient in JNK activation, have constitutive NFκB2 activation and are more resistant to apoptosis (Gardam et al., 2008; Grech et al., 2004).

Interestingly, Zhang and coworkers (Zhang et al., 2007) have provided proof of the direct involvement of dysregulated NFκB2 in the development of SLL/CLL. These authors developed transgenic mice expressing in lymphocytes p80HT, a lymphoma-associated NFκB2 mutant (Kim et al., 2000). These mice displayed a marked expansion of peripheral B cell populations and developed SLL. B cells from these mice were also resistant to apoptosis induced by cytokine deprivation and mitogenic stimulation. However, these authors also developed transgenic mice overexpressing in B cells p52, the active subunit of NFκB2 normally produced upon activation. These mice were predisposed to inflammatory autoimmune disease. Mice with the disease contain high levels of autoantibodies in serum and immune complex glomerulonephitis (Wang et al., 2008). These results place NFκB2 in the crossroad of autoimmunity and CLL and suggest that proteins controlling the transcriptional specificity of NFκB2 might function as a switch for autoimmunity or CLL.

Altogether, our results suggest that in the *Traf2DN/Bcl-2* transgenic mouse model of SLL/CLL, *Traf2*-deficiency might increase the resistance of subsets of B cells to apoptosis induced by specific TNF-family members. It is also conceivable that upon B cell activation (by antigen, for instance), the absence of functional TRAF2 might direct stimulated B cells through alternative maturation pathways, while overexpression of BCL-2 would protect these B cells from apoptotic stimuli involving the intrinsic pathway, ultimately promoting the development of malignancies.

2.4.2 BAFF and APRIL models of CLL/SLL

BAFF (B cell activating factor; TNFSF13b) and APRIL (a proliferation-inducing ligand; TNFSF13) are two closely related TNF family members that bind the members of the TNFR family BCMA (B cell maturation antigen) and TACI (transmembrane activator of the calcium modulator and cyclophilin ligand interactor). BAFF, but not APRIL, can also interact with BAFF-receptor (BAFFR), another TNFR family member, which seems to be the preferential receptor for BAFF (Mackay et al., 2007; Planelles et al., 2008) (Figure 1). BAFF overexpression is causative of autoimmune diseases such as systemic lupus erythematosus (SLE), rheumatoid arthritis and Sjögren's syndrome in both human and mice. Indeed, three different BAFF-transgenic mice were produced independently by three different laboratories, and all three developed SLE-like disease (Gross et al., 2000; Khare et al., 2000; Mackay et al., 1999). Furthermore, BAFF and APRIL have been shown to support chronic lymphocytic leukemia survival in a mechanism that seems to implicate BCMA and TACI and the activation of the canonical NFκB pathway (Endo et al., 2007). Elevated serum levels of APRIL have been found in CLL patients, and high APRIL levels correlate with poor prognosis (Planelles et al., 2007). Both BAFF and APRIL are produced by nurselike cells (Nishio et al., 2005) and BAFF is also produced by proliferating prolymphocytes in the CLL proliferation centers of the lymph nodes (Herreros et al., 2010), suggesting that BAFF might provide autocrine and paracrine protection to CLL cells in the lymph node microenvironment. Altogether, these results suggest that BAFF and APRIL might sustain CLL cell survival (Figure 1).

We have mentioned above that CLL-like cells from the *IgH-Eμ-Tcl-1* transgenic mice have unexpected high proliferation rates compared to non-transformed lymphocytes (Enzler et al., 2009). However, disease progression in these mice was slow, which might be a consequence of the high death rate of the transformed $B220^{low}IgM^{high}CD5^{+}$ cells as demonstrated by TUNEL staining of the spleens of these mice. Enzler and coworkers (Enzler et al., 2009) produced double transgenic *IgH-Eμ-Tcl-1/Baff* mice to investigate whether BAFF could exacerbate the disease. Indeed, these mice developed CLL at a significantly younger age and had more rapid disease progression and shorter survival compared to *IgH-Eμ-Tcl-1* transgenic mice. As expected, BAFF protected CLL cells from apoptosis without having any effect on the proliferation rates of CLL cells.

Another interesting mouse model of CLL overexpressing both BAFF and c-Myc was recently described by Zhang and coworkers (Zhang et al., 2010). Transgenic mice with *c-Myc* under the control of the *IgEα* enhancer (*iMyc*$^{C\alpha}$-tg) were initially generated to enforce c-Myc expression in plasma cells and memory cells (Cheung et al., 2004). Zhang and coworkers (Zhang et al., 2010) asked whether BAFF overexpression in these mice could induce development of CLL, since recent evidence indicates that CLL cells might arise from memory B cells (Klein et al., 2001). Interestingly, male *c-Myc/Baff* double transgenic mice did indeed developed lymphocytosis starting at 3 months of age because of increased blood B-cell number relative to that observed for single transgenic, wild type or female double transgenic mice. By month 8, clonal expansions of $CD3^{-}B220^{low}CD5^{+}$ cells were observed in as many as 78% of male *c-Myc/Baff* mice, but only in 9% of females. Mice also developed splenomegaly, lymphadenopathy and bone marrow infiltration. Histochemical and morphological analyses of the tumor populations were consistent with CLL/SLL. This mouse model of CLL is particularly interesting because is the only mouse model of CLL/SLL that mimics the gender bias observed in human patients, with a higher incidence of the disease in males.

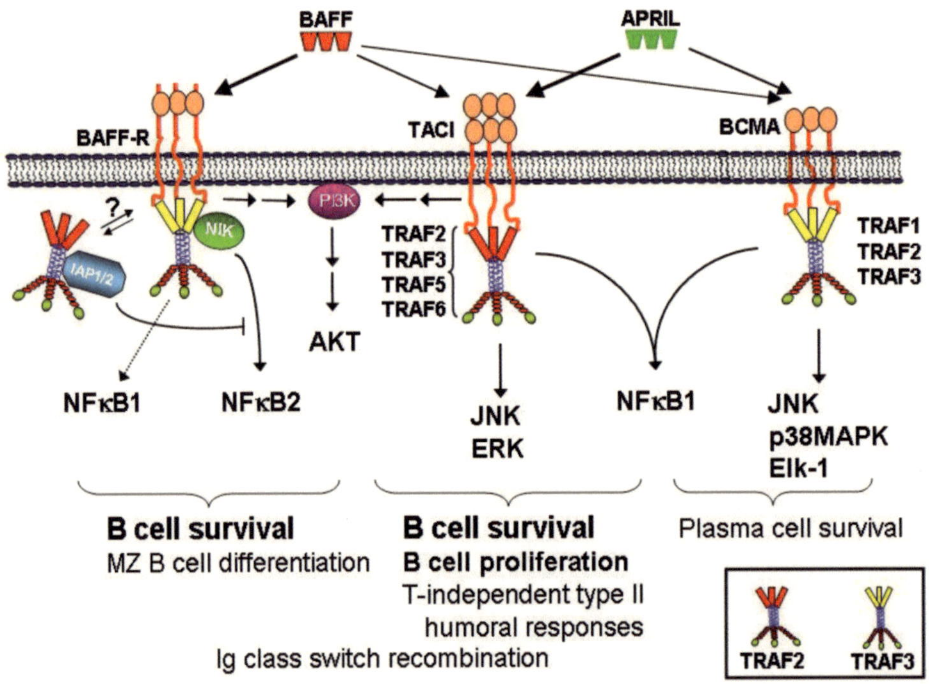

Fig. 1. Schematic representation of the signal transduction pathways and activities induced by APRIL, BAFF and their receptors. BAFF is the main ligand for BAFF-R, but it can also interact as a multimerized ligand with TACI and BCMA. APRIL is the ligand for TACI and BCMA, although it has a higher affinity for TACI. Signaling from all three receptors is mediated by members of the TRAF family. TRAF3 seems to be the only TRAF-family member capable to directly interact with BAFF-R, but TRAF2 is crucial to control the extent of BAFF-R-mediated NFκB2 activation (Gardam et al., 2008; Grech et al., 2004). Different members of the TRAF-family, including TRAF2 and 3, seem to interact with the cytosolic tail of BCMA and TACI and to regulate the activation of the canonical NFκB pathway (NFκB1) and MAPKs. Engagement of BAFF-R and TACI also induces AKT activation. CLL cells seem to express all three receptors, and BAFF and APRIL have been shown to support chronic lymphocytic leukemia survival in a mechanism that seems to implicate the activation of the canonical NFκB pathway (Endo et al., 2007). For additional information, see (Mackay et al., 2007; Planelles et al., 2008; Mackay & Schneider, 2008, 2009; Kimberley et al., 2009).

As stated above, elevated serum levels of APRIL have been found in CLL patients, and high APRIL levels seem to correlate with poor prognosis (Planelles et al., 2007). Planelles and coworkers (Planelles el al., 2004) have shown that transgenic mice with *April* under the control of the *lck* promoter developed progressive hyperplasia in mesenteric lymph nodes and Peyer's patches, disorganization of affected lymphoid tissues, and mucosal and capsular infiltration. Tumor cells will eventually infiltrate non-lymphoid tissues, such as kidney and liver in some of the mice. The expanded B cell population is $B220^{low}IgM^{low}CD5^{+}$ and $CD23^{-}$, which seems to indicate that these cells have a peritoneal B-1 origin. The incidence of the most severe pathologies was low (25%) and there was no evidence that these pathologies caused any reduction in lifespan. Although the authors did not assess whether B cell expansions in the *April*-tg mice were monoclonal or polyclonal, this model demonstrates that APRIL is a survival B cell factor *in vivo* and supports a role for APRIL in CLL progression.

Furthermore, pharmacological inhibition of the IKK-NFκB axis could prevent the pro-survival effect of BAFF overexpression in these mouse models, thus highlighting the role of the canonical NFκB pathway in CLL survival. Interestingly, TCL-1 might function as a transcriptional regulator controlling AP-1 and NFκB activity. Indeed, TCL-1 has been shown to inhibit AP-1 transcriptional activity by interacting with c-Jun, JunB and c-Fos, and to increase NFκB activity by physically interacting with p300/CREB binding protein (Pekarsky et al., 2008). Recent studies on the epigenetic changes occurring in the *Tcl-1* transgenic B cells show that NFκB1-dependent inactivation of *Foxd3* expression is an early epigenetic event causing the silencing of target genes that might be implicated in CLL development (Chen et al., 2009).

Finally, it is interesting to mention that *DLEU7*, a gene in the 13q14 deletion region which is also downregulated in other subtypes of CLL (Ouillette et al., 2008) (see below), seems to inhibit TRAF-mediated NFκB and nuclear factor of activated T cells (NFAT) activation. The mechanism might involve LEU7 interaction with BCMA and TACI (transmembrane activator of the calcium modulator and cyclophilin ligand interactor) (Palamarchuk et al., 2010) thus preventing TRAF-interaction with the activated receptors. The authors proposed that inhibition of *DLEU* expression might increase NFκB activation and apoptosis resistance.

2.5 Mice with deletions of the *DLEU2/miR15a/16-1* cluster

Among the genomic aberrations that are found in CLL patients, the most common (55%) is deletion of 13q14 (Bullrich et al., 1996; Dohner et al., 2000; Kalachikov et al., 1997; Stilgenbauer et al., 2000). In the vast majority (76%) of CLL cases this deletion is monoalellic, and only 24% are biallellic (Dohner et al., 2000). Similar frequencies of this deletion (50%) are also found in mantle cell lymphoma and at lower frequency in DLBCL, multiple myeloma, mature T cell lymphomas (Capello & Gaidano, 2000) and in a variety of solid tumors (Dong et al., 2001) which is indicative of its relevance in disease.

Studies with large cohorts of CLL patients harboring monoalellic 13q14 deletions allowed the identification of a 10 Kb minimal deleted region (MDR) common to all CLL patients (Liu et al., 1997; Migliazza et al., 2001) (Figure 2). In humans, this region contains the noncoding RNA gene *(DLEU)-2*, *miR-15a* and *miR16-1* (Calin et al., 2008), that are expressed as a cluster under the control of the *DLEU2* promoter (Klein & Dalla-Favera, 2010).

The relevance in pathogenesis of this minimal 13q14 deletion has been elegantly demonstrated by Klein and coworkers (Klein et al., 2010). These authors have generated mice that have deletion of either the *MDR* (encompassing the whole *DLEU2* gene including the *miR15a/16-1* cluster in its intron 4) or the *miR15a/16-1* only. Young *MDR*$^{-/-}$ and *miR15a/16-1*$^{-/-}$ mice showed no differences in B cell populations compared to wild-type mice, indicating the lack of involvement of this gene cluster in B cell development. These mice also mounted normal T-dependent antigen responses, suggesting that antigen-driven B cell differentiation is not affected by any of these deletions. However, as these mice grew older (15-18 months), they develop CD5+ B cells lymphoproliferative disorders, the most frequent being CLL/SLL, which could be detected in 27% of *MDR*$^{-/-}$ mice and in 21% of *miR15a/16-1*$^{-/-}$ mice. As many as 5% of these mice developed clonal expansions of B220^{low} CD5^{+} B cells in peripheral blood, closely resembling human monoclonal B cell lymphocytosis. Furthermore, a fraction of *MDR*$^{-/-}$ (9%) and *miR15a/16-1*$^{-/-}$ (2%) mice developed CD5^{null} NHL of splenic and/or lymph node origin, the majority of which were histologically similar to DLBCL, thus resembling Richter's transformation of human CLL patients (Foucar & Rydell, 1980). The rest of NHL lymphomas developed by these mice were similar to plasmacytic lymphomas (Klein et al., 2010).

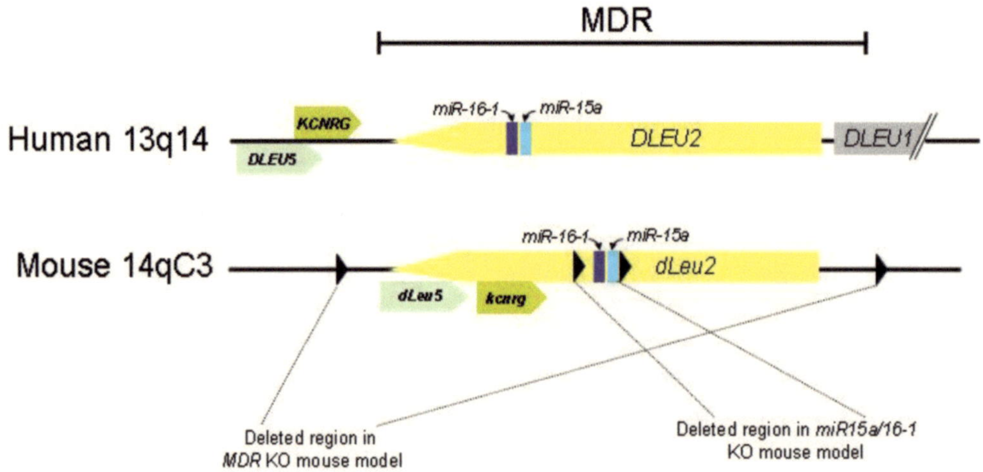

Fig. 2. Schematic representation of the minimal deletion region (MDR) in human 13q14 and the corresponding region in mouse 14qC3. Deleted genomic regions in *MDR*-deficient and *miR15a/16-1*-deficient mice are shown. Adapted from (Klein et al., 2010).

Interestingly, the mice with the *MDR* deletion not only displayed a larger incidence of disease (42% for the *MDR*$^{-/-}$ and 24% for the *MDR*$^{+/-}$), but they also had a reduced lifespan (around 70% of the *MDR*$^{-/-}$ mice and 50% of the *MDR*$^{+/-}$ died by month 20), compared to *miR15a/16-1*$^{-/-}$ mice, which had an overall 26% tumor incidence and no significant lifespan reduction compared to wild-type littermates. Thus, these results support a role for miR15a/16 as tumor suppressor, but also indicate that there might be additional genetic elements within the MDR locus implicated in the etiology of CLL.

The analysis of the genes targeted by miR15a/16-1 was also assessed by Klein and coworkers (Klein et al., 2010) in B cells from the *miR15a/16-1*$^{-/-}$ mice. Their results showed the role of this miR cluster in the regulation of cell proliferation through the control of the expression of cyclins and other genes involved in cell cycle progression, as previously described in a variety of cell types (Bandi et al., 2009; Bonci et al., 2008; Linsley et al., 2007; Liu et al., 2008). Using a green fluorescence protein lentiviral expression system, Salerno and coworkers (Salerno et al., 2009) further demonstrated the direct targeting of Cyclin D1 3′ unstranslated region by miR16.

Of special interest is the role of miR15a/16-1 in the regulation of BCL-2 expression. As stated above, BCL-2 is a pro-survival protein that is upregulated in several lymphoid malignancies, including CLL/SLL (Reed, 2008). Indeed, enforced BCL-2 overexpression in mice predisposes to CLL/SLL (Zapata et al., 2004), although its overexpression alone is not sufficient for CLL development (Katsumata et al., 1992). High levels of BCL-2 are a trademark of CLL but the mechanism underlying BCL-2 overexpression in CLL/SLL remains unclear. Cimmino and coworkers (Cimmino et al., 2005) showed evidence indicating that miR15a/16-1 targeted BCL-2 mRNA, and found an inverse correlation between miRNA15/16 and BCL-2 expression levels. However, other studies (Fulci et al., 2007; Ouillette et al., 2008) failed to find such correlation and showed that down-regulation of both miR15a and 16-1 was not paralleled by any significant increase in BCL-2 levels. In this regard, the studies by Klein and coworkers (Klein et al., 2010) showed that neither deletion of *MDR* or *miR15a/16-1* had any significant effect on BCL-2 expression when compared to that of B cells from wild-type littermates. Upregulation of BCL-2 expression in germinal centers was also unaffected in $MDR^{-/-}$ and $miR15a/16\text{-}1^{-/-}$ mice. Although additional studies are needed to elucidate whether miR15a/16-1 expression might regulate BCL-2 expression in specific cell contexts and physiological situations, it seems unlikely that miR15a/16-1 downregulation accounts for BCL-2 upregulation in CLL.

In summary, these results strongly suggest that the main physiological role of miR15a/16-1 is to regulate cell homeostasis by controlling the expression of proteins implicated in cell cycle progression. However, similar to the *IgH-Eμ-TCL-1* mice, where high CLL proliferation rates were compensated with increased cell death rates (Enzler et al., 2009), efficient transformation of cells bearing the 13q14 deletion might require also the cooperation of pro-survival factors.

2.6 A SV40 T antigen-driven mouse model of CLL

Ter Brugge and coworkers (ter Brugge et al., 2009) reported a new mouse model based on expression of the simian virus 40 (SV40) large T antigen. These authors generated 2 different mouse models introducing the SV40 *T* gene in the immunoglobulin heavy chain locus between the *D* and *J* segments, in opposite transcriptional orientation. SV40 T expression was enforced in each mouse model by either 1 or 2 copies of the *IgH* intronic enhancer *Eμ*. The levels of SV40 *T* expression were higher in the transgenic mice with two copies of the *Eμ* enhancer. Mice carrying two copies of the *Eμ* enhancer developed clonal expansions of mature B cells in blood, lymph nodes, spleen, and bone marrow before the age of 10 months. In contrast only 10% of the mice carrying only one copy of the enhancer developed this malignancy. Expanded B cells were $CD19^{+}IgM^{high}CD5^{+}CD43^{+}$, consistent with CLL. In addition, DNA sequencing analysis determined that V_H regions were either unmutated, with preferential usage of the V_H11, or showed extensive somatic hypermutation and usage of V_HJ558.

SV40 large T protein interacts with numerous cellular proteins and pathways, most notably the Retinoblastoma and p53 pathways (Ahuja et al., 2005; Ali & DeCaprio, 2001), although in this model, p53 expression seems to be deleterious for the transforming activity of the T protein (ter Brugge et al., 2009). Similar to TCL-1 (see above), SV40 large T protein has been shown to induce cell survival via AKT activation (Cacciotti et al., 2005).

2.7 Transplantation models of CLL

2.7.1 Xenograft models

Development of xenograft models of human CLL cells has been a troublesome task as a result of the non-proliferative nature of circulating CLL cells. Initial approaches involved transferring CLL cells from patients into mice with severe combined immunodeficiency (SCID). A percentage of these mice developed tumors, but they were composed by CD5- EBV+ B cells, emulating the EBV-associated lymphoproliferations noted in SCID mice reconstituted with normal human PBL (Kobayashi et al., 1992). Intraperitoneal injections of IL-2 and IL-7 in SCID mice previously inoculated with human CLL failed to improve the efficacy of this type of engraftment (Hummel et al., 1996). Shimoni and coworkers (Shimoni et al., 1997) used lethally irradiated Balb/c or beige/nude/Xid (BNX) mice radioprotected with bone marrow from SCID mice as engraftment recipients for human CLL cells. These authors found that adoptive transfer of low-stage CLL peripheral blood mononuclear cells (PBMCs) (Rai 0) led to marked engraftment of T cells or combined T and CLL cell engraftment, whereas inoculation of high-stage (III-IV) CLL PBMCs led to dominance of CLL cells with negligible involvement of T cells. These authors succeeded in transplanting low-stage CLLs by depleting T cells from the PBMC culture using OKT3 antibody. In contrast, eliminating T cells was not as critical for promoting engraftment of high-stage CLL cells (Shimoni et al., 1999). The authors concluded that autologous T cells can actively suppress the expansion of CLL in the mouse recipient. Indeed, Durig and coworkers (Durig et al., 2007) obtained similar results using sublethally irradiated nonobese diabetes (NOD)/SCID mice as recipients for CLL xenotransplantation. These authors combined intra-peritoneal and intra-venous injections of PBMCs from CLL patients, achieving a highly reproducible splenic and peritoneal engraftment that remained stable for 4-8 weeks. However, these authors also reported that PBMCs from CLL donors with Binet stage A favored T cell engraftment over CLLs. In contrast, predominant engraftment of CLL cells was achieved using PBMCs from CLL patients with Binet stage C.

Recent data, however, put into question the deleterious role of autologous T cells in CLL engraftment. Bagnara and coworkers (Bagnara et al., 2011) have described a novel adoptive transfer model of chronic lymphocytic leukemia in which primary CLL cells proliferate in NSG (NOD/SCID/*IL2Rγ-/-)* mice under the influence of activated CLL-derived T lymphocytes. The NSG recipient mouse strain is a NOD/SCID-derived strain that lacks the IL-2 family common cytokine receptor gamma chain gen (IL2Rγ), rendering mice completely deficient in lymphocytes (including NK cells). The authors have shown that by co-transferring autologous T lymphocytes, activated *in vivo* by alloantigens, the survival and growth of primary CLL cells *in vivo* could be achieved and quantified. However, although T cells are required for CLL survival and proliferation, eventually all human CLL cells disappeared and the animal died after 12 weeks by T cell-dependent graft versus host disease. Although it has some significant limitations, this mouse model should simplify analyzing kinetics of CLL cells *in vivo* and permitting personalized preclinical studies of novel therapeutics.

Kikushige and coworkers (Kikushige et al., 2011) have recently used xenogeneic transplantation of different CLL subpopulations to demonstrate that the propensity to generate clonal B cells is already acquired at the hematopoietic stem cell (HSC) stage. These authors transplanted either mature CLL cells, purified proB cells or purified HSCs from CLL patients into NSG or into NOD/*Rag1-/- IL2Rγ-/-* (NRG) mice. CLL cells or proB cells from patients failed to engraft in any of the xenotransplanted mice, but CLL-HSCs, similar to normal donors HSCs, were able to reconstitute the hematopoietic lineages in the mice. However, contrary to normal donors HSCs, CLL-HSCs differentiation in xenotransplanted mice seemed to be skewed toward B cell lineage and B cell maturation was always restricted to mono- or oligo-clones with CLL-like phenotype, thus suggesting that HSCs could be involved in leukemogenesis even in mature lymphoid tumors.

Finally, Bertilaccio and coworkers (Bertilaccio et al., 2010) have described the engraftement of the CLL cell line MEC1 in *Rag2-/- IL2Rγ-/-* mice This xenograft mouse model has systemic organ involvement, develops very rapidly, allows the measurement of tumor burden, and has 100% engraftment efficiency, thus closely resembling aggressive human disease. This mouse model has also been used to study the role of the Lyn substrate HS1 in CLL (Scielzo et al., 2010).

2.7.2 Allograft models

Nakagawa and coworkers (Nakagawa et al., 2006b) have demonstrated a role for PKCα in the etiology of CLL using a new approach involving allogeneic transplantation. These authors stably expressed a plasmid encoding a dominant-negative PKCα (PKCα-KR) mutant in fetal liver-derived hematopoietic progenitor cells (HPC) from wild-type mice. Interestingly, *in vitro* and *in vivo* expansion of these cells in transplanted *Rag-/-* mice resulted in the generation of a population of B cells expressing $B220^{+}IgM^{low}CD5^{+}CD23^{+}$ resembling human CLL cells. Compared to untransfected cells, these CLL-like cells display enhanced proliferation in the presence of growth factors and stroma and apoptosis resistance, which seems to be mediated by BCL-2 overexpression. Furthermore, other PKC family members did not cause this transformation, thus highlighting the role of PKCα as a tumor suppressor in CLL. This model of "instant transgenesis" is particularly interesting because it allows determining the role of specific signaling molecules during lymphocyte development *in vivo* by introducing a defined gene, such as a wild-type or mutated signaling molecule, into a lymphoid progenitor population by retroviral infection that could be expanded *in vivo* in recipient *Rag -/-* mice (Nakagawa et al., 2006a).

2.8 Mouse models of CLL as preclinical platforms for testing new chemotherapeutic drugs

Preclinical studies of new drug candidates would benefit from the availability of mouse models of CLL that closely recapitulate key aspects of the disease as seen in humans. Indeed, the *IgH-Eμ-Tcl-1* and the *Traf2DN/Bcl-2* transgenic mice have been already used to test the anti-CLL efficacy of new drugs in mice. Thus, the *IgH-Eμ-Tcl-1* transgenic mice were used to assess the efficacy of fludarabine, a drug used as a first line of treatment of CLL patients, in the leukemic mice (Johnson et al., 2006). Fludarabine was shown to be clinically active at low dose in the mice, reducing leukemic burden. However, an emergence of resistance over repeated treatments was observed in the mice, similar to what happens to CLL patients (Johnson et al., 2006).

Furthermore, cells from the *IgH-Eμ-Tcl-1* mice were transplanted into syngeneic mice to test the *in vivo* efficacy of rapamycin, a specific pharmacologic inhibitor of the AKT/mTOR pathway, in the progression of the disease (Zanesi et al., 2006). Treatment with rapamycin significantly prolonged the life of all treated animals compared to untreated mice. However, the delaying effect of rapamycin on mouse CLL was relatively short and, eventually, all mice died from the disease. A similar approach was also used to show the anti-leukemic activity of fosfamatinib disodium (R788), a Syk inhibitor that blocks BCR signaling (Suljagic et al., 2010). R788 effectively reduced proliferation and survival of the malignant cells without affecting normal B lymphocytes. (Suljagic et al., 2010).

Traf2DN/Bcl-2 mice served also as a preclinical platform to test the anti-CLL efficacy of the synthetic triterpenoid 2-Cyano-3,12-Dioxooleana-1,9-Dien-28-Oic Acid (CDDO) and its imidazolide derivative (CDDO-Im). Treating *Traf2DN/Bcl-2* mice that had developed leukemia with liposome-formulated CDDO or CDDO-Im resulted in significant amelioration of CLL/SLL burden by dramatically reducing malignant B cells in blood, spleen and lung, without having any significant effect on the viability of normal B and T cells (Kress et al., 2007).

3. Conclusion

The different genetically modified mice or natural strains described above have provided valuable insights into the molecular mechanisms behind CLL/SLL transformation and progression. They have also demonstrated that it is possible to develop mouse models that share defining characteristics with specific human CLL subsets. Just as an example, *Tcl-1-tg* mice might be counterpart of aggressive CLL, *miR29* tg mice seem to be related to indolent CLL, and the *Traf2DN/Bcl-2-tg* mice might be a good model of refractory disease.

The results and conclusions achieved from the studies with mice might not always be extrapolated to human, and *vice versa*. However, preclinical studies performed in CLL/SLL mouse models of specific CLL subclasses would be a leap forward in our understanding of the biological behavior and specificity of new chemotherapeutic drug families. These studies will help to determine *in vivo* not only the efficacy of the drug, but also to identify potential problems with the therapy, such as lysis shock, high protein binding, first pass effect and non-appropriate biodistribution of the drug that may limit its efficacy.

Future studies in the mouse models described in this chapter and in others still to be developed will expand our understanding of CLL etiology and will provide new tools for fighting the disease.

4. Ackowledgements

We are thankful to Drs. Miguel R. Campanero and Filip Lim for critical reading of the manuscript. We are grateful to the Fondo de Investigaciones Sanitarias (FIS PI080170) and Consejo Superior de Investigaciones Científicas (CSIC JAE Doc/09/021) for its generous support.

5. References

Abrams, S.T., Lakum, T., Lin, K., Jones, G.M., Treweeke, A.T., Farahani, M., Hughes, M., Zuzel, M., & Slupsky, J.R. (2007). B-cell receptor signaling in chronic lymphocytic leukemia cells is regulated by overexpressed active protein kinase CbetaII. Blood *109*, 1193-1201.

Ahuja, D., Saenz-Robles, M.T., & Pipas, J.M. (2005). SV40 large T antigen targets multiple cellular pathways to elicit cellular transformation. Oncogene *24*, 7729-7745.

Ali, S.H., and DeCaprio, J.A. (2001). Cellular transformation by SV40 large T antigen: interaction with host proteins. Semin Cancer Biol *11*, 15-23.

Bagnara, D., Kaufman, M.S., Calissano, C., Marsilio, S., Patten, P.E., Simone, R., Chum, P., Yan, X.J., Allen, S.L., Kolitz, J.E., *et al.* (2011). A novel adoptive transfer model of chronic lymphocytic leukemia suggests a key role for T lymphocytes in the disease. Blood *117*, 5463-5472.

Bandi, N., Zbinden, S., Gugger, M., Arnold, M., Kocher, V., Hasan, L., Kappeler, A., Brunner, T., & Vassella, E. (2009). miR-15a and miR-16 are implicated in cell cycle regulation in a Rb-dependent manner and are frequently deleted or down-regulated in non-small cell lung cancer. Cancer Res *69*, 5553-5559.

Bertilaccio, M.T., Scielzo, C., Simonetti, G., Ponzoni, M., Apollonio, B., Fazi, C., Scarfo, L., Rocchi, M., Muzio, M., Caligaris-Cappio, F., *et al.* (2010). A novel Rag2-/-gammac-/--xenograft model of human CLL. Blood *115*, 1605-1609.

Bertilaccio, M.T., Simonetti, G., Dagklis, A., Rocchi, M., Rodriguez, T.V., Apollonio, B., Mantovani, A., Ponzoni, M., Ghia, P., Garlanda, C., *et al.* (2011). Lack of TIR8/SIGIRR triggers progression of chronic lymphocytic leukemia in mouse models. Blood *118*, 660-669.

Bichi, R., Shinton, S.A., Martin, E.S., Koval, A., Calin, G.A., Cesari, R., Russo, G., Hardy, R.R., & Croce, C.M. (2002). Human chronic lymphocytic leukemia modeled in mouse by targeted TCL1 expression. Proc Natl Acad Sci U S A *99*, 6955-6960.

Bonci, D., Coppola, V., Musumeci, M., Addario, A., Giuffrida, R., Memeo, L., D'Urso, L., Pagliuca, A., Biffoni, M., Labbaye, C., *et al.* (2008). The miR-15a-miR-16-1 cluster controls prostate cancer by targeting multiple oncogenic activities. Nat Med *14*, 1271-1277.

Browning, R.L., Geyer, S.M., Johnson, A.J., Jelinek, D.F., Tschumper, R.C., Call, T.G., Shanafelt, T.D., Zent, C.S., Bone, N.D., Dewald, G.W., *et al.* (2007). Expression of TCL-1 as a potential prognostic factor for treatment outcome in B-cell chronic lymphocytic leukemia. Leukemia research *31*, 1737-1740.

Buggins, A.G., & Pepper, C.J. (2010). The role of Bcl-2 family proteins in chronic lymphocytic leukaemia. Leukemia research *34*, 837-842.

Bullrich, F., Veronese, M.L., Kitada, S., Jurlander, J., Caligiuri, M.A., Reed, J.C., & Croce, C.M. (1996). Minimal region of loss at 13q14 in B-cell chronic lymphocytic leukemia. Blood *88*, 3109-3115.

Cacciotti, P., Barbone, D., Porta, C., Altomare, D.A., Testa, J.R., Mutti, L., & Gaudino, G. (2005). SV40-dependent AKT activity drives mesothelial cell transformation after asbestos exposure. Cancer Res *65*, 5256-5262.

Calin, G.A., Cimmino, A., Fabbri, M., Ferracin, M., Wojcik, S.E., Shimizu, M., Taccioli, C., Zanesi, N., Garzon, R., Aqeilan, R.I., *et al.* (2008). MiR-15a and miR-16-1 cluster functions in human leukemia. Proc Natl Acad Sci U S A *105*, 5166-5171.

Calin, G.A., Liu, C.G., Sevignani, C., Ferracin, M., Felli, N., Dumitru, C.D., Shimizu, M., Cimmino, A., Zupo, S., Dono, M., *et al.* (2004). MicroRNA profiling reveals distinct signatures in B cell chronic lymphocytic leukemias. Proc Natl Acad Sci U S A *101,* 11755-11760.

Capello, D., & Gaidano, G. (2000). Molecular pathophysiology of indolent lymphoma. Haematologica *85,* 195-201.

Chen, S.S., Claus, R., Lucas, D.M., Yu, L., Qian, J., Ruppert, A.S., West, D.A., Williams, K.E., Johnson, A.J., Sablitzky, F., *et al.* (2010). Silencing of the inhibitor of DNA binding protein 4 (ID4) contributes to the pathogenesis of mouse and human CLL. Blood *117,* 862-871.

Chen, S.S., Raval, A., Johnson, A.J., Hertlein, E., Liu, T.H., Jin, V.X., Sherman, M.H., Liu, S.J., Dawson, D.W., Williams, K.E., *et al.* (2009). Epigenetic changes during disease progression in a murine model of human chronic lymphocytic leukemia. Proc Natl Acad Sci U S A *106,* 13433-13438.

Cheung, W.C., Kim, J.S., Linden, M., Peng, L., Van Ness, B., Polakiewicz, R.D., & Janz, S. (2004). Novel targeted deregulation of c-Myc cooperates with Bcl-X(L) to cause plasma cell neoplasms in mice. J Clin Invest *113,* 1763-1773.

Chiorazzi, N., & Ferrarini, M. (2003). B cell chronic lymphocytic leukemia: lessons learned from studies of the B cell antigen receptor. Annu Rev Immunol *21,* 841-894.

Chiorazzi, N., & Ferrarini, M. (2011). Cellular origin(s) of chronic lymphocytic leukemia: cautionary notes and additional considerations and possibilities. Blood *117,* 1781-1791.

Chiron, D., Bekeredjian-Ding, I., Pellat-Deceunynck, C., Bataille, R., & Jego, G. (2008). Toll-like receptors: lessons to learn from normal and malignant human B cells. Blood *112,* 2205-2213.

Cimmino, A., Calin, G.A., Fabbri, M., Iorio, M.V., Ferracin, M., Shimizu, M., Wojcik, S.E., Aqeilan, R.I., Zupo, S., Dono, M., *et al.* (2005). miR-15 and miR-16 induce apoptosis by targeting BCL2. Proc Natl Acad Sci U S A *102,* 13944-13949.

Coll-Mulet, L., & Gil, J. (2009). Genetic alterations in chronic lymphocytic leukaemia. Clin Transl Oncol *11,* 194-198.

Contri, A., Brunati, A.M., Trentin, L., Cabrelle, A., Miorin, M., Cesaro, L., Pinna, L.A., Zambello, R., Semenzato, G., & Donella-Deana, A. (2005). Chronic lymphocytic leukemia B cells contain anomalous Lyn tyrosine kinase, a putative contribution to defective apoptosis. J Clin Invest *115,* 369-378.

Czarneski, J., Lin, Y.C., Chong, S., McCarthy, B., Fernandes, H., Parker, G., Mansour, A., Huppi, K., Marti, G.E., & Raveche, E. (2004). Studies in NZB IL-10 knockout mice of the requirement of IL-10 for progression of B-cell lymphoma. Leukemia *18,* 597-606.

Dameshek, W. (1967). Chronic lymphocytic leukemia - an accumulative disease of immunologically incompetent lymphocytes. Blood *29,* 566-584.

Damle, R.N., Ghiotto, F., Valetto, A., Albesiano, E., Fais, F., Yan, X.J., Sison, C.P., Allen, S.L., Kolitz, J., Schulman, P., *et al.* (2002). B-cell chronic lymphocytic leukemia cells express a surface membrane phenotype of activated, antigen-experienced B lymphocytes. Blood *99,* 4087-4093.

Damle, R.N., Wasil, T., Fais, F., Ghiotto, F., Valetto, A., Allen, S.L., Buchbinder, A., Budman, D., Dittmar, K., Kolitz, J., *et al.* (1999). Ig V gene mutation status and CD38 expression as novel prognostic indicators in chronic lymphocytic leukemia. Blood *94*, 1840-1847.

Dohner, H., Stilgenbauer, S., Benner, A., Leupolt, E., Krober, A., Bullinger, L., Dohner, K., Bentz, M., & Lichter, P. (2000). Genomic aberrations and survival in chronic lymphocytic leukemia. N Engl J Med *343*, 1910-1916.

Dong, J.T., Boyd, J.C., & Frierson, H.F., Jr. (2001). Loss of heterozygosity at 13q14 and 13q21 in high grade, high stage prostate cancer. Prostate *49*, 166-171.

Durig, J., Ebeling, P., Grabellus, F., Sorg, U.R., Mollmann, M., Schutt, P., Gothert, J., Sellmann, L., Seeber, S., Flasshove, M., *et al.* (2007). A novel nonobese diabetic/severe combined immunodeficient xenograft model for chronic lymphocytic leukemia reflects important clinical characteristics of the disease. Cancer Res *67*, 8653-8661.

Endo, T., Nishio, M., Enzler, T., Cottam, H.B., Fukuda, T., James, D.F., Karin, M., & Kipps, T.J. (2007). BAFF and APRIL support chronic lymphocytic leukemia B-cell survival through activation of the canonical NF-kappaB pathway. Blood *109*, 703-710.

Enzler, T., Kater, A.P., Zhang, W., Widhopf, G.F., 2nd, Chuang, H.Y., Lee, J., Avery, E., Croce, C.M., Karin, M., & Kipps, T.J. (2009). Chronic lymphocytic leukemia of Emu-TCL1 transgenic mice undergoes rapid cell turnover that can be offset by extrinsic CD257 to accelerate disease progression. Blood *114*, 4469-4476.

Fabbri, M., Ivan, M., Cimmino, A., Negrini, M., & Calin, G.A. (2007). Regulatory mechanisms of microRNAs involvement in cancer. Expert Opin Biol Ther *7*, 1009-1019.

Fais, F., Ghiotto, F., Hashimoto, S., Sellars, B., Valetto, A., Allen, S.L., Schulman, P., Vinciguerra, V.P., Rai, K., Rassenti, L.Z., *et al.* (1998). Chronic lymphocytic leukemia B cells express restricted sets of mutated and unmutated antigen receptors. J Clin Invest *102*, 1515-1525.

Foucar, K., & Rydell, R.E. (1980). Richter's syndrome in chronic lymphocytic leukemia. Cancer *46*, 118-134.

Fulci, V., Chiaretti, S., Goldoni, M., Azzalin, G., Carucci, N., Tavolaro, S., Castellano, L., Magrelli, A., Citarella, F., Messina, M., *et al.* (2007). Quantitative technologies establish a novel microRNA profile of chronic lymphocytic leukemia. Blood *109*, 4944-4951.

Gardam, S., Sierro, F., Basten, A., Mackay, F., & Brink, R. (2008). TRAF2 and TRAF3 signal adapters act cooperatively to control the maturation and survival signals delivered to B cells by the BAFF receptor. Immunity *28*, 391-401.

Garzon, R., Heaphy, C.E., Havelange, V., Fabbri, M., Volinia, S., Tsao, T., Zanesi, N., Kornblau, S.M., Marcucci, G., Calin, G.A., *et al.* (2009). MicroRNA 29b functions in acute myeloid leukemia. Blood *114*, 5331-5341.

Ghia, P., Chiorazzi, N., & Stamatopoulos, K. (2008). Microenvironmental influences in chronic lymphocytic leukaemia: the role of antigen stimulation. J Intern Med *264*, 549-562.

Grech, A.P., Amesbury, M., Chan, T., Gardam, S., Basten, A., & Brink, R. (2004). TRAF2 differentially regulates the canonical and noncanonical pathways of NF-kappaB activation in mature B cells. Immunity *21*, 629-642.

Gritti, C., Dastot, H., Soulier, J., Janin, A., Daniel, M.T., Madani, A., Grimber, G., Briand, P., Sigaux, F., & Stern, M.H. (1998). Transgenic mice for MTCP1 develop T-cell prolymphocytic leukemia. Blood *92*, 368-373.

Gross, J.A., Johnston, J., Mudri, S., Enselman, R., Dillon, S.R., Madden, K., Xu, W., Parrish-Novak, J., Foster, D., Lofton-Day, C., *et al.* (2000). TACI and BCMA are receptors for a TNF homologue implicated in B-cell autoimmune disease. Nature *404*, 995-999.

Ha, H., Han, D., & Choi, Y. (2009). TRAF-mediated TNFR-family signaling. Curr Protoc Immunol *Chapter 11*, Unit11 19D.

Hamano, Y., Hirose, S., Ida, A., Abe, M., Zhang, D., Kodera, S., Jiang, Y., Shirai, J., Miura, Y., Nishimura, H., *et al.* (1998). Susceptibility alleles for aberrant B-1 cell proliferation involved in spontaneously occurring B-cell chronic lymphocytic leukemia in a model of New Zealand white mice. Blood *92*, 3772-3779.

Hamblin, T.J., Davis, Z., Gardiner, A., Oscier, D.G., & Stevenson, F.K. (1999). Unmutated Ig V(H) genes are associated with a more aggressive form of chronic lymphocytic leukemia. Blood *94*, 1848-1854.

Herling, M., Patel, K.A., Khalili, J., Schlette, E., Kobayashi, R., Medeiros, L.J., & Jones, D. (2006). TCL1 shows a regulated expression pattern in chronic lymphocytic leukemia that correlates with molecular subtypes and proliferative state. Leukemia *20*, 280-285.

Herling, M., Patel, K.A., Weit, N., Lilienthal, N., Hallek, M., Keating, M.J., & Jones, D. (2009). High TCL1 levels are a marker of B-cell receptor pathway responsiveness and adverse outcome in chronic lymphocytic leukemia. Blood *114*, 4675-4686.

Herreros, B., Rodriguez-Pinilla, S.M., Pajares, R., Martinez-Gonzalez, M.A., Ramos, R., Munoz, I., Montes-Moreno, S., Lozano, M., Sanchez-Verde, L., Roncador, G., *et al.* (2010). Proliferation centers in chronic lymphocytic leukemia: the niche where NF-kappaB activation takes place. Leukemia *24*, 872-876.

Herron, L.R., Coffman, R.L., Bond, M.W., & Kotzin, B.L. (1988). Increased autoantibody production by NZB/NZW B cells in response to IL-5. J Immunol *141*, 842-848.

Hofbauer, S.W., Pinon, J.D., Brachtl, G., Haginger, L., Wang, W., Johrer, K., Tinhofer, I., Hartmann, T.N., & Greil, R. (2010). Modifying akt signaling in B-cell chronic lymphocytic leukemia cells. Cancer Res *70*, 7336-7344.

Holler, C., Pinon, J.D., Denk, U., Heyder, C., Hofbauer, S., Greil, R., & Egle, A. (2009). PKCbeta is essential for the development of chronic lymphocytic leukemia in the TCL1 transgenic mouse model: validation of PKCbeta as a therapeutic target in chronic lymphocytic leukemia. Blood *113*, 2791-2794.

Hoyer, K.K., French, S.W., Turner, D.E., Nguyen, M.T., Renard, M., Malone, C.S., Knoetig, S., Qi, C.F., Su, T.T., Cheroutre, H., *et al.* (2002). Dysregulated TCL1 promotes multiple classes of mature B cell lymphoma. Proc Natl Acad Sci U S A *99*, 14392-14397.

Hummel, J.L., Lichty, B.D., Reis, M., Dube, I., & Kamel-Reid, S. (1996). Engraftment of human chronic lymphocytic leukemia cells in SCID mice: in vivo and in vitro studies. Leukemia *10*, 1370-1376.

Jahrsdorfer, B., Wooldridge, J.E., Blackwell, S.E., Taylor, C.M., Griffith, T.S., Link, B.K., & Weiner, G.J. (2005). Immunostimulatory oligodeoxynucleotides induce apoptosis of B cell chronic lymphocytic leukemia cells. J Leukoc Biol *77*, 378-387.

Jiang, Y., Hirose, S., Hamano, Y., Kodera, S., Tsurui, H., Abe, M., Terashima, K., Ishikawa, S., & Shirai, T. (1997). Mapping of a gene for the increased susceptibility of B1 cells to Mott cell formation in murine autoimmune disease. J Immunol *158*, 992-997.

Johnson, A.J., Lucas, D.M., Muthusamy, N., Smith, L.L., Edwards, R.B., De Lay, M.D., Croce, C.M., Grever, M.R., & Byrd, J.C. (2006). Characterization of the TCL-1 transgenic mouse as a preclinical drug development tool for human chronic lymphocytic leukemia. Blood *108*, 1334-1338.

Kalachikov, S., Migliazza, A., Cayanis, E., Fracchiolla, N.S., Bonaldo, M.F., Lawton, L., Jelenc, P., Ye, X., Qu, X., Chien, M., *et al.* (1997). Cloning and gene mapping of the chromosome 13q14 region deleted in chronic lymphocytic leukemia. Genomics *42*, 369-377.

Kanno, K., Okada, T., Abe, M., Hirose, S., & Shirai, T. (1992). CD5+ B cells as precursors of CD5- IgG anti-DNA antibody-producing B cells in autoimmune-prone NZB/W F1 mice. Ann N Y Acad Sci *651*, 576-578.

Katsumata, M., Siegel, R.M., Louie, D.C., Miyashita, T., Tsujimoto, Y., Nowell, P.C., Greene, M.I., & Reed, J.C. (1992). Differential effects of Bcl-2 on B and T lymphocytes in transgenic mice. Proc Natl Acad Sci USA *89*, 11376-11380.

Khare, S.D., Sarosi, I., Xia, X.Z., McCabe, S., Miner, K., Solovyev, I., Hawkins, N., Kelley, M., Chang, D., Van, G., *et al.* (2000). Severe B cell hyperplasia and autoimmune disease in TALL-1 transgenic mice. Proc Natl Acad Sci U S A *97*, 3370-3375.

Kikushige, Y., Ishikawa, F., Miyamoto, T., Shima, T., Urata, S., Yoshimoto, G., Mori, Y., Iino, T., Yamauchi, T., Eto, T., *et al.* (2011). Self-Renewing hematopoietic stem cell is the primary target in pathogenesis of human chronic lymphocytic leukemia. Cancer Cell *20*, 246-259

Kim, K.E., Gu, C., Thakur, S., Vieira, E., Lin, J.C., & Rabson, A.B. (2000). Transcriptional regulatory effects of lymphoma-associated NFKB2/lyt10 protooncogenes. Oncogene *19*, 1334-1345.

Kimberley, F.C., Hahne, M. & Medema, J.P. (2009). April hath put a spring of youth in everything:relevance of APRIL for survival. J.Cell. Physiol. *218*, 1-8.

Kiss, C., Nishikawa, J., Takada, K., Trivedi, P., Klein, G. and Szekely, L. (2003). T cell leukemia 1 oncogenen expression depends on the presence of Epstein-Barr vius in the virus-carrying Burkitt lymphoma lines. Proc Natl Acad Sci USA *100*, 4813-4810

Klein, U., & Dalla-Favera, R. (2010). New insights into the pathogenesis of chronic lymphocytic leukemia. Semin Cancer Biol *20*, 377-383.

Klein, U., Lia, M., Crespo, M., Siegel, R., Shen, Q., Mo, T., Ambesi-Impiombato, A., Califano, A., Migliazza, A., Bhagat, G., *et al.* (2010). The DLEU2/miR-15a/16-1 cluster controls B cell proliferation and its deletion leads to chronic lymphocytic leukemia. Cancer Cell *17*, 28-40.

Klein, U., Tu, Y., Stolovitzky, G.A., Mattioli, M., Cattoretti, G., Husson, H., Freedman, A., Inghirami, G., Cro, L., Baldini, L., *et al.* (2001). Gene expression profiling of B cell chronic lymphocytic leukemia reveals a homogeneous phenotype related to memory B cells. J Exp Med *194*, 1625-1638.

Kobayashi, R., Picchio, G., Kirven, M., Meisenholder, G., Baird, S., Carson, D.A., Mosier, D.E., & Kipps, T.J. (1992). Transfer of human chronic lymphocytic leukemia to mice with severe combined immune deficiency. Leuk Res *16*, 1013-1023.

Kress, C.L., Konopleva, M., Martinez-Garcia, V., Krajewska, M., Lefebvre, S., Hyer, M., McQueen, T., Andreef, M., Reed, J.C., & Zapata, J.M. (2007). Triterpenoids display single agent anti-tumor activity in a transgenic mouse model of chronic lymphocytic leukemia and small lymphocytic lymphoma. PloS ONE *2*, e559.

Lee, S.Y., Reichlin, A., Santana, A., Sokol, K.A., Nussenzweig, M.C., & Choi, Y. (1997). TRAF2 is essential for JNK but not NF-kappaB activation and regulates lymphocyte proliferation and survival. Immunity *7*, 703-713.

Linsley, P.S., Schelter, J., Burchard, J., Kibukawa, M., Martin, M.M., Bartz, S.R., Johnson, J.M., Cummins, J.M., Raymond, C.K., Dai, H., *et al.* (2007). Transcripts targeted by the microRNA-16 family cooperatively regulate cell cycle progression. Mol Cell Biol *27*, 2240-2252.

Liu, Q., Fu, H., Sun, F., Zhang, H., Tie, Y., Zhu, J., Xing, R., Sun, Z., & Zheng, X. (2008). miR-16 family induces cell cycle arrest by regulating multiple cell cycle genes. Nucleic Acids Res *36*, 5391-5404.

Liu, Y., Corcoran, M., Rasool, O., Ivanova, G., Ibbotson, R., Grander, D., Iyengar, A., Baranova, A., Kashuba, V., Merup, M., *et al.* (1997). Cloning of two candidate tumor suppressor genes within a 10 kb region on chromosome 13q14, frequently deleted in chronic lymphocytic leukemia. Oncogene *15*, 2463-2473.

Longo, P.G., Laurenti, L., Gobessi, S., Petlickovski, A., Pelosi, M., Chiusolo, P., Sica, S., Leone, G., & Efremov, D.G. (2007). The Akt signaling pathway determines the different proliferative capacity of chronic lymphocytic leukemia B-cells from patients with progressive and stable disease. Leukemia *21*, 110-120.

Longo, P.G., Laurenti, L., Gobessi, S., Sica, S., Leone, G., & Efremov, D.G. (2008). The Akt/Mcl-1 pathway plays a prominent role in mediating antiapoptotic signals downstream of the B-cell receptor in chronic lymphocytic leukemia B cells. Blood *111*, 846-855.

Mackay, F. & Schneider, P. (2008). TACI, an enigmatic BAFF/APIL receptor, with new unappreciated biochemical and biological properties. Cytokines and Growth Factor Reviews *17*, 263-276.

Mackay, F. & Schneider, P. (2009). Cracking the BAFF code. Nat. Rev. Immunol. *9*, 491-502.

Mackay, F., Schneider, P., Rennert, P., & Browning, J. (2003). BAFF AND APRIL: A Tutorial on B Cell Survival. Annu Rev Immunol *21*, 231-264.

Mackay, F., Silveira, P.A., & Brink, R. (2007). B cells and the BAFF/APRIL axis: fast-forward on autoimmunity and signaling. Curr Opin Immunol *19*, 327-336.

Mackay, F., Woodcock, S.A., Lawton, P., Ambrose, C., Baetscher, M., Schneider, P., Tschopp, J., & Browning, J.L. (1999). Mice transgenic for BAFF develop lymphocytic disorders along with autoimmune manifestations. J Exp Med *190*, 1697-1710.

Marton, S., Garcia, M.R., Robello, C., Persson, H., Trajtenberg, F., Pritsch, O., Rovira, C., Naya, H., Dighiero, G., & Cayota, A. (2008). Small RNAs analysis in CLL reveals a deregulation of miRNA expression and novel miRNA candidates of putative relevance in CLL pathogenesis. Leukemia *22*, 330-338.

Migliazza, A., Bosch, F., Komatsu, H., Cayanis, E., Martinotti, S., Toniato, E., Guccione, E., Qu, X., Chien, M., Murty, V.V., *et al.* (2001). Nucleotide sequence, transcription map, and mutation analysis of the 13q14 chromosomal region deleted in B-cell chronic lymphocytic leukemia. Blood *97*, 2098-2104.

Mott, J.L., Kobayashi, S., Bronk, S.F., & Gores, G.J. (2007). mir-29 regulates Mcl-1 protein expression and apoptosis. Oncogene *26*, 6133-6140.

Mraz, M., Pospisilova, S., Malinova, K., Slapak, I., & Mayer, J. (2009). MicroRNAs in chronic lymphocytic leukemia pathogenesis and disease subtypes. Leuk Lymphoma *50*, 506-509.

Muzio, M., Bertilaccio, M.T., Simonetti, G., Frenquelli, M., & Caligaris-Cappio, F. (2009a). The role of toll-like receptors in chronic B-cell malignancies. Leuk Lymphoma *50*, 1573-1580.

Muzio, M., Scielzo, C., Bertilaccio, M.T., Frenquelli, M., Ghia, P., & Caligaris-Cappio, F. (2009b). Expression and function of toll like receptors in chronic lymphocytic leukaemia cells. Br J Haematol *144*, 507-516.

Nakagawa, R., Mason, S.M., & Michie, A.M. (2006a). Determining the role of specific signaling molecules during lymphocyte development in vivo: instant transgenesis. Nat Protoc *1*, 1185-1193.

Nakagawa, R., Soh, J.W., & Michie, A.M. (2006b). Subversion of protein kinase C alpha signaling in hematopoietic progenitor cells results in the generation of a B-cell chronic lymphocytic leukemia-like population in vivo. Cancer Res *66*, 527-534.

Nishio, M., Endo, T., Tsukada, N., Ohata, J., Kitada, S., Reed, J.C., Zvaifler, N.J., & Kipps, T.J. (2005). Nurselike cells express BAFF and APRIL, which can promote survival of chronic lymphocytic leukemia cells via a paracrine pathway distinct from that of SDF-1alpha. Blood *106*, 1012-1020.

Norton, J.D., Deed, R.W., Craggs, G., & Sablitzky, F. (1998). Id helix-loop-helix proteins in cell growth and differentiation. Trends Cell Biol *8*, 58-65.

Okada, T., Abe, M., Takiura, F., Hirose, S., & Shirai, T. (1990). Distinct surface phenotypes of B cells responsible for spontaneous production of IgM and IgG anti-DNA antibodies in autoimmune-prone NZB x NZW F1 mice. Autoimmunity *7*, 109-120.

Ouillette, P., Erba, H., Kujawski, L., Kaminski, M., Shedden, K., & Malek, S.N. (2008). Integrated genomic profiling of chronic lymphocytic leukemia identifies subtypes of deletion 13q14. Cancer Res *68*, 1012-1021.

Palamarchuk, A., Efanov, A., Nazaryan, N., Santanam, U., Alder, H., Rassenti, L., Kipps, T., Croce, C.M., & Pekarsky, Y. (2010). 13q14 deletions in CLL involve cooperating tumor suppressors. Blood *115*, 3916-3922.

Parker, G.A., Peng, B., He, M., Gould-Fogerite, S., Chou, C.C., & Raveche, E.S. (2000). In vivo and in vitro antiproliferative effects of antisense interleukin 10 oligonucleotides. Methods Enzymol *314*, 411-429.

Pekarsky, Y., & Croce, C.M. (2010). Is miR-29 an oncogene or tumor suppressor in CLL? Oncotarget *1*, 224-227.

Pekarsky, Y., Hallas, C., & Croce, C.M. (2001). The role of TCL1 in human T-cell leukemia. Oncogene *20*, 5638-5643.

Pekarsky, Y., Koval, A., Hallas, C., Bichi, R., Tresini, M., Malstrom, S., Russo, G., Tsichlis, P., & Croce, C.M. (2000). Tcl1 enhances akt kinase activity and mediates its nuclear translocation. Proc Natl Acad Sci (USA) *97*, 3028-3033.

Pekarsky, Y., Palamarchuk, A., Maximov, V., Efanov, A., Nazaryan, N., Santanam, U., Rassenti, L., Kipps, T., & Croce, C.M. (2008). Tcl1 functions as a transcriptional regulator and is directly involved in the pathogenesis of CLL. Proc Natl Acad Sci U S A *105*, 19643-19648.

Pekarsky, Y., Santanam, U., Cimmino, A., Palamarchuk, A., Efanov, A., Maximov, V., Volinia, S., Alder, H., Liu, C.G., Rassenti, L., *et al.* (2006). Tcl1 expression in chronic lymphocytic leukemia is regulated by miR-29 and miR-181. Cancer Res *66*, 11590-11593.

Peng, B., Mehta, N.H., Fernandes, H., Chou, C.C., & Raveche, E. (1995). Growth inhibition of malignant CD5+B (B-1) cells by antisense IL-10 oligonucleotide. Leukemia research *19*, 159-167.

Petlickovski, A., Laurenti, L., Li, X., Marietti, S., Chiusolo, P., Sica, S., Leone, G., & Efremov, D.G. (2005). Sustained signaling through the B-cell receptor induces Mcl-1 and promotes survival of chronic lymphocytic leukemia B cells. Blood *105*, 4820-4827.

Phillips, J.A., Mehta, K., Fernandez, C., & Raveche, E.S. (1992). The NZB mouse as a model for chronic lymphocytic leukemia. Cancer Res *52*, 437-443.

Planelles L., Carvalho-Pinto C.E., Hardenberg G., Smaniotto S., Savino W., Gómez-Caro R., Alvarez-Mon M., de Jong J., Eldering E., Martínez-A. C. *et al.* (2004). April promotes B-1 cell-associated neoplasm. Cancer Cell *6*, 399-408

Planelles, L., Castillo-Gutierrez, S., Medema, J.P., Morales-Luque, A., Merle-Beral, H., & Hahne, M. (2007). APRIL but not BLyS serum levels are increased in chronic lymphocytic leukemia: prognostic relevance of APRIL for survival. Haematologica *92*, 1284-1285.

Planelles, L., Medema, J.P., Hahne, M., & Hardenberg, G. (2008). The expanding role of APRIL in cancer and immunity. Curr Mol Med *8*, 829-844.

Plass, C., Byrd, J.C., Raval, A., Tanner, S.M., & de la Chapelle, A. (2007). Molecular profiling of chronic lymphocytic leukaemia: genetics meets epigenetics to identify predisposing genes. Br J Haematol *139*, 744-752.

Ramachandra, S., Metcalf, R.A., Fredrickson, T., Marti, G.E., & Raveche, E. (1996). Requirement for increased IL-10 in the development of B-1 lymphoproliferative disease in a murine model of CLL. J Clin Invest *98*, 1788-1793.

Raveche, E.S. (1990). Possible immunoregulatory role for CD5 + B cells. Clin Immunol Immunopathol *56*, 135-150.

Raveche, E.S., Salerno, E., Scaglione, B.J., Manohar, V., Abbasi, F., Lin, Y.C., Fredrickson, T., Landgraf, P., Ramachandra, S., Huppi, K., *et al.* (2007). Abnormal microRNA-16 locus with synteny to human 13q14 linked to CLL in NZB mice. Blood *109*, 5079-5086.

Reed, J.C. (2008). Bcl-2-family proteins and hematologic malignancies: history and future prospects. Blood *111*, 3322-3330.

Salerno, E., Scaglione, B.J., Coffman, F.D., Brown, B.D., Baccarini, A., Fernandes, H., Marti, G., & Raveche, E.S. (2009). Correcting miR-15a/16 genetic defect in New Zealand Black mouse model of CLL enhances drug sensitivity. Mol Cancer Ther *8*, 2684-2692.

Sanchez-Aguilera, A., Rattmann, I., Drew, D.Z., Muller, L.U., Summey, V., Lucas, D.M., Byrd, J.C., Croce, C.M., Gu, Y., Cancelas, J.A., *et al.* (2010). Involvement of RhoH GTPase in the development of B-cell chronic lymphocytic leukemia. Leukemia *24*, 97-104.

Santanam, U., Zanesi, N., Efanov, A., Costinean, S., Palamarchuk, A., Hagan, J.P., Volinia, S., Alder, H., Rassenti, L., Kipps, T., *et al.* (2010). Chronic lymphocytic leukemia modeled in mouse by targeted miR-29 expression. Proc Natl Acad Sci U S A *107*, 12210-12215.

Scaglione, B.J., Salerno, E., Balan, M., Coffman, F., Landgraf, P., Abbasi, F., Kotenko, S., Marti, G.E., & Raveche, E.S. (2007). Murine models of chronic lymphocytic leukaemia: role of microRNA-16 in the New Zealand Black mouse model. Br J Haematol *139*, 645-657.

Schroeder, H.W., Jr., & Dighiero, G. (1994). The pathogenesis of chronic lymphocytic leukemia: analysis of the antibody repertoire. Immunol Today *15*, 288-294.

Scielzo, C., Bertilaccio, M.T., Simonetti, G., Dagklis, A., ten Hacken, E., Fazi, C., Muzio, M., Caiolfa, V., Kitamura, D., Restuccia, U., *et al.* (2010). HS1 has a central role in the trafficking and homing of leukemic B cells. Blood *116*, 3537-3546.

Shimoni, A., Marcus, H., Canaan, A., Ergas, D., David, M., Berrebi, A., & Reisner, Y. (1997). A model for human B-chronic lymphocytic leukemia in human/mouse radiation chimera: evidence for tumor-mediated suppression of antibody production in low-stage disease. Blood *89*, 2210-2218.

Shimoni, A., Marcus, H., Dekel, B., Shkarchi, R., Arditti, F., Shvidel, L., Shtalrid, M., Bucher, W., Canaan, A., Ergas, D., *et al.* (1999). Autologous T cells control B-chronic lymphocytic leukemia tumor progression in human-->mouse radiation chimera. Cancer Res *59*, 5968-5974.

Shinohara, H., & Kurosaki, T. (2009). Comprehending the complex connection between PKCbeta, TAK1, and IKK in BCR signaling. Immunol Rev *232*, 300-318.

Stilgenbauer, S., Lichter, P., & Dohner, H. (2000). Genetic features of B-cell chronic lymphocytic leukemia. Rev Clin Exp Hematol *4*, 48-72.

Suljagic, M., Longo, P.G., Bennardo, S., Perlas, E., Leone, G., Laurenti, L., & Efremov, D.G. (2010). The Syk inhibitor fostamatinib disodium (R788) inhibits tumor growth in the Emu- TCL1 transgenic mouse model of CLL by blocking antigen-dependent B-cell receptor signaling. Blood *116*, 4894-4905.

Teitell, M.A. (2005). The TCL1 family of oncoproteins: co-activators of transformation. Nat Rev Cancer *5*, 640-648.

ter Brugge, P.J., Ta, V.B., de Bruijn, M.J., Keijzers, G., Maas, A., van Gent, D.C., & Hendriks, R.W. (2009). A mouse model for chronic lymphocytic leukemia based on expression of the SV40 large T antigen. Blood *114*, 119-127.

Tokado, H., Yumura, W., Shiota, J., Hirose, S., Sato, H., & Shirai, T. (1991). Lupus nephritis in autoimmune-prone NZB x NZW F1 mice and mechanisms of transition of the glomerular lesions. Acta Pathol Jpn *41*, 1-11.

Umland, S.P., Go, N.F., Cupp, J.E., & Howard, M. (1989). Responses of B cells from autoimmune mice to IL-5. J Immunol *142*, 1528-1535.

Virgilio, L., Lazzeri, C., Bichi, R., Nibu, K., Narducci, M.G., Russo, G., Rothstein, J.L., & Croce, C.M. (1998). Deregulated expression of TCL1 causes T cell leukemia in mice. Proc Natl Acad Sci U S A *95*, 3885-3889.

Wang, Z., Zhang, B., Yang, L., Ding, J., & Ding, H.F. (2008). Constitutive production of NF-kappaB2 p52 is not tumorigenic but predisposes mice to inflammatory autoimmune disease by repressing Bim expression. J Biol Chem *283*, 10698-10706.

Wen, X., Zhang, D., Kikuchi, Y., Jiang, Y., Nakamura, K., Xiu, Y., Tsurui, H., Takahashi, K., Abe, M., Ohtsuji, M., *et al.* (2004). Transgene-mediated hyper-expression of IL-5 inhibits autoimmune disease but increases the risk of B cell chronic lymphocytic leukemia in a model of murine lupus. Eur J Immunol *34*, 2740-2749.

Yan, X.J., Albesiano, E., Zanesi, N., Yancopoulos, S., Sawyer, A., Romano, E., Petlickovski, A., Efremov, D.G., Croce, C.M., & Chiorazzi, N. (2006). B cell receptors in TCL1 transgenic mice resemble those of aggressive, treatment-resistant human chronic lymphocytic leukemia. Proc Natl Acad Sci U S A *103*, 11713-11718.

Zanesi, N., Aqeilan, R., Drusco, A., Kaou, M., Sevignani, C., Costinean, S., Bortesi, L., La Rocca, G., Koldovsky, P., Volinia, S., *et al.* (2006). Effect of rapamycin on mouse chronic lymphocytic leukemia and the development of nonhematopoietic malignancies in Emu-TCL1 transgenic mice. Cancer Res *66*, 915-920.

Zapata, J.M., Krajewska, M., Morse, H.C., 3rd, Choi, Y., & Reed, J.C. (2004). TNF receptor-associated factor (TRAF) domain and Bcl-2 cooperate to induce small B cell lymphoma/chronic lymphocytic leukemia in transgenic mice. Proc Natl Acad Sci U S A *101*, 16600-16605.

Zapata, J.M., Lefebvre, S., & Reed, J.C. (2007). Targeting TRAFs for therapeutic intervention. Adv Exp Med Biol *597*, 188-201.

Zhang, B., Wang, Z., Li, T., Tsitsikov, E.N., & Ding, H.F. (2007). NF-kappaB2 mutation targets TRAF1 to induce lymphomagenesis. Blood *110*, 743-751.

Zhang, W., Kater, A.P., Widhopf, G.F., 2nd, Chuang, H.Y., Enzler, T., James, D.F., Poustovoitov, M., Tseng, P.H., Janz, S., Hoh, C., *et al.* (2010). B-cell activating factor and v-Myc myelocytomatosis viral oncogene homolog (c-Myc) influence progression of chronic lymphocytic leukemia. Proc Natl Acad Sci U S A *107*, 18956-18960.

11

Altering microRNA miR15a/16 Levels as Potential Therapy in CLL: Extrapolating from the *De Novo* NZB Mouse Model

Siddha Kasar, Yao Yuan, Chingiz Underbayev, Dan Vollenweider, Matt Hanlon, Victor Chang, Hina Khan and Elizabeth Raveche
University of Medicine and Dentistry of New Jersey, Newark
United States of America

1. Introduction

1.1 Chronic lymphocytic leukemia (CLL)

CLL is a hematological malignancy characterized by accumulation of B-1 cells in peripheral lymphoid organs, bone marrow and peripheral blood. It is the most common lymphoid malignancy in the Western World, accounting for 30% of all leukemias. Although the median age at diagnosis is 73, our ever increasing lifespan has put the lifetime risk of developing CLL at 1 in 210 people (NCI, 2011). In addition, since its first description more than 150 years ago, the etiology of CLL remains largely unknown. Hence, it is imperative to study this largely geriatric and incurable disease in more detail.

Diagnosis is made based on the presence of B-lymphocytosis (>5000/ul of peripheral blood), and in particular the expansion of $CD5^+CD19^+CD20^{dull}CD23^+IgM^{dull}$ B cells [Reviewed by (Hallek et al., 2008)]. The disease is usually asymptomatic and as a result in most cases it is diagnosed during a routine blood test. Clinically CLL is most commonly classified using the modified Rai Staging System or Binet Classification (Hallek et al., 2008). With recent advances in screening procedures, increasing number of patients are been diagnosed at Rai Stage 0 (Shanafelt, 2009). The current treatment protocol adopts the 'wait and watch' policy until the disease progresses or becomes symptomatic since treatment does not offer any survival advantage (Mhaskar et al., 2010). Based on the rate of disease progression, CLL can be classified as either Aggressive or Indolent, with either type exhibiting a characteristic molecular signature. Grossly, aggressive CLL is characterized by high ZAP70 (a kinase not normally expressed in B cells which is detected by flow cytometric techniques) and unmutated IgH V_H whereas indolent is characterized by low ZAP70 and mutated IgH V_H [Reviewed by (Gribben and O'Brien, 2011)].

The circulating B-CLL cells have an apoptosis defect and are hence long lived. Spleen, bone marrow and lymph nodes are believed to be proliferating centers and replenish the peripheral B-CLL cells [Reviewed by (Damle et al., 2010)]. Although traditionally B-CLL was described as accumulation of quiescent B-1 cells in the periphery, recent in vivo kinetic studies using deuterium (Messmer et al., 2005) or deuterated glucose (van Gent et al., 2008) have shown that 0.08-1.76% of new CLL cells are generated per day.

1.2 NZB as a mouse model of CLL

Mouse models are very crucial for the study of human malignancies since unlike in vitro cell culture systems they allow the study of complex interplay of cells involved in tumor formation and maintenance. Currently there are several transgenic mouse models of CLL available, for example: Tcl1 transgenic, TRAF2DN/Bcl2 transgenic, miR155 transgenic [Reviewed by (Pekarsky et al., 2010). Although transgenic models can be used to ascertain the oncogenic potential of candidate genes, they make poor models for a more holistic study of the tumor development and progression since cancer is a multifactorial disorder. Hence, de novo mouse models that can faithfully mimic human malignancy are a better system for the latter purpose. Our lab has long been interested in the study of CLL biology using the NZB mouse model. The disease penetrance is near 100% in these mice indicating the presence of a strong genetic bias. Similar to CLL patients, NZB mice exhibit age associated spontaneous development of $CD5^{+}B220^{dull}IgM^{+}$ B-1 cell malignancy [Reviewed by (Scaglione et al., 2007)]. These mice also exhibit an underlying autoimmunity characterized by the presence of anti-RBC and anti-DNA antibodies and hence are used as a model for Sytemic Lupus Erythematosus (SLE) [Reviewed by (Scaglione et al., 2007)]. The underlying autoimmunity makes these mice an even more faithful model of human CLL since 10-25% of patients develop Autoimmune Hemolytic Anemia (AIHA) and 2% of patients develop autoimmune thrombocytopenia (Kipps and Carson, 1993).

Recent evidence suggests that almost all cases of CLL are preceded by an asymptomatic precursor stage of monoclonal or pauci-clonal B cell lymphocytosis ($<5x10^9/l$) termed MBL (Shim et al., Caporaso et al., 2010, Rawstron et al., 2002). Most subjects possess MBL whose immunophenotype is similar to CLL. Although the incidence of expression of prognostic markers like Zap70 and CD38 was less than that observed in CLL, approximately 70% of MBL cases in families with a history of CLL possess the 13q14 deletion (Lanasa et al., 2011). We have recently shown that NZB mice also exhibit this pre-cursor MBL stage, further validating it as a true model for human CLL (Salerno et al., 2010).

1.3 Genetic abnormalities in CLL

In their seminal review, Hanahan and Weinberg proposed that genetic abnormalities underly the six hallmarks of cancer: Constitutive proliferative signaling, Immunity to tumor suppressors, Apoptosis Evasion, Limitless Replicative Potential, Sustained Angiogenesis and Metastasis (Hanahan and Weinberg, 2000). With the advent of High Throughput DNA Sequencing, this theory has gained further credence and it is now widely accepted that cancer arises due to a series of genetic hits (Reviewed in (Hanahan and Weinberg, 2011)). Some of the frequently observed chromosomal abnormalities in CLL include 11q23 deletions (contains ATM and miR34b/miR34c cluster), trisomy 12 (increase in MDM2), 17p deletions (contains p53) (Dohner et al., 2000). However, the most common chromosomal abnormality observed in CLL patients (50-60%) is 13q14 deletion (contains miR15a/16-1) (Dohner et al., 2000). This region is also deleted in 50% of Mantle Cell Lymphomas and 40% of Multiple Myeloma indicating that it harbors critical tumor suppressor genes (Chang et al., 2004, Chen et al., 2007, Flordal Thelander et al., 2007). Detailed characterization of the 13q region in CLL patients led to the discovery of a 130kb Minimal Deleted Region (MDR) centromeric to the marker D13S272 (Corcoran et al., 1998, Migliazza et al., 2001). Potential CLL-associated tumor suppressor genes in the MDR identified by earlier studies include Exon 1 of Dleu1,

Dleu2, Dleu5, Dleu7 and Kcnrg. However, currently only Dleu2 and Dleu7 have been demonstrated to have tumor suppressive functions in CLL (Klein et al., 2010, Palamarchuk et al., 2010).

1.3.1 Role of 13q14 locus in CLL

In a *Blood* plenary paper, we reported the linkage of three loci - D14Mit160, D18Mit4, and D19Mit6 - to the presence of lymphoproliferative disease (LPD) in NZB mice (Raveche et al., 2007). Due to the homology to human Chr.13, we further analyzed the candidate genes in the D14Mit160 locus and discovered an association between miR15a/16-1 and CLL.

The highly conserved large non-coding RNA, Dleu2, is the host transcript for the biscistronic microRNAs miR15a/16-1 (Calin et al., 2002). It is located within intron 4 of the Dleu2 transcript in mouse (See Fig.1A) and within intron 3 in human (See Fig.1B). Dleu2 has not been shown to encode any protein, yet there is high degree of sequence homology between mouse and human suggesting that it is biologically very important (See Fig.1C). Currently it is unclear whether the full length Dleu2 transcript is functionally important; however critical functions have been assigned to two genes encoded within Dleu2. In addition to miR15a/16-1, Dleu2 transcript also encodes an anti-sense for Dleu5 (also called Rfp2 of Trim13) (Corcoran et al., 2004). Dleu2 is transcribed from the reverse strand while Dleu5 is transcribed from the forward strand in Chr.13 in humans and Chr.14 in mice. In humans, there is partial overlap between Dleu5 and Dleu2 genes leading to the formation of a sense-anti-sense pair. In mice a region of Dleu5 has been duplicated and inserted upstream into Dleu2 giving rise to a sense-anti-sense pair even in the absence of physical overlap. In humans miR15a/16-1 is upstream of Dleu5 antisense whereas in mice it downstream of the Dleu5 antisense. The interaction between Dleu5 and Dleu2 is represented schematically in Fig.1D. Dleu5 protein contains a tripartite Ring finger B-box coiled-coil domain (RBCC) and thus belongs to the RBCC or Trim family of proteins. It is frequently deleted or downregulated in various malignancies. It functions as a novel E3 ubiquitin ligase (Lerner et al., 2007) and can cause proteosomal degradation of MDM2 and ATM thereby enhancing DNA damage induced apoptosis (Joo et al., 2011).

1.4 MicroRNA as oncomiRs or tumor suppressor miRs

microRNA genes are frequently located at cancer associated loci or fragile sites making them vulnerable to genetic lesions (Calin et al., 2004). Similar to other regulatory elements like transcription factors, dysregulation of microRNAs has been implicated in the pathogenesis of different types of cancer. Based on the genes they target, their up or down regulation could have an oncogenic effect. miR17-92 cluster was the first reported oncomiR and its upregulation accelerated lymphoma development in a mouse model of B cell lymphoma [Reviewed by (van Haaften and Agami, 2010)] indicating that it possesses direct oncogenic potential. Since then a number of other microRNAs like miR21, miR155, miR29 etc have been shown to function as oncomiRs in a number of tumor types. On the opposite end of the spectrum are tumor suppressor microRNAs like miR15a/16-1 whose down-regulation is associated with CLL pathogenesis (Calin et al., 2002). The expression of miR15a/16-1 is also frequently reduced in prostrate cancer and exogenously increasing the level of these microRNAs had a therapeutic effect on xenograft models of prostrate cancer (Bonci et al., 2008).

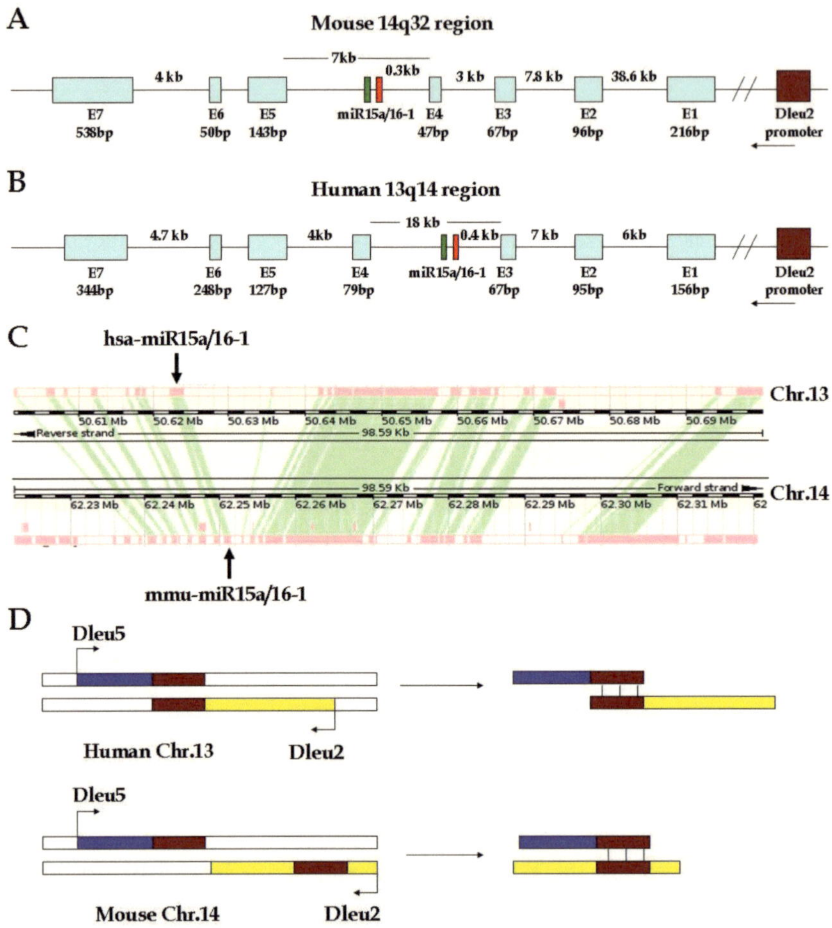

Fig. 1. Genomic Organization of Dleu2 Cluster in Mouse and Humans: Schematic representation of Dleu2 gene in mouse – Transcript ID ENMUST00000152279 (A) and in human – Transcript ID ENST00000416253 (B). In both humans and mice, miR15a/16-1 is found in the large intronic region of this large non-coding RNA (lncRNA), DLEU2. C) Human and mouse Dleu2 genes are aligned against each other. The homologous regions are shown by connecting green bars. D) Schematic representation of sense-anti-sense pairing of Dleu2 and Dleu5 transcripts in human (upper) and mouse (lower).

1.5 Serum microRNAs as biomarkers

MicroRNA levels in serum can serve as noninvasive biomarkers for diagnosis of hepatitis B, cardiovascular diseases, various cancers and a potential host of other diseases. For example, serum levels of miR-141 can be used to differentiate patients with prostate cancer from normal healthy controls with elevated levels of this miRNA in patient's serum (Mitchell et al., 2008). In another study, four miRNAs, miR-21, miR-210, miR-155, and miR-196a, were assayed in plasma and shown to be associated with pancreatic adenocarcinoma thus offering blood-based biomarkers (Wang et al., 2009). In a recent study it was shown that elevated miRNA levels in serum may also offer early CLL detection and differentiation between Zap70 status (Moussay et al., 2011). Earlier studies were mainly focused on serum microRNA levels in solid tumors; however, this study also showed that hematological malignancies also harbor increased serum microRNA levels. The authors further concluded that increased expression of miR-150, miR-29a, miR-222 and miR-195 can be used as a highly sensitive diagnostic test for CLL. Interestingly the level of miR16-1 was elevated in CLL patients as compared to healthy controls. We have observed a similar increase in the plasma level of miR15a in our NZB mouse model as compared to wild type mice. This finding is intriguing since the cellular level of miR15a/16-1 is reduced by up to 50% in NZB mice and CLL patients. The finding that serum levels of miR15a/16-1 are somewhat increased in NZB mice and CLL patients as compared to control was opposite to anticipated. There seems to be a disconnect between the cellular and serum levels of miR15a/16-1. However, enhanced exosomal secretion could be responsible for this disconnect. Exosomes are cargo containing nano-vesicles (30-100 nm) that are secreted by numerous cell types and proteomic studies have shown that they harbor an abundance of microRNAs, mRNAs and proteins characteristic of their particular cellular origin. Exosomes have been shown to transfer both cellular and viral microRNAs that can give rise to pathological consequences like malignant transformation (Meckes et al., 2010, Valadi et al., 2007). Studies have demonstrated that malignant cells have increased microvesicle formation than do non-malignant cells (Ghosh et al., 2010). We speculate that the elevated serum miR15a/16-1 in NZB mice may be the result of increased exosomal packaging of all the microRNAs in the malignant cells, including the reduced level of miR-15a/16.

2. Results

2.1 Mutated miR15a/16-1 loci in CLL patients and NZB mice

We recently reported the presence of a mutation and a deletion in the 3′ flanking region of miR15a/16-1 gene of NZB mouse model of CLL (See Fig.2A) (Raveche et al., 2007). This mutation in NZB is at a nearly identical location as a C to T point mutation found in CLL patients (Calin et al., 2005). However, this mutation is rare in patients (Calin et al., 2005),(Yazici et al., 2009). We have also shown that this mutation and deletion is associated with almost a 50% reduction in the cellular level of mature miR15a/16-1 in the NZB mice (See Fig.2B) and the NZB derived cell line, LNC (See Fig.2C). Although the expression of miR15a/16-1 is reduced in both B-1 and B-2 cells in the NZB (as compared to non-NZB strain), pathologic consequences are observed only in the B-1 cells. A number of targets have been validated for miR15a/16-1; however, targeting of critical anti-apoptotic and cell cycle regulatory proteins like Bcl-2 and Cyclin D1 respectively is of particular importance in CLL pathogenesis (Salerno et al., 2009). Thus, the reduced expression of miR15a/16-1 confers an anti-apoptotic phenotype to the cells. Recently a transgenic mouse having conditional knock-out of the entire MDR region or the miR15a/16-1 region was generated (Klein et al., 2010). 42% of the MDR-/- mice and 26% of the miR15a/16-/- mice developed a lymphoproliferative disorder at 15 to 18 months of age. Moreover, CD19-cre driven knockout gave rise to an apoptosis defect in the B cells. In summary these findings show that the miR15a/16-1 locus plays a critical tumor suppressive role in CLL. Therefore, we hypothesized that increasing the miR15a/16-1 levels can serve as a novel therapeutic strategy for CLL.

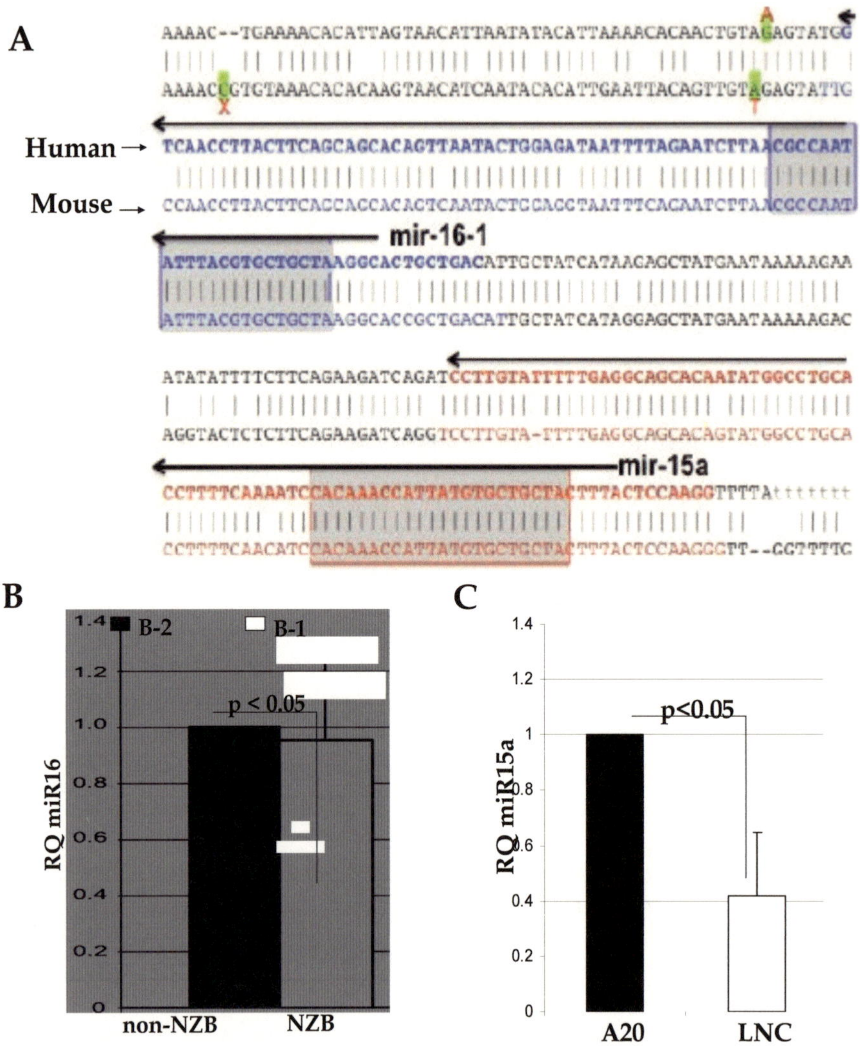

Fig. 2. Identification of Point Mutation and Deletion in miR15a/16-1 Flanking Region: A) Wild type sequence of human (top row) and mouse (bottom row) miR15a/16-1 and its flanking region is shown. The mature miR15a sequence is in red and mature miR16-1 sequence is in blue. Sequencing of this region led to the discovery of an A to T point mutation and deletion of C (40bp upstream of miR16-1) in NZB mice. A homologous A to G point mutation was found in a subset of CLL patients. The substituted nucleotide is written below the corresponding wild type base and the deletion is indicated by an 'X'. B) Spleen cells from NZB and non-NZB mice were sorted into B-2 (IgM+B220+) and B-1 (IgM+B220dull). The expression of mature miR16 in the sorted cells was measured using TaqMan miR-16 Assay according to manufacture's instructions. Data from three independent sorts was analyzed using student's t test ($p<0.05$). C) The expression of mature miR15a was compared between the NZB derived cell line LNC and a non-NZB derived B cell line A20 using TaqMan miR-15a Assay. Data from three independent experiments was analyzed using student's t test ($p<0.05$).

MicroRNAs are usually present in intergenic regions and may possess their own promoter or use the host gene promoter. Whether miR15a/16-1 is transcribed from its own promoter or from Dleu2 promoter or a combination of both, is controversial. However, data from our lab supports that it depends on the Dleu2 promoter since there is a strong positive correlation between the level of Dleu2 and miR15a/16-1 transcripts. RNA pol II transcribes the host gene to form a long primary transcript (pri-miR). In the nucleus the pri-miR transcript is processed to a 60-70nt long stem loop precursor transcript (pre-miR) by the RNase III enzyme Drosha. The pre-miR is then exported to the cytoplasm via Exportin 5 where it is further cleaved by Dicer to give the 22nt long mature microRNA duplex. Preliminary data from our lab suggests that the mutation and deletion leads to defective processing of pri-miR15a/16-1 to mature miR15a/16-1. We speculate that the mutation and deletion may lead to the formation of an unstable stem loop structure or inhibit the binding of Drosha.

2.2 In vitro miR15a/16 upregulation in NZB derived malignant CLL cell line

We hypothesized that the reduced miR15a/16-1 levels observed in CLL lead to an apoptosis defect. Our lab has previously developed the cell line LNC (CLL cell line derived from a NZB mouse lymph node) (Peng et al., 1994). LNC cells make a great in vitro system for studying the effect of mutated miR15a/16-1 loci since they have retained the NZB miR15a/16-1 genotype. Similar to the NZB mice, as compared to a non-NZB B cell line, the level of mature miR15a/16-1 in LNC cells is reduced by as much as 50% (See Fig.2C). In order to test our hypothesis, we employed 1) microRNA mimics or 2) replication incompetent lentiviruses; to artificially increase the level of mature miR15a/16-1.

2.2.1 Effect of miR15a/16 mimics on LNC

microRNA mimics are commercially available double stranded RNA oligonucleotides that resemble endogenous mature microRNA molecules. They are commonly used to transiently increase the expression of microRNA in vitro and more recently in vivo as well (Trang et al., 2011). Transfection of miR15a or miR16 mimics led to a significant increase in the percentage of cells in G1 and a decrease in the S phase as compared to negative control mimics (See Fig.3A). miR15a/16-1 targets cyclin D1 and hence we hypothesized that the observed cell cycle arrest could be in part attributed to cyclin D1 degradation. microRNAs have been shown to reduce target gene expression either by mRNA decay or instabilty or by translational repression. microRNAs can interfere with protein translation by blocking initiation or elongation stage, as well as by promoting pre-mature termination and co-translational protein degradation [Reviewed in (Huntzinger and Izaurralde, 2011)]. Although we did not see a difference in the mRNA level of cyclin D1, we observed a reduction in the protein levels in NZB cell line expressing high level of miR15a/16 (See Fig.3B). Thus, miR15a/16-1 seems to interfere with translation of cyclin D1 mRNA and not cause mRNA degradation. However, since the effect of microRNA mimics is transient, we then derived stable LNC sub-lines having increased miR15a/16 levels using a lentiviral approach.

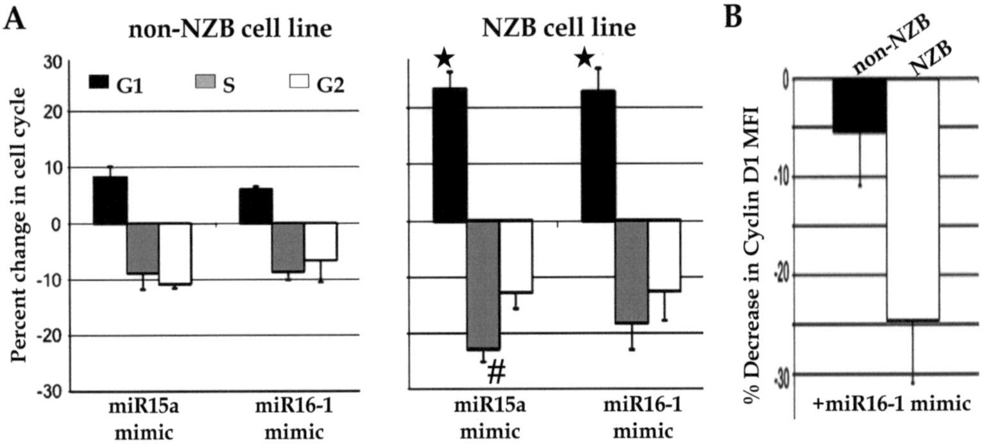

Fig. 3. Growth Inhibitory Effect of miR15a and miR16-1 mimics: NZB cell line and non-NZB cell line were transfected with 3ug of mmu-miR15a or mmu miR16-1 mimic or a non-targeting negative control mimic (Dharmacon) using Amaxa Nucleofection and analyzed 24hrs later. A) The transfected cells were stained with hypotonic prodium iodide and acquired on BD FACS Calibur to analyze the cell cycle distribution. Y-axis is the change in the percentage of cells in different cell cycle phases relative to the negative control mimic. As compared to a non-NZB cell line, a significant increase in cells in G1 (★ $p<0.05$) and a significant decrease in cells in the S phase (# $p<0.05$) was observed. Similar results were obtained with both miR15a and miR16-1 mimic. B) Cyclin D1 protein level was measured using intracellular flow cytometry. The percent decrease in mean fluorescence intensity (MFI) of cyclin D1 in miR16-1 mimic treated cells relative to the negative control mimic is plotted on the Y-aixs.

2.2.2 Effect of stable miR15a/16 increase using lentivirus

HIV-1 derived lentiviruses as a tool for stable delivery of genetic material were first described by Naldini et al (Naldini et al., 1996a, Naldini et al., 1996b). They are a type of retrovirus and can be used to target up to 8kb of genetic material to a broad variety of cell types (proliferating as well as quiescent). Lentiviruses are safer gene delivery vehicles than earlier viral vectors like adenovirus, gamma-retrovirus and adeno-associated viral vectors. Lentiviruses are less immunogenic than adenoviruses [Reviewed by (Nayak and Herzog, 2010)]. Early gene therapy trials for the treatment of X-linked SCID utilized gamma-retroviruses to deliver the therapeutic gene to patient stem cells ex vivo. Two out of the nine children treated successfully developed T cell Acute Lymphoblastic Leukemia (T-ALL) 3 years post treatment due to insertional activation of the LMO2 proto-oncogene (Hacein-Bey-Abina et al., 2003). Gamma retroviruses primarily integrate into 5′ region of genes and the strong enhancers present in the viral LTR can hyper-activate the adjoining gene promoters leading to tumorigenesis [Reviewed by (Bushman et al., 2005)]. In contrast, inspite of greater integration load lentiviruses did not enhance tumorogenesis since they target other areas of gene rich regions (Montini et al., 2006). The lentivirus employed in our experiments is Self-Inactivating (SIN) and hence its LTR lacks strong viral promoters, thereby further reducing the risk of insertional gene activation (Zufferey et al., 1998). Owing to their broad tropism they pose a potential biosafety hazard. However the 3rd generation of lentiviruses has been engineered to be replication incompetent and the amount of HIV genome has been reduced to 20%.

We utilized a custom made lentiviral vector encoding miR15a/16-1 from System Biosciences, to stably increase the expression of these two microRNAs in vitro and later in vivo. The lentiviral vector also has a puromycin resistance and a GFP expression cassette for selection of transduced cells. LNC cells were transduced overnight with miR15a/16-GFP-puro lentivirus (miR lentivirus) or an empty GFP-puro lentivirus (GFP lentivirus) at an MOI of 10 in the presence of 4ug/ml polybrene. The miR lentivirus transduced cells were then sorted on the basis of GFP (See Fig.4A, left) and maintained in media containing puromycin to obtain stable sub-lines (GFP low and GFP hi) (See Fig.4A, right). The cells transduced with miR-lenti exhibited 50% increase in the sub-G1 or apoptotic population as compared to those transduced with GFP-lenti (See Fig.4C). The sub-lines were characterized further for the expression for miR15a and its effects on cell cycle. The expression of miR15a was significantly higher in GFP low and GFP hi as compared to untransduced LNC cells (See Fig.4B). A strong positive correlation exists between intensity of the GFP signal and miR15a/16-1 expression. The sub-lines also exhibit a significant reduction in the percentage of cells in the S phase indicating reduced proliferation in response to increase miR15a/16-1 levels (data not shown).

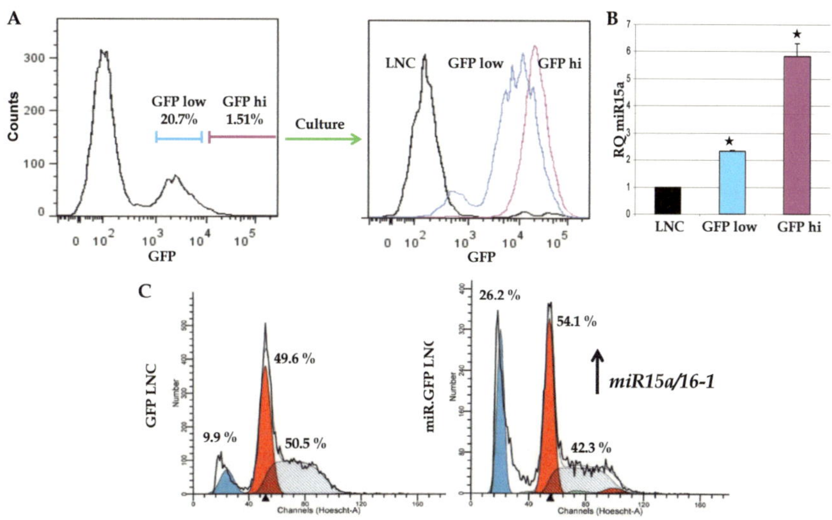

Fig. 4. In vitro Effects of Lentiviral Delivery of miR15a/16 Levels: The NZB derived B cell line LNC was transduced with lentivirus encoding bicistronic miR15a/16-1 (miR lentivirus) under the control of a CMV promoter or with a control empty lentivirus (GFP lentivirus). A) 48hrs post transduction of the miR lentivirus, cells were sorted based on GFP expression into GFP low and GFP hi populations according to the gating strategy indicated (left). The cells were then cultured and the GFP expression was measured using the BD LSR II instrument (right). Thus, two stable LNC sub-lines - GFP low and GFP hi - were established. B) The expression of miR15a was compared between LNC and the two new sub-lines using TaqMan microRNA Assay ($p<0.05$). C) 48hrs post transduction cells were stained with Hoescht dye and their cell cycle was analyzed. A considerable increase in the sub-G1 peak is observed in the miR lentivirus transduced cells (right) as compared to the GFP lentivirus transduced cells (left).

2.3 Potential Triggers for regulation of miR15a/16 and B-1 clonal expansion

A single microRNA can critically regulate a number of genes in a cell type specific manner. Hence they can serve as very efficient effectors for master regulators like c-Myc. A single genetic hit involving this network could potentially lead to tumorigenesis since it can simultaneously disrupt multiple pathways. A recent report by Chang et al, gives credence to this theory since they showed that c-Myc induced expression of miR17-92 cluster and a more global repression of other microRNAs led to the development of B cell lymphomas (Chang et al., 2008). An increased c-Myc transcript level is associated with disease progression and severity in CLL patients (Halina et al., 2010). Interestingly miR15a/16 expression is negatively regulated by c-Myc via repression of the Dleu2 promoter (Lerner et al., 2009). However little is known about other transcription factors that can regulate microRNA transcription.

2.3.1 miR15a/16-1 Increase as a Consequence of BSAP knockdown

BSAP is a transcription factor considered to be a key regulator of B-lymphocyte development and is encoded by the PAX-5 gene. It plays a critical role in early B-cell lymphopoiesis and for progression beyond the pro-B-cell stage [Reviewed by (Cobaleda et al., 2007) (Nutt et al., 1998)] On the other hand, overproduction of BSAP in a late B-cell line was shown to suppress differentiation into plasma cells (Nera et al., 2006, Morrison et al., 1998). Malignant B-1 cells have been found to have increased BSAP levels (Chong et al., 2001). As normal B cells have been shown to react to IL-2 stimulation by BSAP downregulation continued BSAP expression in CLL could explain their blocked differentiation stage (Wallin et al., 1999).

We have previously shown that BSAP levels are higher in LNC cells as compared to a non-NZB cell line and normal B-1 cell. BSAP knockdown gives rise to a growth inhibitory effect in LNC cells but not in non-NZB cell line (Chong et al., 2001). A recent report showed that BSAP negatively regulates the promoter of Dleu2, the host gene for miR15a/16 in a lymphoma cell line Myc5 (Chung et al., 2008). However, since gene regulation is highly cell type specific, we first wanted to test whether a similar loop exists between BSAP and miR15a/16 in our system, especially due to the presence of the mutated miR15a/16 locus. siRNA mediated knockdown of BSAP (See Fig.5A) led to an increase in the level of mature miR15a/16 in LNC cells (See Fig.5B). Next we wanted to examine whether this increase in miR15a/16-1 expression was sufficient to give rise cell cycle arrest. Indeed, we observe an increase in the percentage of cells in the G2 phase in the siRNA treated cells as compared to the controls (See Fig.5C).

2.4 In vivo augmentation of miR15a/16 via lentivirus in NZB mice with CLL

Having successfully demonstrated the inhibition of malignant cell growth in vitro by increasing miR15a/16 levels by different strategies, we next wanted to test its therapeutic potential in vivo. In the current clinical trials involving lentiviruses, they are only used for adoptive transfer of ex vivo transduced cells or for intra-tumoral delivery. This is a serious drawback in the treatment of systemic diseases like leukemias. To overcome this caveat we attempted to employ lentivirus for systemic delivery of miR15a/16 in our murine model of B-CLL.

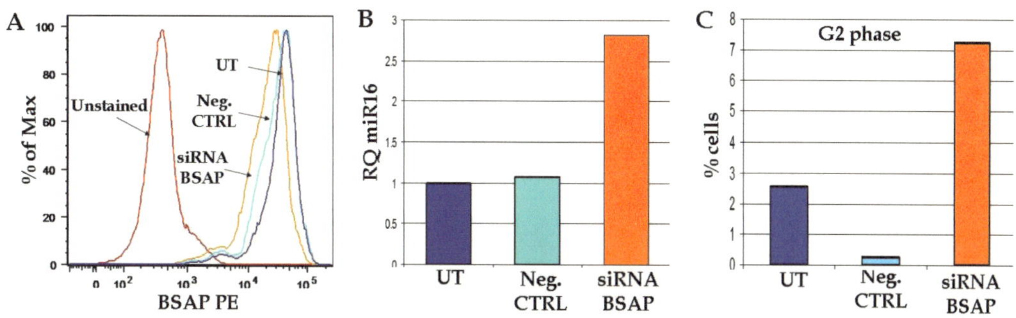

Fig. 5. In vitro effects of BSAP Silencing: NZB derived B cell line, LNC was transfected with 200nM siRNA against BSAP or with 200nM negative control siRNA using HiPerFect (Qiagen) according to manufacturer's instructions or were transfected (UT) and analyzed 24hrs later. A) Cells were stained with BSAP-PE antibody (eBiosciences) and acquired on BD LSR II. Single color PE histograms of different treatment groups have been overlayed. B) The levels of miR16-1 were measured using TaqMan MicroRNA Assay (Applied Biosystems). The reduced expression of BSAP observed by flow cytometry translated into increased miR16-1 expression in the siRNA treated groups. C) Cells were stained with hypotonic PI and the cell cycle distribution was assessed. Shown above is the percentage of cells in G2 phase of the cell cycle in the different treatment groups. Data is from a representative experiment. Similar trends were observed in the replicates.

Aged NZB mice were injected with lentivirus at day 0 and sacrificed on day 8 for the short term group or administered a second dose on day 24 and sacrificed on day 29 for the long term group. We were able to successfully increase the expression of miR15a/16 in NZB mice following intravenous (i.v) and intraperitoneal (i.p) injections of the lentiviral prep. Interestingly, the expression of miR15a/16 is elevated only in the transduced B-1 population. This could be due to cell type specific regulation of microRNA levels. In line with the in vitro data, systemic delivery of miR15a/16 led to a considerable reduction in the percentage of B-1 cells in the spleen as compared to control lentivirus treated mice both in the short term and long term study (See Fig.6A). Similar reduction was observed in the peritoneal cavity of these mice (Data not shown). In order to confirm that the lentiviral delivery led to an increase in miR15a/16-1 expression, we sorted the cells into B-1/GFP+ and B-2/GFP+ and quantified the levels of miR15a/16-1 using 100 cell RT-PCR. The expression of miR15a/16-1 was significantly increased in mice injected with miR-lentivirus as compared to those injected with the control lentivirus (See Fig.6B). Interestingly only B-1/GFP+ cells and not B2/GFP+ cells exhibited an increase in the miR15a/16-1 levels. B-1 cells were preferentially transduced in comparison to other cell types like B-2 and T cells (Data not shown).

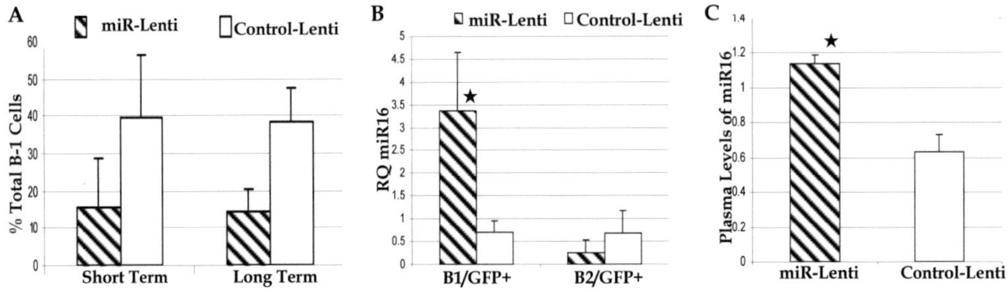

Fig. 6. In vivo effects of miR15a/16 increases on CLL in NZB mice: A) Percentage of total B-1 cells in the short term (n=3 per group) and in the long term (n=4 per group). B-1 cells were gated as $CD5^{dull}B220^{+/dull}$. B) Spleen cells from the short term treatment were sorted into B1 ($CD5^{dull}B220^{+/dull}$) and B-2 ($CD5^{-}B220^{+}$) and then further sorted based on GFP expression. 100 cell RT-PCR was performed to quantitate the level of miR16 in the sorted cells. n=3 per group, ★ B1/GFP+ from miR-Lenti Vs B1/GFP+ from Control-lenti, $p<0.05$. C) Mice were bled retro-orbitally into EDTA tubes; RNA was extracted using Trizol-LS reagent and used to perform TaqMan miR16 Expression Assay (Applied Biosystems). n=3 per group. ★ miR16 in miR-Lenti group Vs control-Lenti group, $p<0.05$.

With the advent of microRNA based therapy, it is critical to devise means to study its pharmacokinetic properties. Just before sacrificing, plasma was collected and miR16 levels were measured in the short term group. Even 8 days post injection, the level of miR16 was significantly elevated in the miR-Lenti mice as compared to the control-Lenti mice (See Fig.6C).

2.5 Alteration of miR15a/16 in human CLL using BSAP knockdown

Next, we wanted to extrapolate the findings from the mouse model presented above to patient cells. CLL patient PBMCs were purified using Ficoll-Hypaque Density Gradient Centrifugation. Malignant B-1 cells isolated from patient blood are quiescent and BSAP was knocked down using siRNA and its effects were studied at 24, 48, 72 and 96hrs. The reduced levels of BSAP protein translated into increased miR15a/16-1 as well as an increase in the percentage of cells undergoing apoptosis (See Fig.7). However, although the BSAP levels were greatly reduced even at 96 hrs post transfection, the miR15a/16 levels returned to baseline after 48hrs (data not shown), indicating the presence of a compensatory mechanism for maintaining lower levels of miR15a/16. Moreover, the microRNA levels peaked at different time points in different patients.

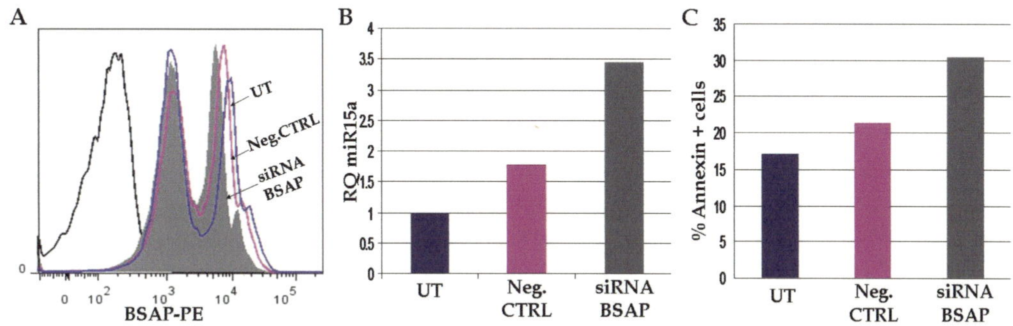

Fig. 7. Effect of Increasing miR15a/16-1 in Ex Vivo CLL Cells: 2x10⁶ patient PBMCs were transfected with BSAP siRNA or negative control siRNA using Human B cell Nucleofection kit (Lonza) or were untransfected (UT) and analyzed at different time-points.A) PBMCs were stained with BSAP-PE antibody and acquired on BD LSR II. B) Total RNA was extracted using Trizol and used to measuring the level of miR15a by TaqMan miR15a Assay (Applied Biosystems). C) Cells were stained with Annexin-V PE (BD Biosciences) and apoptosis was measured as the percentage of Annexin-V+ cells.

3. Conclusion

NZB mice faithfully mimic human CLL in phenotype, disease development and progression. The mutation and deletion in NZB mice leads to a significant reduction in the cellular level of mature miR15a/16-1 as compared to wild type mice. Similar reduction in miR15a/16-1 is observed in 50-60% of CLL patients [Reviewed by (Pekarsky et al., 2010)]. Yet patients harboring 13q14 deletions alone exhibit a more indolent disease as compared to patients having 17p and or 11q deletions in combination with 13q deletions. Moreover, in comparison to patients having a normal FISH profile, patients having 13q14 deletions have a shorter survival period that correlates with the percentage of nuclei with the deletion (Van Dyke et al., 2010, Chena et al., 2008).

We have also explored the therapeutic potential of systemic lentiviral delivery of miR15a/16-1 in the NZB mouse model of CLL. We propose that in addition to the direct cytotoxic effect of lentivirus mediated miR15a/16-1 increase; other indirect mechanisms may be responsible for the reduced percentage of B-1 cells post treatment. We observed a significant increase in the level of plasma miR16 in miR-Lenti mice as compared to control-lenti mice. However, the transduction efficiency was only 5-10%. This is consistent with reports from other labs that B cells and T cells are not amenable to efficient lentiviral transduction [Reviewed by (Frecha et al., 2010)]. We speculate that the few cells that were transduced secreted miR16 into circulation that was taken up by the non-transduced cells leading to their apoptosis. Another possibility is that the lentivirus transduced and killed supporting cells thereby reducing the amount of growth factors.

BSAP negatively regulates the Dleu2 gene promoter (Chung et al., 2008), and hence we hypothesized that its knockdown would lead to enhanced transcription of Dleu2 and in turn of miR15a/16-1. Although the mutation and deletion slows down the processing of pri-miR15a/16-1, its effect can be compensated by correspondingly increasing the transcription of its host gene. This strategy holds true even in CLL patients since although 13q14 region is frequently deleted, the size of the deleted region varies and may or may not include miR15a/16-1 (Mosca et al., 2010). In addition the deletion is usually heterozygous and does not affect all the malignant cells.

miR15a/16-1 levels seem to be very tightly regulated in CLL cells. BSAP knockdown (removing the repressor of the miR-15a/16 host gene) in ex vivo patient cells gave rise to an initial increase in miR15a/16-1 levels and apoptosis (See Fig.7). However, the miR15a/16-1 levels were decreased shortly thereafter. This initial transient increased miR15a/16-1 levels could lead to the repression of an activator like p53. Fabri et al showed that p53 and miR15a/16-1 form a feedback inhibition loop (Fabbri et al., 2011). p53 acts as a transactivator of miR15a/16-1 and increases its expression. However, p53 is a target of miR15a/16-1 and is degraded in the presence of increased miR15a/16-1. Future studies will involve the transfection with BSAP siRNA followed by p53 knock-in at 48hrs to see whether miR15a/16-1 levels can be elevated for longer time.

In conclusion, we have successfully demonstrated that miR15a/16-1 levels can be modulated by different strategies - mimics, lentiviral delivery of the microRNAs and BSAP knockdown (removal of a repressor) - both in vitro and in vivo/ex vivo (See Section 2.2, 2.3, 2.4, 2.6). We have also presented evidence that increasing the level of miR15a/16-1 in B-CLL cells leads to cell cycle arrest (See Fig.3A, 5C), reduced proliferation (See Fig.4C) and increased apoptosis (See Fig.5C, 8C), which in effect leads to reduced malignancy (See Fig.6A). Future studies will be directed at further exploring the therapeutic potential of exogenous miR15a/16-1 delivery alone or in combination with siRNA BSAP using novel delivery vehicles like lipidoids that have been shown to be very efficient for systemic in vivo delivery (Goldberg et al., 2011). microRNAs have multiple targets and the net outcome of their up-regulation is very difficult to predict and may give rise to serious side-effects. However, we have shown here that exogenous increase of miR15a/16-1 has a net positive effect on disease outcome. These findings validate miR15a/16-1 as a promising therapeutic target for the treatment of CLL.

4. Acknowledgements

These studies were supported by a grant from NIH R01CA129826 (ESR) and are in partial fulfillment of the PhD requirements for (SK)

5. References

Bonci, D., Coppola, V., Musumeci, M., Addario, A., Giuffrida, R., Memeo, L., D'urso, L., Pagliuca, A., Biffoni, M., Labbaye, C., Bartucci, M., Muto, G., Peschle, C. & De Maria, R. (2008) The miR-15a-miR-16-1 cluster controls prostate cancer by targeting multiple oncogenic activities. *Nat Med,* 14, 1271-7.

Bushman, F., Lewinski, M., Ciuffi, A., Barr, S., Leipzig, J., Hannenhalli, S. & Hoffmann, C. (2005) Genome-wide analysis of retroviral DNA integration. *Nat Rev Microbiol,* 3, 848-58.

Calin, G. A., Dumitru, C. D., Shimizu, M., Bichi, R., Zupo, S., Noch, E., Aldler, H., Rattan, S., Keating, M., Rai, K., Rassenti, L., Kipps, T., Negrini, M., Bullrich, F. & Croce, C. M. (2002) Frequent deletions and down-regulation of micro- RNA genes miR15 and miR16 at 13q14 in chronic lymphocytic leukemia. *Proc Natl Acad Sci U S A,* 99, 15524-9.

Calin, G. A., Ferracin, M., Cimmino, A., Di Leva, G., Shimizu, M., Wojcik, S. E., Iorio, M. V., Visone, R., Sever, N. I., Fabbri, M., Iuliano, R., Palumbo, T., Pichiorri, F., Roldo, C., Garzon, R., Sevignani, C., Rassenti, L., Alder, H., Volinia, S., Liu, C. G., Kipps, T. J., Negrini, M. & Croce, C. M. (2005) A MicroRNA signature associated with prognosis and progression in chronic lymphocytic leukemia. *N Engl J Med,* 353, 1793-801.

Calin, G. A., Sevignani, C., Dumitru, C. D., Hyslop, T., Noch, E., Yendamuri, S., Shimizu, M., Rattan, S., Bullrich, F., Negrini, M. & Croce, C. M. (2004) Human microRNA genes are frequently located at fragile sites and genomic regions involved in cancers. *Proc Natl Acad Sci U S A,* 101, 2999-3004.

Caporaso, N. E., Marti, G. E., Landgren, O., Azzato, E., Weinberg, J. B., Goldin, L. & Shanafelt, T. (2010) Monoclonal B cell lymphocytosis: clinical and population perspectives. *Cytometry B Clin Cytom,* 78 Suppl 1, S115-9.

Chang, H., Li, D., Zhuang, L., Nie, E., Bouman, D., Stewart, A. K. & Chun, K. (2004) Detection of chromosome 13q deletions and IgH translocations in patients with multiple myeloma by FISH: comparison with karyotype analysis. *Leuk Lymphoma,* 45, 965-9.

Chang, T. C., Yu, D., Lee, Y. S., Wentzel, E. A., Arking, D. E., West, K. M., Dang, C. V., Thomas-Tikhonenko, A. & Mendell, J. T. (2008) Widespread microRNA repression by Myc contributes to tumorigenesis. *Nat Genet,* 40, 43-50.

Chen, L., Li, J., Xu, W., Qiu, H., Zhu, Y., Zhang, Y., Duan, L., Qian, S. & Lu, H. (2007) Molecular cytogenetic aberrations in patients with multiple myeloma studied by interphase fluorescence in situ hybridization. *Exp Oncol,* 29, 116-20.

Chena, C., Avalos, J. S., Bezares, R. F., Arrossagaray, G., Turdo, K., BISTMANS, A. & SLAVUTSKY, I. (2008) Biallelic deletion 13q14.3 in patients with chronic lymphocytic leukemia: cytogenetic, FISH and clinical studies. *Eur J Haematol,* 81, 94-9.

Chong, S. Y., Zhang, M., Lin, Y. C., Coffman, F., Garcia, Z., Ponzio, N. & Raveche, E. S. (2001) The growth-regulatory role of B-cell-specific activator protein in NZB malignant B-1 cells. *Cancer Immunol Immunother,* 50, 41-50.

Chung, E. Y., Dews, M., Cozma, D., Yu, D., Wentzel, E. A., Chang, T. C., Schelter, J. M., Cleary, M. A., Mendell, J. T. & Thomas-Tikhonenko, A. (2008) c-Myb oncoprotein is an essential target of the dleu2 tumor suppressor microRNA cluster. *Cancer Biol Ther,* 7, 1758-64.

Cobaleda, C., Schebesta, A., Delogu, A. & Busslinger, M. (2007) Pax5: the guardian of B cell identity and function. *Nat Immunol,* 8, 463-70.

Corcoran, M. M., Hammarsund, M., Zhu, C., Lerner, M., Kapanadze, B., Wilson, B., Larsson, C., Forsberg, L., Ibbotson, R. E., Einhorn, S., Oscier, D. G., Grander, D. & Sangfelt, O. (2004) DLEU2 encodes an antisense RNA for the putative bicistronic RFP2/LEU5 gene in humans and mouse. *Genes Chromosomes Cancer,* 40, 285-97.

Corcoran, M. M., Rasool, O., Liu, Y., Iyengar, A., Grander, D., Ibbotson, R. E., Merup, M., Wu, X., Brodyansky, V., Gardiner, A. C., Juliusson, G., Chapman, R. M., Ivanova, G., Tiller, M., Gahrton, G., Yankovsky, N., Zabarovsky, E., Oscier, D. G. & Einhorn,

S. (1998) Detailed molecular delineation of 13q14.3 loss in B-cell chronic lymphocytic leukemia. *Blood,* 91, 1382-90.

Damle, R. N., Calissano, C. & Chiorazzi, N. (2010) Chronic lymphocytic leukaemia: a disease of activated monoclonal B cells. *Best Pract Res Clin Haematol,* 23, 33-45.

Dohner, H., Stilgenbauer, S., Benner, A., Leupolt, E., Krober, A., Bullinger, L., Dohner, K., Bentz, M. & Lichter, P. (2000) Genomic aberrations and survival in chronic lymphocytic leukemia. *N Engl J Med,* 343, 1910-6.

Fabbri, M., Bottoni, A., Shimizu, M., Spizzo, R., Nicoloso, M. S., Rossi, S., Barbarotto, E., Cimmino, A., Adair, B., Wojcik, S. E., Valeri, N., Calore, F., Sampath, D., Fanini, F., Vannini, I., Musuraca, G., Dell'aquila, M., Alder, H., Davuluri, R. V., Rassenti, L. Z., Negrini, M., Nakamura, T., Amadori, D., Kay, N. E., Rai, K. R., Keating, M. J., Kipps, T. J., Calin, G. A. & Croce, C. M. (2011) Association of a microRNA/TP53 feedback circuitry with pathogenesis and outcome of B-cell chronic lymphocytic leukemia. *JAMA,* 305, 59-67.

Flordal Thelander, E., Ichimura, K., Collins, V. P., Walsh, S. H., Barbany, G., Hagberg, A., Laurell, A., Rosenquist, R., Larsson, C. & Lagercrantz, S. (2007) Detailed assessment of copy number alterations revealing homozygous deletions in 1p and 13q in mantle cell lymphoma. *Leuk Res,* 31, 1219-30.

Frecha, C., Levy, C., Cosset, F. L. & Verhoeyen, E. (2010) Advances in the field of lentivector-based transduction of T and B lymphocytes for gene therapy. *Mol Ther,* 18, 1748-57.

Ghosh, A. K., Secreto, C. R., Knox, T. R., Ding, W., Mukhopadhyay, D. & Kay, N. E. (2010) Circulating microvesicles in B-cell chronic lymphocytic leukemia can stimulate marrow stromal cells: implications for disease progression. *Blood,* 115, 1755-64.

Goldberg, M. S., Xing, D., Ren, Y., Orsulic, S., Bhatia, S. N. & Sharp, P. A. (2011) Nanoparticle-mediated delivery of siRNA targeting Parp1 extends survival of mice bearing tumors derived from Brca1-deficient ovarian cancer cells. *Proc Natl Acad Sci U S A,* 108, 745-50.

Gribben, J. G. & O'brien, S. (2011) Update on Therapy of Chronic Lymphocytic Leukemia. *Journal of Clinical Oncology,* 29, 544-550.

Hacein-Bey-Abina, S., Von Kalle, C., Schmidt, M., Mccormack, M. P., Wulffraat, N., Leboulch, P., Lim, A., Osborne, C. S., Pawliuk, R., Morillon, E., Sorensen, R., Forster, A., Fraser, P., Cohen, J. I., De Saint Basile, G., Alexander, I., Wintergerst, U., Frebourg, T., Aurias, A., Stoppa-Lyonnet, D., Romana, S., Radford-Weiss, I., Gross, F., Valensi, F., Delabesse, E., Macintyre, E., Sigaux, F., Soulier, J., Leiva, L. E., Wissler, M., Prinz, C., Rabbitts, T. H., Le Deist, F., Fischer, A. & Cavazzana-Calvo, M. (2003) LMO2-Associated Clonal T Cell Proliferation in Two Patients after Gene Therapy for SCID-X1. *Science,* 302, 415-419.

Halina, A., Artur, P., Barbara, M. K., Joanna, S. & Anna, D. (2010) Alterations in TP53, cyclin D2, c-Myc, p21WAF1/CIP1 and p27KIP1 expression associated with progression in B-CLL. *Folia Histochem Cytobiol,* 48, 534-41.

Hallek, M., Cheson, B. D., Catovsky, D., Caligaris-Cappio, F., Dighiero, G., Dohner, H., Hillmen, P., Keating, M. J., Montserrat, E., Rai, K. R. & Kipps, T. J. (2008) Guidelines for the diagnosis and treatment of chronic lymphocytic leukemia: a report from the International Workshop on Chronic Lymphocytic Leukemia updating the National Cancer Institute-Working Group 1996 guidelines. *Blood,* 111, 5446-56.

Hanahan, D. & Weinberg, R. A. (2000) The hallmarks of cancer. *Cell,* 100, 57-70.

Hanahan, D. & Weinberg, R. A. (2011) Hallmarks of cancer: the next generation. *Cell,* 144, 646-74.

Huntzinger, E. & Izaurralde, E. (2011) Gene silencing by microRNAs: contributions of translational repression and mRNA decay. *Nat Rev Genet,* 12, 99-110.

Joo, H. M., Kim, J. Y., Jeong, J. B., Seong, K. M., Nam, S. Y., Yang, K. H., Kim, C. S., Kim, H. S., Jeong, M., An, S. & Jin, Y. W. (2011) Ret finger protein 2 enhances ionizing radiation-induced apoptosis via degradation of AKT and MDM2. *Eur J Cell Biol,* 90, 420-31.

Kipps, T. J. & Carson, D. A. (1993) Autoantibodies in chronic lymphocytic leukemia and related systemic autoimmune diseases. *Blood,* 81, 2475-87.

Klein, U., Lia, M., Crespo, M., Siegel, R., Shen, Q., Mo, T., Ambesi-Impiombato, A., Califano, A., Migliazza, A., Bhagat, G. & Dalla-Favera, R. (2010) The DLEU2/miR-15a/16-1 cluster controls B cell proliferation and its deletion leads to chronic lymphocytic leukemia. *Cancer Cell,* 17, 28-40.

Lanasa, M. C., Allgood, S. D., Slager, S. L., Dave, S. S., Love, C., Marti, G. E., Kay, N. E., Hanson, C. A., Rabe, K. G., Achenbach, S. J., Goldin, L. R., Camp, N. J., Goodman, B. K., Vachon, C. M., Spector, L. G., Rassenti, L. Z., Leis, J. F., Gockerman, J. P., Strom, S. S., Call, T. G., Glenn, M., Cerhan, J. R., Levesque, M. C., Weinberg, J. B. & Caporaso, N. E. (2011) Immnuophenotypic and gene expression analysis of monoclonal B-cell lymphocytosis shows biologic characteristics associated with good prognosis CLL. *Leukemia.*

Lerner, M., Corcoran, M., Cepeda, D., Nielsen, M. L., Zubarev, R., Ponten, F., Uhlen, M., Hober, S., Grander, D. & Sangfelt, O. (2007) The RBCC gene RFP2 (Leu5) encodes a novel transmembrane E3 ubiquitin ligase involved in ERAD. *Mol Biol Cell,* 18, 1670-82.

Lerner, M., Harada, M., Loven, J., Castro, J., Davis, Z., Oscier, D., Henriksson, M., Sangfelt, O., Grander, D. & Corcoran, M. M. (2009) DLEU2, frequently deleted in malignancy, functions as a critical host gene of the cell cycle inhibitory microRNAs miR-15a and miR-16-1. *Exp Cell Res,* 315, 2941-52.

Meckes, D. G., Jr., Shair, K. H., Marquitz, A. R., Kung, C. P., Edwards, R. H. & Raab-Traub, N. (2010) Human tumor virus utilizes exosomes for intercellular communication. *Proc Natl Acad Sci U S A,* 107, 20370-5.

Messmer, B. T., Messmer, D., Allen, S. L., Kolitz, J. E., Kudalkar, P., Cesar, D., Murphy, E. J., Koduru, P., Ferrarini, M., Zupo, S., Cutrona, G., Damle, R. N., Wasil, T., Rai, K. R., Hellerstein, M. K. & Chiorazzi, N. (2005) In vivo measurements document the dynamic cellular kinetics of chronic lymphocytic leukemia B cells. *J Clin Invest,* 115, 755-64.

Mhaskar, A. R., Quinn, G., Vadaparampil, S., Djulbegovic, B., Gwede, C. K. & Kumar, A. (2010) Timing of first-line cancer treatments - early versus late - a systematic review of phase III randomized trials. *Cancer Treat Rev,* 36, 621-8.

Migliazza, A., Bosch, F., Komatsu, H., Cayanis, E., Martinotti, S., Toniato, E., Guccione, E., Qu, X., Chien, M., Murty, V. V., Gaidano, G., Inghirami, G., Zhang, P., Fischer, S., Kalachikov, S. M., Russo, J., Edelman, I., Efstratiadis, A. & Dalla-Favera, R. (2001) Nucleotide sequence, transcription map, and mutation analysis of the 13q14 chromosomal region deleted in B-cell chronic lymphocytic leukemia. *Blood,* 97, 2098-104.

Mitchell, P. S., Parkin, R. K., Kroh, E. M., Fritz, B. R., Wyman, S. K., Pogosova-Agadjanyan, E. L., Peterson, A., Noteboom, J., O'briant, K. C., Allen, A., Lin, D. W., Urban, N., Drescher, C. W., Knudsen, B. S., Stirewalt, D. L., Gentleman, R., Vessella, R. L., Nelson, P. S., Martin, D. B. & Tewari, M. (2008) Circulating microRNAs as stable blood-based markers for cancer detection. *Proc Natl Acad Sci U S A,* 105, 10513-8.

Montini, E., Cesana, D., Schmidt, M., Sanvito, F., Ponzoni, M., Bartholomae, C., Sergi Sergi, L., Benedicenti, F., Ambrosi, A., Di Serio, C., Doglioni, C., Von Kalle, C. & Naldini, L. (2006) Hematopoietic stem cell gene transfer in a tumor-prone mouse model uncovers low genotoxicity of lentiviral vector integration. *Nat Biotechnol,* 24, 687-96.

Morrison, A. M., Nutt, S. L., Thevenin, C., Rolink, A. & Busslinger, M. (1998) Loss- and gain-of-function mutations reveal an important role of BSAP (Pax-5) at the start and end of B cell differentiation. *Semin Immunol,* 10, 133-42.

Mosca, L., Fabris, S., Lionetti, M., Todoerti, K., Agnelli, L., Morabito, F., Cutrona, G., Andronache, A., Matis, S., Ferrari, F., Gentile, M., Spriano, M., Callea, V., Festini, G., Molica, S., Deliliers, G. L., Bicciato, S., Ferrarini, M. & Neri, A. (2010) Integrative genomics analyses reveal molecularly distinct subgroups of B-cell chronic lymphocytic leukemia patients with 13q14 deletion. *Clin Cancer Res,* 16, 5641-53.

Moussay, E., Wang, K., Cho, J. H., Van Moer, K., Pierson, S., Paggetti, J., Nazarov, P. V., Palissot, V., Hood, L. E., Berchem, G. & Galas, D. J. (2011) MicroRNA as biomarkers and regulators in B-cell chronic lymphocytic leukemia. *Proc Natl Acad Sci U S A,* 108, 6573-8.

Naldini, L., Blomer, U., Gage, F. H., Trono, D. & Verma, I. M. (1996a) Efficient transfer, integration, and sustained long-term expression of the transgene in adult rat brains injected with a lentiviral vector. *Proc Natl Acad Sci U S A,* 93, 11382-8.

Naldini, L., Blomer, U., Gallay, P., Ory, D., Mulligan, R., Gage, F. H., Verma, I. M. & Trono, D. (1996b) In vivo gene delivery and stable transduction of nondividing cells by a lentiviral vector. *Science,* 272, 263-7.

Nayak, S. & Herzog, R. W. (2010) Progress and prospects: immune responses to viral vectors. *Gene Ther,* 17, 295-304.

NCI (2011) SEER Stat Fact Sheets: Chronic Lymphocytic Leukemia.

Nera, K. P., Kohonen, P., Narvi, E., Peippo, A., Mustonen, L., Terho, P., Koskela, K., Buerstedde, J. M. & Lassila, O. (2006) Loss of Pax5 promotes plasma cell differentiation. *Immunity,* 24, 283-93.

Nutt, S. L., Morrison, A. M., Dorfler, P., Rolink, A. & Busslinger, M. (1998) Identification of BSAP (Pax-5) target genes in early B-cell development by loss- and gain-of-function experiments. *EMBO J,* 17, 2319-33.

Palamarchuk, A., Efanov, A., Nazaryan, N., Santanam, U., Alder, H., Rassenti, L., Kipps, T., Croce, C. M. & Pekarsky, Y. (2010) 13q14 deletions in CLL involve cooperating tumor suppressors. *Blood,* 115, 3916-22.

Pekarsky, Y., Zanesi, N. & Croce, C. M. (2010) Molecular basis of CLL. *Seminars in Cancer Biology,* 20, 370-376.

Peng, B., Sherr, D. H., Mahboudi, F., Hardin, J., Wu, Y. H., Sharer, L. & Raveche, E. S. (1994) A cultured malignant B-1 line serves as a model for Richter's syndrome. *J Immunol,* 153, 1869-80.

Raveche, E. S., Salerno, E., Scaglione, B. J., Manohar, V., Abbasi, F., Lin, Y. C., Fredrickson, T., Landgraf, P., Ramachandra, S., Huppi, K., Toro, J. R., Zenger, V. E., Metcalf, R.

A. & Marti, G. E. (2007) Abnormal microRNA-16 locus with synteny to human 13q14 linked to CLL in NZB mice. *Blood,* 109, 5079-86.

Rawstron, A. C., Green, M. J., Kuzmicki, A., Kennedy, B., Fenton, J. A., Evans, P. A., O'connor, S. J., Richards, S. J., Morgan, G. J., Jack, A. S. & Hillmen, P. (2002) Monoclonal B lymphocytes with the characteristics of "indolent" chronic lymphocytic leukemia are present in 3.5% of adults with normal blood counts. *Blood,* 100, 635-9.

Salerno, E., Scaglione, B. J., Coffman, F. D., Brown, B. D., Baccarini, A., Fernandes, H., Marti, G. & Raveche, E. S. (2009) Correcting miR-15a/16 genetic defect in New Zealand Black mouse model of CLL enhances drug sensitivity. *Mol Cancer Ther,* 8, 2684-92.

Salerno, E., Yuan, Y., Scaglione, B. J., Marti, G., Jankovic, A., Mazzella, F., Laurindo, M. F., Despres, D., Baskar, S., Rader, C. & Raveche, E. (2010) The New Zealand black mouse as a model for the development and progression of chronic lymphocytic leukemia. *Cytometry B Clin Cytom,* 78 Suppl 1, S98-109.

Scaglione, B. J., Salerno, E., Balan, M., Coffman, F., Landgraf, P., Abbasi, F., Kotenko, S., Marti, G. E. & Raveche, E. S. (2007) Murine models of chronic lymphocytic leukaemia: role of microRNA-16 in the New Zealand Black mouse model. *Br J Haematol,* 139, 645-57.

Shanafelt, T. D. (2009) Predicting clinical outcome in CLL: how and why. *Hematology Am Soc Hematol Educ Program,* 421-9.

Shim, Y. K., Middleton, D. C., Caporaso, N. E., Rachel, J. M., Landgren, O., Abbasi, F., Raveche, E. S., Rawstron, A. C., Orfao, A., Marti, G. E. & Vogt, R. F. Prevalence of monoclonal B-cell lymphocytosis: a systematic review. *Cytometry B Clin Cytom,* 78 Suppl 1, S10-8.

Trang, P., Wiggins, J. F., Daige, C. L., Cho, C., Omotola, M., Brown, D., Weidhaas, J. B., Bader, A. G. & Slack, F. J. (2011) Systemic Delivery of Tumor Suppressor microRNA Mimics Using a Neutral Lipid Emulsion Inhibits Lung Tumors in Mice. *Mol Ther,* 19, 1116-22.

Valadi, H., Ekstrom, K., Bossios, A., Sjostrand, M., Lee, J. J. & Lotvall, J. O. (2007) Exosome-mediated transfer of mRNAs and microRNAs is a novel mechanism of genetic exchange between cells. *Nat Cell Biol,* 9, 654-9.

Van Dyke, D. L., Shanafelt, T. D., Call, T. G., Zent, C. S., Smoley, S. A., Rabe, K. G., Schwager, S. M., Sonbert, J. C., Slager, S. L. & Kay, N. E. (2010) A comprehensive evaluation of the prognostic significance of 13q deletions in patients with B-chronic lymphocytic leukaemia. *Br J Haematol,* 148, 544-50.

Van Gent, R., Kater, A. P., Otto, S. A., Jaspers, A., Borghans, J. A., Vrisekoop, N., Ackermans, M. A., Ruiter, A. F., Wittebol, S., Eldering, E., Van Oers, M. H., Tesselaar, K., Kersten, M. J. & Miedema, F. (2008) In vivo dynamics of stable chronic lymphocytic leukemia inversely correlate with somatic hypermutation levels and suggest no major leukemic turnover in bone marrow. *Cancer Res,* 68, 10137-44.

Van Haaften, G. & Agami, R. (2010) Tumorigenicity of the miR-17-92 cluster distilled. *Genes Dev,* 24, 1-4.

Wallin, J. J., Rinkenberger, J. L., Rao, S., Gackstetter, E. R., Koshland, M. E. & Zwollo, P. (1999) B cell-specific activator protein prevents two activator factors from binding to the immunoglobulin J chain promoter until the antigen-driven stages of B cell development. *J Biol Chem,* 274, 15959-65.

Wang, J., Chen, J., Chang, P., Leblanc, A., Li, D., Abbruzzesse, J. L., Frazier, M. L., Killary, A. M. & Sen, S. (2009) MicroRNAs in plasma of pancreatic ductal adenocarcinoma patients as novel blood-based biomarkers of disease. *Cancer Prev Res (Phila),* 2, 807-13.

Yazici, H., Zipprich, J., Peng, T., Akisik, E. Z., Tigli, H., Isin, M., Akisik, E. E., Terry, M. B., Senie, R. T., Li, L., Peng, M., Liu, Z., Dalay, N. & Santella, R. M. (2009) Investigation of the miR16-1 (C > T) + 7 Substitution in Seven Different Types of Cancer from Three Ethnic Groups. *J Oncol,* 2009, 827532.

Zufferey, R., Dull, T., Mandel, R. J., Bukovsky, A., Quiroz, D., Naldini, L. & Trono, D. (1998) Self-inactivating lentivirus vector for safe and efficient in vivo gene delivery. *J Virol,* 72, 9873-80.

Part 4

CLL Prognosis

12

Prognostic Factors in Chronic Lymphoid Leukemia and Identification of New Clinically Relevant Molecular Markers

José-Ángel Hernández[1], Marcos González[2] and Jesús-María Hernández[2]
[1]Hospital Universitario Infanta Leonor, Madrid,
[2]Hospital Clínico Universitario, Salamanca,
Spain

1. Introduction

Chronic lymphocytic leukemia (CLL) is a hematological malignancy with significant clinical heterogeneity, due in part to the genetic alterations that leukemic cells present in each patient (Chiorazzi et al, 2005). CLL has a highly variable clinical course. Traditionally, it has been considered that about one-third of patients will never require treatment, as they will have prolonged survival and they will die from causes unrelated to the disease. In another third of cases, after an indolent phase disease progression occurs. In the remaining third of patients early treatment is required because of the aggressiveness of the disorder. However, due to the routine performance of blood counts in the population, the number of asymptomatic patients is increasing and, conversely, those who require initial treatment account for fewer than 15% of cases (Hernandez et al, 2010). Since the first descriptions of the disease, researchers have attempted to establish prognostic factors with which to make a risk assessment of disease progression and probability of death. The ultimate aim is to try and apply a targeted and early treatment that increases overall survival and quality of life in patients with more aggressive forms, and to determine reliably the cases who do not need further treatment. (Dighiero & Hamblin, 2008).

Historically, there have been two distinct phases in the analysis of prognostic factors in CLL. Until the late 1980s, most prognostic factors were related to clinical presentation, cellular morphology, the pattern of infiltration of the bone marrow and lymphocyte progression over a period of time. Some of these are no longer considered relevant. Since the 1990s several prognostic factors associated with the immunophenotypic profile, cytogenetic features and mutational status of the immunoglobulin heavy chain (IGVH) have been added (Moreno & Montserrat, 2008). However, nomograms and predictors that include common clinical and pathological factors are still valid.

2. Prognostic factors in CLL

2.1 Clinical characteristics

In most published series, male patients have a more aggressive clinical course and worse survival than women with CLL (Catovsky et al, 1989). More than 30 years ago, Rai and Binet established two staging systems by which patients could be classified into low-, intermediate- and high-risk groups according to the presence or absence of certain clinical features (lymphadenopathy, visceromegalies, anemia and thrombocytopenia) (Binet et al, 1981; Rai et al, 1975). Nowadays, both clinical staging systems are widely used because of their simplicity and applicability. Different stages can be defined: early (Rai 0, Binet A), intermediate (Rai I-II, Binet B) and advanced (Rai III-IV, Binet C). These stages have a median overall survival (OS) of 10-12, 7 and 1.5-4 years, respectively (Tables 1 and 2). The Rai and Binet clinical stages have several limitations: a) they are unable to predict which patients from the initial stages will progress; b) they do not considerer tumor burden; c) they do not take into account the mechanism of cytopenias and d) they do not predict the response to therapy. At present, over 80% of cases are diagnosed in early stage A (0), since very often the diagnosis is made in the context of a routine analysis or of comorbidities that are unrelated to CLL.

Stage	Clinical features	Overall survival (years)
0	Blood and bone marrow lymphocytosis*	10
I	Lymphocytosis and large lymph nodes	7
II	Lymphocytosis and splenomegaly and/or hepatomegaly with or without large lymph nodes	7
III	Lymphocytosis and anemia** (hemoglobin level < 11 g/dL) with or without large lymph nodes, splenomegaly or hepatomegaly	1,5-4
IV	Lymphocytosis and thrombocytopenia** (platelet count < 100 x 10^9/L) with or without anemia, large lymph nodes, splenomegaly or hepatomegaly	1,5-4

*Lymphocyte count > 5 x 10^9/L in peripheral blood and > 30% of nucleated cells in bone marrow aspiration count.**Immune anemias or thrombocytopenias are excluded.

Table 1. Rai clinical stage system.

Stage	Clinical features	Overall survival (years)
A	Lymphocytosis in peripheral blood and bone marrow* and < 3 lymphoid regions involved**. No anemia, no thrombocytopenia	12
B	Lymphocytosis in peripheral blood and bone marrow* and ≥ 3 lymphoid regions involved **, with or without splenomegaly and/or hepatomegaly. No anemia, no thrombocytopenia	7
C	Lymphocytosis * with anemia*** (hemoglobin level < 11 g/dL in male and < 10 g/dL in female) or thrombocytopenia*** (platelet count < 100 x 10^9/L)	2-4

*Lymphocyte count > 5 x 10^9/L in peripheral blood and > 30% of nucleated cells in bone marrow aspiration count. **Each cervical, axillary and inguinal area can be unilateral or bilateral. Splenomegaly and hepatomegaly are one lymphoid region (5 areas). ***Immune anemias or thrombocytopenias are excluded.

Table 2. Binet clinical stage system.

2.2 Morphological features

Prolymphocytic transformation of CLL carries a worse prognosis, as well as atypical CLL (> 15% cell morphology is not compatible with the CLL, such as the presence of cleaved nuclei lymphocytes) compared with the typical morphology of CLL. It has recently been reported that patients with more than 30% of nuclear shadows (smudge cells) in the differential count are more likely to have a mutated IGVH pattern and, therefore, a longer time to treatment and better survival (Nowakowski et al, 2007).

The pattern of bone marrow infiltration may be nodular, interstitial, mixed (the most common type) and diffuse. In practice, we have to consider the first three as non-diffuse, because there are prognostic differences between patients with diffuse vs non-diffuse pattern. Patients treated with fludarabine schedules often show a persistent nodular pattern after therapy (nodular partial response), which represents a higher quality response than a partial one. The group at the Hospital Clinic, Barcelona, showed that the presence of a diffuse pattern of bone marrow infiltration is associated with a worse prognosis (Montserrat & Rozman, 1987). However, this prognostic factor was not independently confirmed by others, when new genetic markers were included in the analysis (Geisler et al, 1996).

2.3 Markers of proliferation or tumor burden and markers of angiogenesis

A lymphocyte doubling time (LDT) less than 6 months or an increase in lymphocyte count > 50% in 2 months is associated with a worse prognosis because they indicate an increased activity of the disease (Viñolas et al, 1987). In any case, LDT should only be recommended to initiate the treatment of CLL or to establish the prognosis with elevated lymphocyte counts (> 30 x 10^9/L). Despite their limitations, including the changes that occur during the course of the disease, LDT is a simple and inexpensive method, that is still interpreted in most clinical trials and clinical practice as an indication to start treatment.

Elevation of serum levels of lactate dehydrogenase (LDH), β2 microglobulin (B2M), thymidine kinase (TK) and soluble CD23 also indicate a high tumor burden (Hallek et al, 1996; Sarfati et al, 1996). Of these, LDH, contrary to what is observed in other lymphoproliferative disorders, is of minor relevance, although it is used in clinical practice due to the simplicity of its determination.

Elevated levels of TK are correlated with increased proliferation and predict the progression of CLL. In patients with early-stage CLL, high TK levels are correlated with the expression of CD38, ZAP-70, poor prognostic cytogenetic abnormalities and unmutated IGVH status. Moreover, serum TK levels have an independent value in the differentiation of CLL patients in early stages according to progression-free survival (PFS). Two limitations of the use of TK as a prognostic factor are the variation between laboratories, as well as their levels can be increased in patients with viral infections. However, its prognostic value in early-stage CLL has been fully established.

High levels of serum B2M, a protein that binds to the class I major histocompatibility complex, is one of the most important prognostic factors in some of the reported series. Moreover, their levels are correlated with the expression of CD38 and ZAP-70. Recently, the MD Anderson Cancer Center has proposed a prognostic nomogram that includes age, sex, absolute lymphocyte count, the number of lymphoid areas involved and B2M (Wierda et al,

2007). Furthermore, this group has also confirmed that low levels of B2M are independently associated with better complete responses (CR) rates, disease-free survival (DFS) and OS in patients treated with fludarabine-based schemes, with or without the addition of rituximab. The prognostic value of B2M in patients with impaired renal function is limited. Nevertheless, B2M is currently one of the most important prognostic factors for evaluating patients with advanced-stage CLL.

High levels and/or duplication of soluble CD23 also predicts a worse outcome for patients with CLL, with progression of patients in early stages and decreased survival.

Finally, the rise in the microvascular density and high levels of growth factor (VEGF) are also associated with poor prognosis (Ferrajoli et al, 2001).

2.4 Diagnostic imaging

Changes in abdominal computed tomography is a predictor of progression in patients with early-stage CLL, so its inclusion in the initial diagnostic tests can provide clinically relevant information (Muntañola et al, 2007). Even so, there are controversies regarding its value as a prognostic factor.

2.5 Immunophenotypic markers expression

2.5.1 Expression of CD38

CD38 is expressed in various hematopoietic cells and progenitors, thymus cells, T cells and activated B cells in later stages of differentiation. Determining the expression of CD38 is a useful tool and the results are easily analyzed to determine the prognosis of patients with CLL. However, because it is not a unique antigen of the proliferating cell in CLL it should not be analyzed independently, but along with the CD19 or CD20 and CD5, due to the aforementioned expression in other mononuclear cells. CD38 has been proposed as a prognostic marker in CLL, which has led to CD38 being proposed as a prognostic marker in CLL, indicating a more aggressive disease (Damle et al, 1999; Ghia et al, 2003). However, there is no consensus about the cutoff of positivity. Some authors suggest this to be 7%, although most choose levels above 30%. Different levels of CD38 expression can be observed over the course of the illness, during which its prognostic relevance diminishes. In fact, CD38 expression is not a perfect marker that can be a surrogates for IGVH mutational status, although it is associated with an increased incidence of organomegaly, bad prognosis cytogenetics, high B2M serum level and worse PFS and OS (Hamblin et al, 2002).

2.5.2 Expression of ZAP-70

The chain-associated protein zeta 70 (ZAP-70) is an intracellular tyrosine kinase Syk family/ZAP, which is associated with the zeta chain of the T cell receptor (TCR). Its expression is normally restricted to T and NK cells, which initiate the signaling pathways of T cells, resulting in the activation, differentiation and proliferation of effector cell functions in response to TCR stimulation. B cells of CLL may variably express this marker, but its positivity is one of the most powerful prognostic factors for predicting the course of the disease. The expression of ZAP-70 can be performed by various molecular techniques such as western blot, immunohistochemistry, RT-PCR, microarray expression and flow cytometry. One of the weaknesses of its determination by flow cytometry is the lack of reproducibility of the results. Several research groups have attempted to standardize the methodology in recent years (Letestu et al, 2006). It is likely that once it has been determined, along with other clinical and biological markers, it will help clinicians to assess the prognosis in newly diagnosed CLL patients more reliably. Results published by the Barcelona group, with a 20 % cutoff of ZAP-70, determined by flow cytometry (a higher level of expression indicates a worse prognosis) demonstrated significant differences in the OS and PFS of patients with CLL (Crespo et al, 2003). Unlike the case with CD38, ZAP-70 expression seems to be better than IGVH mutational status in predicting the time to receive the first treatment. The concordance between ZAP-70 expression and IGVH mutational status is 75-90% (Rassenti et al, 2004). When the positivity of ZAP70 and CD38 expression are combined, the time to treatment is 30 months, while it is 130 months in cases where both markers are negative.

However, the expression of both CD38 and ZAP-70 has proved controversial in the scientific community regarding its prognostic value for the next reasons: a) different results may be obtained with the same samples in different laboratories (indicating lack of validity and reproducibility of the techniques used), b) there may be temporal variations in the expression of CD38, c) it is difficult to establish the correct cutoff point for the expression of CD38 (<vs> 7% <vs> 30%) and ZAP-70 (the most widely accepted value being 20%), d) a careful separation of T cells for the determination of ZAP-70 by flow cytometry techniques is mandatory, which has meant that, even recently, several experts in this area have tried to systematize the method of determination, and e) a 20-30% discrepancy in the results of ZAP-70 provided by immunophenotyping by flow cytometry and IGVH mutational status has been described.

The CD49d antigen, whose expression is associated with a worse prognosis, has acquired a special significance in recent years (Gattei et al, 2008).

2.6 IGVH mutational status

One of the most important genetic parameters to establish the prognosis of patients with CLL is the mutational status of VH genes. Somatic mutations of the VH gene region of the heavy chain of immunoglobulins are present in about half of all CLL cases. In 1999, two research groups reported the importance of this observation as a predictor of disease progression, with survival of 8 years in cases of patients with CLL and unmutated pattern *vs* 24 years in those with mutated status (Damle et al, 1999; Hamblin et al, 1999). Unmutated cases originate from cells in the pregerminal center and clearly have a worse prognosis than mutated CLL cells also arising from the postgerminal center. The definition of non-mutated *vs* mutated pattern resides in a cutoff point, defined arbitrarily as a homology greater than 98% (non-mutated) gene most similar to the germline (Schroeder & Dighiero, 1994).

Patients with CLL and an unmutated status have an unfavorable course and progress more rapidly, as opposed to patients exhibiting a mutated state, whose survival is much better (Figures 1, 2). Unmutated CLL patients have a greater tendency to acquire poor prognostic cytogenetic abnormalities. It has also been observed that, irrespective of mutational status, some VH regions are associated with specific clinical features and different geographical incidences (Ghia et al, 2005). This is the case for IGHV3-21 usage, whose involvement provides a worse prognosis regardless of mutational status and, characteristically, is less prevalent in southern European countries, as confirmed by the results of an Italian group, who even showed that it is less frequent in southern than in northern Italy. This poorer clinical behavior of patients with IGHV3-21 may be explained because of the complementarity determining regions (HCDR3) are shorter and it is possible that the stimulatory influence of some unknown antigen leads to CLL progression. Other genes from the IGHV3 family, the most frequently used subgroup in CLL, are associated with prognosis. Thus, IGHV3-23 is related with a bad prognosis. On the other hand, IGHV3-72 and IGHV3-30 usages indicate good clinical outcomes, including spontaneous regression in anecdotal cases (Dal-Bo et al, 2011). Moreover, the involvement of the IGHV1-69 family, although it does not seem to have a lower survival compared to patients expressing other unmutated genes, and the IGHV4-39 usage occurs mainly in unmutated cases, while the IGHV4-34 and most cases of IGHV3 contain mutated cases. Patients with unmutated state have a poor prognosis if an autologous transplantation is performed, although the graft versus leukemia effect may counteract the therapeutic resistance of these patients if an allogeneic transplant is offered. The rearrangements of IGHV3-48 and IGHV3-53 are also associated with poor prognosis.

IGVH mutational status and cytogenetic abnormalities identified by FISH have a major impact on the survival of patients with CLL, but while cytogenetic changes during the course of the disease are relatively common, IGVH mutational status remains constant over time. One of the limitations of its use is the high cost of testing, due to its laboriousness and the expertise required.

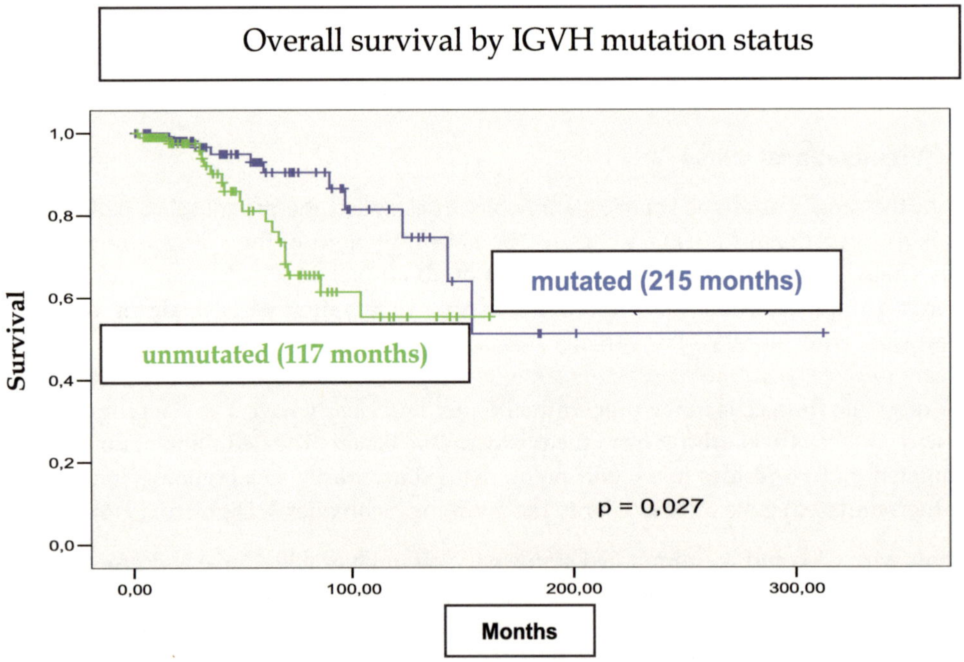

Fig. 1. Overall survival of the Salamanca University series of 226 patients with CLL by IGVH mutation status.

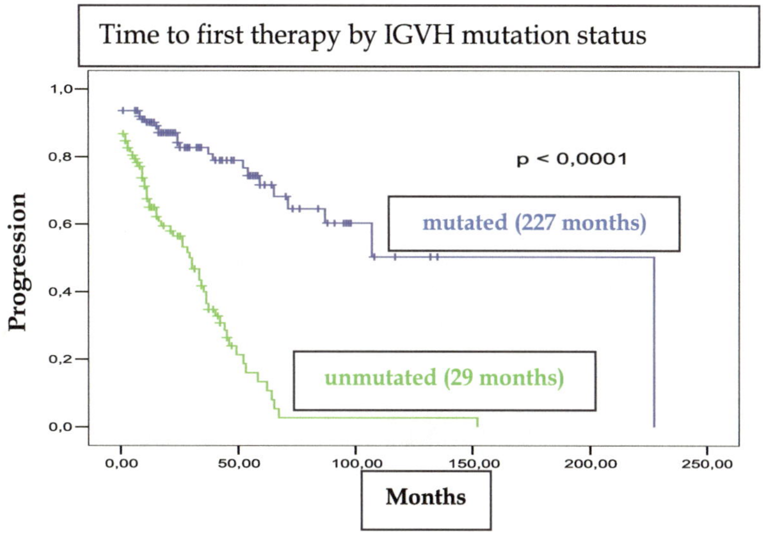

Fig. 2. Time to first therapy of the Salamanca University series of 226 patients with CLL by IGVH mutation status.

2.7 Cytogenetics and fluorescence in situ hybridization (FISH)

In 2000, the University of Ulm Group published their results from 325 patients with CLL concerning the relationship of various cytogenetic abnormalities, determined by FISH, with survival (Dohner et al, 2000). Using a panel of eight FISH probes, they analyzed the losses in 6q, 11q, 13q and 17p, the trisomies of 3q26, 8q24 and 12q13 and 14q32 translocations. They found that 82% of patients had chromosomal abnormalities, some of which were of prognostic relevance. In order of frequency, loss of 13q14 was the most frequent (present in 55% of cases), followed by loss of 11q22-23 (18%), trisomy of chromosome 12 (16%), loss of 17p13 (7%) and loss of 6q21 (6%). Only 57 patients (18%) had no abnormalities according to FISH, while 67 and 26 patients had two or more cytogenetic abnormalities, respectively. Median survival of patients with 17p-, 11q-, trisomy 12, normal cytogenetics and 13q- as a single alteration were 32, 79, 114, 111 and 133 months, respectively. In addition, patients with 17p- had the shortest interval before first treatment (9 months), whereas this period was longest in those with 13q- (92 months). In the Cox regression of overall survival time, patients with 17p deletion had a hazard ratio eight times that of other patients, whereas for those with 11q loss the hazard ratio was somewhat less than 3. These results have been reproduced in several series (Figure 3) (Tables 3, 4).

It is of note that some of the cytogenetic changes are related to characteristics of the disease: patients with 11q- tend to be younger and have marked lymphadenopathy, while those with 17p- are resistant to standard treatments, including that with fludarabine. 17p and 11q deletions were independently associated with other prognostic factors, such as IGVH mutation state, and the patients with these deletions had an adverse clinical outcome with progression of CLL and decreased survival (Krober et al, 2006). The British Group recently reported that patients with a more than 20% loss of function of TP53, a gene located on 17p, have a worse prognosis than those with a lower percentage loss (Gonzalez et al, 2011).

On the other hand, although it has customarily been considered that patients with del (13q) have a better prognosis, those with a high number of losses and/or the size of the deletion is greater have a worse prognosis in terms of time to receive the first treatment and survival, as shown recently by four independent groups (Figures 4, 5) (Dal Bo et al, 2011). Our genomic expression profile (GEP) studies have shown that those cases with a high number of losses of 13q have a higher expression of genes related to proliferation and reduced expression of apoptosis-related genes (Hernandez et al, 2009).

The 14q32/IGH translocation is present in 5-7% of CLL cases. Patients with IGH rearrangements can be classified in the intermediate prognosis group, as occurs with 6q deletion CLL patients (Cavazzini et al, 2008).

Clonal evolution may be observed during the course of CLL with the acquisition of new cytogenetic abnormalities (Stilgenbauer et al, 2007). These cytogenetic aberrations occur in 20-45% of patients and are associated with the presence of unmutated state and/or ZAP-70 expression. Therefore, FISH analysis should be done to diagnose CLL, before starting treatment and during relapse.

Finally, it has recently been shown that the presence of chromosomal translocations is associated with poor prognosis in CLL patients and that the length of telomeres is a prognostic factor related to mutation status (Sellmann et al, 2011).

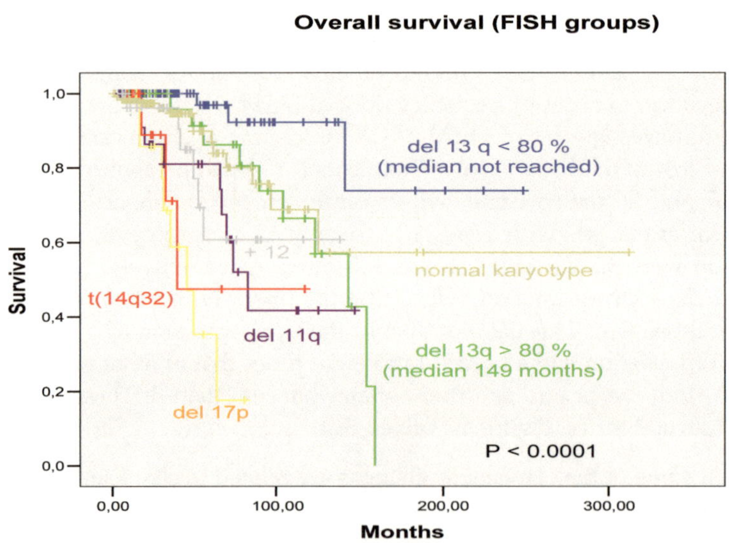

Fig. 3. Overall survival of the Salamanca University series of 350 patients with CLL by FISH group.

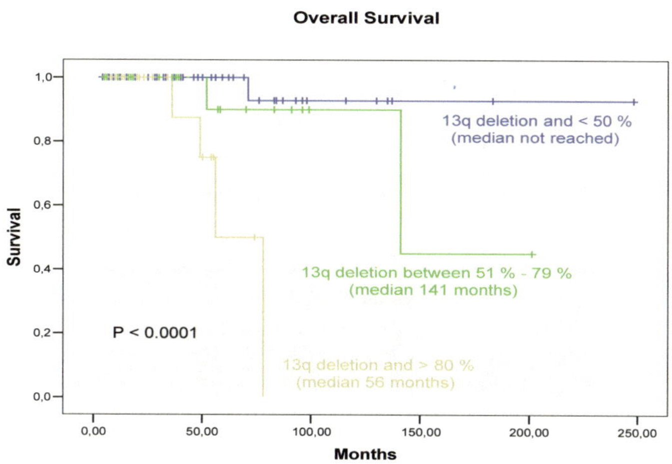

Fig. 4. Overall survival of the Salamanca University series of 109 patients with 13q deletion as unique alteration at diagnosis. A high number of losses in 13q is associated with a worse prognosis.

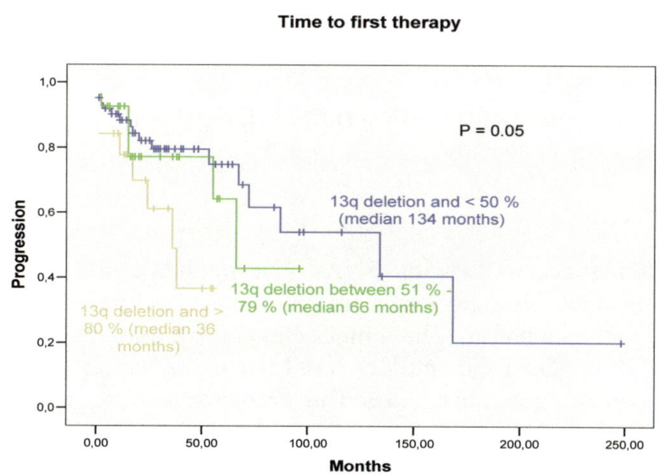

Fig. 5. Time to first therapy of the Salamanca University series of 109 patients with 13q deletion as unique alteration at diagnosis. A high number of losses in 13q is associated with a worse prognosis.

Study	$13q^-$	$13q^-$ as unique alteration	$11q^-$	+12	$17p^-$	Mutated status	Unmutated status
Ulm University	55	36	18	16	7	56	44
CLL1[1]	59	40	10	13	4	41	59
CLL4[2]	53	34	21	11	3	69	31
CLL3[3]	52	27	22	12	3	68	32
CLL2H[4]	48	14	32	18	27	81	19
Salamanca University[5]	46	36	9	12	4	56	44

*Results indicate percentages. 1. Patients in Binet A clinical stage without classical indication of therapy. 2. Patients aged < 65 years and Binet B and C clinical stages, included in randomized clinical trial (fludarabine *vs* fludarabine + cyclophosphamide). 3. Patients aged < 60 years and Binet B and C clinical stages, included in a clinical trial of autologous transplantation. 4. Patients refractory to fludarabine included in a clinical trial of subcutaneous alemtuzumab. 5. t(14q32) in 6 % of patients.

Table 3. Incidence of genomic aberrations and IGVH mutational status in several series of the CLL German Study Group and our series from the Salamanca University*

Variable	Hazard ratio (95% CI*)
Deletion 17p	7.03 (3.23-15.3)
IGVH1-69 usage	2.60 (1.04-6.44)
Deletion 11q	2.52 (1.29-4.90)
Normal cytogenetics	0.47 (0.23-0.97)
Deletion 13q as unique aberration	0.34 (0.18-0.64)
Mutated IGVH status	0.43 (0.20-0.91)

*CI: confidence interval.

Table 4. Cox regression analysis of overall survival in the series of CLL patients of the CLL patients of the Salamanca University

2.8 MicroRNAs

MicroRNAs (miRNA) are a class of RNAs that modulate the expression of post-transcriptional genes. miRNAs are small, non-coding RNAs involved in cancer genesis, apoptosis and the cell metabolism. These molecules show a role in CLL pathogenesis and prognosis (Calin et al, 2005). So, miR-29 has been described as a tumor-suppressing molecule that targets oncogenes like TCL1. This oncogene is overexpressed in CLL and is associated with an unmutated IGVH status, a high level of ZAP-70 expression and high-risk cytogenetics. In CLL patients, TCL1 protein expression is inversely correlated with miR-29 and miR-81 expression. Recently, it has been confirmed that the expression of miR-29 and miR-223 are correlated with poor prognosis. These two miRNAs, ZAP-70 and lipoprotein lipase (LPL) are the four variables comprising a new progressive prognostic score from 0 to 4 with the median TFS decreased from 312 months in the very good prognosis group to 12 months in the poor prognosis group. Also, high and low levels of expression of miR-21 and miR-181b, respectively, have been reported as risk prognostic factors, and miR-15a and miR-

16 expression is related to IGVH mutation status. Finally, a correlation between 17p deletion, TP53 and miR-34a has been reported. It seems likely that miRNA research will be increasingly influential in determining the prognosis of CLL, and some of these molecules may prove to be surrogate markers in this disorder (Ward et al, 2011).

2.9 Lipoproteinlipase (LPL) and ADAM 29 gene expression

Recently, several studies have demonstrated the importance of LPL expression, such as that of the principal RNA prognostic marker. A comparative study of RNA-based markers in CLL revealed LPL to be a powerful predictor of clinical outcome. In the initial report the LPL/ADAM29 expression ratio was described as a strong prognosis indicator in CLL, that enabled a better assessment than ZAP-70 in advances stages of CLL (Oppezzo et al, 2005).

2.10 Genomic expression profiles

Another area of development is the analysis of gene expression by RNA microarrays, which has led to improved diagnosis and classification of the neoplasms of leukemia patients. Although little information is currently available, the discovery through the analysis of microarray gene expression of a group of genes associated with survival of patients reflects the potential of this technology to detect new markers that may be prognostically relevant. In 2001, it was demonstrated the association between gene expression and mutational pattern and the existence of a homogeneous phenotype related to memory B cells in patients with CLL (Klein et al, 2001; Rosenwald et al, 2001). Subsequently, it was observed that the study of gene expression profiles showed a common molecular signature in patients with CLL, what contributed to the identification of markers of progression or it was different in mutated and unmutated CLL. In addition, genes that are significantly more highly expressed are located in the corresponding aberrant chromosomal regions, indicating the existence of a genetic effect of dose, which may have a pathogenic role in CLL. Significant differences in gene expression according to sex were also found, which suggests that differences in molecular signatures relating to IGVH mutational status may be related to the sex of the patient (Haslinger et al, 2004). Several genes have been implicated in the pathogenesis and prognosis of CLL. Other research lines related to the DNA methylation and the phosphorylation of receptor and adaptor proteins are providing an increasing amount of information about this disease and could have a prognostic role (Prieto-Sanchez et al, 2006). Even so, more work remains to be done in this field (Codony et al, 2009).

2.11 Treatment response and prognosis

The quality, depth and length of the response in the CLL treatment are of great prognostic importance. The achievement of a complete or a nodular partial response predicts better DFS and OS. In addition, some therapy schedules, mainly those based on immunochemotherapy (i.e., FCR combination) might overcome the dismal prognosis of patients with CLL and del (11q). On the other hand, negative minimal residual disease (MRD) improves the outcome of CLL patients, in terms of PFS, TTT and OS. Nevertheless, MRD assessment is not recommended in clinical practice, although it might be of great value in the coming years (Cramer & Hallek, 2011).

2.12 Comorbidities and prognosis

Performance status, physical fitness and comorbidities are important features in the selection of therapy and thereby in the prognosis of patients with CLL (Zenz et al, 2010). In this context, patients with CLL are divided in three groups: a) Fit or 'Go go' patients, for whom a standard treatment can be administered with the aim of achieving the best response, such as FCR; b) 'Slow go' patients, who should be treated with modified therapies in order to control the disease; c) Unfit or 'No go' patients, who should receive palliative care.

2.13 Other prognostic factors

2.13.1 Bcl2 and other immunophenotypic markers

Patients who are CD71+ and Bcl2+ have a shorter PFS and OS than those who are CD71- and Bcl2. In a recent paper, the independent prognostic value of bcl-2 was confirmed within ZAP-70 negative patients (Del Poeta et al, 2010). Other immunophenotypic markers, such as soluble CD20, have been investigated as potential prognostic factors in CLL.

2.13.2 CD26; CD44

CD26 antigen is strongly upregulated in activated B cells. CD26-positive patients show a shorter time to treatment and this positivity is correlated with ZAP-70 expression or IGVH mutational status (Cro et al, 2009). On the other hand, high levels of soluble CD44 predict the risk of illness progression in patients with early-stage CLL.

2.13.3 Circulating endothelial cells (CECs)

In patients with CLL, as occurs in other malignancies, CECs are increased and are correlated with an aggressive clinical outcome. In a recent report, the gene expression profile in patients with higher levels of CECs indicated increased cell survival and proliferation, diminished cell adhesion to the extracellular matrix, and enhanced proangiogenic function. CECs might be considered a biological marker for new targeted antiangiogenic therapies (Rigolin et al, 2010).

2.13.4 CLLU1 expression

High CLLU1 expression levels are associated with shorter OS in patients younger than 70 years of age. CLLU1 expression analysis adds prognostic information in risk prediction in CLL patients with the exception of those who have an unmutated IGVH status (Josefsson et al, 2007).

2.13.5 Interleukin (IL) 6, IL-8 and IL-10

IL-6 is a strong predictor of shorter survival in CLL patients with advanced disease. Furthermore, high levels of IL-8 are associated with shorter OS (Wierda et al, 2003). Finally, IL-10 levels are elevated in patients with CLL and are correlated with adverse clinical and biological characteristics of the disease and with shorter survival. The role of several IL inhibitors in the treatment of patients with CLL is currently being explored (Fayad et al, 2001) .

2.13.6 Matrix metalloproteinase-9 (MMP9)

MMP9 is involved in migration and tissue invasion in patients with CLL. The combined macromolecular cell surface complex formed by CD38, CD49d, CD44 and MMP9 is associated with a dismal prognosis, and, recently, it has been suggested as a novel therapeutic target (Buggins et al, 2011).

2.13.7 PEG10 expression

The overexpression of the paternally expressed gene 10 (PEG10) is observed in high-risk CLL patients, defined by high levels of LPL mRNA expression. Recently, PEG10 has been proposed as a new marker in CLL by Austrian and German researchers (Kainz et al, 2007).

2.13.8 Telomerase activity and telomere length

Several reports have illustrated the role of telomerase activity and telomere length in cancer prognosis. In CLL, short telomeres and high telomerase activity are associated with poor prognosis (Sellmann et al, 2011). Telomerase inhibitors are being investigated as novel targeted therapies in CLL.

2.13.9 TOSO/FCMR expression

Recently, the overexpression of the new gene TOSO (or FC mu receptor [FCMR, FAIM3/TOSO]) has been shown to be associated with the Binet clinical stage, IGVH mutation status, age and time to treatment in CLL. Furthermore, a high level of expression of TOSO is an independent predictor of shorter SLT in CLL (Hancer et al, 2011). However, no correlation has been found between the expression of TOSO and ZAP-70 or CD38. On the other hand, overexpression of FCMR seems to promote chromosomal abnormalities.

2.13.10 Tumor necrosis factor (TNF) alpha

MD Anderson Clinical Cancer investigators reported several years ago a correlation between elevated TNF-alpha levels and advanced clinical stage patients, high B2M levels and lower hemoglobin and platelet counts (Ferrajoli et al, 2002).

2.13.11 Rel A DNA binding

Researchers from Cardiff University recently demonstrated the importance of the NF-kappa B subunit Rel A in CLL (Hewamana et al, 2009). Rel A DNA binding appears to be strongly associated with advanced Binet stage, time to first therapy and survival. In addition, it seems to have the unique capacity to predict the duration of response to therapy.

3. Conclusions

A wide variety of prognostic factors have been studied in CLL, but clinical staging according to Binet or Rai systems, LTD and B2M are the main clinical and biological prognostic markers. Cytogenetics, using FISH (especially using the del (17p) probe), and expression of CD38 and ZAP-70 as surrogate markers for the IgVH mutational status are used routinely worldwide, although CD38 and ZAP-70 are not mandatory in clinical practice. New markers such as LPL, miR29c and TCL7 predict OS in CLL. On the other hand, the evaluation of patient physical fitness and the assessment of the response to therapy are critical elements.

Recently, sequencing the CLL genome and advances in computing and robotics have produced a revolution in general genetics and CLL (Puente et al, 2011). The combination of these methodologies has led to the development of microarray technology, enabling thousands of genes to be analyzed simultaneously. In CLL patients, the gene expression profile indicates that significantly differentiated genes are located in regions with chromosomal aberrations. However, the evidence linking specific genetic alterations using FISH or mutational status to the results of arrays is still not very consistent.

4. References

Binet, JL.; Auquier, A.; Dighiero, G., et al. (1981). A new prognostic classification of chronic lymphocytic leukemia derived from a multivariate survival analysis. *Cancer*, Vol.48, No.4, pp. 198-206, ISSN 0008-543X.

Buggins, AG.; Levi, A.; Gohil, S., et al. (2011). Evidence for a macromolecular complex in poor prognosis CLL that contains CD38, CD49d, CD44 and MMP-9. *Br J Haematol*, Vol.154, No.2, pp. 216-222, ISSN 1365-2141.

Calin, GA.; Ferracin, M.; Cimmino, A., et al. (2005). A microRNA signature associated with prognosis and progression in chronic lymphocytic leukemia. *N Engl J Med*, Vol.353, No.17, pp. 1793-1801. ISSN 1533-4406.

Catovsky, D.; Fooks, J. & Richards, S. (1989). Prognostic factors in chronic lymphocytic leukaemia: the importance of age, sex and response to treatment in survival. A report from the MRC CLL 1 trial. MRC Working Party on Leukaemia in Adults. *Br J Haematol*, Vol.72, No.2, pp. 141-149. ISSN 0007-1048.

Cavazzini, F.; Hernández, JA.; Gozzetti, A., et al. (2008). Chromosome 14q32 translocations involving the immunoglobulin heavy chain locus in chronic lymphocytic leukemia identify a disease subset with poor prognosis. *Br J Haematol*, Vol.142, No.4, pp. 529-537. ISSN 1365-2141.

Chiorazzi, N.; Rai, KR. & Ferrarini, M. (2005). Chronic lymphocytic leukemia. *N Engl J Med*, Vol.352, No.8, pp. 804-815. ISSN 1533-4406.

Codony, C.; Crespo, M.; Abrisqueta, P., et al. (2009). Gene expression profiling in chronic lymphocytic leukaemia. *Best Pract Res Clin Haematol*, Vol.22, No.2, pp. 211-22.ISSN 1532-1924.

Cramer, P. & Hallek, M. (2011). Prognostic factors in chronic lymphocytic leukemia-what do we need to know?. *Nat Rev Clin Oncol*, Vol.8, No.1, pp. 38-47. ISSN 1759-4782.

Crespo, M.; Bosch, F.; Villamor, N., et al. (2003). ZAP-70 expression as a surrogate for immunoglobulin-variable-region mutations in chronic lymphocytic leukemia. *N Engl J Med*, Vol.348, No.18, pp. 1764-1775. ISSN 1533-4406.

Cro, L.; Morabito, F.; Zucal, N., et al. (2009). CD26 expression in mature B-cell neoplasia: its possible role as a new prognostic marker in B-CLL. *Hematol Oncol*, Vol.27, No.3, pp. 140-7. ISSN 1099-1069.

Dal Bo, M.; Rossi, FM.; Rossi, D., et al. (2011a). 13q14 deletion size and number of deleted cells both influence prognosis in chronic lymphocytic leukemia. *Genes, Chromosomes Cancer*, Vol.50, No.8, pp. 633-643. ISSN 1098-2264.

Dal-Bo, M; Del Giudice, I; Bomben, R., et al. (2011b). B-cell receptor, clinical course and prognosis in chronic lymphocytic leukaemia: the growing saga of the IGHV3 subgroup gene usage. *Br J Haematol*, Vol.153, No.1, pp. 3-14. ISSN 1365-2141.

Damle, RN.; Wasil, T.; Fais, F., et al. (1999). Ig V gene mutation status and CD38 expression as novel prognostic indicators in chronic lymphocytic leukemia. *Blood*, Vol.94, No.6, pp. 1840-1847. ISSN 0006-4971.

Del Poeta, G.; Del Principe, MI.; Maurillo, L., et al. (2010). Spontaneous apoptosis and proliferation detected by BCL-2 and CD71 proteins are important progression indicators within ZAP-70 negative chronic lymphocytic leukemia. *Leuk Lymphoma*, Vol.51, No.1, pp. 95-106. ISSN 1029-2403.

Dighiero, G. & Hamblin, TJ. (2008). Chronic lymphocytic leukaemia. *Lancet*, Vol.371, No.9617, pp. 1017-1029. ISSN 1474-547X.

Dohner, H.; Stilgenbauer, S.; Benner, A., et al. (2000). Genomic aberrations and survival in chronic lymphocytic leukemia. *N Engl J Med*, Vol.343, No.26, pp. 1910-1916. ISSN 0028-4793.

Fayad, L; Keating, MJ.; Reuben, JM., et al. (2001). Interleukin-6 and interleukin-10 levels in chronic lymphocytic leukemia: correlation with phenotypic characteristics and outcome. *Blood*, Vol.97, No.1, pp. 256-263. ISSN 0006-4971.

Ferrajoli, A; Keating, MJ; Manshouri, T., et al. (2002). The clinical significance of tumor necrosis factor-alpha plasma level in patients having chronic lymphocytic leukemia. *Blood*, Vol.100, No.4, pp. 1215-1219. ISSN 0006-4971.

Ferrajoli, A.; Manshouri, T.; Estrov, Z., et al. (2001). High levels of vascular endothelial growth factor receptor-2 correlate with shortened survival in chronic lymphocytic leukemia. *Clin Cancer Res*, Vol.7, No.4, pp. 795-799. ISSN 1078-0432.

Gattei, V.; Bulian, P.; Del Principe, MI., et al. (2008). Relevance of CD49d protein expression as overall survival and progressive disease prognosticator in chronic lymphocytic leukemia. *Blood*, Vol.111, No.2, pp. 865-873. ISSN 0006-4971.

Geisler, CH.; Hou-Jensen, K.; Jensen, OM., et al. (1996). The bone-marrow infiltration pattern in B-cell chronic lymphocytic leukemia is not an important prognostic factor. Danish CLL Study Group. *Eur J Haematol*, Vol.57, No. 4, pp. 292-300. ISSN: 0902-4441.

Ghia, P.; Guida, G.; Stella, S., et al. (2003). The pattern of CD38 expression defines a distinct subset of chronic lymphocytic leukemia (CLL) patients at risk of disease progression. *Blood*, Vol.101, No.4, pp. 1262-1269. ISSN 0006-4971.

Ghia, P.; Stamatopoulos, K.; Belessi, C., et al. (2005). Geographic patterns and pathogenetic implications of IGHV gene usage in chronic lymphocytic leukemia: the lesson of the IGHV3-21 gene. *Blood*, Vol.105, No. 4, pp. 1678-1685. ISSN 0006-4971.

Gonzalez, D,; Martínez, P., Wade, R., et al. (2011). Mutational status of the TP53 gene as a predictor of response and survival in patients with chronic lymphocytic leukemia: results from the LRF CLL4 trial. *J Clin Oncol*, Vol.29, No.16, pp. 2223-2229. ISSN 1527-7755.

Haferlach, T.; Kohlmann, A.; Schnittger, S., et al. (2005) Global approach to the diagnosis of leukemia using gene expression profiling. *Blood*, Vol.106, No.4, pp. 1189-1198. ISSN 0006-4971.

Hallek, M.; Wanders, L.; Ostwald, M., et al. (1996). Serum beta(2)-microglobulin and serum thymidine kinase are independent predictors of progression-free survival in chronic lymphocytic leukemia and immunocytoma. *Leuk Lymphoma*, Vol.22, No.5-6, pp. 439-447. ISSN 1042-8194.

Hamblin, TJ.; Davis, Z.; Gardiner, A., et al. (1999). Unmutated Ig V(H) genes are associated with a more aggressive form of chronic lymphocytic leukemia. *Blood*, Vol.94, No.6, pp. 1848-1854. ISSN 0006-4971.

Hamblin, TJ.; Orchard, JA.; Ibbotson, RE, et al. (2002). CD38 expression and immunoglobulin variable region mutations are independent prognostic variables in chronic lymphocytic leukemia, but CD38 expression may vary during the course of the disease. *Blood*, Vol. 99, No.3, pp. 1023-1029. ISSN 0006-4971.

Hancer, VS.; Diz-Kucukkaya, R. & Aktan M. (2011). Overexpression of Fc mu receptor (FCMR, TOSO) gene in chronic lymphocytic leukemia patients. *Med Oncol.* 2011 Jan 25. [Epub ahead of print]. ISSN 1559-131X.

Haslinger, C.; Schweifer, N.; Stilgenbauer, S., et al. (2004). Microarray gene expression profiling of B-cell chronic lymphocytic leukemia subgroups defined by genomic aberrations and VH mutation status. *J Clin Oncol*, Vol.22, No.19, pp. 3937-3949. ISSN 0732-183X.

Hernández, JA.; González, M. & Hernández, JM. (2010). Chronic lymphoid leukemia. *Med Clin (Barc)*, Vol.135, No.4, pp. 172-178. ISSN 0025-7753.

Hernández, JA.; Rodríguez, AE.; González, M., et al. (2009). A high number of losses in 13q14 chromosome is associated with a worse outcome and biological differences in patients with B chronic lymphoid leukemia. *Haematologica*, Vol.94, No.3, pp. 364-371. ISSN 1592-8721.

Hernandez, JM.; Mecucci, C.; Criel, A., et al. (1995). Cytogenetic analysis of B cell chronic lymphoid leukemias classified according to morphologic and immunophenotypic (FAB) criteria. *Leukemia*, Vol.9, No.12, pp. 2140-2146. ISSN 0887-6924.

Hewamana, S.; Lin, TT.; Rowntree, C., et al. (2009). Rel a is an independent biomarker of clinical outcome in chronic lymphocytic leukemia. *J Clin Oncol*, Vol.27, No.5, pp. 763-769. ISSN 1527-7755.

Josefsson, P.; Geisler, CH.; Leffers, H., et al. (2007). CLLU1 expression analysis adds prognostic information to risk prediction in chronic lymphocytic leukemia. *Blood*, Vol.109, No.11, pp. 4973-4979. ISSN 0006-4971.

Kainz, B.; Shehata, M.; Bilban, M., et al. (2007). Overexpression of the paternally expressed gene 10 (PEG10) from the imprinted locus on chromosome 7q21 in high-risk B-cell chronic lymphocytic leukemia. *Int J Cancer*, Vol.121, No.9, pp. 1984-1993. ISSN 0020-7136.

Klein, U.; Tu, Y.; Stolovitzky, GA., et al. (2001). Gene expression profiling of B cell chronic lymphocytic leukemia reveals a homogeneous phenotype related to memory B cells. *J Exp Med*, Vol.194, No.11, pp. 1625-1638. ISSN 0022-1007.

Krober, A.; Bloehdorn, J.; Hafner, S., et al. (2006). Additional genetic high-risk features such as 11q deletion, 17p deletion, and V3-21 usage characterize discordance of ZAP-70 and VH mutation status in chronic lymphocytic leukemia. *J Clin Oncol*, Vol.24, No.6, pp. 969-975. ISSN 1527-7755.

Lai, R.; O'Brien, S.; Maushouri, T., et al. (2002). Prognostic value of plasma interleukin-6 levels in patients with chronic lymphocytic leukemia. *Cancer*, Vol.95, No.5, pp. 1071-1075. ISSN 0008-543X.

Letestu, R.; Rawstron, A.; Ghia, P.; et al. (2006). Evaluation of ZAP-70 expression by flow cytometry in chronic lymphocytic leukemia: A multicentric international harmonization process. *Cytometry B Clin Cytom*, Vol.70, No.4, pp. 309-314. ISSN 1552-4949.

Molica, S.; Vitelli, G.; Levato, D., et al. (2003). Increased serum levels of matrix metalloproteinase-9 predict clinical outcome of patients with early B-cell chronic lymphocytic leukaemia. *Eur J Haematol*, Vol.70, No.6, pp. 373-378. ISSN 0902-4441.

Montserrat, E. New prognostic markers in CLL. (2006). *Hematology Am Soc Hematol Educ Program*, pp. 279-284. ISSN 1520-4391.

Montserrat, E. & Rozman, C. (1987). Bone marrow biopsy in chronic lymphocytic leukemia: a review of its prognostic importance. *Blood Cells*, Vol.12, No.2, pp. 315-326. ISSN 0340-4684.

Moreno, C. & Montserrat, E. (2008). New prognostic markers in chronic lymphocytic leukemia. *Blood Rev*, Vol.22, No.4, pp. 211-219. ISSN 0268-960X.

Muntañola, A.; Bosch, F.; Arguis, P., et al. (2007). Abdominal computed tomography predicts progression in patients with Rai stage 0 chronic lymphocytic leukemia. *J Clin Oncol*, Vol.25, No.12, pp. 1576-1580. ISSN 1527-7755.

Nowakowski, GS.; Hoyer, JD.; Shanafelt, TD., et al. (2007). Using smudge cells on routine blood smears to predict clinical outcome in chronic lymphocytic leukemia: a universally available prognostic test. *Mayo Clin Proc*, Vol.82, No.4, pp. 449-453. ISSN 0025-6196.

Oppezzo, P.; Vasconcelos, Y.; Settegrana, C., et al. (2005). The LPL/ADAM29 expression ratio is a novel prognosis indicator in chronic lymphocytic leukemia. *Blood*, Vol.106, No.2, pp. 650-7. ISSN 0006-4971.

Orfao, A.; Gonzalez, M.; San Miguel, JF., et al. (1989). B-cell chronic lymphocytic leukaemia: prognostic value of the immunophenotype and the clinico-haematological features. *Am J Hematol*, Vol.31, No.1, pp. 26-31. ISSN 0361-8609.

Prieto-Sanchez, RM.; Hernandez, JA.; Garcia, JL., et al. (2006). Overexpression of the *VAV* proto-oncogene product is associated with b-cell chronic lymphocytic leukaemia displaying loss on 13q. *Br J Haematol*,Vol.133, No.6, pp. 642-645. ISSN 0007-1048.

Puente, XS.; Pinyol, M.; Quesada, V., et al. (2011). Whole-genome sequencing identifies recurrent mutations in chronic lymphocytic leukemia. *Nature*, Vol.475, No.7354, pp. 101-105. ISSN 1476-4687.

Rai, KR.; Sawitsky, A.; Cronkite, EP., et al. (1975). Clinical staging of chronic lymphocytic leukemia. *Blood*, Vol.46, No.2, pp. 219-234. ISSN 0006-4971.

Rassenti, LZ.; Huynh, L.; Toy, TL., et al. (2004). ZAP-70 compared with immunoglobulin heavy-chain gene mutation status as a predictor of disease progression in chronic lymphocytic leukemia. *N Engl J Med*, Vol.351, No.9, pp. 893-901. ISSN 1533-4406.

Rigolin, GM.; Maffei, R.; Rizzotto, L., et al. (2010). Circulating endothelial cells in patients with chronic lymphocytic leukemia:clinical-prognostic and biologic significance. *Cancer*, Vol.116, No.8, pp. 1926-1937. ISSN 0008-543X.

Rosenwald, A.; Alizadeh, AA.; Widhopf, G., et al. (2001). Relation of gene expression phenotype to immunoglobulin mutation genotype in B cell chronic lymphocytic leukemia. *J Exp Med*, Vol.194: No.11, pp. 1639-1647. ISSN 0022-1007.

Sarfati, M.; Chevret, S.; Chastang, C., et al. (1996). Prognostic importance of serum soluble CD23 level in chronic lymphocytic leukemia. *Blood*, Vol.88, No.11, pp. 4259-4264. ISSN 0006-4971.

Schroeder, HW. Jr. & Dighiero, G. (1994). The pathogenesis of chronic lymphocytic leukemia: analysis of the antibody repertoire. *Immunol Today*, Vol.15, No.6, pp. 288-294. ISSN 0167-5699.

Sellmann, L.; de Beer, D.; Bartels, M., et al. (2011). Telomeres and prognosis in patients with chronic lymphocytic leukaemia. *Int J Hematol*, Vol.93, No.1, pp. 74-82. ISSN 1865-3774.

Stilgenbauer, S.; Sander, S.; Bullinger, L., et al. (2007). Clonal evolution in chronic lymphocytic leukemia: acquisition of high-risk genomic aberrations associated with unmutated VH, resistance to therapy, and short survival. *Haematologica*, Vol.92, No.9, pp. 1242-1245. ISSN 1592-8721.

Viñolas, N.; Reverter, JC.; Urbano-Ispizua, A., et al. (1987). Lymphocyte doubling time in chronic lymphocytic leukemia: an update of its prognostic significance. *Blood Cells*, Vol.12, No.2, pp. 457-470. ISSN 0340-4684.

Ward, BP.; Tsongalis, GJ. & Kaur,P. (2011). MicroRNAs in chronic lymphocytic leukemia. *Exp Mol Pathol*, Vol. 9, No.2, pp. 173-178. ISSN 1096-0945.

Wierda, WG.; Johnson, MM.; Do, KA., et al. (2003). Plasma interleukin 8 level predicts for survival in chronic lymphocytic leukaemia. *Br J Haematol*, Vol.120, No.3, pp. 452-456. ISSN 0007-1048.

Wierda, WG.; O'Brien, S.; Wang, X., et al. (2007). Prognostic nomogram and index for overall survival in previously untreated patients with chronic lymphocytic leukemia. *Blood*, Vol.109, No.11, pp. 4679-4685. ISSN 0006-4971.

Yi, S.; Yu, Z.; Zhou, K., et al. (2011). TOSO is overexpressed and correlated with disease progression in Chinese patients with chronic lymphocytic leukemia. *Leuk Lymphoma*, Vol.52, No.1, pp. 72-78. ISSN 1029-2403.

Zenz, T.; Fröling, S.; Mertens, D., et al. (2010). Moving from prognostic to predictive factors in chronic lymphocytic leukaemia (CLL). *Best Pract Res Clin Haematol*, Vol.23, No.1, pp. 71-84.ISSN 1532-1924.

13

Genetics of Chronic Lymphocytic Leukemia: Practical Aspects and Prognostic Significance

N. Put[1], I. Wlodarska[1], P. Vandenberghe[1] and L. Michaux[1,2]
[1]*Center for Human Genetics, Catholic University of Leuven, Leuven*
[2]*Department of Hematology, University Hospital UCL Saint-Luc, Brussels, Belgium*

1. Introduction

B-cell chronic lymphocytic leukemia (CLL) is a mature B-cell neoplasm. Affecting mainly the elderly, CLL represents the most common hematological malignancy in Western countries, and 6-7% of non Hodgkin's lymphomas.

The disease course is heterogenous. Clinical staging systems (i.e. Rai and Binet) are used for estimating the tumor burden and prognosis and for making therapeutic decisions in individual patients. However, the evolution, even in the early stages, remains highly variable with at least 50% of cases showing early or late progression. Since the large majority of newly diagnosed cases present with early or intermediate stage, it is important to assess the risk profile within this group.

Several biological variables have been proposed for the prognostic stratification of early stage CLL, including chromosomal abnormalities [as assessed by karyotyping or fluorescent *in situ* hybridization (FISH)], expression of CD38, the proportion of ZAP-70-positive cells, somatic hypermutation of the variable part of the B-cell receptor gene (*IGVH*) and *VH* 3-21 usage. In addition, acquisition of particular chromosomal aberrations could be relevant, i.e. a 17p deletion appearing during the disease course confers resistance to alkylating agents and purine analogs, underscoring the need for defining the genetic patterns of disease evolution.

Here, chromosomal aberrations in CLL will be reviewed. First, the different techniques to detect abnormalities will be described. Second, the CLL-associated (cyto)genetic abnormalities and their relevance for clinical practice will be discussed, with a focus on the role of these aberrations in disease onset, progression, and on their prognostic significance.

2. Cytogenetic techniques

Numerous studies have shown that the presence, number, and type of chromosomal aberrations represent an independent predictor of prognosis in CLL (Döhner *et al*, 2000; Juliusson *et al*, 1990; Mayr *et al*, 2006; Van Den Neste *et al*, 2007). Therefore, cytogenetic analysis is now routinely performed in this disease. Different techniques are available to detect chromosomal abnormalities. Conventional cytogenetic analysis (CCA) can be performed, but is hampered by the poor mitotic index of CLL lymphocytes *in vitro*.

Although several mitogens have been used to overcome this problem, alternative approaches allowing analysis of nondividing cells are available, i.e. interphase FISH is widely used and has become the standard technique. In addition multiplex ligation-dependent probe amplification (MLPA) (Coll-Mulet *et al*, 2008; Fabris *et al*, 2011) and more recently analysis by means of different array-platforms (Gunn *et al*, 2008; Hagenkord *et al*, 2010) have been investigated in research and routine setting.

2.1 Conventional cytogenetic analysis

CCA or chromosome banding analysis (CBA) examines the patient's chromosomes in a sample of cells. Counting the number of chromosomes and evaluating their structural aberrations (banding patterns) results in the construction of a karyogram and karyotype. The resolution is determined by the number of bands seen in a haploid set of chromosomes (300-850 bands, each band contains approximately 5-10 megabase of DNA) (Shaffer *et al*, 2009). The work-flow of the technical procedure is shown in Fig 1. Peripheral blood is the preferred tissue for CCA in CLL, but bone marrow, lymph node, spleen or effusions can be analyzed as well.

Since CLL is a malignancy of mature B-cells, these cells are often arrested at the G_0G_1 phase of the cell cycle and do not divide spontaneously. They accumulate primarily as a result of lack of apoptosis, rather than by accelerated cell division (Chiorazzi, 2007). As a consequence, CLL lymphocytes have a poor mitotic index *in vitro*. Therefore longer culture duration has been introduced, i.e. 72 hours instead of 24-48 hours, and several stimulating agents have been added to the culture medium. Mitogens and agents such as 12-O-tetradecanoylphorbol-13-acetate (TPA), the lectine phyotohemagglutinin (PHA), lipopolysaccharide (LPS) and pokeweed mitogen (PWM), the cytokine interleukin-2 (IL-2) and Epstein-Barr virus, have been used to improve the yield of aberrant metaphases. However, abnormal karyotypes were revealed in only 40–50% of cases (Juliusson *et al*, 1990). These low abnormality detection rates can be attributed to a lack of aberrant metaphases, i.e. proliferation disadvantage of the aberrant B-cell clone, and to the presence of cryptic deletions escaping the low resolution of CCA. Recently, improved culture methods have been introduced, i.e. CD40 ligand (CD40L)-induced cell cycle stimulation, and the immunostimulatory CpG oligonucleotide (DSP30) (Dicker *et al*, 2006; Haferlach *et al*, 2007; Mayr *et al*, 2006; Put *et al*, 2009a; Struski *et al*, 2009).

2.1.1 TPA

Before the introduction of DSP30, the phorbol ester TPA was considered to be the stimulating agent of choice to improve the mitotic index of CLL cells. TPA stimulates slowly proliferating immature B-cells by activating protein kinase C. This results in phosphorylation of downstream proteins, maturation of these cells towards a plasmacytoid phenotype and inhibition of apoptosis (Barragan *et al*, 2002). However, the induction of cells in G_2 and metaphase is weak (2-10%) (Carlsson *et al*, 1988; Stephenson *et al*, 1991).

In addition, TPA has been shown to induce the IL-2 receptor and CLL colony formation. The addition of the cytokine IL-2 to TPA stimulated CLL cell cultures was reported to directly stimulate CLL proliferation, even in absence of T-lymphocytes (Touw and Lowenberg, 1985). Although the latter findings provide evidence for the addition of IL-2 to TPA cultures, it is not mandatory for successful CCA (Put *et al*, 2009a; Struski *et al*, 2009).

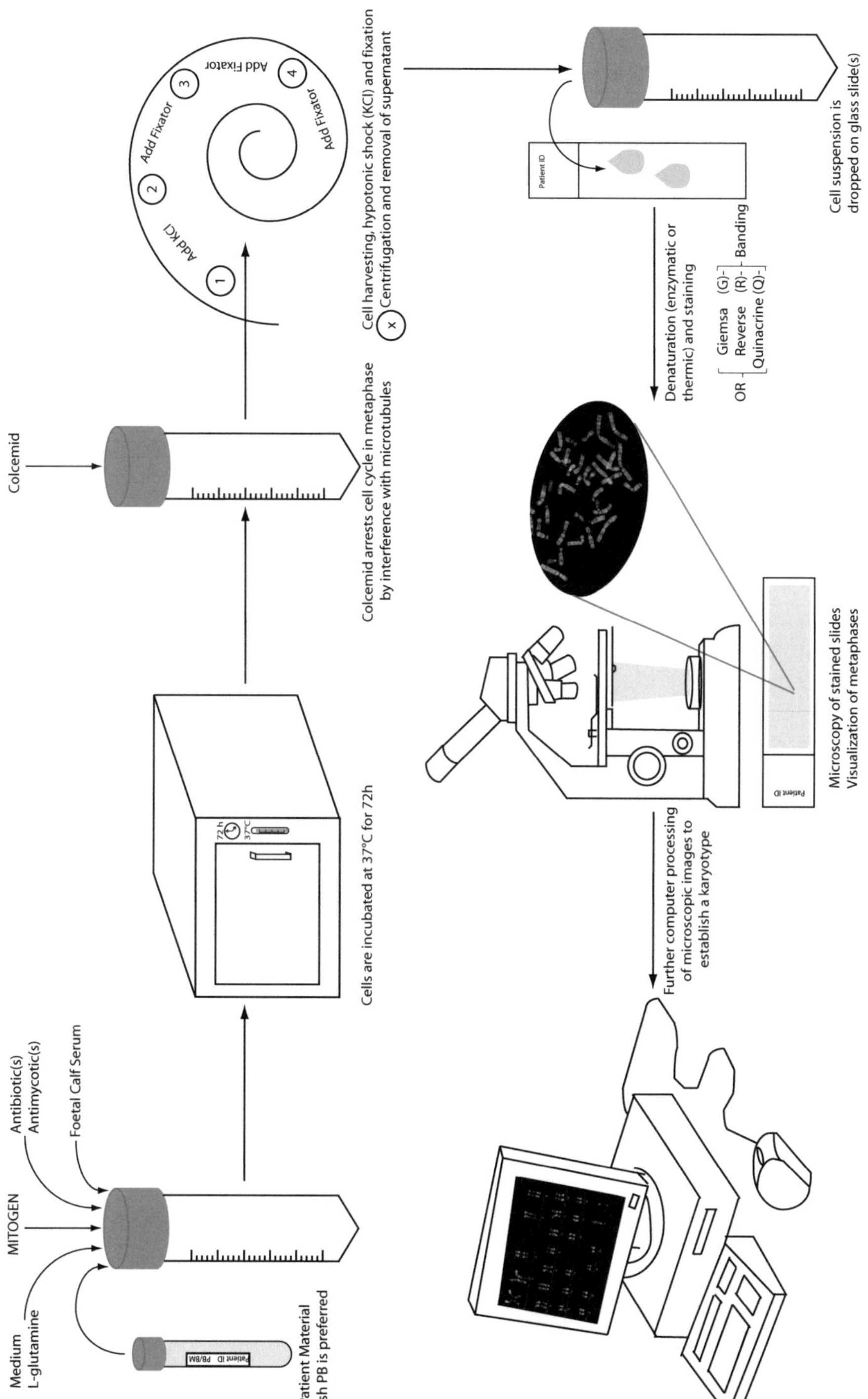

Fig. 1. Conventional cytogenetic analysis: summarized procedure
PB, peripheral blood; BM, bone marrow; CLL, chronic lymphocytic leukemia

2.1.2 CD40-ligand (CD40L)

As metaphase induction by TPA is weak and aberration detection is inferior compared with FISH, efforts were made to improve culture methods. In contrast to the environment of lymph node proliferation centers, *in vitro* cultures do not protect the lymphocytes from apoptotic and cytotoxic triggers. The addition of CD40 was able to induce an antiapoptotic profile in CLL cells (Hallaert *et al*, 2008) and therefore it could improve the generation of metaphases. CD40 is an antigen expressed on the surface of normal and malignant B-cells and induces cell cycle progression after activation by its ligand (Buhmann *et al*, 2002). CD40L-induced cell cycle stimulation resulted in a threefold increase in generation of metaphases compared with stimulation with B-cell mitogens such as TPA, LPS and PWM. In addition, the success rate of CCA and aberration detection rate were higher in the CD40L cultures (93% vs. 78% and 89% vs. 22%, respectively) (Buhmann *et al*, 2002). However, this technique is labor-intensive and expensive, and therefore not applicable for routine analysis.

2.1.3 DSP30

At the present time, the best CCA results in CLL are obtained with the addition of CpG oligodinucleotides (ODN) and IL-2 to the culture medium. ODN containing a CpG motif, such as DSP30, stimulate cells of the immune system via the Toll-like receptor 9 (TLR9). In humans, the only cell types known to express TLR9 are B-cells and plasmacytoid dendritic cells (Hornung et al., 2002). It has been established that CpG stimulates a broad spectrum of B-cell malignancies, i.e. CLL (Jahrsdorfer *et al*, 2005). CpG induces proliferation in normal B-cells; however, proliferation is weaker and followed by increased apoptosis in CLL cells (Jahrsdorfer *et al*, 2005). The lower proliferative response to CpG-ODN in CLL cells compared with normal B-cells can be overcome by addition of IL-2. Indeed, compared with normal B-cells, CpG causes a stronger induction of the IL-2 receptor α chain (CD25) in CLL, resulting in higher numbers of IL-2 receptors with a stronger affinity. Costimulation with CpG and IL-2 might alter IL-2 signaling in CLL cells in addition to increase cytokine production and surface molecule expression (Decker et al., 2000a).

The use of CpG/IL-2 improves proliferation capacity of CLL cells, and therefore it enables karyotyping in more cases (79-98%). Moreover, the technique yields detection rates of aberrations comparable with interphase FISH (81–83%) (Dicker et al., 2006; Haferlach et al., 2007). Other groups confirmed an improvement of the aberration detection rate in CpG/IL-2 (i.e. an increase of 9-13% of cases with aberrations) compared with TPA stimulated cultures (Put *et al*, 2009a; Struski *et al*, 2009). Moreover, the detection of translocations and del(13q) in particular, has been found to be superior after CpG/IL-2 stimulation compared with TPA (Put *et al*, 2009a).

The influence of CpG/IL-2 on quality of banding and metaphase generation is not clear (Put *et al*, 2009a; Struski *et al*, 2009).

Another question to address is whether abnormalities found after CpG/IL-2 stimulation might be related to activation-induced cytidine deaminase (AID). CpG stimulation of CLL and normal B-cells induces expression of AID, an enzyme that is linked to the development of genetic abnormalities (Capolunghi et al., 2008). However, culturing B-cells of healthy blood donors with CpG/IL-2 did not induce clonal abnormalities, thus validating CpG/IL-2 as a tool for the cytogenetic analysis of CLL (Dicker *et al*, 2006; Put *et al*, 2009a; Wu *et al*, 2008).

In conclusion, CpG/IL-2 should be preferred for routine CCA of CLL. However, as neither conventional cytogenetics nor CLL-specific FISH can detect all aberrations, both techniques should be complementarily applied.

2.2 FISH

FISH uses labeled DNA probes directed to selected targets and has a higher resolution than standard cytogenetics (approximately 40 Kb - 1 Mb, depending on the size of the FISH-probes vs. 10 Mb, respectively). Moreover, it can be used on metaphases and on nondividing cells. Sample types that may be used for FISH include in most cases peripheral blood or bone marrow, but also lymph node, spleen or effusions. Either uncultured fresh or frozen cells, cultured fixed cells, or paraffin-embedded tissue sections can be investigated.

The procedure is summarized in Fig 2. Interphase FISH yields high rates of detection of abnormalities, i.e. 80% (Döhner *et al*, 2000). However, this technique provides only partial information confined to the chromosomal loci examined, whereas CCA gives an overview of all microscopically visible aberrations.

Although FISH is a very sensitive technique, one should consider certain shortcomings. As already mentioned, a limited number of probes is applied. For this reason FISH can underestimate genomic complexity. False-positive and false-negative interpretations occur in 5% of FISH assays (Smoley *et al*, 2010). Wrong results may be due to i.e. inadequate cut-offs, co-hybridization or poor hybridization of probes, background signals, difficulties in visualizing probe signals in different planes of the nucleus, inadequate probes [in case of microdeletions or microduplications, i.e. *ATM* or *miR-15a/16-1*, in which the probe may be too large or not covering the deletion]. Lack of proliferation of the aberrant clone can occur when FISH is performed on cultured material. Furthermore, complex and cryptic translocations may generate special patterns of FISH signals that do not match the normal, expected signal pattern.

In clinical practice, FISH is performed for the regions 17p13 (*TP53)*, 11q13 (*ATM)*, chromosome 12 and 13q14 (*RB1* and *miR15.a/16.1*). The panel can be extended with probes for the regions 6q21 and 14q32 (*IGH*). Of interest, particular aberrations detected by FISH (discussed in section 3.1), e.g. loss of 17p13, were identified as major prognostic markers in CLL.

Hence abnormalities detected by FISH may guide patient monitoring and therapeutic decisions. Moreover FISH analysis is recommended for pretreatment evaluation and before subsequent, second- or third-line treatment (Hallek *et al*, 2008).

2.3 MLPA

Since FISH is a quite laborious, time-consuming and expensive technique, MLPA has been developed as an alternative tool. This technique relies on the comparative quantitation of specifically bound probes that are amplified by polymerase chain reaction (PCR) with universal primers. The latter allows simultaneous processing of multiple samples and has proven to be accurate and reliable for identifying deletions, duplications, and amplifications (Coll-Mulet *et al*, 2008). The procedure is summarized in Fig 3. (Schouten *et al*, 2002) and an example of MLPA results is shown in Fig 4. In a study comparing FISH and MLPA on 100 samples of untreated early stage (Binet A) CLL patients, a high degree of concordance between both techniques was observed (95%). Seven aberrations were not detected by

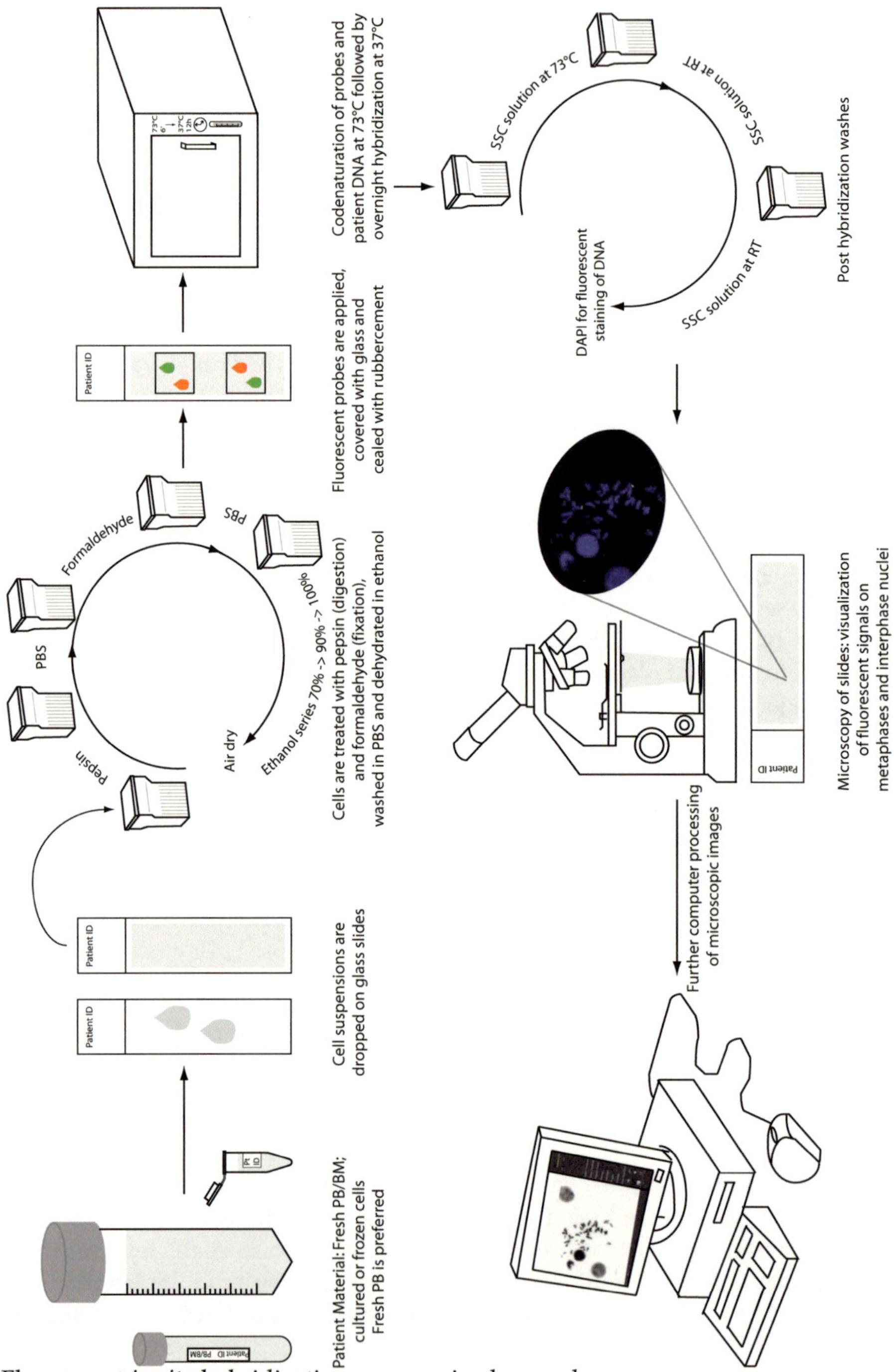

Fig. 2. Fluorescent *in situ* hybridization: summarized procedure
PB, peripheral blood; BM, bone marrow; PBS, phosphate buffered saline; SSC, saline-sodium citrate (SSC) buffer; DAPI, 4',6-diamidino-2-phenylindole

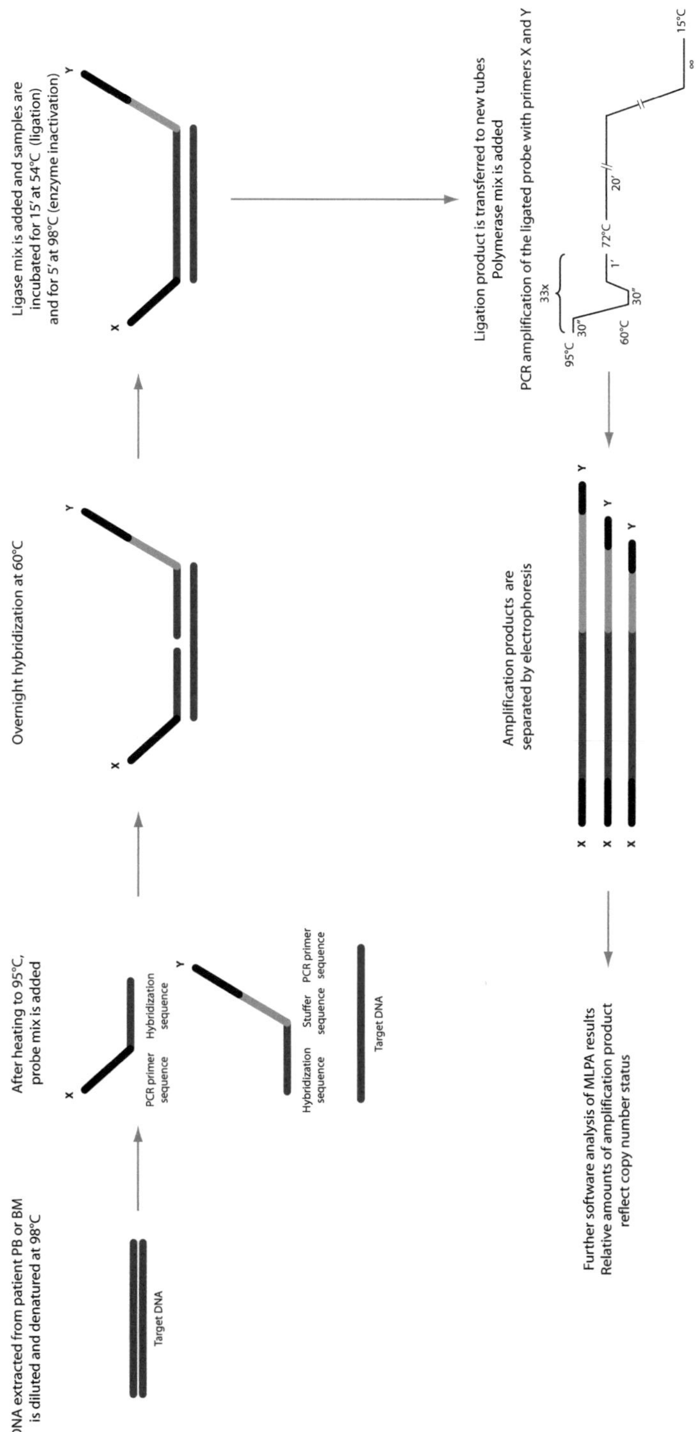

Fig. 3. Multiplex ligation-dependent probe amplification (MLPA): summarized procedure
PB, peripheral blood; BM, bone marrow

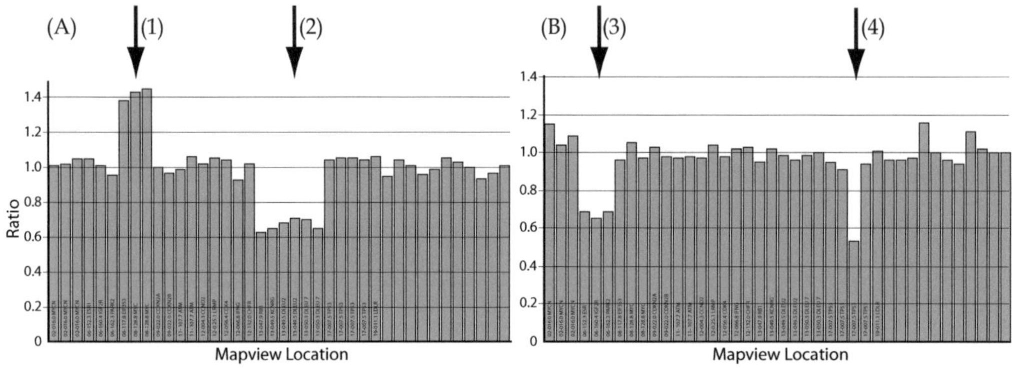

Fig. 4. Example of MLPA analysis performed in two cases of CLL (A and B).
Arrows indicate the unbalanced regions: (1) gain of 8q24 and (2) loss of 13q14 in case A, and (3) loss of 6q25 and (4) loss of exon 5 of *TP53* on 17p13 in case B. (Courtesy of M. Jarosova)

MLPA, probably due to the low percentage of leukemic cells (<30%) carrying the aberration (Fabris *et al,* 2011). The sensitivity may even be lower if no B-cell pre-enrichment is performed (i.e. aberrations not detected when the percentage of leukemic cells <50%). Moreover MLPA fails to detect concomitant mono- and biallelic losses at 13q (Fabris *et al,* 2011). However, the availability of multiple probes in MLPA allows the identification of genetic aberrations which are not incorporated in the standard FISH probe panel. In conclusion, MLPA can be used alone or in association with FISH to detect both recurrent and less frequent lesions in CLL.

2.4 Comparative genomic hybridization and single nucleotide polymorphism arrays

Very recently (2000s), comparative genomic hybridization arrays (aCGH) and single nucleotide polymorphism (SNP)-arrays have been validated as reliable tools to investigate global genetic abnormalities in CLL with a higher resolution (i.e. 200 basepairs - 10 kilobases), compared with FISH and conventional cytogenetics. Therefore, it allows to detect new, cytogenetically cryptic, recurrent chromosomal changes, such as microdeletions.

However, aCGH has shortcomings as it detects genomic imbalances, but not balanced aberrations. In contrast with aCGH, SNP-arrays have the additional advantage of detecting copy number neutral loss of heterozygosity (cnLOH) or uniparental disomy (UPD). LOH results from the loss of normal function of one allele of a gene in which the other allele has already been inactivated, whereas UPD is a cnLOH in which all copies of an allele are derived from one parent and no copies from the other parent are present. Until now, the application of aCGH and SNP-arrays is restricted to research setting, but may possibly be implemented in routine analysis of CLL in the near future. As many platforms from different companies are available and each platform has its own technical specifications, Fig 5. gives only a brief and general overview of the technique. In the next paragraphs, we will focus in detail on the main results.

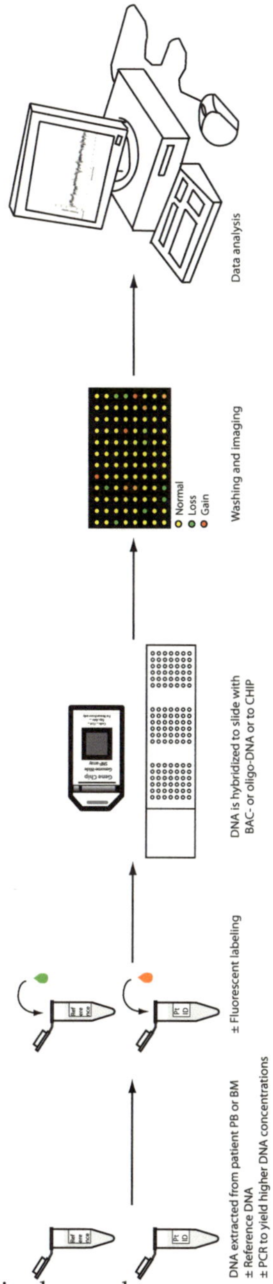

Fig. 5. Array-technology: summarized procedure.
PB, peripheral blood; BM, bone marrow; BAC, bacterial artificial chromosome

2.5 Next generation sequencing

Next-generation sequencing (NGS, also known as massively parallel sequencing) technologies have a higher throughput than traditional sequencing methods. It allows millions of sequencing reactions to happen in parallel, using different approaches, either by creating micro-reactors and/or attaching DNA molecules to solid surfaces or beads. Unlike previous methods NGS generates millions of short reads (21-400 base pairs) and does not require amplification as sequencing can be performed from a single DNA molecule. The short reads can be quantified, allowing accurate copy number assessment. Moreover, with approaches that sequence both ends of a DNA molecule (paired end massively parallel sequencing), it has become possible to detect balanced and unbalanced somatic rearrangements (i.e. fusion genes) in a genome-wide fashion. Since each type of NGS has specific artefacts, one should be aware of this phenomenon and new findings should be interpreted with caution (Reis-Filho, 2009). In addition, the high cost of the technique limits its use in (routine) practice.

3. Cytogenetic and molecular abnormalities in CLL prognosis

3.1 Five prognostically important FISH-categories

A landmark interphase FISH-study of 325 mainly untreated CLL patients identified five prognostically important hierarchical categories: 17p deletion (with or without concomitant lesions), 11q deletion (with no concomitant 17p deletion), 12 trisomy (with neither concomitant 17p- nor 11q deletion), none of these aberrations, and 13q deletion as the sole abnormality (Fig 6. and Fig 7.). Median survival times for patients in these five groups were 32, 79, 114, 111, and 133 months, respectively and the treatment-free survival was 9, 13, 33, 49 and 92 months, respectively (Döhner *et al*, 2000).

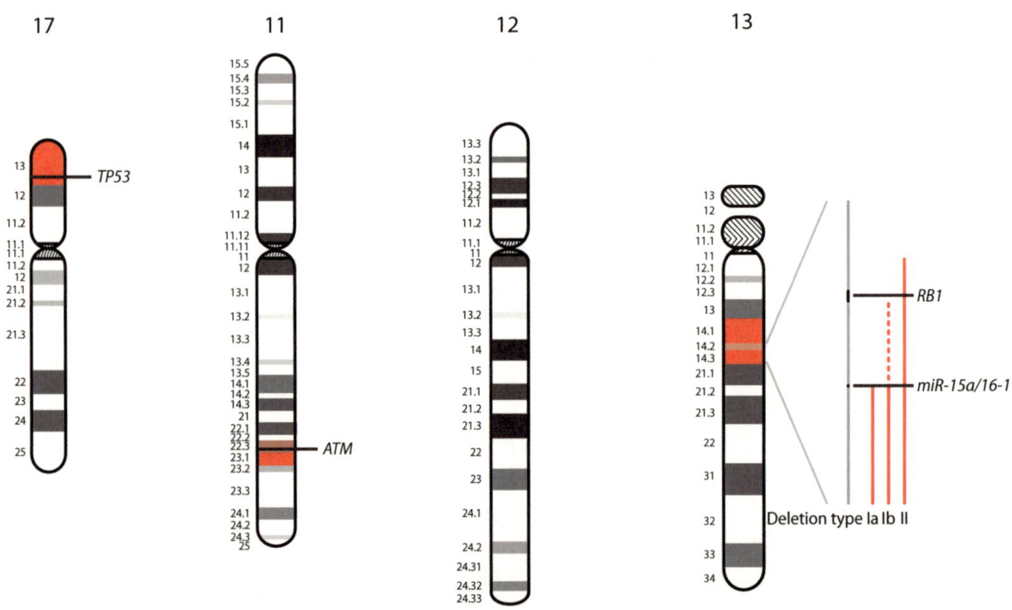

Fig. 6. Idiogram of G-banded chromosomes involved in prognostically important aberrations, at 550-band level.
Commonly deleted regions are indicated in red (caveat: deletions may be larger or smaller). Del(13q) type Ib can vary in length, as indicated by the dashed line.

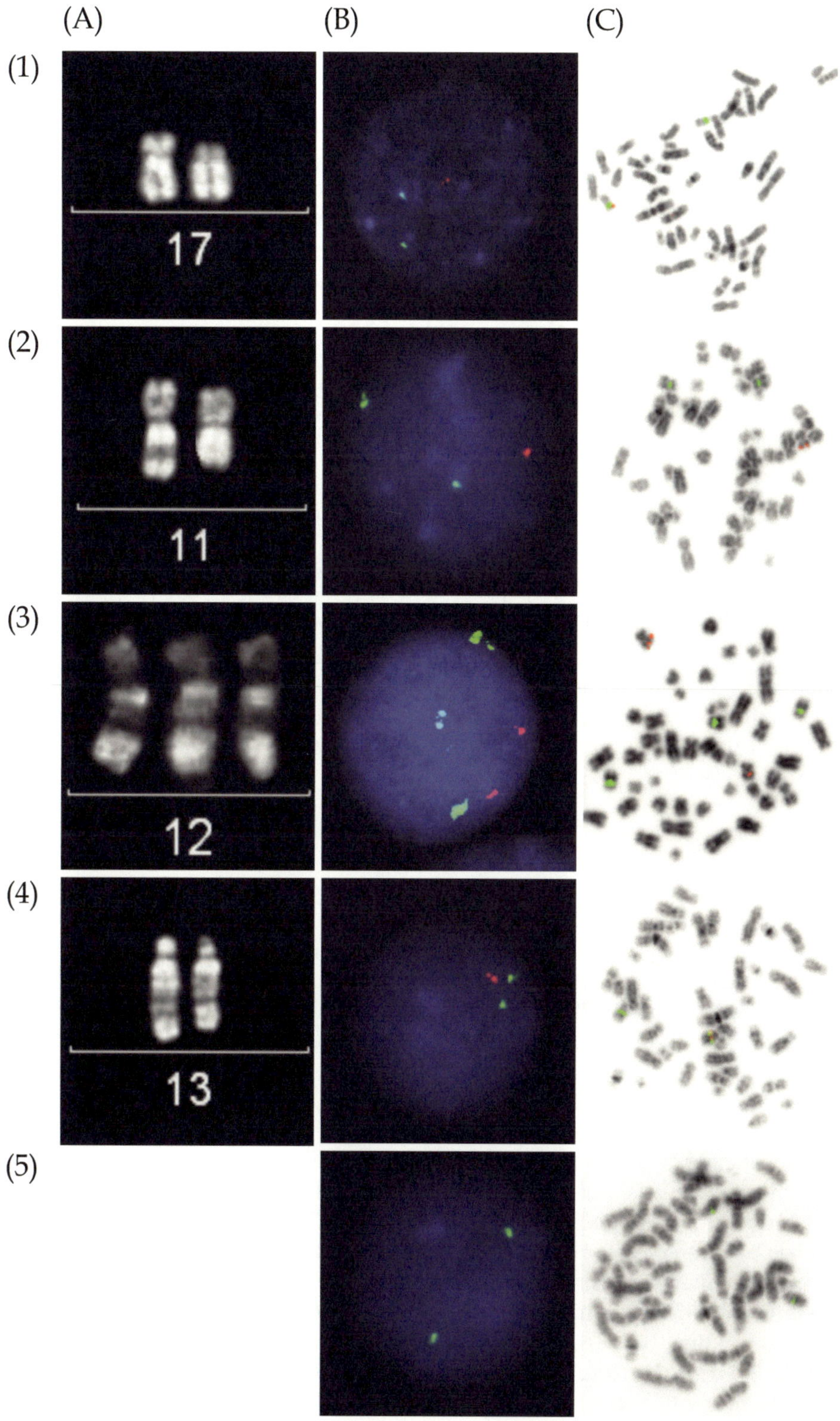
(A)
(B)
(C)
(1)
17
(2)
11
(3)
12
(4)
13
(5)

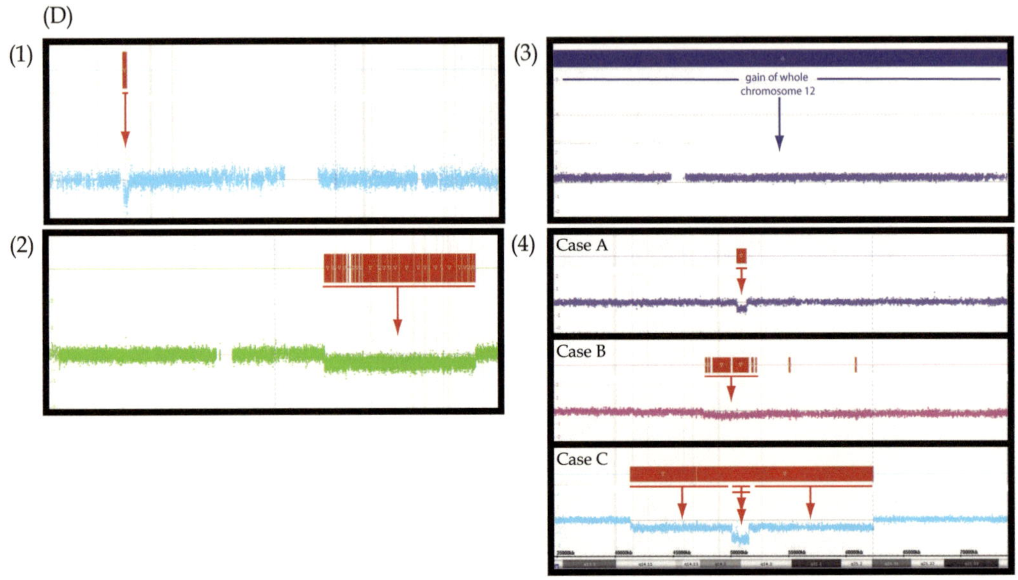

Fig. 7. Examples of the four prognostically important aberrations in CLL, namely del(17p) (1), del(11q) (2), trisomy 12 (3) and del(13q) (4, 5), as observed by CCA (A), interphase FISH (B), metaphase FISH (C) and the Affymetrix 2.7M array platform (D). Applied FISH-probes are specific for *TP53* (red) and centromere 17 (CEP17) (green) (1), for *ATM* (red) and centromere 12 (green) (2+3), for *RB1* (green) and D13S319 (red) (4+5). Note a monoallelic loss of *TP53* (B1, C1, D1 red arrow), monoallelic loss of *ATM* (B2, C2, D2 red arrow), trisomy 12 (B3, C3, D3 blue arrow), a monoallelic (B4, C4, D4 cases A+B+C, single red arrows) and biallelic del(13q) in (B5, C5, D4 case C, double red arrow).

3.1.1 17p deletions

Patients with a deletion of 17p have worst outcome. The del(17p) is found in 3-8% of previously untreated patients, although higher incidences up to 45% have been reported in patients with relapsed or refractory CLL, as a consequence of clonal selection (Cramer and Hallek, 2011; Zenz *et al*, 2011). Del(17p) usually encompasses the *TP53* locus at 17p13. A gene-dosage effect of *TP53* has been reported. About 80-90% of the cases harbor a biallelic inactivation of *TP53* (i.e. deletion of one copy and mutation of the remaining copy), but also the monoallelic inactivation of *TP53* is an adverse prognostic marker (Cramer and Hallek, 2011; Zenz *et al*, 2011). The tumor suppressor p53 plays an essential role in inducing apoptosis or cell cycle arrest after DNA damage. Since therapy with purine nucleoside analogues (e.g. fludarabine) and alkylating agents (e.g. chlorambucil) is based on p53-dependent mechanisms, CLL patients with deletion 17p or inactivating mutations of *TP53* are refractory to such chemotherapy (Van Bockstaele *et al*, 2008) and have impaired survival. A threshold of > 20-25% interphase nuclei harboring the del(17p) has been reported to correlate with adverse survival (Catovsky *et al*, 2007; Tam *et al*, 2009). Because of the very poor prognosis, risk-adapted treatment for this subgroup has been developed. Current treatment approaches (in clinical trials) use agents acting independently of p53 (e.g. alemtuzumab, high dose steroids) or allogeneic stem cell transplantation for fit patients (Zenz *et al*, 2011). In the future, optimization of the therapeutic strategies hopefully may improve outcome for this poor prognostic subgroup.

3.1.2 11q deletions

Deletions of 11q have been associated with adverse outcome. It is found in about 20% of the patients with CLL (Van Bockstaele *et al*, 2008; Zenz *et al*, 2011). The minimally deleted region (MDR) at 11q22.3-q23.1 harbors the *ATM* (ataxia telangiectasia mutated) gene. ATM is a protein that acts upstream of p53 in the DNA damage response pathway. Mutations of *ATM* have been reported in 12% of patients with CLL and in 30% of patients with del(11q) (Zenz *et al*, 2011). As not all patients with del(11q) have an *ATM* mutation (and vice versa), haplo-insufficiency of ATM or the presence of other tumor suppressor genes in the MDR can be suspected. In the patients with del(11q), the biallelic inactivation of *ATM* leads to a worse clinical outcome (Cramer and Hallek, 2011). Of note, rarely the del(11q) does not encompass *ATM*, but affects the telomerically located *FDX* locus (Heim and Mitelman, 2009). Patients with del(11q) are generally younger, have more B-symptoms and more advanced clinical stages. Furthermore, the del(11q) is typically associated with extensive lymphadenopathy (Cramer and Hallek, 2011; Van Bockstaele *et al*, 2008).

3.1.3 Trisomy 12

An intermediate outcome has been described for patients with trisomy 12. While progression free survival (PFS) may be shorter (PFS rate at 3 years of 48-83%), overall survival (OS) is rather favorable (OS rates at 3 years of 86-96%). Trisomy 12 has been associated with atypical morphology or immunophenotype (i.e. stronger surface immunoglobulin and FMC7 expression) (Zenz *et al*, 2011). The aberration is observed in 10-30% of patients (Van Bockstaele *et al*, 2008; Zenz *et al*, 2011). This variation probably reflects differences in patient selection. Partial trisomy 12q was reported in 10-20% of the cases and a minimal common gained region has been confined to 12q13 (Heim and Mitelman, 2009).

The critical genes involved in the trisomy 12 are yet unknown. Small duplications of 12q have been reported and in particular the murine double minute 2 gene (*MDM2*) located at 12q15 has been found amplified in CLL (Merup *et al*, 1997). Overexpression of the MDM2 protein was also observed in CLL and this was significantly more frequent in the advanced rather than the earlier stages (Watanabe *et al*, 1996). The MDM2 SNP309 in B-CLL has been suggested to be an unfavorable prognostic marker; however the results of several recent publications are conflicting (Willander *et al*, 2010). The CLL upregulated gene 1 (*CLLU1*) located at 12q22 was overexpressed exclusively in CLL and its expression was shown to have a strong prognostic significance in patients younger than 70 years, namely higher expression was associated with shorter overall survival (Josefsson *et al*, 2007). However overexpression of *CLLU1* occurs irrespectively of trisomy 12 or other large chromosomal rearrangements (Buhl *et al*, 2006).

Recurrent association of trisomy 12 with *IG*-aberrations, such as t(14;19)(q32;q13), t(14;18)(q32;q21) and del(14)(q24q32), and with trisomy 18 and/or trisomy 19, has been observed in a subset of cases (Heim and Mitelman, 2009). Trisomy 12 with concomitant *TP53* mutations is rare.

3.1.4 13q deletions

Although deletions of 13q are often cytogenetically cryptic, they represent the most frequently observed FISH-aberration in CLL, with a prevalence of 40-60% (Van Bockstaele *et al*, 2008). Only when present as a solitary aberration (by FISH), the del(13q) implies a favorable prognosis. Higher percentages (that is > 65% or > 80%) of interphase FISH nuclei showing the del(13q) have been associated with shorter overall survival and time to first treatment (Hernandez *et al*, 2009; Van Dyke *et al*, 2010). The MDR located at 13q14 contains *miR-15a* and *miR-16-1*. These microRNAs are small non-coding RNA genes that regulate gene expression. The *miR-15a/16-1* cluster seems to negatively regulate the expression of multiple genes involved in proliferation and apoptosis (Klein and Dalla-Favera, 2010). Deletion of the MDR-region in mice models suggested that this lesion is sufficient for lymphomagenesis. In some CLL cases without del(13q), downregulation of *miR-15a* and *miR-16-1* has been described, suggesting an epigenetic mechanism suppressing the miR-cluster (Klein and Dalla-Favera, 2010). Mutations in the miR-cluster appear to be very rare (Zenz *et al*, 2011). The del(13q) is most frequently heterozygous (monoallelic, 76% of cases), but can be homozygous (biallelic, 24% of cases). While the former is suggested to be an early event, the latter probably occurs at a later stage. A gene dosage-effect of *miR-15a/16-1* has been reported (Zenz *et al*, 2011). In addition, SNP-arrays showed that the extent of the deletion (Fig 6) is associated with disease characteristics, for example del(13q) type II (long, involving *RB1*, related with disease progression) and del(13q) type I (short, not involving *RB1*, related with disease progression only when associated with other aberrations) (Malek *et al*, 2010; Zenz *et al*, 2011).

3.2 Other cytogenetic aberrations

Several other recurrent genomic aberrations have been described in CLL, such as del(6q), del(14)(q24.1q32.33) involving *IGH* (Pospisilova *et al*, 2007), t(1;6)(p35;p25) involving *MUM1/IRF4* (Michaux *et al*, 2005), total or partial trisomy 3, trisomy 8, trisomy 18 and 19 and changes leading to gains of 2p24-25, 3q26-27, and 8q24. These aberrations are rare in CLL (prevalence < 5-10%). Most of the genes involved are not yet identified and their prognostic relevance remains to be investigated (Heim and Mitelman, 2009; Van Bockstaele *et al*, 2008).

3.3 Translocations

Translocations have been reported in up to 34-42% of patients with CLL (Mayr *et al*, 2006; Van Den Neste *et al*, 2007). Balanced translocations are relatively rare, but unbalanced non-reciprocal aberrations are frequent and are often observed within complex karyotypes. Although translocations are heterogenous in CLL, many breakpoints are located in regions showing recurrent loss, like 13q14 and 17p13 (Heim and Mitelman, 2009). Chromosomal translocations in general may have a negative impact on response to therapy and survival, especially when unbalanced (Mayr *et al*, 2006; Van Den Neste *et al*, 2007). Balanced translocations, especially those involving immunoglobulin (*IG*) genes, are recurrent, but uncommon (i.e. 5%) (Haferlach *et al*, 2007). Recurrent partners include *BCL2, BCL3, BCL11A* and *MYC* (Table 2). In published reports (Cavazzini *et al*, 2008; Nowakowski *et al*, 2007), at least part of the cases have unknown partner genes. In most studies, CLL cases with translocations involving *IG* are analyzed as a single group (Cavazzini *et al*, 2008; Juliusson *et al*, 1990). However, the partner gene that becomes overexpressed as a result of the translocation, may be relevant for the outcome. The best described is the *BCL3* gene involved in the t(14;19), often associated with atypical morphology, unmutated *IGVH* genes and inferior prognosis (Cavazzini *et al*, 2008; Chapiro *et al*, 2008; Martin-Subero *et al*, 2007; Nowakowski *et al*, 2007). Similarly, translocations involving *MYC* have been associated with loss (i.e. monosomy) of 17, del(11q) complex karyotype, additional unbalanced translocations and poor prognosis (Put *et al*, 2011). In contrast, translocations involving *BCL2* are associated with mutated *IGVH* genes, trisomy 12, absence of del(11q) and more favorable outcome (Put *et al*, 2009b).

Translocation[a,b]	Partner Gene	Morphology	*IGVH*	Associated changes	Prognosis
t(2;14)(p16;q32)	*BCL11a*	Atypical	U > M	Trisomy 12	Uncertain
t(8;14)(q24;q32)	*MYC*	PL / PT	U ≈ M	Monosomy 17p Del(11q) Complex karyotype Unbalanced translocations	Poor
t(14;18)(q32;q21)	*BCL2*	Typical	M > U	Trisomy 12 Absence of del(11q)	Favorable
t(14;19)(q32;q21)	*BCL3*	Atypical	U > M	Trisomy 12	Poor

PL, prolymphocyte; PT, prolymphocytic transformation; U, unmutated; M, mutated
[a]*IG*-translocations involve most frequently *IGH* located on 14q32. Variant translocations involve either *IGK* on 2p12 or *IGL* on 22q11
[b] To date, most cases with t(11;14)(q13;q32), involving *CCND1*, are diagnosed as mantle cell lymphoma; however, rare cases of t(11;14)-positive CLL might exist.

Table 1. Overview of translocations involving immunoglobulin (*IG*)-genes in CLL

3.4 Genomic complexity

Cytogenetic complexity is defined as the presence of three or more clonal chromosomal aberrations. CCA was found to be superior in the detection of complexity, compared with FISH (Haferlach *et al*, 2007), probably due to the limited number of investigated loci in the latter approach. Complexity is found in a minority of the cases with CLL (10-30%) (Haferlach *et al*, 2007; Kujawski *et al*, 2008). A highly significant association was observed between complex aberrant karyotypes and 17p deletions, unmutated *IGVH* and expression of CD38 (Haferlach *et al*, 2007). In addition, particular aberrations (i.e. translocations involving *MYC*) have also been associated with a complex aberrant karyotype (Put *et al*, unpublished data). Prognostically, patients with complex genomic changes appear to have more aggressive disease. Similarly, genomic complexity detected by SNP-arrays (≥ 3 genetic lesions) has been associated with poor outcome (Kujawski *et al*, 2008). An impaired apoptotic DNA double-strand break response and multiple genomic deletions, including del(17p), del(11q), and del(13q) type II were identified as independent strong predictors of genomic complexity in CLL. Moreover, a strong independent effect of aberrant p53 function on genomic complexity and a modest effect of decreased ATM function have been observed (Ouillette *et al*, 2010). Such multiple independent gene defects in CLL may contribute to genomic instability. In addition, telomere dysfunction as a consequence of telomere erosion may also drive genomic instability during the progression of CLL (Lin *et al*, 2010). Indeed, short telomeres have been associated with a high risk of genomic aberrations and genetic complexity (Roos *et al*, 2008).

3.5 Clonal evolution

Clonal evolution (CE) represents the acquisition of new or additional cytogenetic aberrations during disease course. As a consequence, CCA or FISH should not only be used for initial prognostication of patients with CLL, but also at the time of disease progression or before therapy initiation [FISH is mandatory in this setting for detection of del(17p)]. Initially, CE as evaluated by sequential CCA, was considered infrequent, i.e. in 16% of CLL patients (Oscier *et al*, 1991). Later studies reported higher frequencies of 25-43% (Fegan *et al*, 1995; Finn *et al*, 1998; Haferlach *et al*, 2007). Interphase FISH studies (Table 2) revealed CE in 27% and 17% after a median follow-up of more than 5 years and 42.3 months, respectively (Shanafelt *et al*, 2006;

Stilgenbauer *et al*, 2007). Interestingly, CE occurred more frequently among cases with unmutated *IGVH* status (Shanafelt *et al*, 2006; Stilgenbauer *et al*, 2007). However, another study did not find a correlation between CE and unmutated *IGVH*, expression of CD38 and ZAP70 on one hand, but the combination of all three prognostic factors correlated highly significantly with CE and with a shift from lower to higher FISH risk category (Berkova *et al*, 2009). Patients with CE showed progression to more advanced stages, greater need for therapy and a higher hazard ratio for death. Moreover, CE was identified as an independent factor for survival (Stilgenbauer *et al*, 2007). As a consequence, CCA or FISH should not only be used for initial prognostication of patients with CLL, but also at the time of disease progression or before therapy initiation [FISH is mandatory in this setting for detection of del(17p)]

Reference	CLL Patients (n)	Follow-up (months)	CE: patients (n)	CE: previously treated patients (n)	CE: abnormalities	Other findings
Shanafelt *et al*, 2006	108[a]	67 (23-136)	18 (11%)	13 (71%)	del(13q) (72%) > del(17p) (22%) > del(11q) (6%)	CE not confined to unmutated *IGVH* (association ns) Correlation between ZAP70+ and CE CE more frequent after 50 months compared with before 24 months (27% vs. <2%, respectively)
Stilgenbauer *et al*, 2007	64	42 (23-73)	11 (17%)	1 (9%)	del(17p) (36%) > del(13q) = del(6q) (27%) > del(11q) (18%) > +8q24 (9%)	CE confined to unmutated *IGVH* CE correlates with progressive clinical stages, greater need for therapy, higher hazard ratio for death CE as independent factor for survival
Berkova *et al*, 2009	97	66 (22-304)	25 (26%)	7 (28%)	del(13q) (64%) > del(17p) = del(11q) (16%) > trisomy 12 (4%)	Combination of unmutated *IGVH*, CD38+ and ZAP70+ correlates highly significantly with CE and with a shift from lower to higher FISH risk category
Loscertales *et al*, 2010	81	67 (16-111)	17 (21%)	13 (76%)	del(17p) (53%) > del(11q) (35%)	CE not confined to unmutated *IGVH* del(17p) observed in untreated patients

N, number; CE, clonal evolution; ns, not significant,
[a]Sequential samples were available in 108/159 patients.

Table 2. Overview of clonal evolution investigated by FISH

3.6 Molecular karyotyping

The introduction of aCGH and SNP-arrays enables to investigate CLL at a resolution, greatly surpassing this of conventional cytogenetics. Different array-platforms were validated as a powerful, cost-effective tool for clinical risk assessment in CLL (Table 3) (Gunn *et al*, 2008; Hagenkord *et al*, 2010; O'Malley *et al*, 2011). Of note, the sensitivity of these platforms varies and is related to i.e. the resolution of the array. For example, the Affymetrix SNP6.0 array was found to be superior to the 250K array in detecting small aberrations of uncertain significance and equivalent to the 250K array in detecting clinically relevant lesions. Since the cost of the 250K array is lower, it is preferred for routine use. In contrast, the 10K array is not suitable for routine clinical use due to its low resolution (Hagenkord *et al*, 2010).

New recurrent cytogenetic abnormalities were detected by aCGH and SNP-arrays. In Table 3 an overview of selected publications on array-applications in CLL is shown, describing known prognostically important lesions and new molecular cytogenetic findings (Grubor et al, 2009;

Gunn et al, 2008; Gunn et al, 2009; Gunnarsson et al, 2008; Gunnarsson et al, 2010; Gunnarsson et al, 2011; Hagenkord et al, 2010; Kay et al, 2010; Kujawski et al, 2008; Lehmann et al, 2008; O'Malley et al, 2011; Ouillette et al, 2010; Ouillette et al, 2011; Pfeifer et al, 2007; Rinaldi et al, 2011). Other recent studies using array-platforms revealed new insights in the disease: i.e. the genome of CLL appeared to be quite stable over time (Brown et al, 2010); disease progression has been associated with large, but not small copy number alterations (Gunnarsson *et al*, 2010), genomic complexity, 13q deletion in the presence of other aberrations, and 13q deletion type II (that is, deletions involving *RB1*) (Malek *et al*, 2010).

Reference	Array	Patients (n)	17	11	12	13	Other highlighted abnormalities	LOH/CN LOH	Remarks
Pfeifer *et al*, 2007	10K and 50K Affymetrix	70	5.7%	12.8%	12.8%	51.4%	Gain of 2p16 (n=4; *REL, BCL11a*)	14 patients with 24 large CN LOH > 10 Mb	Recombination hot spots on both sides of *mir15a/16-1* Slower lymphocyte growth kinetics for monoallelic vs. biallelic del(13q14)
Lehman *et al*, 2008	50K Affymetrix	56	5%	9%	7%	59%	Loss of 6q21 (n=4; *AIM1*)	4 patients with UPD	Genetic abnormalities of chr 13 (including UPD) are very common events in early stage CLL
Ouillette *et al*, 2008	50K Affymetrix	171	NA	NA	NA	48%	NA	5 patients with CN LOH of 13q14: 4 with extensive LOH but copy loss restricted to a small area at ~D13S319 and 1 without any LOH-associated copy loss (UPD)	Del(13q14) is heterogeneous Type Ia lesions are uniform with one breakpoint close to the *mir15a/16-1* cluster Type I lesions correlate with higher *LATS2* RNA levels *PHLPP* RNA is absent in 50% of del(13q14) 15% CLL have reduced *mir15a/16-1* expression
Kujawski *et al*, 2008	50K Affymetrix	178	7-13%[a]	8-13%[a]	14-28%[a]	46-28%[a,b]	≥ 2, ≥2.5, or ≥3 genomic lesions in 35%, 19%, and 15% of patients, respectively	10 patients with UPD	Genomic complexity as an independent risk factor for short TTT in multivariate analysis
Gunn *et al*, 2008	44K Agilent	174	4.6%	11%	13%	47%	Gain of 2p (n=5; *NMYC in 5/5, REL and BCL11a* in 4/5 cases). del(5q) (n=3), del(2q) (n=2), del(8p) (n=2), gain of 8q (n=3), gain of whole-chr 19 (n=1) and 22 (n=3).	NA	Genomic instability (i.e. ≥3 loci not investigated by FISH panels) was observed in 21% of the cases.
Gunnarsson *et al*, 2008	32K BAC, 185K Agilent, 250K Affymetrix, and 317K Illumina	10	20%	10%	20%	40%	NA	Concordance of large regions; smaller regions escaping detection	All platforms detect large CNAs, however findings are discrepant for small CNAs
Gunn *et al*, 2009	CA1000 microarrays BAC array (Combimatrix Molecular Diagnostics)	187	NA	NA	NA	NA	Loss of 22q11 (n=28; *ZNF280A, ZNF280B, GGTLC2, and PRAME*)	NA	
Grubor *et al*, 2009	85K and 390K NimbleGen (ROMA)	58	5%	10%	17%	40%	Loss of 8p21.2-p12 (n=2; *TRIM35), 2q37.1 (n=2; SP100/110/140), 9p21.3 [n2; CDKN2A (P16-INK4)] and 18q23 (n=2; NFATC1)*	NA	CNA differences between CD38+ and CD38− cell fractions (3/4 cases)

Table 3. Overview of selected publications on genomic array-applications in CLL

Kay *et al*, 2010	1M Agilent	48	6.3%	12.5%	23%	52%	Loss of 3p21, 8p11, 10q24, 11q22, 14q24 (all aberrations present in n≥3)	NA	Higher genomic complexity (> 15 CNAs or ≥66 Mb length) associated with shorter PFS, poor response to therapy Loss of p53 function [in pt with del(17p) or del(13q)] was associated with a complex genome
Hagenkord *et al*, 2010	10K, 250K and SNP 6.0 Affymetrix	33	NA	NA	NA	55%	Atypical loss of 11q (n=5; not including *ATM*) and 13q (n=1; not including *mir15a/16-1*)	4 patients with UPD: at 17p13 (n=1), 11q22 (n=1), and13q14 (n=2)	
Gunnarsson *et al*, 2010	250K Affymetrix	203	4.4%	13%	11%	54%	Loss of 4p (n=3), 8p (n=3), gain of 8q (n=5), combination of gain of 2p (2p24.3) and loss of 11q (n=5)	All CN regions included a homozygous del(13q)	Genomic complexity (increasing number of CNAs >5 Mb) as a poor-prognostic marker, although a complex genome often included del(17p) and del(11q)
Gunnarsson *et al*, 2011	250K Affymetrix	369+59[c]	4%	10%	10.5%	55%	Acquisition of aberrations of 6q, 8p, 9p and 10q (i.e. clonal evolution) were exclusively associated with UM *IGHV*	CN LOH on 13q in 3.5%, most with homozygous del(13q)	Genomic complexity (associated with poor prognostic aberrations) and large 13q deletions correlate with inferior outcome CE correlates with poor prognostic markers and commonly includes the known recurrent aberrations
O'Malley *et al*, 2011	HemeScan® BAC (Combimatrix Molecular Diagnostics)	55	11%	9%	25%	46%	Loss of 6q (n=3), 8p (n=4), 10q (n=2), 14q32 (n=14), 18q (n=4) and gain of 10q (n=2)	NA	
Rinaldi *et al*, 2011	SNP 6.0 Affymetrix	148	10%	10%	19%[d]	50%	Gains at 2p25.3-p22.3 (n=5; *NMYC*), 2p22.3 (n=5), 2p16.2-p14 (n=5; *REL*), 8q23.3-q24.3 (n=7; *MYC*), losses at 8p23.1-p21.2 (n=7), 8p21.2 (n=7), 17p13.3-p11.2 (n=15), and 17p12-p11.2 (n=22)	NA	Gains at 2p and 8q and *TP53* inactivation showed prognostic significance (multivariate analysis, confirmed in a hierarchical model) Gains at 2p determined a higher risk of Richter transformation. Gains at 2p and 8q proposed as relevant novel genomic regions for prognostic stratification
Ouillette *et al*, 2011	SNP 6.0 Affymetrix	255	10%	10%	17%	51%	Loss at chr 6 (n=7), 8p (n=7), 10q (n=10), 14q (n=9), 18q (n=8), gains at 8q (n=5), 17q (n=6), and 18p (n=6). Recurrent biallelic losses on chr 9 (n=2; *P16/ CDKN2A*) and chr X (n=2).	In the group of CLL with elevated array-based genomic complexity, 3 patients had acquired 17p-UPD	≥3 subchromosomal aCNA were detected in 20% of the cases. Genomic complexity was identified as an independent and powerful marker for the identification of CLL patients with aggressive disease and short survival

Table 3 (continued).
17, Del(17p); 11, Del(11q); 12, Trisomy 12; 13, Del(13q); NA, not available; LOH, loss of heterozygosity; CN, copy number neutral; UPD, uniparental disomy; UM, unmutated; M, mutated; *IGVH*, immunoglobulin heavy chain mutational status; CGH, comparative genomic hybridization; TTT, time to treatment; CNA, copy number alteration; PFS, progression-free survival; CE, clonal evolution;
[a]Untreated – treated patients, respectively;
[b]Solitary del(13q) only;
[c]At diagnosis + at follow-up, respectively;
[d]Lowest frequency of (partial) gain of 12q

3.7 Next generation sequencing

Whole genome sequencing of cases with CLL led to the discovery of several genes, previously unsuspected to be involved in this disease. For example, combining NGS and copy number analysis in 5 patients, < 20 clonal genomic alterations/case and recurrent mutations of *NOTCH1, TGM7, BIRC3,* and *PLEKHG5* were observed (Fabbri *et al,* 2011). Lesions of *MYD88, BIRC3,* and *PLEKHG5* are all linked to alteration of the NF-κβ pathway. In a screening cohort of 48 CLL cases, *NOTCH1* mutations were found in 8.3% of CLL cases at diagnosis and were associated with aggressive disease (i.e. higher frequency of *NOTCH1* mutations were associated with Richter transformation and refractoriness to chemotherapy, in 31.0% and 20.8% of the cases, respectively). Moreover *NOTCH1* mutation at diagnosis emerged as an independent risk factor for poor survival (Fabbri *et al,* 2011). Another NGS and exome sequencing study identified four genes that were recurrently mutated, namely *NOTCH1, XPO1* predominantly in CLL with unmutated *IGVH,* and *MYD88* and *KLHL6* in CLL with mutated *IGVH* status (Puente *et al,* 2011). *NOTCH1, XPO1* and *MYD88* mutations are suspected to be oncogenic changes, contributing to disease progression, based on their patterns of mutation and functional analyses, (Puente *et al,* 2011). In conclusion, NGS appears to be a highly effective technique in identifying new genetic lesions and future studies are promising to contribute to an improved understanding of disease onset and evolution.

4. The origin of cytogenetic abnormalities

Genomic imbalances, such as gains and losses of chromosome segments or whole chromosomes (aneuploidy), are more frequently observed than translocations in CLL. However, in the following paragraphs we will focus mainly on the origin of translocations, in particular translocations involving *IG* loci, as the underlying mechanisms are quite specific for lymphoid malignancies, i.e. CLL.

4.1 The origin of aneuploidy and structural aberrations

Aneuploidy may arise due to defects in segregation of chromosomes during cell division, including multipolar spindles, but also abnormal kinetochore-spindle interactions, premature chromatid separation, centrosome amplification, and abnormal cytokinesis. Defects of centrosome function in particular have been suggested to be involved in a wide variety of human malignancies. Centrosomes have central role in organizing microtubuli and the mitotic spindle. An aberrant number, size, shape of the centrosome, as well as aberrant phosphorylation of centrosome proteins, may missegregate chromosomes, resulting in aneuploid cells. In addition, errors in the separation of sister chromatids could also be a cause of aneuploidy. Finally, checkpoint controls are expected to be abrogated in order to enable unequal chromosome segregation during cell cycle progression (Gollin, 2004; Schwab, 2001).

Structural chromosomal instability results from chromosome breakage and rearrangement due to defects in the cell cycle checkpoints, the DNA damage response and/or loss of telomere integrity (Gollin, 2004). When a chromatid break occurs, an unprotected chromosomal end will probably fuse with either another broken chromatid or its sister chromatid to produce a dicentric chromosome. During the anaphase, the two centromeres are pulled to opposite poles, forming a bridge that breaks, resulting in more unprotected chromosomal ends, thus resulting in breakage-fusion-bridge cycles. Telomere mechanics, defects in DNA damage response and cell cycle checkpoint may play important roles in the development and maintenance of chromosomal instability (Gollin, 2004).

4.2 The origin of translocations

Recurrent translocations in CLL often involve *IG* loci. These translocations may follow DNA double strand breaks (DSBs) that are generated during V(D)J recombination (i.e. recombination of Variable, Diversity, and Joining segments of *IG*-genes) and somatic hypermutation (SHM) in developing B-cells and in the context of class switch recombination (CSR) in activated mature B-cells. DSBs in the partner loci may be generated by off-target VDJ recombination, CSR activities or may result from more general factors, such as oxidative metabolism or genotoxic agents. Misrepair of these DSBs can promote oncogenic translocations. When a translocation involves oncogenes or tumor suppressor genes, it can be positively selected in the context of neoplastic transformation. Selection likely plays the main role in the appearance of most clonal translocations in tumors (Gostissa *et al*, 2011).

4.2.1 VDJ recombination and RAG-mediated DSB

The complete VDJ recombination involves RAG-mediated cleavage, which generates DSBs, and the DSB repair pathway "classical nonhomologous DNA end-joining" (C-NHEJ). The latter promotes chromosomal integrity and suppresses the formation of translocations. In the absence of C-NHEJ, DSBs still can be joined by alternative end-joining (A-EJ), a process that contributes to oncogenic chromosomal translocations (Gostissa *et al*, 2011; Nussenzweig and Nussenzweig, 2010).

4.2.2 SHM, CSR and AID-mediated DSB

Although representing different processes, SHM and CSR are both initiated by AID (Gostissa *et al*, 2011; Perez-Duran *et al*, 2007). SHM generates point mutations, small deletions and insertions in variable region exons. This occurs in the germinal centers (GCs) and allows the selection of B-cells that express higher affinity B-cell receptors. CSR can also occur within the GC, as well as in extrafollicular regions (Gostissa *et al*, 2011).

AID initiates both SHM and CSR in B-cells by deaminating cytosines on the DNA of *IG* genes. The generated lesion can be processed into a mutation (SHM) or a DSB followed by a recombination reaction (CSR) (Perez-Duran *et al*, 2007). CSR requires the generation of AID-initiated DSBs. In contrast, SHM generally does not require DSBs. The latter are only occasionally generated as by-products of AID activity (Gostissa *et al*, 2011). It has been suggested that AID may have a dual role; initiating chromosomal translocations on one hand and generating secondary hits by mutagenesis on the other (Perez-Duran *et al*, 2007). Aberrant SHM and involvement of AID were reported to be involved in mutations of *TP53* (Malcikova et al, 2008), *MYC*, *PAX5* and *RhoH* (Reiniger et al, 2006). Moreover, AID activity has been linked to the generation of DSBs involved in translocations in both *IG* and non-*IG* loci (Gostissa *et al*, 2011). While AID was shown to initiate the formation of translocations and mutations, ATM, p53 and ARF provide surveillance mechanisms to prevent these aberrations (Perez-Duran *et al*, 2007).

AID expression results from interaction with an activated microenvironment. In a study of CLL patients with unmutated *IGVH*, high AID expression was found exclusively in the small subset of cells with ongoing CSR (Palacios *et al*, 2010). In addition, in CLL and small lymphocytic lymphoma, AID expression has been associated with unfavorable clinical course and with adverse biological parameters, i.e. higher proliferation rate, deletion of *ATM* and *TP53* (Leuenberger *et al*, 2010). AID expression has been considered to be predictive for CLL with unmutated *IGVH* status (Palacios *et al*, 2010). However, in other reports the association of AID expression and *IGVH* mutational status is considered controversial (Leuenberger *et al*, 2010).

4.2.3 Combined action of RAG and AID

In conclusion, RAG and AID can generate DSBs leading to translocations via VDJ recombination and CSR, respectively. RAG and AID are usually expressed in distinct B-cell developmental compartments. Activity of RAG has been observed in developing bone marrow B-cells, whereas AID activity has been found in peripheral mature B-cells. Breakpoint sequences can provide information regarding the developmental stage at which the translocation occurred (Gostissa *et al*, 2011; Nussenzweig and Nussenzweig, 2010). However, collaboration between RAG and AID in generating translocations has been reported. RAG induced DSBs can persist in the absence of ATM, an essential DNA damage checkpoint regulator, or in absence of the NHEJ factor XRCC4, leading to abnormal or delayed repair of RAG-mediated DSBs. In addition, AID may facilitate off-target DSB formation by RAG. As a consequence RAG and AID-mediated DSBs may coexist and become partners in translocation formation (Nussenzweig and Nussenzweig, 2010). Finally, not all DSBs that are precursors of translocations in lymphomas appear to be initiated by RAG or AID (Gostissa *et al*, 2011). The mechanism(s) involved herein remain largely unknown.

4.2.4 Oncogene activation

Most recurrent translocations activate oncogenes, either by generating oncogenic fusion proteins or by deregulating oncogene expression by linking it to strong transcriptional control elements. The *IGH* locus contains two known major transcriptional enhancer regions: the intronic enhancer (iEμ), which promotes optimal VDJ recombination in developing B-cells and the IGH 3' regulatory region (IGH3'RR), which modulates CSR in mature B-cells by long-range (over 100 kb) activation of certain promoters. The IgH3'RR does not gain full enhancer activity until late in B-cell development. It was reported that iEμ has low oncogenic activity, suggesting that VDJ-mediated translocations that retain iEμ near the translocation breakpoint may arise in early B-cell developmental stages but remain oncogenically silent until the IgH3'RR becomes fully active at the mature B-cell stage. Alternatively, the development of mature B-cell tumors from cells carrying VDJ-mediated translocations might reflect the time required for the accumulation of secondary mutations necessary for transformation. Another explanation is that translocations may be generated directly in mature B-cells, either by persisting VDJ breaks arisen at the pro-B-cell stage or by RAG-mediated breaks in peripheral B-cells (Gostissa *et al*, 2011).

5. Acknowledgements

N. Put is supported by Fonds voor Wetenschappelijk Onderzoek (FWO) Vlaanderen - Research Foundation Flanders. P. Vandenberghe is a senior clinical investigator of FWO Vlaanderen. We thank E. Van Den Neste and A. Hagemeijer for critical reading of this manuscript.

6. References

Barragan, M., Bellosillo, B., Campas, C., Colomer, D., Pons, G. & Gil, J. (2002) Involvement of Protein Kinase C and Phosphatidylinositol 3-Kinase Pathways in the Survival of B-Cell Chronic Lymphocytic Leukemia Cells. *Blood,* Vol.99, No.8, (Apr) 2969-2976

Berkova, A., Zemanova, Z., Trneny, M., Schwarz, J., Karban, J., Cmunt, E., et al. (2009) Clonal Evolution in Chronic Lymphocytic Leukemia Studied by Interphase Fluorescence in-Situ Hybridization. *Neoplasma,* Vol.56, No.5, (Febr) 455-458

Brown, J.R., Hanna, M., Tesar, B., Werner, L., Reynolds, H., Fernandes, S.M., et al. (2010) High Resolution Genomic Analysis in CLL Demonstrates Genomic Stability in Untreated Patients and Novel Markers of Progression in Treated Patients. *ASH Annual Meeting Abstracts,* Vol.116, No.21, (Nov) 2426

Buhl, A.M., Jurlander, J., Jorgensen, F.S., Ottesen, A.M., Cowland, J.B., Gjerdrum, L.M., et al. (2006) Identification of a Gene on Chromosome 12q22 Uniquely Overexpressed in Chronic Lymphocytic Leukemia. *Blood,* Vol.107, No.7, (Apr) 2904-2911

Buhmann, R., Kurzeder, C., Rehklau, J., Westhaus, D., Bursch, S., Hiddemann, W., et al. (2002) CD40L Stimulation Enhances the Ability of Conventional Metaphase Cytogenetics to Detect Chromosome Aberrations in B-Cell Chronic Lymphocytic Leukaemia Cells. *Br J Haematol,* Vol.118, No.4, (Sep) 968-975

Carlsson, M., Totterman, T.H., Matsson, P. & Nilsson, K. (1988) Cell Cycle Progression of B-Chronic Lymphocytic Leukemia Cells Induced to Differentiate by TPA. *Blood,* Vol.71, No.2, (Feb) 415-421

Catovsky, D., Richards, S., Matutes, E., Oscier, D., Dyer, M.J., Bezares, R.F., et al. (2007) Assessment of Fludarabine Plus Cyclophosphamide for Patients with Chronic Lymphocytic Leukaemia (the LRF CLL4 Trial): A Randomised Controlled Trial. *Lancet,* Vol.370, No.9583, (Jul) 230-239

Cavazzini, F., Hernandez, J.A., Gozzetti, A., Russo Rossi, A., De Angeli, C., Tiseo, R., et al. (2008) Chromosome 14q32 Translocations Involving the Immunoglobulin Heavy Chain Locus in Chronic Lymphocytic Leukaemia Identify a Disease Subset with Poor Prognosis. *Br J Haematol,* Vol.142, No.4, (Aug) 529-537

Chapiro, E., Radford-Weiss, I., Bastard, C., Luquet, I., Lefebvre, C., Callet-Bauchu, E., et al. (2008) The Most Frequent t(14;19)(q32;q13)-Positive B-Cell Malignancy Corresponds to an Aggressive Subgroup of Atypical Chronic Lymphocytic Leukemia. *Leukemia,* Vol.22, No. (May) 2123-2127

Chiorazzi, N. (2007) Cell Proliferation and Death: Forgotten Features of Chronic Lymphocytic Leukemia B Cells. *Best Pract Res Clin Haematol,* Vol.20, No.3, (Sep) 399-413

Coll-Mulet, L., Santidrian, A.F., Cosialls, A.M., Iglesias-Serret, D., de Frias, M., Grau, J., et al. (2008) Multiplex Ligation-Dependent Probe Amplification for Detection of

Genomic Alterations in Chronic Lymphocytic Leukaemia. *Br J Haematol,* Vol.142, No.5, (Sep) 793-801

Cramer, P. & Hallek, M. (2011) Prognostic Factors in Chronic Lymphocytic Leukemia-What Do We Need to Know? *Nat Rev Clin Oncol,* Vol.8, No.1, (Jan) 38-47

Dicker, F., Schnittger, S., Haferlach, T., Kern, W. & Schoch, C. (2006) Immunostimulatory Oligonucleotide-Induced Metaphase Cytogenetics Detect Chromosomal Aberrations in 80% of CLL Patients: A Study of 132 CLL Cases with Correlation to Fish, *IGVH* Status, and CD38 Expression. *Blood,* Vol.108, No.9, (November 2006) 3152-3160

Döhner, H., Stilgenbauer, S., Benner, A., Leupolt, E., Krober, A., Bullinger, L., et al. (2000) Genomic Aberrations and Survival in Chronic Lymphocytic Leukemia. *N Engl J Med,* Vol.343, No.26, (Dec) 1910-1916

Fabbri, G., Rasi, S., Rossi, D., Trifonov, V., Khiabanian, H., Ma, J., et al. (2011) Analysis of the Chronic Lymphocytic Leukemia Coding Genome: Role of *NOTCH1* Mutational Activation. *J Exp Med,* Vol.208, No.7, (Jul) 1389-1401

Fabris, S., Scarciolla, O., Morabito, F., Cifarelli, R.A., Dininno, C., Cutrona, G., et al. (2011) Multiplex Ligation-Dependent Probe Amplification and Fluorescence in Situ Hybridization to Detect Chromosomal Abnormalities in Chronic Lymphocytic Leukemia: A Comparative Study. *Genes Chromosomes Cancer,* Vol.50, No.9, (Jun) 726-734

Fegan, C., Robinson, H., Thompson, P., Whittaker, J.A. & White, D. (1995) Karyotypic Evolution in CLL: Identification of a New Sub-Group of Patients with Deletions of 11q and Advanced or Progressive Disease. *Leukemia,* Vol.9, No.12, (Dec) 2003-2008

Finn, W.G., Kay, N.E., Kroft, S.H., Church, S. & Peterson, L.C. (1998) Secondary Abnormalities of Chromosome 6q in B-Cell Chronic Lymphocytic Leukemia: A Sequential Study of Karyotypic Instability in 51 Patients. *Am J Hematol,* Vol.59, No.3, (Nov) 223-229

Gollin, S.M. (2004) Chromosomal Instability. *Curr Opin Oncol,* Vol.16, No.1, (Jan) 25-31

Gostissa, M., Alt, F.W. & Chiarle, R. (2011) Mechanisms That Promote and Suppress Chromosomal Translocations in Lymphocytes. *Annu Rev Immunol,* Vol.29, (Apr) 319-350

Grubor, V., Krasnitz, A., Troge, J.E., Meth, J.L., Lakshmi, B., Kendall, J.T., et al. (2009) Novel Genomic Alterations and Clonal Evolution in Chronic Lymphocytic Leukemia Revealed by Representational Oligonucleotide Microarray Analysis (ROMA). *Blood,* Vol.113, No.6, (Feb) 1294-1303

Gunn, S.R., Bolla, A.R., Barron, L.L., Gorre, M.E., Mohammed, M.S., Bahler, D.W., et al. (2009) Array CGH Analysis of Chronic Lymphocytic Leukemia Reveals Frequent Cryptic Monoallelic and Biallelic Deletions of Chromosome 22q11 That Include the *PRAME* Gene. *Leuk Res,* Vol.33, No.9, (Sep) 1276-1281

Gunn, S.R., Mohammed, M.S., Gorre, M.E., Cotter, P.D., Kim, J., Bahler, D.W., et al. (2008) Whole-Genome Scanning by Array Comparative Genomic Hybridization as a Clinical Tool for Risk Assessment in Chronic Lymphocytic Leukemia. *J Mol Diagn,* Vol.10, No.5, (Sep) 442-451

Gunnarsson, R., Isaksson, A., Mansouri, M., Goransson, H., Jansson, M., Cahill, N., et al. (2010) Large but Not Small Copy-Number Alterations Correlate to High-Risk Genomic Aberrations and Survival in Chronic Lymphocytic Leukemia: A High-

Resolution Genomic Screening of Newly Diagnosed Patients. *Leukemia,* Vol.24, No.1, (Jan) 211-215

Gunnarsson, R., Mansouri, L., Isaksson, A., Goransson, H., Cahill, N., Jansson, M., et al. (2011) Array-Based Genomic Screening at Diagnosis and Follow-up in Chronic Lymphocytic Leukemia. *Haematologica,* Vol.96, No.8, (Aug), 1161-1169

Gunnarsson, R., Staaf, J., Jansson, M., Ottesen, A.M., Goransson, H., Liljedahl, U., et al. (2008) Screening for Copy-Number Alterations and Loss of Heterozygosity in Chronic Lymphocytic Leukemia--a Comparative Study of Four Differently Designed, High Resolution Microarray Platforms. *Genes Chromosomes Cancer,* Vol.47, No.8, (Aug) 697-711

Haferlach, C., Dicker, F., Schnittger, S., Kern, W. & Haferlach, T. (2007) Comprehensive Genetic Characterization of CLL: A Study on 506 Cases Analysed with Chromosome Banding Analysis, Interphase FISH, IGV(H) Status and Immunophenotyping. *Leukemia,* Vol.21, No.12, (December 2007) 2442-2451

Hagenkord, J.M., Monzon, F.A., Kash, S.F., Lilleberg, S., Xie, Q. & Kant, J.A. (2010) Array-Based Karyotyping for Prognostic Assessment in Chronic Lymphocytic Leukemia: Performance Comparison of 10K2.0, 250K Nsp, and SNP6.0 arrays *J Mol Diagn,* Vol.12, No.2, (Mar) 184-196

Hallaert, D.Y., Jaspers, A., van Noesel, C.J., van Oers, M.H., Kater, A.P. & Eldering, E. (2008) c-Abl Kinase Inhibitors Overcome CD40-Mediated Drug Resistance in CLL: Implications for Therapeutic Targeting of Chemoresistant Niches. *Blood,* Vol.112, No.13, (Dec) 5141-5149

Hallek, M., Cheson, B.D., Catovsky, D., Caligaris-Cappio, F., Dighiero, G., Dohner, H., et al. (2008) Guidelines for the Diagnosis and Treatment of Chronic Lymphocytic Leukemia: A Report from the International Workshop on Chronic Lymphocytic Leukemia Updating the National Cancer Institute-Working Group 1996 Guidelines. *Blood,* Vol.111, No.12, (Jun) 5446-5456

Heim, S. & Mitelman, F. (Eds.) (2009) *Cancer Cytogenetics.* Wiley-Blackwell, ISBN 978-0-470-18179-9, Hoboken, N.J. Hoboken, N.J.

Hernandez, J.A., Rodriguez, A.E., Gonzalez, M., Benito, R., Fontanillo, C., Sandoval, V., et al. (2009) A High Number of Losses in 13q14 Chromosome Band Is Associated with a Worse Outcome and Biological Differences in Patients with B-Cell Chronic Lymphoid Leukemia. *Haematologica,* Vol.94, No.3, (Mar) 364-371

Jahrsdorfer, B., Muhlenhoff, L., Blackwell, S.E., Wagner, M., Poeck, H., Hartmann, E., et al. (2005) B-Cell Lymphomas Differ in Their Responsiveness to CpG Oligodeoxynucleotides. *Clin Cancer Res,* Vol.11, No.4, (Feb) 1490-1499

Josefsson, P., Geisler, C.H., Leffers, H., Petersen, J.H., Andersen, M.K., Jurlander, J., et al. (2007) *CLLU1* Expression Analysis Adds Prognostic Information to Risk Prediction in Chronic Lymphocytic Leukemia. *Blood,* Vol.109, No.11, (Jun) 4973-4979

Juliusson, G., Oscier, D.G., Fitchett, M., Ross, F.M., Stockdill, G., Mackie, M.J., et al. (1990) Prognostic Subgroups in B-Cell Chronic Lymphocytic Leukemia Defined by Specific Chromosomal Abnormalities. *N Engl J Med,* Vol.323, No.11, (Sep) 720-724

Kay, N.E., Eckel-Passow, J.E., Braggio, E., Vanwier, S., Shanafelt, T.D., Van Dyke, D.L., et al. (2010) Progressive but Previously Untreated CLL Patients with Greater Array CGH Complexity Exhibit a Less Durable Response to Chemoimmunotherapy. *Cancer Genet Cytogenet,* Vol.203, No.2, (Dec) 161-168

Klein, U. & Dalla-Favera, R. (2010) New Insights into the Pathogenesis of Chronic Lymphocytic Leukemia. *Semin Cancer Biol,* Vol.20, No.6, (Dec) 377-383

Kujawski, L., Ouillette, P., Erba, H., Saddler, C., Jakubowiak, A., Kaminski, M., et al. (2008) Genomic Complexity Identifies Patients with Aggressive Chronic Lymphocytic Leukemia. *Blood,* Vol.112, No.5, (Sep) 1993-2003

Lehmann, S., Ogawa, S., Raynaud, S.D., Sanada, M., Nannya, Y., Ticchioni, M., et al. (2008) Molecular Allelokaryotyping of Early-Stage, Untreated Chronic Lymphocytic Leukemia. *Cancer,* Vol.112, No.6, (Mar) 1296-1305

Leuenberger, M., Frigerio, S., Wild, P.J., Noetzli, F., Korol, D., Zimmermann, D.R., et al. (2010) AID Protein Expression in Chronic Lymphocytic Leukemia/Small Lymphocytic Lymphoma Is Associated with Poor Prognosis and Complex Genetic Alterations. *Mod Pathol,* Vol.23, No.2, (Feb) 177-186

Lin, T.T., Letsolo, B.T., Jones, R.E., Rowson, J., Pratt, G., Hewamana, S., et al. (2010) Telomere Dysfunction and Fusion During the Progression of Chronic Lymphocytic Leukemia: Evidence for a Telomere Crisis. *Blood,* Vol.116, No.11, (Sep) 1899-1907

Malcikova, J., Smardova, J., Pekova, S., Cejkova, S., Kotaskova, J., Tichy, B., et al. (2008) Identification of Somatic Hypermutations in the *TP53* Gene in B-Cell Chronic Lymphocytic Leukemia. *Mol Immunol,* Vol.45, No.5, (Mar) 1525-1529

Malek, S., Parkin, B., Collins, R., Shedden, K. & Ouillette, P. (2010) The Prognostic Importance of Various 13q14 Deletions in CLL. *ASH Annual Meeting Abstracts,* Vol.116, No.21, (Nov) 3587

Martin-Subero, J.I., Ibbotson, R., Klapper, W., Michaux, L., Callet-Bauchu, E., Berger, F., et al. (2007) A Comprehensive Genetic and Histopathologic Analysis Identifies Two Subgroups of B-Cell Malignancies Carrying a t(14;19)(q32;q13) or Variant BCL3-Translocation. *Leukemia,* Vol.21, No.7, (Jul) 1532-1544

Mayr, C., Speicher, M.R., Kofler, D.M., Buhmann, R., Strehl, J., Busch, R., et al. (2006) Chromosomal Translocations Are Associated with Poor Prognosis in Chronic Lymphocytic Leukemia. *Blood,* Vol.107, No.2, (Jan) 742-751

Merup, M., Juliusson, G., Wu, X., Jansson, M., Stellan, B., Rasool, O., et al. (1997) Amplification of Multiple Regions of Chromosome 12, Including 12q13-15, in Chronic Lymphocytic Leukaemia. *Eur J Haematol,* Vol.58, No.3, (Mar) 174-180

Michaux, L., Wlodarska, I., Rack, K., Stul, M., Criel, A., Maerevoet, M., et al. (2005) Translocation t(1;6)(p35.3;p25.2): A New Recurrent Aberration in "Unmutated" B-CLL. *Leukemia,* Vol.19, No.1, (Jan) 77-82

Nowakowski, G.S., Smoley, S., Schwager, S., Zent, C.S., Call, T.G., Shanafelt, T.D., et al. (2007) Presence of Immunoglobulin Heavy Chain Gene (*IGH*) Translocations in Chronic Lymphocytic Leukemia Is Related to Poor Prognosis. *ASH Annual Meeting Abstracts,* Vol.110, No.11, (Nov) 2067

Nussenzweig, A. & Nussenzweig, M.C. (2010) Origin of Chromosomal Translocations in Lymphoid Cancer. *Cell,* Vol.141, No.1, (Apr) 27-38

O'Malley, D.P., Giudice, C., Chang, A.S., Chang, D., Barry, T.S., Hibbard, M.K., et al. (2011) Comparison of Array Comparative Genomic Hybridization (aCGH) to FISH and Cytogenetics in Prognostic Evaluation of Chronic Lymphocytic Leukemia. *Int J Lab Hematol,* Vol.33, No.3, (Jun) 238-244

Oscier, D., Fitchett, M., Herbert, T. & Lambert, R. (1991) Karyotypic Evolution in B-Cell Chronic Lymphocytic Leukaemia. *Genes Chromosomes Cancer,* Vol.3, No.1, (Jan) 16-20

Ouillette, P., Collins, R., Shakhan, S., Li, J., Peres, E., Kujawski, L., et al. (2011) Acquired Genomic Copy Number Aberrations and Survival in Chronic Lymphocytic Leukemia. *Blood,* Vol. 118, No.11, (Sep) 3051-3061

Ouillette, P., Fossum, S., Parkin, B., Ding, L., Bockenstedt, P., Al-Zoubi, A., et al. (2010) Aggressive Chronic Lymphocytic Leukemia with Elevated Genomic Complexity Is Associated with Multiple Gene Defects in the Response to DNA Double-Strand Breaks. *Clin Cancer Res,* Vol.16, No.3, (Feb) 835-847

Palacios, F., Moreno, P., Morande, P., Abreu, C., Correa, A., Porro, V., et al. (2010) High Expression of AID and Active Class Switch Recombination Might Account for a More Aggressive Disease in Unmutated CLL Patients: Link with an Activated Microenvironment in Cll Disease. *Blood,* Vol.115, No.22, (Jun) 4488-4496

Perez-Duran, P., de Yebenes, V.G. & Ramiro, A.R. (2007) Oncogenic Events Triggered by AID, the Adverse Effect of Antibody Diversification. *Carcinogenesis,* Vol.28, No.12, (Dec) 2427-2433

Pfeifer, D., Pantic, M., Skatulla, I., Rawluk, J., Kreutz, C., Martens, U.M., et al. (2007) Genome-Wide Analysis of DNA Copy Number Changes and LOH in CLL Using High-Density SNP Arrays. *Blood,* Vol.109, No.3, (Feb) 1202-1210

Pospisilova, H., Baens, M., Michaux, L., Stul, M., Van Hummelen, P., Van Loo, P., et al. (2007) Interstitial Del(14)(q) Involving *IGH*: A Novel Recurrent Aberration in B-NHL. *Leukemia,* Vol.21, No.9, (Sep) 2079-2083

Puente, X.S., Pinyol, M., Quesada, V., Conde, L., Ordonez, G.R., Villamor, N., et al. (2011) Whole-Genome Sequencing Identifies Recurrent Mutations in Chronic Lymphocytic Leukaemia. *Nature,* Vol.475, No.7354, (Jul) 101-105

Put, N., Konings, P., Rack, K., Jamar, M., Van Roy, N., Libouton, J.M., et al. (2009a) Improved Detection of Chromosomal Abnormalities in Chronic Lymphocytic Leukemia by Conventional Cytogenetics Using CpG Oligonucleotide and Interleukin-2 Stimulation: A Belgian Multicentric Study. *Genes Chromosomes Cancer,* Vol.48, No.10, (Oct) 843-853

Put, N., Meeus, P., Chatelain, B., Rack, K., Boeckx, N., Nollet, F., et al. (2009b) Translocation t(14;18) Is Not Associated with Inferior Outcome in Chronic Lymphocytic Leukemia. *Leukemia,* Vol.23, No.6, (Jun) 1201-1204

Reiniger, L., Bodor, C., Bognar, A., Balogh, Z., Csomor, J., Szepesi, A., et al. (2006) Richter's and Prolymphocytic Transformation of Chronic Lymphocytic Leukemia Are Associated with High mRNA Expression of Activation-Induced Cytidine Deaminase and Aberrant Somatic Hypermutation. *Leukemia,* Vol.20, No.6, (Jun) 1089-1095

Put ,N., Van Roosbroeck, K., Konings, P., Meeus, P., Brusselmans, C., Rack, K., Gervais ,C., Nguyen-Khac, F., Chapiro, E., Radford-Weiss, I., Struski, S., Dastugue, N., Gachard, N., Lefebvre, C., Barin ,C., Eclache, V., Fert-Ferrer, S., Laibe, S., Mozziconacci ,MJ., Quilichini ,B., Poirel, HA., Wlodarska, I., Hagemeijer, A., Moreau, Y., Vandenberghe ,P., Michaux, L.; on behalf of the BCGHo and the GFCH. (2011) Chronic lymphocytic leukemia and prolymphocytic leukemia with MYC translocations: a subgroup with an aggressive disease course.*Ann Hematol*, (Dec). [Epub ahead of print]

Reis-Filho, J.S. (2009) Next-Generation Sequencing. *Breast Cancer Res,* Vol.11 Suppl 3, No.S12, (Dec) 1-7

Rinaldi, A., Mian, M., Kwee, I., Rossi, D., Deambrogi, C., Mensah, A.A., et al. (2011) Genome-Wide DNA Profiling Better Defines the Prognosis of Chronic Lymphocytic Leukaemia. *Br J Haematol,* Vol.154, No.5, (Sep), 590-599

Roos, G., Krober, A., Grabowski, P., Kienle, D., Buhler, A., Dohner, H., et al. (2008) Short Telomeres Are Associated with Genetic Complexity, High-Risk Genomic Aberrations, and Short Survival in Chronic Lymphocytic Leukemia. *Blood,* Vol.111, No.4, (Feb) 2246-2252

Schouten, J.P., McElgunn, C.J., Waaijer, R., Zwijnenburg, D., Diepvens, F. & Pals, G. (2002) Relative Quantification of 40 Nucleic Acid Sequences by Multiplex Ligation-Dependent Probe Amplification. *Nucleic Acids Res,* Vol.30, No.12, (Jun), 1-13

Schwab, M. (Ed.) (2001) *Encyclopedic Reference of Cancer.* Springer, ISBN 978-3-5403-3443-9, Berlin-Heidelberg, New York

Shaffer, L.G., Slovak, M.L. & Campell, L.J. (Eds.) (2009) *ISCN 2009: An International System for Human Cytogenetic Nomenclature.* Karger, ISBN 978-3-8055-8985-7, Basel

Shanafelt, T.D., Witzig, T.E., Fink, S.R., Jenkins, R.B., Paternoster, S.F., Smoley, S.A., et al. (2006) Prospective Evaluation of Clonal Evolution During Long-Term Follow-up of Patients with Untreated Early-Stage Chronic Lymphocytic Leukemia. *J Clin Oncol,* Vol.24, No.28, (Oct) 4634-4641

Smoley, S.A., Van Dyke, D.L., Kay, N.E., Heerema, N.A., Dell' Aquila, M.L., Dal Cin, P., et al. (2010) Standardization of Fluorescence in Situ Hybridization Studies on Chronic Lymphocytic Leukemia (CLL) Blood and Marrow Cells by the CLL Research Consortium. *Cancer Genet Cytogenet,* Vol.203, No.2, (Dec) 141-148

Stephenson, C.F., Desai, Z.R. & Bridges, J.M. (1991) The Proliferative Activity of B-Chronic Lymphocytic Leukaemia Lymphocytes Prior to and after Stimulation with TPA and PHA. *Leuk Res,* Vol.15, No.11, 1005-1012

Stilgenbauer, S., Sander, S., Bullinger, L., Benner, A., Leupolt, E., Winkler, D., et al. (2007) Clonal Evolution in Chronic Lymphocytic Leukemia: Acquisition of High-Risk Genomic Aberrations Associated with Unmutated *VH,* Resistance to Therapy, and Short Survival. *Haematologica,* Vol.92, No.9, (Sep) 1242-1245

Struski, S., Gervais, C., Helias, C., Herbrecht, R., Audhuy, B. & Mauvieux, L. (2009) Stimulation of B-Cell Lymphoproliferations with CpG-Oligonucleotide DSP30 Plus IL-2 Is More Effective Than with TPA to Detect Clonal Abnormalities. *Leukemia,* Vol.23, No.3, (Mar) 617-619

Tam, C.S., Shanafelt, T.D., Wierda, W.G., Abruzzo, L.V., Van Dyke, D.L., O'Brien, S., et al. (2009) De Novo Deletion 17p13.1 Chronic Lymphocytic Leukemia Shows Significant Clinical Heterogeneity: The M. D. Anderson and Mayo Clinic Experience. *Blood,* Vol.114, No.5, (Jul) 957-964

Touw, I. & Lowenberg, B. (1985) Interleukin 2 Stimulates Chronic Lymphocytic Leukemia Colony Formation in Vitro. *Blood,* Vol.66, No.1, (Jul) 237-240

Van Bockstaele, F., Verhasselt, B. & Philippe, J. (2008) Prognostic Markers in Chronic Lymphocytic Leukemia: A Comprehensive Review. *Blood Rev,* Vol.23, No.1, (Jan) 25-47

Van Den Neste, E., Robin, V., Francart, J., Hagemeijer, A., Stul, M., Vandenberghe, P., et al. (2007) Chromosomal Translocations Independently Predict Treatment Failure, Treatment-Free Survival and Overall Survival in B-Cell Chronic Lymphocytic Leukemia Patients Treated with Cladribine. *Leukemia,* Vol.21, No.8, (Aug) 1715-1722

Van Dyke, D.L., Shanafelt, T.D., Call, T.G., Zent, C.S., Smoley, S.A., Rabe, K.G., et al. (2010) A Comprehensive Evaluation of the Prognostic Significance of 13q Deletions in Patients with B-Chronic Lymphocytic Leukaemia. *Br J Haematol,* Vol.148, No.4, (Feb) 544-550

Watanabe, T., Ichikawa, A., Saito, H. & Hotta, T. (1996) Overexpression of the *MDM2* Oncogene in Leukemia and Lymphoma. *Leuk Lymphoma,* Vol.21, No.5-6, (May) 391-397

Willander, K., Ungerback, J., Karlsson, K., Fredrikson, M., Soderkvist, P. & Linderholm, M. (2010) *MDM2* SNP309 Promoter Polymorphism, an Independent Prognostic Factor in Chronic Lymphocytic Leukemia. *Eur J Haematol,* Vol.85, No.3, (Sep) 251-256

Wu, X., Nowakowski, G.S., Smoley, S.A., Arendt, B.A., Peterson, M.A., van Dyke, D., et al. (2008) Cytogenetic Analysis of Normal Human B Cells Following CpG Stimulation: Implications for Interpretation of CpG Induced CLL Metaphase Analysis. *ASH Annual Meeting Abstracts,* Vol.112, No.11, (Nov) 3124

Zenz, T., Mertens, D., Dohner, H. & Stilgenbauer, S. (2011) Importance of Genetics in Chronic Lymphocytic Leukemia. *Blood Rev,* Vol.25, No.3, (May) 131-137

Part 5

CLL Therapy

14

Immune Response and Immunotherapy in Chronic Lymphocytic Leukemia

Leticia Huergo-Zapico[1], Ana P. Gonzalez-Rodríguez[2], Juan Contesti[3], Azahara Fernández-Guizán[1], Andrea Acebes Huerta[1], Alejandro López-Soto[1] and Segundo Gonzalez[1]
[1]*Functional Biology Department, Instituto Universitario Oncologico del Principado de Asturias (IUOPA), University of Oviedo, Oviedo,*
[2]*Hematology Department, Hospital Universitario Central de Asturias, Oviedo*
[3]*Hematology Department, Hospital Cabueñe, Gijón,*
Spain

1. Introduction

The contribution of the immune system to the pathogenesis of chronic lymphocytic leukemia (CLL) is receiving increasing attention in recent years. This interest has been supported by population studies, which have shown the increase of cancer risk in immunodeficient individuals (Grulich *et al., 2007;* Smyth *et al., 2006;* Swann *et al., 2007),* and experimental studies, which have shown that deficiencies in key immunological molecules and cells increase the susceptibility to develop several types of solid tumors and hematological malignancies (Smyth *et al., 2006;* Swann *et al., 2007).* Additionally, the interest in the study of tumor immunology has been boosted by the increasing use of immunotherapy in the treatment of cancer, particularly in CLL. In this chapter, we review the role of the immune system in the elimination of CLL, the mechanisms that leukemia cells use to evade the immune response, and finally, we analyze the basis of the use of immunotherapy in the treatment of CLL patients.

2. Immune surveillance of cancer

The immune system is able to prevent cancer development by eliminating cancer cells prior to tumors becoming clinically detectable or by attenuating tumor growth and progression (Smyth *et al., 2006;* Swann *et al., 2009*). Both T cells and Natural Killer (NK) cells play a critical role in cancer immune surveillance (**Figure 1**). T cells are able to recognize tumor antigens, which differentiate cancer cells from their nontransformed counterparts. Several tumor antigens have been described such as mutation of oncogenic proteins (e.g. p53), over-expressed cellular antigens (such as HER-2), viral antigens, differentiation antigens and aberrantly expressed antigens (Smyth *et al., 2006;* Swann *et al., 2007*). Cytotoxic CD8 T cells and helper CD4 T cells may recognize transformed cells bearing these tumor antigens presented as peptides by MHC class I and class II molecules, respectively.

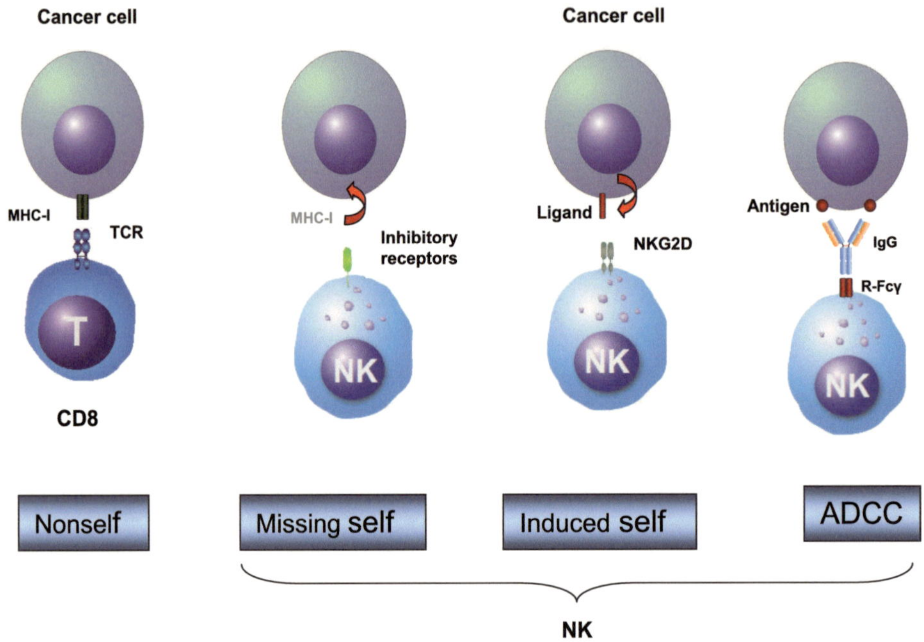

Fig. 1. Mechanisms of cancer immune surveillance. T Cell Receptor (TCR) expressed by CD8 T cells is able to recognize tumor antigens presented as peptides by the Major Histocompatibility Complex class I proteins (MHC-I) (nonself recognition). NK cells use several mechanisms to recognize tumor cells. NK cells use inhibitory receptors to differentiate "*self*" from "*missing self*". The impairment of MHC class I expression observed in some tumor cells impairs the recognition by CD8 T cells. Nevertheless, MHC class I molecules have an inhibitory effect on the activation of NK cells. Consequently, the lack of expression of MHC class I molecules (*missing self*) promotes the activation of NK cells and the lysis of the target cell. NK cells also express activating receptors, such as NKG2D, which is able to recognize several ligands induced in transformed cells (*induced self*). NK cells also express the FcγRIII receptor (also named CD16), which is able to recognize tumor cells that have been bound by specific IgG antibodies. This mechanism of recognition is termed Antibody-Dependent Cell-Mediated Cytotoxicity (ADCC).

NK cells do not directly recognize tumor antigens, but instead, they recognize changes in cells caused by transformation. Several mechanisms of cancer recognition by NK cells have been described (Gonzalez *et al., 2011).* NK cells use a set of inhibitory receptors, such as killer cell immunoglobulin-like receptors (KIRs), to differentiate and eliminate cancer cells that lack MHC class I expression ("missing self" recognition) (Figure 1) (Gonzalez *et al., 2011).* NK cells also express activating receptors which recognize stress-induced molecules expressed on tumor cells ("induced self" recognition). The activating receptor NKG2D plays a pivotal role in the immune response against cancer. This receptor is expressed by NK cells, γδT cells and CD8 T cells, and recognizes several tumor-associated ligands named MICA, MICB and ULBP1-5 molecules. NKG2D ligands are restrictedly expressed in healthy cells, but they are induced in stressed and transformed cells, allowing the elimination of these cells by the immune system (Das *et al.,* 2001; Raulet et al., 2003; Bauer et al., 1999; Lopez-Larrea et al., 2008; Bahram et al., 1994 ; Cosman et al., 2001; González et al., 2008; Guerra et al., 2008). NK cells may also lyse target cells that have been bound by specific IgG antibodies. They are able to recognize the Fc region of the antibody through FcγRIII receptor (also named CD16). This mechanism of recognition is termed Antibody-Dependent Cell-Mediated Cytotoxicity (ADCC) and it is an important mechanism of action against tumors of therapeutic monoclonal antibodies, such as rituximab and alemtuzumab (Figure 1). These mechanisms of anti-tumor immune response may protect the host in the early stages of tumor initiation; however during cancer progression, tumors develop a plethora of mechanisms of immune evasion. Consequently, the anti-tumor response is ineffective in advanced tumors (Smyth *et al., 2006;* Swann *et al., 2007*).

3. Immune surveillance of chronic lymphocytic leukemia

There is little information related to the role of the immune response in the early stages of CLL progression. Nevertheless, it has widely been reported that the amounts of CD8 and CD4 T cells and NK cells are significantly elevated at diagnosis of the disease. The expansion of cytotoxic CD8 T cells is higher than CD4 T cells, and many CLL patients showed an inversion of CD4/CD8 ratio (Gonzalez-Rodriguez et al., 2010). Similar expansions of immune cells have been observed in other hematological malignancies and this increase of immune cells has been associated with a better prognosis of patients. Thus, higher absolute lymphocyte count predicts higher survival in lymphoma, acute myeloblastic leukemia and myeloma (Cox et al., 2008; Siddiqui et al., 2006; Porrata et al., 2007, 2009; Ray-Coquard et al., 2009; De Angulo et al., 2008; Behl et al. 2006, 2007; Ege et al., 2008). NK cell count has also been associated with clinical outcome in patients with diffuse large B-cell lymphoma (Plonquet et al., 2007). The expansion of immune cells observed in CLL and in other hematological malignancies may be compared to the expansion of tumor infiltrating lymphocytes in epithelial tumors. In several types of cancer, the presence of tumor infiltrating lymphocytes, mainly NK and CD8 T cells, has also been associated with the anti-tumor response and was found to be a better predictor of patient survival than traditional histopathological methods used to stage tumors (Dunn et al., 2004; Clemente et al., 1996; Scanlan et al., 2004; Rollins et al., 2006; Moore OS et al., 1949; Clark et al., 1969; Pagès et al., 2005)

In agreement with an anti-tumor role of the immune system, the expansion of NK and T cells has been associated with the time to treatment in CLL (Palmer et al., 2008). Furthermore, the relative numbers of CD8 and CD4 T cells at diagnosis are independent predictors for survival, and higher CD8 count is associated with significantly higher median time of survival of CLL patients (Gonzalez-Rodriguez et al., 2010). This suggests that the expansion of immune cells observed at diagnosis of CLL patients may be due, at least in part, to the expansion of anti-tumor immune cells. However, the analysis of the functionality of these cells is still lacking. Early studies showed that the expanded CD8 T cells have an activated phenotype and cytotoxic function and appear to have restricted clonality, which were originally interpreted as evidence of an autologous T cell response against leukemia cells. Furthermore, a subset of γδT cells with anti-tumor activity is one type of the immune cells expanded in CLL patients (Poggi et al., 2004). These T cells express the activating receptor NKG2D, which is able to mediate the lysis of CLL cells expressing NKG2D ligands (*"induced self" recognition*) (**Figure 1**). Leukemia cells from most patients lack NKG2D ligands expression and are highly resistant to NK cell-mediated lysis, but NKG2D ligands expression may be induced in leukemia cells by treatment with trans-retinoic acid or histone deacetilases (HDACs) inhibitors, rendering leukemia cells susceptible to lysis by immune cells (Kato et al., 2007; Del Giudice et al., 2009). The expansion of γδT cells has been associated with a better prognosis of CLL patients, supporting the hypothesis that the increase of T cells observed at diagnosis of CLL patients may be due, at least in part, to the expansion of anti-tumor T cells.

The activation of the immune system in CLL patients has not only been associated with improved prognosis, but also with tumor regression. The natural history of stage A disease is generally indolent or only slowly progressive. However, it is less known that CLL may undergo spontaneous regression (Del Giudice et al., 2009). There are no data about the functional role of the immune system in these remissions; however the activation of immune system has been associated with spontaneous remissions in other types of cancers (Smyth et al., 2006; Swann et al., 2007). This suggests that the activation of the anti-tumor immune response may have a significant impact on the progression of CLL, however further analyses about the functionality of immune cells in CLL are clearly warranted.

The role of immune system in CLL is further highlighted by the analysis of cancer risk in immunodeficient individuals. However, the deficiency of CD8 T cells is not compatible with life and most of the studies about the role of other immune deficiencies on cancer susceptibility are nonpopulation-based and of small sample size, making difficult to draw definite conclusions. Nevertheless, primary immune deficiency patients have been associated with a marked increased risk of cancer. Some types of cancers appear to be associated with specific forms of immunodeficiency including stomach cancer with common variable immune deficiency (CVID) (Kinlen et al., 1985; Mellemkjaer et al., 2002), leukemia with ataxia-telangiectasia (Morrell *et al.,* 1986), and nonmelanocytic skin cancer with cartilage-hair hypoplasia (Taskinen *et al.,* 2008). In a recent population-based study, the association of antibody deficiency with an increasing risk of leukemia, non-Hodgkin lymphoma and gastric cancer has been described (Vajdic et al., 2010). In agreement with clinical data, deficiencies in T cells and NK cells have also been associated with increased susceptibility of cancer in a diversity of experimental models of cancer (Smyth et al., 2006; Swann et al., 2007).

Nevertheless, the most compelling evidence about the potential role of the immune system in the pathogenesis of CLL is the increasing use of immunotherapy in the treatment of this disease. This highlights the capacity of the activation of the immune system to eliminate CLL cells and the potential role of immune system to cure this disease. Thus, the therapeutic effect of allogeneic hematopoietic stem cell transplantation in CLL relies on the ability of the immune cells of the graft to recognize and eliminate leukemia cells (Mehta et al., 1996; Ritgen et al., 2008). Similarly, the therapeutic use of immunomodulatory drugs, such as lenalidomide, is not directly based on a cytotoxic effect on CLL cells, but instead, lenalidomide exerts its therapeutic effect through the stimulation of the immune system.

4. Immune defects in chronic lymphocytic leukemia patients

In spite of the existence of compelling evidences about the ability of the immune system to eliminate nascent tumors, when the immune system is unable to eliminate all cancer cells, it sculpts or edits the phenotype of cancer cells, eliminating the most immunogenic ones and selecting the less immunogenic tumor cells, which are able to evade or suppress the immune response. The consequence of this process, named cancer immunoediting, is the development of numerous mechanisms of immune evasion and immune suppression in advanced tumors (Smyth et al., 2006; Swann et al., 2007). Accordingly, there is a progressive acquisition of a wide variety of immune defects in the course of the progression of CLL. As a result, patients progressively acquire a immunodeficiency status, which increases the incidence of opportunistic infections and the development of secondary neoplasias (Hamblin et al., 2008). The corollary of immune defects also includes the development of several autoimmune reactions. CLL patients have a 5-10% risk of development of an autoimmune complication, which primarily cause cytopaenia (Zent et al., 2010). The most common autoimmune disease affecting CLL patients is hemolytic anemia, with a lower frequency of immune thrombocytopenia and pure red blood cell aplasia and only rarely, autoimmune granulocytopaenia.

Practically all components of the immune system are impaired in CLL patients. The most obvious and well-known immune defect is hypogammaglobulinemia, which is present in up to 85% of patients (Hamblin *et al.,* 1987). Hypogammaglobulinemia is observed in other lymphoid malignancies, but the impairment of the humoral immune response is far greater in CLL. The clinical consequence of hypogammaglobulinemia is the increase of susceptibility of CLL patients to infection with extracellular bacterias, commonly affecting respiratory tract, skin and urinary tract, and the reactivation of some latent virus infections, mainly belonging to *Herpesviridae* family.

The defects in the humoral immunity are accompanied by several abnormalities in the cellular immune response, including quantitative and qualitative alterations of NK cells, CD4 and CD8 T cells, dendritic cells, neutrophils, monocytes and cytokines. The activity of NK cells against leukemia cells is frequently reduced and lymphoid neoplasms are quite resistant to NK cell-mediated cytotoxicity (Foa et al., 1984; Jewell et al., 1992; Kato et al., 2007). All effector mechanisms of NK cells analyzed are impaired in some degree in advanced CLL patients (Katrinakis et al., 1996; Caligaris-Cappio et al., 1999; Wierda et al., 1999). A partial down-regulation of MHC class I molecules, which allow leukemic cells to escape from cytotoxic T cell attack, has been reported (Demanet et al., 2004). However, the "missing self" recognition by NK cells (**Figure 1**) is limited in CLL by the aberrant expression of HLA-G in leukemia cells. HLA-G is a non classical MHC class I molecule that is physiologically expressed on fetal derived placental cells. Classical MHC class I molecules (HLA-A, -B and -C) are not expressed in fetal placental cells, but HLA-G inhibits NK cells activation against placental cells by interacting with several inhibitory receptors expressed by NK cells and cytotoxic T lymphocytes. Likewise, the aberrant expression of HLA-G on leukemia cells impairs the anti-leukemia immune response mediated by these cells. Accordingly, the expression of HLA-G on leukemia cells correlated with progression free survival and the level of immunosuppression of CLL patients (Nückel et al., 2005; Erikci et al., 2009).

There are also defects on the expression of NKG2D and its ligands in CLL (Gasser et al., 2005; Groh et al., 1996, 1999; Diefenbach et al., 2001; Cerwenka et al., 2001; González et al., 2006). The expression of NKG2D ligands in leukemia cells is low or absent in most of patients, which confers them with a high resistance to lysis by immune cells (Poggi et al., 2004). Furthermore, leukemia cells may also counter the anti-tumor activity of NKG2D by shedding some of its soluble ligands. Serum levels of soluble MICA, MICB and ULBP2 are significantly increased in

CLL patients and are associated with a poor treatment-free survival (Nückel et al., 2010). The shedding of soluble MICA has been described in many types of cancer and elevated levels of soluble MICA correlated with advanced stage tumors, metastasis and poor prognosis (Salih et al. 2002, 2003; Raffaghello et al., 2004; Rebmann et al., 2007), because soluble MICA impairs the recognition of cancer cells by immune cells and suppress the immune response (Groh et al., 2002, 2006). Of relevance, some of the immune defects observed in CLL patients may be reversible. For instance, leukemia cells which express low levels of NKG2D ligands may be rendered susceptible to immune cells when are treated with trans-retinoic acid or histone deacetylase inhibitors inhibitors, which restored the expression of NKG2D ligands on leukemia cells (**Salih et** al., 2002). This clearly suggests that therapeutic approaches that can bypass the immune evasion mechanisms of CLL patients may have therapeutic application in this disease.

T cell function is also impaired in CLL. There are defects on antigen presentation (Cantwell et al., 1997), T cell activation, in differentiation and function of CD4 T cells and defects in the cytotoxic activity of CD8 cells that are caused by direct contact with leukemia cells (Gorgun et al., 2005; Rossi et al., 1996; Junevik et al., 2007; Mackus et al., 2003). Regulatory T cells, a specialized subpopulation of T cells which suppresses the activation of the immune system and thereby maintains tolerance to self antigens, are increased in number in CLL and this increase is more significantly in most advanced patients (Beyer *et al.,* 2006). It is not yet clear whether inhibitory T cells may promote the tolerance of leukemia cells by the immune system and may contribute to the immune deficiency. Nevertheless, it is noticeable that this population is exquisitely sensitive to treatment with fludarabine. It has been proposed that the elimination of these inhibitory T cells might be one of the mechanisms that favors the development of autoimmune hemolytic anemia after treatment of CLL patients with fludarabine (Hamblin *et al.,* 2006).

The defects of cellular immunity observed in CLL increase the susceptibility of patients to virus infections, opportunistic infections and second malignancies, and may contribute to impair the anti-leukemia immune response. Additionally, the use of chemotherapy agents may complicate the clinical course of CLL since may exacerbate the pre-existing immunodeficiency. Nevertheless, the development of drugs and therapeutic strategies that can either bypass immune evasion mechanisms or rescue immune suppressor pathways may significantly benefit CLL patients. Thus, the increasing understanding of the molecular and cellular events underlying the immune dysfunction in CLL is of key importance in the development of novel immune-based therapies.

5. Immunotherapy

CLL is generally considered as an incurable disease, but it frequently progresses slowly. Early-stage CLL is, in general, not treated since there are no clear evidences that early therapeutic intervention improves survival time or quality of life. Instead, the disease is monitored over time to detect changes in disease progression. Determining when to start the treatment and by what means is often difficult. The National Cancer Institute Working Group has issued guidelines for treatment (Cheson et al., 1996; Hallek et al., 1996).

Until recently, chemotherapy has been the keystone of treatment of CLL. Alkylating agents have been considered the first line in the treatment of CLL patients for a long time. They can induce complete responses, but it is not considered curative. Chlorambucil slows disease progression, but does not prolong survival (Dighiero et al., 1998; Eichhorst et al., 2006; Hallek, 2010) (**Figure 2**). The purine analogue fludarabine was shown to give superior response rates to chlorambucil as primary therapy (Steurer et al., 2006; Rai et al., 2000), but there are no evidences that the early use of fludarabine improves overall survival. Treatment combinations of Fludarabine with the alkylating agent Cyclophosphamide (FC) result in higher response rates, in longer median progression-free survival and longer treatment-free survival than single agents (Maloney et al., 1999). Thus far, no difference in median overall survival has been observed.

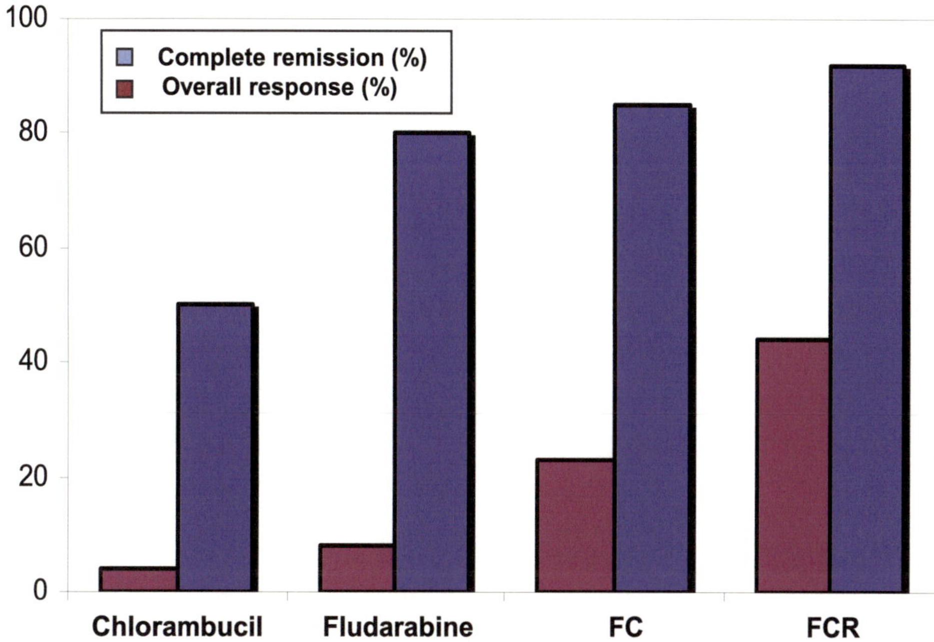

Fig. 2. Chronic lymphocytic leukemia therapy. The figure shows rates of complete remissions and overall response in CLL first line treatment. (F=Fludarabine, C=Cyclophosphamide, R= Rituximab).

In spite of the fact that chemotherapy provides benefits for CLL patients, it is palliative, and treated patients frequently develop recurrent disease. Likewise treatment induces myelosuppression and selection of chemotherapy resistant clones. Additionally, it can worsen immune function, increasing the immunodeficiency status of CLL patients. Prognosis for patients treated with chemotherapy regimens remains poor, prompting the development of new targeted agents. In line with this idea, the activation of the immune system to fight against CLL cells has opened new vistas in the treatment of CLL. Immunotherapy may potentially provide curative treatment and some immunotherapeutic approaches may mitigate disease complications caused by the defects of the immune system observed in CLL patients. In this sense, monoclonal antibodies, allogeneic hematopoietic stem cell transplantation and immunomodulatory drugs have successfully been used in the treatment of CLL. Immune-based therapy represents an exciting mode of treatment since it may be able to eliminate leukemia cells without myelosuppression.

5.1 Monoclonal antibodies

Monoclonal antibodies have the ability to target specific antigens expressed preferentially on the surface of malignant cells. Due to their specificity, the therapeutic efficacy of monoclonal antibodies is not generally associated with a high non-specific toxicity. Thus, they are increasingly being used in the treatment of hematological malignancies and solid tumors. In CLL, the use of **rituximab**, a chimeric murine/human monoclonal antibody directed against CD20, has improved the treatment of patients. Unlike other B cells antigens, CD20 is neither shedded nor internalized in resting normal B cells. Therefore it is an ideal target for antibody-based therapy in mature B cell malignancies. Rituximab treatment induces a significant reduction in B cell count within 3 days followed by a slow recovery over 9-12 months (Maloney et al., 1997; Onrust et al., 1999). The mechanism of B cell killing has not completely been elucidated, but rituximab acts through Antibody-Dependent Cell-Mediated Cytotoxicity, complement-mediated cytotoxicity, the activation of macrophages, and direct apoptosis of leukemia cells both caspase dependent and independent (Jaglowski et al., 2010) (**Figure 3**).

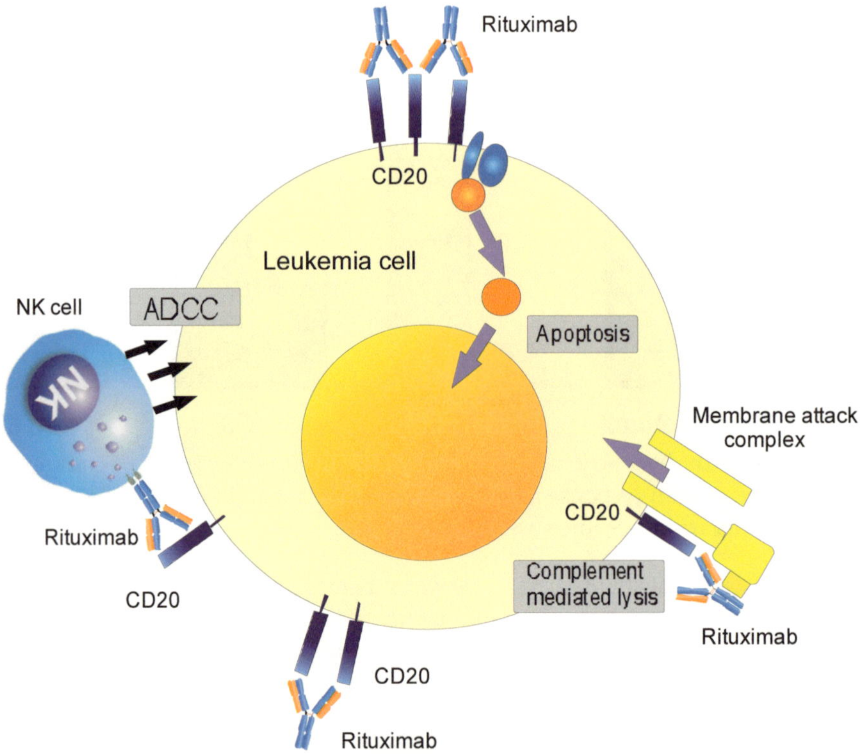

Fig. 3. Mechanism of action of rituximab. Rituximab is a monoclonal antibody directed against CD20 antigen, which is expressed on the surface of B cells. The recognition of the Fc portion of rituximab through the FcγRIII receptor mediates the lysis of leukemia cells by NK cells; a process named Antibody-Dependent Cell-Mediated Cytotoxicity (ADCC). The Fc portion of rituximab also induces the activation of the classical pathway of complement. The activation of complement cascade forms a transmembrane channel, which causes the osmotic lysis of the leukemia cell. Rituximab may also cause a direct apoptosis of CD20 cells.

The efficacy of rituximab monotherapy in CLL is lower than in other B cell malignancies. The resistance to rituximab is frequently associated with a low CD20 expression. Nevertheless, the addition of rituximab to chemotherapy has proven to be very efficacious therapy for CLL. Treatment combinations of Fludarabine, Cyclophosphamide and Rituximab (FCR) obtain the highest response, but they are not still considered curative (Byrd et al., 2005; Tam et al., 2008; Wierda et al., 2005) (**Figure 2**). FCR therapy shows superiority for response rates and progression-free survival when compared to FC chemotherapy (Hallek et al., 2009; Robak et al., 2008), and it is becoming the first-line choice for younger patients (Casak et al., 2011). Additionally, rituximab represents one of the most active therapies for the treatment of autoimmune complications of CLL not responding to initial steroid treatment. The use of monoclonal antibodies for purging of leukemia cells *ex vivo* also improves the results of autologous stem cell transplantation (Gribben et al., 2005; Montillo et al., 2006).

The therapeutic efficacy of rituximab is minimally hampered by non-specific toxicity; however it has been associated with adverse events such as immunosuppression, reactivation of latent virus and infusion-related. Combination with chemotherapy may be associated with more profound immunosuppression. Management of these adverse events is a critical component of the treatment strategy for CLL since they can greatly affect the quality of life of patients and the ability to tolerate this therapy.

Alemtuzumab, a CD52-target humanized monoclonal antibody, has demonstrated benefits in the treatment of CLL patients (Gribben et al., 2009). CD52 is a protein highly expressed on both normal and malignant lymphocytes (B and T cells) and it is also found in other immune cells such as monocytes, macrophages and eosinophils; but it is not expressed on hematopoietic progenitors. The administration of alemtuzumab results in a severe lymphopenia with a reduction in both B and T cells, but it also affects other healthy CD52-expressing immune cells, which likely exacerbate the pre-existing immunodeficiency. After treatment, there is a slow recovery of immune cells, except for B cells, which remain at low level at 18 months. Alemtuzumab acts through Antibody-Dependent Cell-Mediated Cytotoxicity (Crowe et al., 1992) (**Figure 1**), complement-mediated cytotoxicity (Golay et al., 2004; Zent et al., 2004), and induces direct cell death through a mechanism that is independent of p53 status and caspase activation (Mone et al., 2006), and is effective in patients with deletion (17p)(13.1).

A significant difference between the efficacy of alemtuzumab and rituximab is based on the fact that the level of CD52 expression in normal and malignant B cells is far greater than the level of CD20 expression in CLL cells. The high expression of CD52 may contribute to the improved clinical activity of alemtuzumab as a single-agent compared to rituximab in CLL (Ashraf et al., 2007). Alemtuzumab is currently approved for first-line treatment of CLL, and it is a good option for symptomatic patients, previously untreated patients and relapsed patients with poor prognostic features (Keating et al., 2002; Osterborg et al., 1996; Lundin et al., 2002 ; Hillmen et al., 2007).

New monoclonal antibodies directed against CD20, such as ofatumumab and GA101, have been developed. **Ofatumumab** and rituximab bind to different epitopes, and, in theory, ofatumumab has greater capacity of activation of complement-dependent cytotoxicity than rituximab (Teeling et al., 2004). *In vitro* studies have demonstrated that ofatumumab is significantly more effective than rituximab at lysing CLL cells and B cell lines, especially those with low CD20 copy numbers. It is currently approved for treating CLL patients who are refractory to fludarabine and alemtuzumab.

The novel third generation humanized monoclonal antibody **GA101** also binds with high affinity to CD20, and as a result it promotes greater induction of Antibody-Dependent Cell-Mediated Cytotoxicity (Jaglowski et al., 2010) and induces more efficient NK cell activation than rituximab (Bologna et al., 2011). The development of new monoclonal antibodies is probably the best demonstration of the therapeutic efficacy that these agents have obtained in CLL and other hematological malignancies.

5.2 Hematopoietic stem cell transplantation

About 20% of patients who need treatment develop an aggressive disease despite early institution of intensive chemotherapy. Efforts to develop curative treatment for these CLL patients have focused on autologous and allogeneic hematopoietic stem cell transplantation (Dreger et al., *2009).* Both approaches show some methodological similarities, but the bases of both treatments are significantly different. Most patients may achieve a complete molecular response followed by **autologous stem cell transplantation**, a lower-risk form of treatment using the patient's own blood cells, which restores the hematopoietic system after an intensive chemotherapy regimen. The increase of the dose chemotherapy regimen is the base of the efficacy of autografting, and consequently, it is not an immune-based therapy. This therapy is not curative and subsequent clinical progression is inevitable (Provan et al., 1996; Milligan et al., 2005). The results of a phase 3 randomized European Group for Blood and Marrow Transplantation trial of autologous stem cell transplantation show the reduction of the risk of progression of CLL by more than 50%, but it does not have an effect on overall survival (Michallet et al., 2011), and it is particularly concerning the high incidence of myelodysplastic syndrome (9-12%) (Kharfan-Dabaja et al., 2007). Therefore, it is necessary to look for other solutions of treatment in this disease different from the chemotherapy and to move toward alternative non-chemotherapy-based treatment approaches.

Allogeneic stem cell transplantation offers a chance of definite cure of CLL, but is only feasible in a minority of patients. The basis of therapeutic response of allogeneic stem cell transplantation relies on the ability of immune cells of the graft to recognize and eliminate leukemia cells, a process known as graft-versus-leukemia effect (GvL) (Mehta et al., 1996; Ritgen et al., 2008) (**Figure 4**). Thus, allogeneic stem cell transplantation is a cellular-based immunotherapy completely different from autografting. The immunology of allogeneic stem cell transplantation is different from other types of transplants, such as heart or kidney transplants, because the graft, in addition to stem cells, contains and generates mature immune cells including T cells, NK cells and dendritic cells. These cells repopulate the recipient's immune system, restoring the response to infections and eliminating leukemia cells. The donor immune cells exert its graft-versus-leukemia effect through T cell-mediated alloreaction against the histocompatibility antigens displayed on leukemia cells. However, as histocompatibility antigens are shared by all cells of individual, recipient tissues may also be attacked by donor's immune system causing graft-versus-host-disease (GvHD) (rejection), a life-threatening condition. For this reason, matching donor and recipient HLA molecules is crucial to minimize graft-versus-host-disease. Mismatches in HLA-A, -B, -C and HLA class II alleles are significant risk factors for graft-versus-host-disease. Due to the high number of HLA alleles is quite difficult to find a HLA-matched unrelated donor, but nearly 25% of siblings share both HLA haplotypes, because all HLA genes are closely linked in a small region of chromosome 6, known as Major Histocompatibility Complex (MHC). However, even in HLA-matched recipient and donor, graft-versus-host-disease may occur due to minor histocompatibility antigens, which are derived from differences between donor and recipient in other polymorphic genes different from HLA, differences in the level of expression of proteins or are derived from genome differences between male and female (such as H-Y antigens encoded by Y chromosome, which is absent in females).

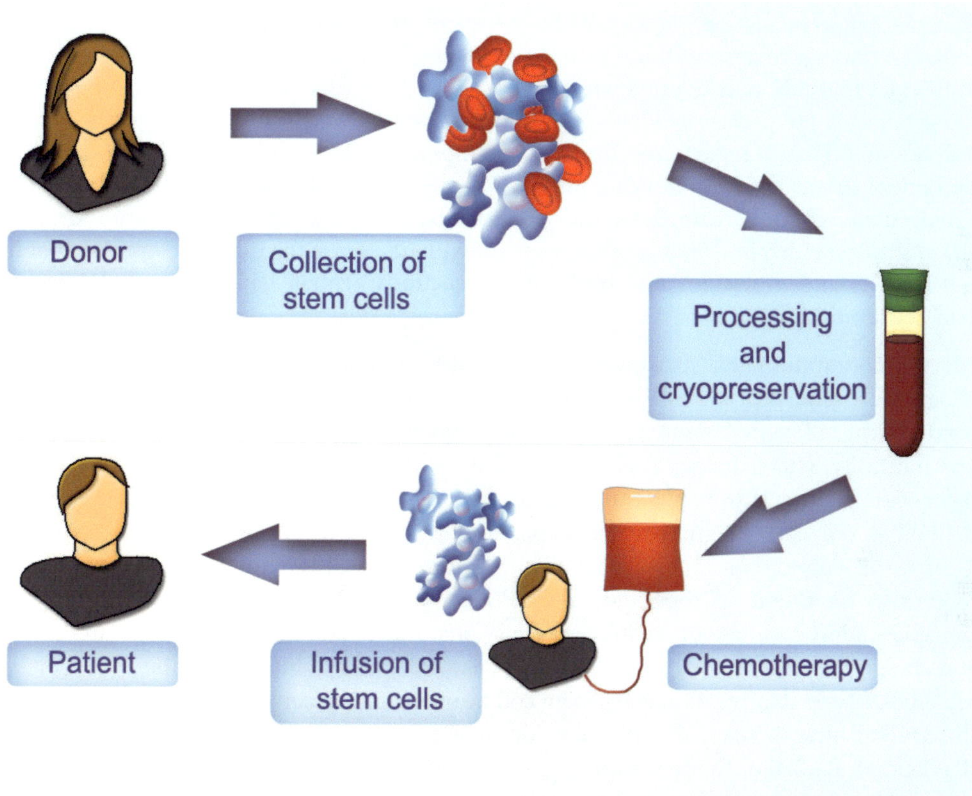

Fig. 4. Allogeneic stem cell transplantation. Hematopoietic stem cells are collected from the bone marrow or blood of the donor. Bone marrow or blood is taken to the processing laboratory where stem cells are concentrated and may be freezed (cryopreservation). High dose chemotherapy and/or radiation are given to the patient. To restore the patient's immune system, thawed or fresh stem cells are infused into the patient. The donor immune cells eliminate leukemia cells (graft-versus-leukemia) through a T cell-mediated alloreaction against patient's histocompatibility antigens displayed on leukemia cells.

If a HLA-matched sibling is not available, the use of unrelated umbilical blood units or an unrelated matched donor are viable options. Umbilical blood units offer the advantage that a higher number of mismatches in HLA antigens does not preclude transplant feasibility since naïve T cells in cord blood are less able to cause graft-versus-host-disease than mature donor T cells in bone marrow or peripheral blood, however graft-versus-leukemia is also less intense. Family donors, who matched a HLA haplotype, but fully mismatched the other ("haploidentical") is another option to obtain hemopoietic stem cells. The haploidentical transplant recipients have high risk of T-cell mediated graft-versus-host-disease (Velardi et al., 2010). This is controlled by an extensive immunosuppressive intensity in the conditioning regimen and extensive T cell depletion of the graft to prevent graft-versus-host-disease. The immune suppression and the depletion of T cells might be expected to result in weak or no graft-versus-leukemia effect, as it is conventionally achieved through T cell-mediated alloreactivity directed against recipient's histocompatibility antigens. Surprisingly, another immune cell influences the outcome of allogeneic stem cell transplantation in a favorable way. In these transplants, NK cell-mediated alloreactivity may control leukemia relapse without causing graft-versus-host-disease. This alloreaction is due to the fact that NK cells express specific inhibitory receptors, such as KIR or CD94/NKG2, for groups of HLA class I alleles. Inhibitory receptors and HLA class I genes structure individual NK cell repertoires during development. To establish a self-tolerance, each individual selects NK cells carrying inhibitory receptor combinations for their self HLA class I molecules. NK cells from those individuals that express inhibitory receptors for a HLA class I group, which is absent on allogeneic transplants, sense the missing expression of their self HLA class I molecules and mediate alloreactions against leukemia cells by "missing self" recognition (Figure 1).

Several nonrandomized prospective trials have demonstrated the potential efficacy of allogeneic stem cell transplantation in CLL; however even with reduced-intensity conditioning allogeneic stem cell transplantation is associated with significant morbidity and mortality. Nevertheless, it is a reasonable treatment option for poor-risk CLL patients. Allogeneic stem cell transplantation can overcome treatment resistance of poor-risk CLL defined as purine analogue refractoriness, early relapse after purine analogue combination therapy or autologous stem cell transplantation, and CLL with p53 deletion/mutation requiring treatment (Dreger et al., 2007). Nonmyeloablative allogeneic stem cell transplantation resulted in sustained remissions and prolonged survival in patients who had chemotherapy-refractory CLL (Sorror et al., 2008) and in high risk patients (Schetelig et al., 2008). Myeloablative allogeneic stem cell transplantation consistently results in a plateau in survival after 1 year, and the development of undetectable minimal residual disease (Pavletic et al., 2005). Evidence for graft-versus-leukemia in CLL can result in a complete and durable suppression of the leukemic clone (Ritgen et al., 2008; Rondón et al., 1996; Dreger et al., 2005; Farina et al., 2009; Sorror et al., 2005; Gribben et al., 2005). A prospective clinical trial is currently being performed in patients with high-risk CLL. This trial will finish in 2012 and will probably give us some guidance when and how to use allogeneic stem cell transplantation in poor-risk CLL.

In summary, there is convincing evidence that allogeneic stem cell transplantation can provide long-term disease control and possibly cure in selected patients with CLL, including those with a biologically highly unfavorable risk profile. Even patients who relapsed after allogeneic transplant may achieve durable remission following **donor lymphocyte infusion** without further chemotherapy or radiation chemotherapy (Hoogendoorn et al., 2007; Schetelig et al., 2003; Delgado et al., 2006; Marina et al., 2010). This further highlights the capacity of the donor-derived immunity in eradicating tumors (Marina et al., 2010).

5.3 Immune modulating drugs

Lenalidomide is a new immunomodulatory drug used in the treatment of CLL that is receiving considerable interest. It is a small molecular analog of thalidomide that was originally selected based on its ability to effectively inhibit tumor necrosis factor α (TNF-α) production. The mechanism of action of lenalidomide is complex and not yet fully understood. In CLL, lenalidomide has not a direct anti-tumor effect by inducing of apoptosis, but it has a significant anti-angiogenic and immune effects. It represents an exciting drug since it is able to eliminate CLL cells without immunosuppression.

Lenalidomide is clinically used in combination with dexamethasone in patients with multiple myeloma who have received prior therapy, in myelodysplasic syndrome, and in addition, there are current clinical trials analyzing the therapeutic effect of this drug in other types of cancers. In CLL, lenalidomide is clinically effective as a single agent in relapsed and refractory patients (Ferrajoli et al., 2008 ; Chanan-Khan et al., 2006), and ongoing trials are demonstrating that lenalidomide is clinically active as first-line CLL therapy (Chen et al., 2010). The responses achieved with lenalidomide are durable, even in patients with high-risk disease, with poor risk cytogenetics and with high-risk cytogenetics [del(11q)(q22.3) or del(17p)(p13.1)] (Sher et al., 2010).

The immunomodulatory mechanism of action of lenalidomide in CLL is poorly understood. Lenalidomide improves the humoral and cellular immune response of CLL patients (**Figure 5**). Lenalidomide treatment is associated with a significant increase in immunoglobulin

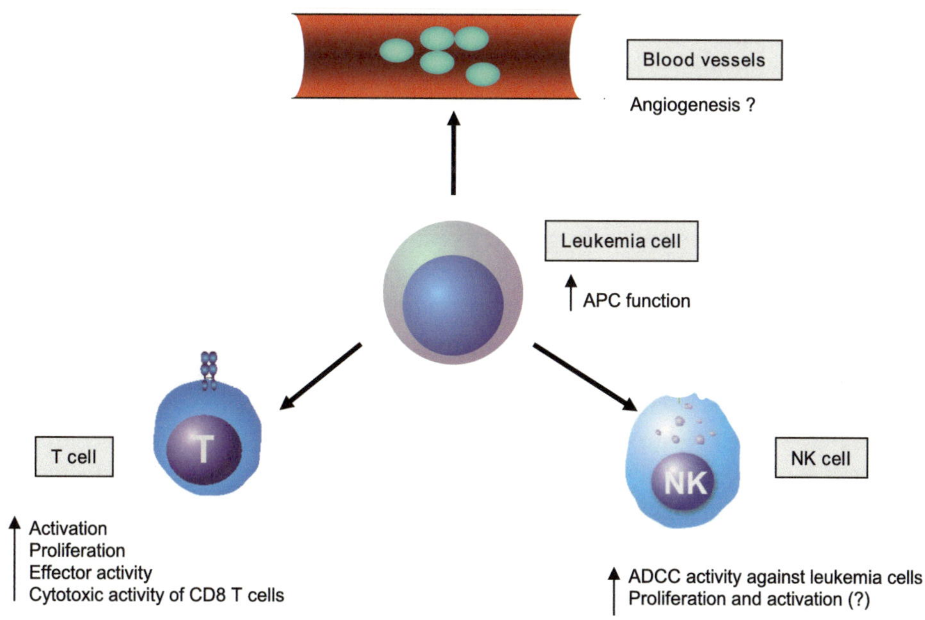

Fig. 5. Mechanism of action of lenalidomide in chronic lymphocytic leukemia. Lenalidomide does not have a direct cytotoxic effect on leukemia cells. Lenalidomide favors antigen presentation, activation, proliferation and functional activity of T cells. It also enhances Antibody-Dependent Cell-Mediated Cytotoxicity (ADCC) against rituximab-exposed leukemia cells. Other effects on angiogenic status remain to be elucidated.

levels. For instance, IgG levels were normalized in 7 out of 12 (58%) CLL patients with hypogammaglobulinemia (Badoux et al., 2009). Lenalidomide enhances antigen presentation to T cells (Aue et al., 2009; Chanan-Khan et al., 2006) and increases proliferation, activation and effector activity of T cells, which as mentioned before is impaired in CLL patients (Ramsay et al., 2008). Thalidomide and lenalidomide also have a significant immunomoudulatory effect on NK cells. In some experimental models, the antitumor effect of lenalidomide was mediated by NK cell stimulation (Awan et al., 2010). There is little information about the effect of lenalidomide on NK cells *in vivo*. Nevertheless, lenalidomide treatment increased the number of NK cells in CLL patients and increased Antibody-Dependent Cell-Mediated Cytotoxicity against leukemia cells (Wu et al., 2008). Lenalidomide induces a unique and previously uncharacterized immune response called tumor flare reaction associated with immune mediated antitumor response. Tumor flare reaction with lenalidomide appears to be disease-specific to CLL, may reflect clinical manifestation of tumor cell activation and correlates with clinical response (Chanan-Khan et al., 2010). Combination of lenalidomide with rituximab may act synergistically if the timing and sequencing strategies are optimized. An exciting new therapeutic strategy may be targeting tumor cell with chemotherapy or monoclonal antibodies and the microenvironment with lenalidomide (Ramsay et al., 2009).

6. Conclusion

In spite of the existence of little information about the role of the immune system in the pathogenesis of CLL, the current data clearly support the hypothesis that the activation of the anti-tumor immune response, particularly in the early stages of the disease, may have a significant impact on tumor progression. However, CLL patients progressively acquire a wide variety of immune evasion mechanisms. As a result, patients acquire a progressive immunodeficiency status, which increases the incidence of opportunistic infections and the development of secondary neoplasias. Chemotherapy has been the keystone of treatment of CLL, but it is palliative and may worsen the immunodeficiency status of patients. Nevertheless, the development of drugs and therapeutic strategies that can either bypass the immune evasion mechanisms or rescue immune suppressor pathways may significantly benefit CLL patients. Thus, immunotherapy may provide curative treatment and may mitigate disease complications caused by the defects of the immune system observed in CLL patients. In this sense, monoclonal antibodies, allogeneic hematopoietic stem cell transplantation and immunomodulatory drugs have successfully been used in the treatment of CLL. Immune-based therapy represents an exciting mode of treatment since it may be able to eliminate leukemia cells without inducing immune suppression. The elucidation of the molecular and cellular events underlying the immune dysfunction in CLL is of key importance to further develop novel immune-based therapies. It is presumably that a deeper knowledge of the immune response in CLL may open new frontiers in the treatment of these patients.

7. Acknowledgement

This work was supported by the Spanish grant of Fondo de Investigaciones Sanitarias (Institute Carlos III) PS09/00420.

8. References

Ashraf, U, Elefante AN, Cruz R, Wallace PK, Czuczman MS,Hernandez-llizaliturri FJ Emergence of rituximab-fludarabine resistance is associated with changes in CD20 antigen expression and improved response to alemtuzumab therapy in patients with chronic lymphocytic leukemia (chronic lymphocytic leukaemia). Blood 2007;110, 612a (abstract 2054).

Aue G, Njuguna N, Tian X, Soto S, Hughes T, Vire B, Keyvanfar K, Gibellini F, Valdez J, Boss C, Samsel L, McCoy JP Jr, Wilson WH, Pittaluga S, Wiestner A. Lenalidomide-induced upregulation of CD80 on tumor cells correlates with T-cell activation, the rapid onset of a cytokine release syndrome and leukemic cell clearance in chronic lymphocytic leukemia. Haematologica. 2009;94(9):1266-73.

Awan FT, Johnson AJ, Lapalombella R, Hu W, Lucas M, Fischer B, Byrd JC. Thalidomide and lenalidomide as new therapeutics for the treatment of chronic lymphocytic leukemia. Leuk Lymphoma. 2010;51(1):27-38.

Badoux, X., Reuben, J., Lee, B., Jorgensen, J., Estrov, Z., Yerrow, K. Ferrajoli, A. (2009). Lenalidomide therapy is associated with normalization of lymphocyte populations and increase in immunoglobulin levels in elderly patients with chronic lymphocytic leukemia [Abstract 10.31]. *Haematologica, 94*(3, Suppl.), S94.

Bahram S, Bresnahan M, Geraghty DE, Spies T. A second lineage of mammalian major histocompatibility complex class I genes, Proc Natl Acad Sci USA 1994; 91:6259-63.

Bauer S, Groh V, Wu J, Steinle A, Phillips JH, Lanier LL, Spies T. Activation of NK cells and T cells by NKG2D, a receptor for stress-inducible MICA. Science 1999; 285: 727-9.

Behl D, Porrata LF, Markovic SN, Letendre L, Pruthi RK, Hook CC, et al. Absolute lymphocyte count recovery after induction chemotherapy predicts superior survival in acute myelogenous leukemia. Leukemia. 2006;20:29-34.

Behl D, Ristow K, Markovic SN, Witzig TE, Habermann TM, Colgan JP,et al. Absolute lymphocyte count predicts therapeutic efficacy of rituximab therapy in follicular lymphomas. Br J Haematol. 2007;137:409-15.

Beyer M, Kochanek M, Darabi K, et al. Reduced frequencies and suppressive function of CD4+ $CD25^{hi}$ regulatory T cells in patients with chronic lymphocytic leukemia after therapy with fludarabine. Blood 2006;106:2018-2025.

Bologna L, Gotti E, Manganini M, Rambaldi A, Intermesoli T, Introna M, Golay J. Mechanism of Action of Type II, Glycoengineered, Anti-CD20 Monoclonal Antibody GA101 in B-Chronic Lymphocytic Leukemia Whole Blood Assays in Comparison with Rituximab and Alemtuzumab. J Immunol. 2011 Feb 4.

Byrd JC, Rai K, Peterson BL, Appelbaum FR, Morrison VA, Kolitz JE, Shepherd L, Hines JD, Schiffer CA, Larson RA. Addition of rituximab to fludarabine may prolong progression-free survival and overall survival in patients with previously untreated chronic lymphocytic leukemia: an updated retrospective comparative analysis of CALGB 9712 and CALGB 9011. Blood. 2005;105(1):49-53.

Caligaris-Cappio F, Hamblin TJ. B-cell chronic lymphocytic leukemia: a bird of a different feather. J Clin Oncol. 1999;17:399-408.

Cantwell M, Hua T, Pappas J, Kipps TJ. Acquired CD40-ligand deficiency in chronic lymphocytic leukemia. Nat Med. 1997;3:984-9.

Casak SJ, Lemery SJ, Shen YL, Rothmann MD, Khandelwal A, Zhao H, Davis G, Jarral V, Keegan P, Pazdur R. U.S. Food and drug administration approval: rituximab in combination with fludarabine and cyclophosphamide for the treatment of patients with chronic lymphocytic leukemia. Oncologist. 2011;16(1):97-104.

Cerwenka A, Baron JL, Lanier LL. Ectopic expression of retinoic acid early inducible-1 gene (RAE-1) permits natural killer cell-mediated rejection of a MHC class I-bearing tumor in vivo. Proc Natl Acad Sci USA 2001; 98:11521-11526.

Chanan-Khan A, Miller KC, Lawrence D, Padmanabhan S, Miller A, Hernandez-Illatazurri F, Czuczman MS, Wallace PK, Zeldis JB, Lee K. Tumor flare reaction associated with lenalidomide treatment in patients with chronic lymphocytic leukemia predicts clinical response. Cancer. 2010 Nov 29.

Chanan-Khan A, Miller KC, Musial L, Lawrence D, Padmanabhan S, Takeshita K, Porter CW, Goodrich DW, Bernstein ZP, Wallace P, Spaner D, Mohr A, Byrne C, Hernandez-Ilizaliturri F, Chrystal C, Starostik P, Czuczman MS. Clinical efficacy of lenalidomide in patients with relapsed or refractory chronic lymphocytic leukemia: results of a phase II study. J Clin Oncol. 2006;24(34):5343-9.

Chanan-Khan A, Porter CW. Immunomodulating drugs for chronic lymphocytic leukaemia. Lancet Oncol. 2006;7(6):480-8.

Chen CI, Bergsagel PL, Paul H, Xu W, Lau A, Dave N, Kukreti V, Wei E, Leung-Hagesteijn C, Li ZH, Brandwein J, Pantoja M, Johnston J, Gibson S, Hernandez T, Spaner D, Trudel S. Single-Agent Lenalidomide in the Treatment of Previously Untreated Chronic Lymphocytic Leukemia. J Clin Oncol. 2010 Dec 28.

Cheson BD, Bennett JM, Grever M, et al. (1996). "National Cancer Institute-sponsored Working Group guidelines for chronic lymphocytic leukemia: revised guidelines for diagnosis and treatment". Blood 87 (12): 4990–7.

Clark WH Jr, From L, Bernardino EA, Mihm MC. The histogenesis and biologic behavior of primary human malignant melanomas of the skin. Cancer Res 1969;29:705-27.

Clemente CG, Mihm MC Jr, Bufalino R, Zurrida S, Collini P, Cascinelli N. Prognostic value of tumor infiltrating lymphocytes in the vertical growth phase of primary cutaneous melanoma. Cancer 1996;77:1303-10

Cosman D, Mullberg J, Sutherland CL, Chin W, Armitage R, Fanslow W, Kubin M, Chalupny NJ. ULBPs, novel MHC class I-related molecules, bind to CMV glycoprotein UL16 and stimulate NK cytotoxicity through the NKG2D receptor. Immunity 2001; 14: 123-33.

Cox MC, Nofroni I, Ruco L, Amodeo R, Ferrari A, La Verde G, et al. Low absolute lymphocyte count is a poor prognostic factor in diffuse-large-B-cell-lymphoma. Leuk Lymphoma. 2008;49:1745-51.

Crowe JS, Hall VS, Smith MA, Cooper HJ, Tite JP. Humanized monoclonal antibody CAMPATH-1H: myeloma cell expression of genomic constructs, nucleotide sequence of cDNA constructs and comparison of effector mechanisms of myeloma and Chinese hamster ovary cell-derived material. Clin Exp Immunol. 19927(1):105-10.

Das H, Groh V, Kuijl C, Sugita M, Morita CT, Spies T, Bukowski JF. MICA engagement by human Vgamma2Vdelta2 T cells enhances their antigen-dependent effector function. Immunity 2001; 15:83-93.

De Angulo G, Yuen C, Palla SL, Anderson PM, Zweidler-McKay PA. Absolute lymphocyte count is a novel prognostic indicator in ALL and AML: implications for risk stratification and future studies. Cancer. 2008;112:407-15.

Del Giudice I, Chiaretti S, Tavolaro S, De Propris MS, Maggio R, Mancini F, Peragine N, Santangelo S, Marinelli M, Mauro FR, Guarini A, Foà R. Spontaneous regression of chronic lymphocytic leukemia: clinical and biologic features of 9 cases. Blood. 2009;114:638-46.

Delgado J, Thomson K, Russell N, et al. Results of alemtuzumab-based reduced-intensity allogeneic transplantation for chronic lymphocytic leukemia: a British Society of Blood and Marrow Transplantation Study. Blood 2006;107(4):1724-1730

Demanet C, Mulder A, Deneys V, Worsham MJ, Maes P, Claas FH, Ferrone S. Down-regulation of HLA-A and HLA-Bw6, but not HLA-Bw4, allospecificities in leukemic cells: an escape mechanism from CTL and NK attack? Blood. 2004;103(8):3122-30.

Diefenbach A, Jensen ER, Jamieson AM, Raulet DH. Rae1 and H60 ligands of the NKG2D receptor stimulate tumor immunity. Nature 2001; 413, 165-171.

Dighiero G, Maloum K, Desablens B, Cazin B, Navarro M, Leblay R, Leporrier M, Jaubert J, Lepeu G, Dreyfus B, Binet JL, Travade P. Chlorambucil in indolentchronic lymphocytic leukemia. French Cooperative Group on Chronic Lymphocytic Leukemia. N Engl J Med. 1998;338(21):1506-14.

Dreger P, Brand R, Milligan D, et al. Reduced-intensity conditioning lowers treatment-related mortality of allogeneic stem cell transplantation for chronic lymphocytic leukemia: a population-matched analysis. Leukemia 2005;19(6):1029-1033.

Dreger P, Corradini P, Kimby E, et al. Indications for allogeneic stem cell transplantation in chronic lymphocytic leukemia: the EBMT transplant consensus. Leukemia. 2007;21:12–17.

Dreger P. Allotransplantation for chronic lymphocytic leukemia Hematology 2009.

Dunn, GP, Old, LJ, Schreiber, RD. The three Es of cancer immunoediting. Annu Rev Immunol 2004; 22:329-60.

Ege H, Gertz MA, Markovic SN, Lacy MQ, Dispenzieri A, Hayman SR, Kumar SK, Porrata LF. Prediction of survival using absolute lymphocyte count for newly diagnosed patients with multiple myeloma: a retrospective study. Br J Haematol. 2008;141(6):792-8.

Eichhorst BF, Busch R, Hopfinger G, Pasold R, Hensel M, Steinbrecher C, Siehl S, Jäger U, Bergmann M, Stilgenbauer S, Schweighofer C, Wendtner CM, Döhner H, Brittinger G, Emmerich B, Hallek M; German chronic lymphocytic leukaemia Study Group. Fludarabine plus cyclophosphamide versus fludarabine alone in first-line therapy of younger patients with chronic lymphocytic leukemia. Blood. 2006;107(3):885-91.

Erikci AA, Karagoz B, Ozyurt M, Ozturk A, Kilic S, Bilgi O. HLA-G expression in B chronic lymphocytic leukemia: a new prognostic marker? Hematology. 2009;14:101-5.

Farina L, Carniti C, Dodero A, et al. Qualitative and quantitative polymerase chain reaction monitoring of minimal residual disease in relapsed chronic lymphocytic leukemia: early assessment can predict long-term outcome after reduced intensity allogeneic transplantation. Haematologica 2009;94(5):654-662.

Ferrajoli A, Lee BN, Schlette EJ, O'Brien SM, Gao H, Wen S, Wierda WG, Estrov Z, Faderl S, Cohen EN, Li C, Reuben JM, Keating MJ. Lenalidomide induces complete and partial remissions in patients with relapsed and refractory chronic lymphocytic leukemia. Blood. 2008;111(11):5291-7.

Foa R, Lauria F, Lusso P, Giubellino MC, Fierro MT, Ferrando ML, et al. Discrepancy between phenotypic and functional features of natural killer T-lymphocytes in B-cell chronic lymphocytic leukaemia. Br J Haematol. 1984;58:509-16.

Gasser S, Orsulic S, Brown EJ, Raulet DH. The DNA damage pathway regulates innate immune system ligands of the NKG2D receptor. Nature 2005; 436:1186-90.

Golay J, Manganini M, Rambaldi A, Introna M. Effect of alemtuzumab on neoplastic B cells. Haematologica. 2004;89(12):1476-83.

Gonzalez S, Gonzalez-Rodríguez AP, Lopez-Soto A, Huergo-Zapico L, Lopez-Larrea C, Suarez-Alvarez B. Conceptual aspects of self and nonself discrimination. 2011, 2(1):1-7.

González S, Groh V, Spies T. Immunobiology of human NKG2D and its ligands. Curr To Microbiol Immunol 2006; 298:121-38.

González S, López-Soto A, Suárez-Álvarez B, López-Vázquez A, López-Larrea C. NKG2D ligands: key targets of the immune response. Trends Immunol 2008; 14:179-89.

Gonzalez-Rodriguez AP, Contesti J, Huergo-Zapico L, Lopez-Soto A, Fernández-Guizán A, Acebes-Huerta A, Gonzalez-Huerta AJ, Gonzalez E, Fernandez-Alvarez C, Gonzalez S. Prognostic significance of CD8 and CD4 T cells in chronic lymphocytic leukemia. Leuk Lymphoma. 2010;51(10):1829-36

Gorgun G, Holderried TA, Zahrieh D, Neuberg D, Gribben JG. Chronic lymphocytic leukemia cells induce changes in gene expression of CD4 and CD8 T cells. J Clin Invest. 2005;115:1797-805.

Gribben JG, Hallek M. Rediscovering alemtuzumab: current and emerging therapeutic roles. Br J Haematol. 2009;144(6):818-31.

Gribben JG, Zahrieh D, Stephans K, Bartlett-Pandite L, Alyea EP, Fisher DC, Freedman AS, Mauch P, Schlossman R, Sequist LV, Soiffer RJ, Marshall B, Neuberg D, Ritz J, Nadler LM. Autologous and allogeneic stem cell transplantations for poor-risk chronic lymphocytic leukemia. Blood. 2005;106(13):4389-96.

Gribben JG, Zahrieh D, Stephans K, et al. Autologous and allogeneic stem cell transplantations for poor-risk chronic lymphocytic leukemia. Blood 2005;106(13):4389-4396

Groh V, Bahram S, Bauer S, Herman A, Beauchamp M, Spies T. Cell stress-regulated human major histocompatibility complex class I gene expressed in gastrointestinal epithelium. Proc Natl Acad Sci USA 1996; 93:12445-50.

Groh V, Rhinehart R, Secrist H, Bauer S, Grabstein KH, Spies T. Broad tumor-associated expression and recognition by tumor-derived gamma delta Tcells of MICA and MICB. Proc Natl Acad Sci USA 1999; 96:6879-6884.

Groh V, Smythe K, Dai Z, Spies T. Fas-ligand-mediated paracrine T cell regulation by the receptor NKG2D in tumor immunity. Nat Immunol 2006; 7:755-762.

Groh V, Wu J, Yee C, Spies T. Tumor-derived soluble MIC ligands impair expression of NKG2D and T-cell activation. Nature 2002; 419:734-738.

Grulich AE, van Leeuwen MT, Falster MO, Vajdic CM. Incidence of cancers in people with HIV/AIDS compared with immunosuppressed transplant recipients: a meta-analysis. Lancet 2007;370(9581):59-67.

Guerra N, Tan YX, Joncker NT, Choy A, Gallardo F, Xiong N, Knoblaugh S, Cado D, Greenberg NM, Raulet DH. NKG2D-deficient mice are defective in tumor surveillance in models of spontaneous malignancy. Immunity 2008; 28:571-80.

Hallek M, Cheson BD, Catovsky D, Caligaris-Cappio F, Dighiero G, Döhner H, Hillmen P, Keating MJ, Montserrat E, Rai KR, Kipps TJ; International Workshop on Chronic Lymphocytic Leukemia. Guidelines for the diagnosis and treatment of chronic lymphocytic leukemia: a report from the International Workshop on Chronic Lymphocytic Leukemia updating the National Cancer Institute-Working Group 1996 guidelines. Blood. 2008;111(12):5446-56.

Hallek M, Therapy of chronic lymphocytic lekemia. Best Pract Res Clin Haematol. 2010;23(1):85-96.

Hallek, M, Fingerle-Rowson G, Fink A-M, Busch R, Mayer J, Hensel M, Hopfinger G, Hess G, von Gruenhagen U et al. First-Line Treatment with Fludarabine (F), Cyclophosphamide (C), and Rituximab (R) (FCR) Improves Overall Survival (OS) in Previously Untreated Patients (pts) with Advanced Chronic Lymphocytic Leukemia (chronic lymphocytic leukaemia): Results of a Randomized Phase III Trial On Behalf of An International Group of Investigators and the German chronic lymphocytic leukaemia Study Group. Blood. ASH Annual Meeting Abstracts 2009; 114 (22): 535.

Hamblin AD, Hamblin TJ. The immunodeficiency of chronic lymphocytic leukaemia. Br Med Bull. 2008;87:49-62.

Hamblin TJ. Autoimmune complications of chronic lymphocytic leukemia. Semin Oncol 2006;33:230-239.

Hamblin TJ.. Chronic lymphocytic leukaemia. Balliere's Clin Haematol 1987;1:449-491.

Hillmen, P., Skotnicki, A.B., Robak, T., Jaksic, B., Dmoszynska, A., Wu, J., Sirard, C. & Mayer, J. (2007) Alemtuzumab compared with chlorambucil as first-line therapy for chronic lymphocytic leukemia. Journal of Clinical Oncology 2007;25:5616–5623.

Hoogendoorn M, Jedema I, Barge RM, et al. Characterization of graft-versus-leukemia responses in patients treated for advanced chronic lymphocytic leukemia with donor lymphocyte infusions after in vitro T-cell depleted allogeneic stem cell transplantation following reduced-intensity conditioning. Leukemia 2007;21(12):2569-2574

Jaglowski SM, Alinari L, Lapalombella R, Muthusamy N, Byrd JC. The clinicalapplication of monoclonal antibodies in chronic lymphocytic leukemia. Blood. 2010;116(19):3705-14.

Jaglowski SM, Byrd JC. Rituximab in chronic lymphocytic leukemia. Semen Hematol. 2010;47(2):156-69.

Jewell AP, Worman CP, Giles FJ, Goldstone AH, Lydyard PM. Resistance of chronic lymphocytic leukaemia cells to interferon-alpha generated lymphokine activated killer cells. Leuk Lymphoma. 1992;7:473-80.

Junevik K, Werlenius O, Hasselblom S, Jacobsson S, Nilsson-Ehle H, Andersson PO. The expression of NK cell inhibitory receptors on cytotoxic T cells in B-cell chronic lymphocytic leukaemia (B-chronic lymphocytic leukaemia). Ann Hematol. 2007;86:89-94.

Kato N, Tanaka J, Sugita J, Toubai T, Miura Y, Ibata M, et al. Regulation of the expression of MHC class I-related chain A, B (MICA, MICB) via chromatin remodeling and its impact on the susceptibility of leukemic cells to the cytotoxicity of NKG2D-expressing cells. Leukemia. 2007;21:2103-8.

Kato N, Tanaka J, Sugita J, Toubai T, Miura Y, Ibata M, Syono Y, Ota S, Kondo T, Asaka M, Imamura M. Regulation of the expression of MHC class I-related chain A, B (MICA, MICB) via chromatin remodeling and its impact on the susceptibility of leukemic cells to the cytotoxicity of NKG2D-expressing cells. Leukemia. 2007;21(10):2103-8.

Katrinakis G, Kyriakou D, Papadaki H, Kalokyri I, Markidou F, Eliopoulos GD. Defective natural killer cell activity in B-cell chronic lymphocytic leukaemia is associated with impaired release of natural killer cytotoxic factor(s) but not of tumour necrosis factor-alpha. Acta Haematol. 1996;96:16-23.

Keating MJ, Flinn I, Jain V, Binet JL, Hillmen P, Byrd J, Albitar M, Brettman L, Santabarbara P, Wacker B,Rai KR..Therapeutic role of alemtuzumab (Campath-1H) in patients who have failed fludarabine: results of a large international study. Blood 2002;9:3554–3561.

Kharfan-Dabaja MA, Kumar A, Behera M, Djulbegovic B. Systematic review of high dose chemotherapy and autologous haematopoietic stem cell transplantation for chronic lymphocytic leukaemia: what is the published evidence? Br J Haematol. 2007;139(2):234-42.

Kinlen LJ, Webster AD, Bird AG, Haile R, Peto J, Soothill JF, Thompson RA. Prospective study of cancer in patients with hypogammaglobulinaemia. Lancet 1985;1(8423):263-266.

leukemia include nonmutated B-cell antigens. Cancer Res. 2010 Feb 15;70(4):1344-55.

leukemia include nonmutated B-cell antigens. Cancer Res. 2010 Feb 15;70(4):1344-55.

Lopez-Larrea C, Suarez-Alvarez B, Lopez-Soto A, Lopez-Vazquez A, Gonzalez S. The NKG2D receptor: sensing stressed cells. Trends Mol Med 2008; 14:179-89.

Lundin J., Kimby E., Bjorkholm M, Broliden, PA, Celsing F, Hjalmar V, Mollgard L, Rebello P, Hale G, Waldmann H, Mellstedt H, Osterborg A. Phase II trial of subcutaneous anti-CD52 monoclonal antibody alemtuzumab (Campath-1H) as first-line treatment for patients with B-cell chronic lymphocytic leukemia (B-chronic lymphocytic leukaemia). Blood 2002;100:68–773.

Mackus WJ, Frakking FN, Grummels A, et al. Expansion of CMV-specific CD8 + CD45RA + CD27- T cells in B-cell chronic lymphocytic leukemia. Blood 2003;102:1057-1063.

Mackus WJ, Frakking FN, Grummels A, Gamadia LE, De Bree GJ, Hamann D, et al. Expansion of CMV-specific CD8+CD45RA+CD27- T cells in B-cell chronic lymphocytic leukemia. Blood. 2003;102:1057-63.

Maloney DG, Grillo-López AJ, Bodkin DJ, White CA, Liles TM, Royston I, Varns C, Rosenberg J, Levy R.IDEC-C2B8: results of a phase I multiple-dose trial in patients with relapsed non-Hodgkin's lymphoma. J Clin Oncol. 1997;15(10):3266-74.

Marina O, Hainz U, Biernacki MA, Zhang W, Cai A, Duke-Cohan JS, Liu F, Brusic V,

Mehta J, Powles R, Singhal S, Iveson T, Treleaven J, Catovsky D. Clinical and hematologic response of chronic lymphocytic and prolymphocytic leukemia persisting after allogeneic bone marrow transplantation with the onset of acute graft-versus-host disease: possible role of graft-versus-leukemia. Bone Marrow Transplant. 1996;17(3):371-5.

Mellemkjaer L, Hammarstrom L, Andersen V, Yuen J, Heilmann C, Barington T, Bjorkander J, Olsen JH. Cancer risk among patients with IgA deficiency or common variable immunodeficiency and their relatives: a combined Danish and Swedish study. Clin Exp Immunol 2002;130(3):495-500

Michallet M, Dreger P, Sutton L, Brand R, Richards S, van Os M, Sobh M, Choquet S, Corront B, Dearden C, Gratwohl A, Herr W, Catovsky D, Hallek M, de Witte T, Niederwieser D, Leporrier M, Milligan D; on behalf of the EBMT Chronic Leukemia Working Party. Autologous hematopoietic stem cell transplantation in chronic lymphocytic leukemia: results of European intergroup randomized trial comparing autografting versus observation. Blood. 2011; 117(5):1516-1521.

Milligan DW, Fernandes S, Dasgupta R, Davies FE, Matutes E, Fegan CD, McConkey C, Child JA, Cunningham D, Morgan GJ, Catovsky D; National Cancer Research Institute Haematological Studies Group. Results of the MRC pilot study show autografting for younger patients with chronic lymphocytic leukemia is safe and achieves a high percentage of molecular responses. Blood. 2005; 105(1):397-404.

Mone AP, Cheney C, Banks AL, Tridandapani S, Mehter N, Guster S, Lin T, Eisenbeis CF, Young DC, Byrd JC. Alemtuzumab induces caspase-independent cell death in human chronic lymphocytic leukemia cells through a lipid raft-dependent mechanism. Leukemia. 2006;20(2):272-9.

Montillo M, Tedeschi A, Miqueleiz S, Veronese S, Cairoli R, Intropido L, RicciF, Colosimo A, Scarpati B, Montagna M, Nichelatti M, Regazzi M, Morra E. Alemtuzumab as consolidation after a response to fludarabine is effective in purging residual disease in patients with chronic lymphocytic leukemia. J Clin Oncol. 2006;24(15):2337-42.

Moore OS Jr, Foote FW Jr. The relatively favourable prognosis of medullary carcinoma of the breast. Cancer 1949;2:635-42.

Morrell D, Cromartie E, Swift M. Mortality and cancer incidence in 263 patients with ataxia-telangiectasia. J Natl Cancer Inst 1986;77(1):89-92.

Neuberg D, Kutok JL, Alyea EP, Canning CM, Soiffer RJ, Ritz J, Wu CJ. Serologic markers of effective tumor immunity against chronic lymphocytic

Nückel H, Rebmann V, Dürig J, Dührsen U, Grosse-Wilde H. HLA-G expression is associated with an unfavorable outcome and immunodeficiency in chronic lymphocytic leukemia. Blood. 2005;105:1694-8.

Nückel H, Switala M, Sellmann L, Horn PA, Dürig J, Dührsen U, Küppers R, Grosse-Wilde H, Rebmann V. The prognostic significance of soluble NKG2D ligands in B-cell chronic lymphocytic leukemia Leukemia. 2010;24(6):1152-9.

Onrust SV, Lamb HM, Balfour JA. Rituximab. Drugs. 1999;58(1):79-88; discussion 89-90.

Osterborg A., Fassas AS, Anagnostopoulos A, Dyer MJ, Catovsky D, Mellstedt H. Humanized CD52 monoclonal antibody Campath-1H as first-line treatment in chronic lymphocytic leukaemia. British Journal of Haematology 1996;93:151–153.

Pagès F, Berger A, Camus M, Sanchez-Cabo F, Costes A, Molidor R, et al. Effector memory T cells, early metastasis, and survival in colorectal cancer. N Engl J Med 2005; 353:2654–66.

Palmer S, Hanson CA, Zent CS, et al. Prognostic importance of T and NK-cells in a consecutive series of newly diagnosed patients with chronic lymphocytic leukemia. Br J Haematol 2008; 141:607-614.

Pavletic SZ, Khouri IF, Haagenson M, King RJ, Bierman PJ, Bishop MR, Carston M, Giralt S, Molina A, Copelan EA, Ringdén O, Roy V, Ballen K, Adkins DR, McCarthy P, Weisdorf D, Montserrat E, Anasetti C. Unrelated donor marrow transplantation for B-cell chronic lymphocytic leukemia after using myeloablative conditioning: results from the Center for International Blood and Marrow Transplant research. J Clin Oncol. 2005;23(24):5788-94.

Plonquet A, Haioun C, Jais JP, Debard AL, Salles G, Bene MC, Feugier P, Rabian C, Casasnovas O, Labalette M, Kuhlein E, Farcet JP, Emile JF, Gisselbrecht C, Delfau-Larue MH; Groupe d'étude des lymphomes de l'adulte Peripheral blood natural killer cell count is associated with clinical outcome in patients with aaIPI 2-3 diffuse large B-cell lymphoma. Ann Oncol. 2007;18(7):1209-15.

Poggi A, Venturino C, Catellani S, Clavio M, Miglino M, Gobbi M, Steinle A, Ghia P, Stella S, Caligaris-Cappio F, Zocchi MR.Vdelta1 T lymphocytes from B-chronic lymphocytic leukaemia patients recognize ULBP3 expressed on leukemic B cells and up-regulated by trans-retinoic acid. Cancer Res. 2004;64(24):9172-9.

Porrata LF, Ristow K, Habermann TM, Witzig TE, Inwards DJ, Markovic SN. Absolute lymphocyte count at the time of first relapse predicts survival in patients with diffuse large B-cell lymphoma. Am J Hematol. 2009;84:93-7.

Porrata LF, Ristow K, Witzig TE, Tuinistra N, Habermann TM, Inwards DJ et al. Absolute lymphocyte count predicts therapeutic efficacy and survival at the time of radioimmunotherapy in patients with relapsed follicular lymphomas. Leukemia. 2007;21:2554-6.

Provan D, Bartlett-Pandite L, Zwicky C, Neuberg D, Maddocks A, Corradini P, Soiffer R, Ritz J, Nadler LM, Gribben JG. Eradication of polymerase chaín reaction-detectable chronic lymphocytic leukemia cells is associated with improved outcome after bone marrow transplantation. Blood. 1996; 88(6):2228-35.

Raffaghello L, Prigione I, Airoldi I, Camoriano M, Levreri I, Gambini C, Pende D, Steinle A, Ferrone S, Pistoia V. Downregulation and/or release of NKG2D ligands as immune evasion strategy of human neuroblastoma. Neoplasia 2004; 6:558-68.

Rai KR, Peterson BL, Appelbaum FR, et al. (2000). "Fludarabine compared with chlorambucil as primary therapy for chronic lymphocytic leukemia". N. Engl. J. Med. 343 (24): 1750–7.

Ramsay AG, Gribben JG. Immune dysfunction in chronic lymphocytic leukemia T cells and lenalidomide as an immunomodulatory drug. Haematologica. 2009;94(9):1198-202.

Ramsay AG, Johnson AJ, Lee AM, Gorgün G, Le Dieu R, Blum W, Byrd JC, Gribben JG. Chronic lymphocytic leukemia T cells show impaired immunological synapse formation that can be reversed with an immunomodulating drug. J Clin Invest. 2008;118(7):2427-37.

Raulet DH. Roles of the NKG2D immunoreceptor and its ligands. Nat Rev Immunol 2003; 3:781-90.

Ray-Coquard I, Cropet C, Van Glabbeke M, Sebban C, Le Cesne A, Judson I,et al; European Organization for Research and Treatment of Cancer Soft Tissue and Bone Sarcoma Group. Lymphopenia as a prognostic factor for overall survival in advanced carcinomas, sarcomas, and lymphomas. Cancer Res. 2009 ;69:5383-91.

Rebmann V, Schütt P, Brandhorst D, Opalka B, Moritz T, Nowrousian MR, Grosse-Wilde H.Soluble MICA as an independent prognostic factor for the overall survival and progression-free survival of multiple myeloma patients. Clin Immunol 2007; 123:114-20.

Ritgen M, Böttcher S, Stilgenbauer S, Bunjes D, Schubert J, Cohen S, Humpe A, Hallek M, Kneba M, Schmitz N, Döhner H, Dreger P; German chronic lymphocytic leukaemia

Study Group. Quantitative MRD monitoring identifies distinct GVL response patterns after allogeneic stem cell transplantation for chronic lymphocytic leukemia: results from the Gchronic lymphocytic leukaemiaSG chronic lymphocytic leukaemia3X trial. Leukemia. 2008;22:1377–1386.

Robak T, Moiseev SI, Dmoszynska A, Solal-Céligny P, Warzocha K, Loscertales J et al. Rituximab, Fludarabine, and Cyclophosphamide (R-FC) Prolongs Progression Free Survival in Relapsed or Refractory Chronic Lymphocytic Leukemia (chronic lymphocytic leukaemia) Compared with FC Alone: Final Results from the International Randomized Phase III REACH Trial. Blood. ASH Annual Meeting Abstracts. 2008; 112 (11):1.

Rollins BJ. Inflammatory chemokines in cancer growth and progression. Eur J Cancer 2006;42:760-7.

Rondón G, Giralt S, Huh Y, Khouri I, Andersson B, Andreeff M, Champlin R. Graft-versus-leukemia effect after allogeneic bone marrow transplantation for chronic lymphocytic leukemia. Bone Marrow Transplant. 1996 Sep;18(3):669-72.

Rossi E, Matutes E, Morilla R, Owusu-Ankomah K, Heffernan AM, Catovsky D. Zeta chain and CD28 are poorly expressed on T lymphocytes from chronic lymphocytic leukemia. Leukemia. 1996;10:494-7.

Salih HR, Antropius H, Gieseke F, Lutz SZ, Kanz L, Rammensee HG, Steinle A. Functional expression and release of ligands for the activating immunoreceptor NKG2D in leukemia. Blood 2003; 102:1389-1396.

Salih HR, Rammensee HG, Steinle A. Cutting edge: down-regulation of MICA on human tumors by proteolytic shedding. J Immunol 2002; 169:4098-4102.

Scanlan MJ, Simpson AJ, Old LJ. The cancer/testis genes: review, standardization, and commentary. Cancer Immun 2004;4:1.

Schetelig J, Thiede C, Bornhauser M, et al. Evidence of a graft-versus-leukemia effect in chronic lymphocytic leukemia after reduced-intensity conditioning and allogeneic stem-cell transplantation: the Cooperative German Transplant Study Group. J Clin Oncol 2003;21(14):2747-2753.

Schetelig J, van Biezen A, Brand R, et al. Allogeneic hematopoietic cell transplantation for chronic lymphocytic leukemia with 17p deletion: a retrospective EBMT analysis. J Clin Oncol. 2008;5094–5100.

Sher T, Miller KC, Lawrence D, Whitworth A, Hernandez-Ilizaliturri F, CzuczmanMS, Miller A, Lawrence W, Bilgrami SA, Sood R, Wood MT, Block AW, Lee K, Chanan-Khan AA. Efficacy of lenalidomide in patients with chronic lymphocytic leukemia with high-risk cytogenetics. Leuk Lymphoma. 2010;51(1):85-8.

Siddiqui M, Ristow K, Markovic SN, Witzig TE, Habermann TM, Colgan JP, et al. Absolute lymphocyte count predicts overall survival in follicular lymphomas. Br J Haematol. 2006;134:596-601.

Smyth MJ, Dunn GP, Schreiber RD. Cancer immunosurveillance and immunoediting: the roles of immunity in suppressing tumor development and shaping tumor immunogenicity. Adv Immunol. 2006;90:1-50.

Sorror ML, Maris MB, Sandmaier BM, et al. Hematopoietic cell transplantation after nonmyelo-ablative conditioning for advanced chronic lymphocytic leukemia. J Clin Oncol 2005;23(16):3819-3829.

Sorror ML, Storer BE, Sandmaier BM, Maris M, Shizuru J, Maziarz R, Agura E, Chauncey TR, Pulsipher MA, McSweeney PA, Wade JC, Bruno B, Langston A, Radich J, Niederwieser D, Blume KG, Storb R, Maloney DG. Five-year follow-up of patients with advanced chronic lymphocytic leukemia treated with allogeneic hematopoietic cell transplantation after nonmyeloablative conditioning. J Clin Oncol. 2008;26(30):4912-20.

Steurer M, Pall G, Richards S, Schwarzer G, Bohlius J, Greil R. Purine antagonists for chronic lymphocytic leukaemia. Cochrane database of systematic reviews (Online) 2006; 3: CD004270.

Swann JB, Smyth MJ. Immune surveillance of tumors. J Clin Invest. 2007;117(5):1137-46.

Tam CS, O'Brien S, Wierda W, Kantarjian H, Wen S, Do KA, Thomas DA, Cortes J, Lerner S, Keating MJ. Long-term results of the fludarabine, cyclophosphamide, and rituximab regimen as initial therapy of chronic lymphocytic leukemia. Blood. 2008;112(4):975-80.

Taskinen M, Ranki A, Pukkala E, Jeskanen L, Kaitila I, Makitie O. Extended follow-up of the Finnish cartilage-hair hypoplasia cohort confirms high incidence of non-Hodgkin lymphoma and basal cell carcinoma. Am J Med Genet A 2008;146A(18):2370-2375.

Teeling JL, French RR, Cragg MS, van den Brakel J, Pluyter M, Huang H, Chan C, Parren PW, Hack CE, Dechant M, Valerius T, van de Winkel JG, Glennie MJ. Characterization of new human CD20 monoclonal antibodies with potent cytolytic activity against non-Hodgkin lymphomas. Blood. 2004;104(6):1793-800.

Totterman TH, Carlsson M, Simonsson B, Bengtsson M, Nilsson K. T-cell activation and subset patterns are altered in B-chronic lymphocytic leukaemia and correlate with the stage of the disease. Blood. 1989;74:786-92.

Vajdic CM, Mao L, van Leeuwen MT, Kirkpatrick P, Grulich AE, Riminton S. Are antibody deficiency disorders associated with a narrower range of cancers than other forms of immunodeficiency? Blood. 2010;116(8):1228-34.

Velardi A. Natural Killer cells and allogeneic haematopoietic cell transplantation. Natural Killer cells. Basic science and clinical application. London 2010, Pag543-53.

Wierda W, O'Brien S, Wen S, Faderl S, Garcia-Manero G, Thomas D, Do KA, Cortes J, Koller C, Beran M, Ferrajoli A, Giles F, Lerner S, Albitar M, Kantarjian H,Keating M. Chemoimmunotherapy with fludarabine, cyclophosphamide, and rituximabfor relapsed and refractory chronic lymphocytic leukemia. J Clin Oncol. 2005;23(18):4070-8.

Wierda WG, Kipps TJ. Chronic lymphocytic leukemia. Curr Opin Hematol. 1999;6:253-61.

Wu L, Adams M, Carter T, Chen R, Muller G, Stirling D, Schafer P, Bartlett JB. Lenalidomide enhances natural killer cell and monocyte-mediated antibody-dependent cellular cytotoxicity of rituximab-treated CD20+ tumor cells. Clin Cancer Res. 2008;14(14):4650-7.

Zent CS, Chen JB, Kurten RC, Kaushal GP, Lacy HM, Schichman SA. Alemtuzumab (CAMPATH 1H) does not kill chronic lymphocytic leukemia cells in serum free medium. Leuk Res. 2004;28(5):495-507.

Zent CS, Kay NE. Autoimmune complications in chronic lymphocytic leukaemia. Best Pract Res Clin Haematol. 2010;23(1):47-59.

15

In Vitro Sensitivity Testing in the Assessment of Anti-CLL Drug Candidates

Günter Krause, Mirjam Kuckertz, Susan Kerwien, Michaela Patz and Michael Hallek
Department I of Internal Medicine, University of Cologne, Center of Integrated Oncology Köln Bonn, Germany

1. Introduction

Chronic lymphocytic leukemia (CLL) is characterized by the accumulation of morphologically mature, but immuno-incompetent B-lymphocytes in the bone marrow, peripheral blood, spleen and lymphoid organs. With an annual incidence of about 2-3/ 100000 in the general population (Hamblin, 2009), CLL represents a frequent leukemia type. Since CLL mostly affects persons of advanced age, the incidence among persons above 65 years reaches ten times this frequency (Eichhorst et al., 2009). Moreover CLL follows a remarkably heterogeneous course, emphasizing the need for personalized treatment approaches. Despite recent advances in CLL therapy, the disease still remains incurable and new treatment options need to be developed (Hallek et al., 2008). New insights into CLL biology have started to result in new targeted, sometimes patient group-specific treatment approaches (Pleyer et al., 2009; Zenz et al., 2010). Candidate substances for pre-clincial assays are mostly molecularly targeted drugs, i.e. either small molecules interfering with intracellular signaling (Wickremasinghe et al., 2011) or mononoclonal antibodies (Jaglowski et al., 2010). As examples we will discuss in this chapter the pre-clinical assessment of protein and lipid kinase inhibitors and of monoclonal antibodies.

Since candidate substances with a potential for treating CLL become available at an increasing pace, there is a growing need for comprehensive laboratory assessment of these substances. For this purpose the effects of these drug candidates on fresh CLL lymphocytes are compared by means of viability and cytotoxicity assays with the aim of selecting suitable candidates for further development. In addition viability and cytotoxicity assays on CLL cells serve to prepare candidate substances for clinical trials and to determine, which subgroups of patients respond best, in the sense of personalized medicine. This endeavor constitutes the small excerpt of the drug discovery process immediately preceding clinical trials (Collins & Workman, 2006). Since it links laboratory investigation and clinical application it can be understood as translational research, which is further underscored by patient samples being subjected to cultivation and observation in the laboratory.

B lymphocytes freshly isolated from peripheral blood of CLL patients constitute a readily available source for the pre-clinical *in vitro* assessment of drugs and combinations with therapeutic potential for treating CLL. Due to the epidemiological features of CLL as a frequent chronic leukemia, with many patients living with the disease for extended periods, a continuous supply of blood samples can be made available and used in a meaningful manner by performing pre-clinical assays, which, according to the concept of translational medicine, in turn could lead to improved therapies. Drug assessment on fresh CLL samples can be performed rapidly and relatively conveniently by comparing untreated and treated *in vitro* cultures.

On the other hand, primary cultures of B cells freshly isolated from the peripheral blood of CLL patients often may represent an insufficient model for predicting clinical drug efficacy, since they are known to behave differently from CLL lymphocytes in their *in vivo* environment. This is evident from the obviously contrasting behavior of CLL cells *in vivo* and during *in vitro* culture. Whereas accumulation of CLL cells *in vivo* is thought to occur due to resistance towards apoptosis and a certain degree of cell proliferation, *in vitro* cultures spontaneously undergo apoptosis and show low viability and almost completely absent proliferation. Because this contrasting behaviour of CLL cells *in vitro* and *in vivo* can be attributed to a lack of the appropriate micro-environment during laboratory culture, the value of drug assessment on CLL lymphocytes *ex vivo* can be greatly enhanced by mimicking certain micro-environmental stimuli.

Commonly used cytotoxicity and viability assays are compiled in this chapter and will be discussed in the context of the assessment of potential anti-CLL drugs. On the level of individual susceptibility it is well established for chemotherapeutic agents that sensitivity of tumor cells *in vitro* corresponds to the probability of clinical response (Bosanquet et al., 2009). Therefore one would expect also for targeted drugs that *in vitro* assays enable to some degree the comparison of the efficacies of different agents and the prediction of the response of molecularly defined subgroups of CLL patients. As examples for correlations of molecularly defined patient subgroups with treatment susceptibility *in vitro* we name here the clearly higher dasatinib sensitivity of CLL samples with unmutated IgHV genes as compared to mutated ones (Veldurthy et al., 2008) or the correlation of the B cell depletion induced by CD20 antibodies with antigen expression on the surface of CLL cells (Patz et al., 2011).

In this chapter we review the pros and cons of pre-clinical drug assessment in comparatively simple *ex vivo* assays. The predictability of treatment out-come from *in vitro* cultures of CLL lymphocytes must be considered, since there are known limitations of the assay system, which can, however, be overcome to a certain degree by linking the results to investigations of target and cell type specificity.

2. Performing cytotoxicity assays on CLL samples

In the course of the pre-clinical assessment of anti-CLL drug candidates, *in vitro* cultures of CLL lymphocytes are treated with test substances. Subsequently dose-dependent treatment effects on the viability of CLL cells are recorded by means of established proliferation and cytotoxicity assays. These assays yield a first measure of drug potency for CLL lymphocytes, but certainly need to be rigidly controlled and standardized. Moreover they should be accompanied by biochemical assays in order to assure cell type and target specificity. Such comprehensive approaches will allow the design of meaningful drug combinations, which then are to be subjected to another round of *in vitro* sensitivity assays.

Cytotoxicity assays play a pivotal role in pre-clinical drug testing (Kepp et al., 2011) and many of them are suitable for assessing treatment effects on fresh CLL cells (*Table 1*). Some of these assays are based on absolute cell counts or less laborious surrogate parameters determining total cellular activities e.g. in colorimetric or fluorimetric non-clonogenic microculture assays (Lindhagen et al., 2008). In contrast, flow cytometric assays usually yield percentages of cells with certain properties within the investigated cell population unless they are standardized for the examined volume, e.g. by absolute counting beads.

Method	Technological platform	parameters
cell counting	light microscope	trypan blue exclusion
metabolic activity	absorbance reader	tetrazolium salt reduction
ATP consumption	luminometer	luciferase activity
intracellular esterase activity	fluorimeter	conversion of non-fluorescent fluorescein diacetate
DNA replication	absorbance reader flow cytometry	bromo-deoxyuridine incorporation
phosphatidylserine exposure	flow cytometry	annexin V-binding
membrane disintegration	flow cytometry	staining with DNA intercalating dye
$\Delta\psi m$ dissipation	flow cytometry	fluorescent dye, e.g. DiOC6
morphology	flow cytometry	forward scatter / side scatter
production of reactive oxygen species	flow cytometry	fluorigenic substrate, e.g. CM-H2-DCF-DA
caspase activation	flow cytometry immunoblotting	fluorescent substrates detection of cleaved fragments

Table 1. Selected cytotoxicity and viability assays commonly used with CLL samples.

2.1 Flow cytometric cell death and viability assays

Flow cytometric assessment of phosphatidylserine exposure and membrane disintegration is among the viability and cytotoxicity assays most frequently applied for monitoring drug effects on CLL cells. Percentages of cell populations undergoing cell death can be determined by monitoring the loss of membrane asymmetry in early phases of apoptosis and subsequent membrane disruption (*Fig. 1*). This can be achieved by staining cells, e.g. B lymphocytes, with fluorescently labeled annexin V, which binds to phosphatidylserine with high affinity (Koopman et al., 1994). Phosphatidylserine exposure accompanies early phases of apoptosis, before membrane disintegration of the cytoplasma membrane allows access of DNA intercalating dies to the nucleus. Counter-staining with DNA intercalating dyes originally served the distinction of apoptotic from necrotic cells. Analysis of annexin V binding or DNA staining can be replaced for staining with dyes indicating mitochondrial membrane potential, e.g. 3,3′-dihexyloxacarbocyanine iodide (DiOC6) (Stanglmaier et al.,

2004; Veldurthy et al., 2008), or reactive oxygen species, e.g. the fluorogenic chloromethyl-2,7-dichlorodihydrofluorescein-diacetate (CM-H_2-DCF-DA) (Lilienthal et al., 2011). Usually populations of CLL cells with phosphatidylserine exposure coincide with those showing typical morphological signs of apoptosis, i.e. reduced size and increased granularity as indicated by forward-scatter (FSC) and side-scatter (SSC) in the flow cytometer. Concerns have been raised about a possible over-estimation of drug effects due to flow cytometry artefacts. For instance, the widely used determination of phosphatidylserine exposure was claimed to over-estimate apoptosis induction in the extraordinarily fragile CLL cells due to *in vitro* handling during sample preparation for flow cytometry (Groves et al., 2009). Similarly antibody effects on CLL samples determined by flow cytometry were suspected of being misinterpreted owing to cell aggregation (Golay et al., 2010). These concerns can be overcome by parallel biological effect monitoring in several different assay systems as controls.

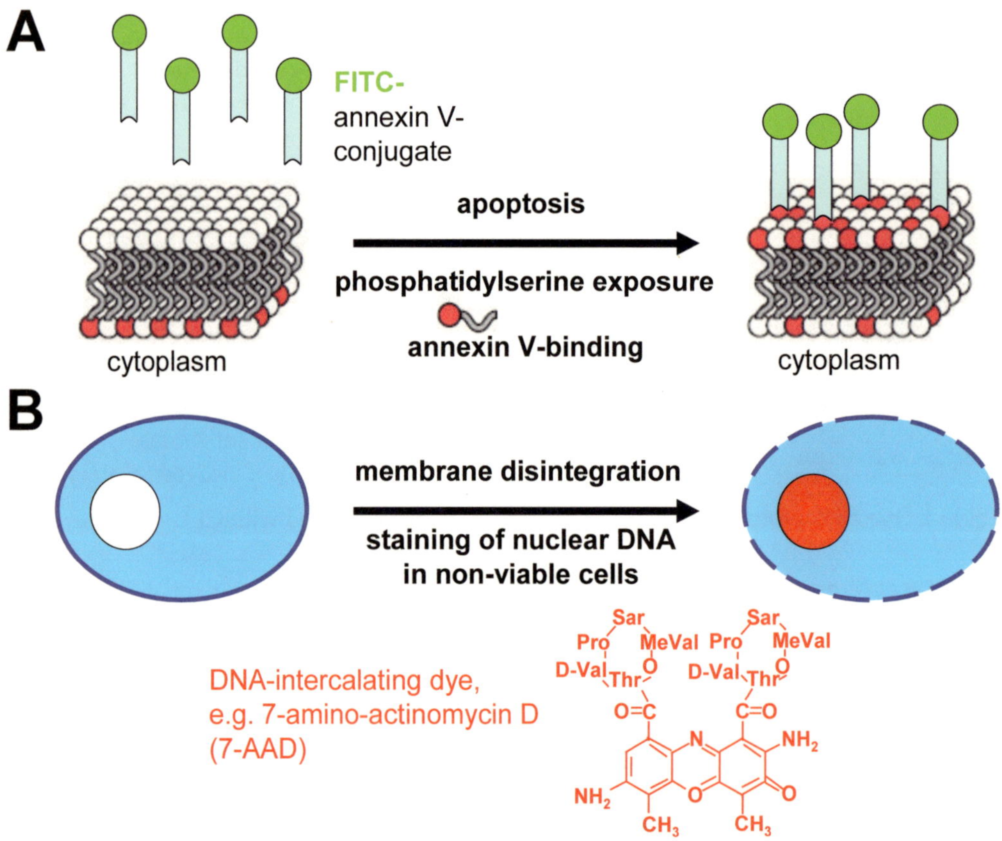

Fig. 1. Principle of a widely used assay for the determination of the percentages of apoptotic cells. The flow cytometric assessment of phosphatidylserine exposure (A) and membrane disintegration (B) can be performed simultaneously.
Part (A) adapted from Zhang et al., 1997 and Pharmingen, 1998.

2.2 Concentration dependence

Investigation of the dose-dependency of drug effects is an important confirmation of any observations that by far surpasses the importance of repeated measurements. In addition, the shape of dose response curves sometimes can provide mechanistic clues, e.g. in the case of saturation effects. When drugs are investigated for CLL that previously have been pre-clinically developed or admitted for the treatment of other cancers, it is possible to consider achievable plasma concentrations for the *in vitro* assessment. Biological effect measurements obtained at multiple concentrations can be conveniently summarized by concentrations inhibiting 50 % (IC_{50}). These IC_{50} concentrations can be a useful manner of comparing the effects of different drugs or diverging sensitivities of different samples. In the case of saturation effects, as in the dose response of CLL lymphocytes to dasatinib (Veldurthy et al., 2008), it might be more appropriate to indicate the individual saturation levels of response rather than extrapolating IC_{50} concentrations. Moreover, investigators must not be misled by the convenience of such tabulated values to regard them as sample-specific constants and therefore to apply them to different assay types, since IC_{50} concentrations strictly depend on the type of assay performed (Krause & Hallek, 2011).

3. Mimicking micro-environmental interactions

Considering the micro-environment of CLL cells may improve predictions of clinical drug efficacy from *in vitro* assays on fresh CLL samples. Regarding their resistance to apoptosis CLL cells in culture behave entirely differently from the situation *in vivo*, owing to dependence on their micro-environment. Therefore it is necessary to simulate certain micro-environmental stimuli for drug assessment *in vitro*, for instance following the approaches described in the following subchapters. A number of ligand/receptor pairs have been identified that activate CLL cells (*Fig.* 2) (Munk Pedersen & Reed, 2004), among them the chemokine stroma-derived factor 1, nowadays referred to as CXCL12 and its receptor CXCR4 on CLL cells, that belongs to the class of G-protein-coupled 7-transmembrane domain receptors (Burger & Kipps, 2006) and VCAM-1 (CD106) expressed on the surface of stroma cells that interacts with the integrin VAL-4 (CD49a) on CLL cells (Burger et al., 2009). The strict dependence of CLL cells on the interactions with their environment is also apparent from the absence of good cell line models for CLL.

3.1 B cell receptor stimulation

Like for normal lymphocytes, also the fate of CLL cells is to a high degree determined by B cell receptor (BCR) stimulation (Stevenson & Caligaris-Cappio, 2004). According to the degree of somatic hypermutation in rearranged antigen receptor genes, subgroups of CLL clones with immunoglobulin heavy chain variable region (IgHV) genes can be distinguished that reflect progressing B cell development stages corresponding to naïve or memory B cells. Usually the threshold separating these molecularly defined prognostic subgroups is set at 2 % sequence divergence of rearranged IgHV genes from the closest germline sequences. The CLL subgroups with unmutated or mutated IgHV genes have a widely different prognosis indicated by 24 versus 8 years median overall survival after diagnosis (Hamblin et al., 1999). High expression of zeta-assoziated protein 70 (ZAP-70) and of CD38 serve as surrogate markers of unmutated IgHV genes (Crespo et al., 2003; Hamblin et al., 2002).

Antigen contact for CLL cells can be mimicked *in vitro* by crosslinking surface IgM by means of anti-IgM antibodies. Long lasting stimulation of the BCR leads to prolonged survival of CLL cells (Deglesne et al., 2006). This can be achieved by using soluble anti-IgM or anti-IgM-coated surfaces.

3.2 CD40 stimulation

The CD40 molecule expressed on the surface of CLL cells belongs to the tumor necrosis factor family and participates in antigen recognition as a co-receptor. Its cognate ligand, CD40 ligand (CD40L), also known as CD154, is expressed on the surface of activated T lymphocytes. Engagement of CD40 on CLL lymphocytes mimics the micro-environment inside lymph nodes and leads to protection against DNA damaging substances, e.g. chemotherapeutic agents. CD40L stimulation of CLL cells can be provided by co-culture with fibroblasts expressing recombinant CD154. For instance co-culture with CD40L expressing fibroblasts protects CLL cells from DNA damaging agents, but this effect can be partly reversed by the kinase inhibitor dasatinib (Hallaert et al., 2008). The sensitivity of CLL cells for the Bcl-2 antagonist ABT737 is decreased by a factor of 1000, if the CLL cells are co-cultivated with fibroblasts expressing CD40L (Vogler et al., 2009).

3.3 Stroma cell-derived soluble factors and cell surface interactions

The soluble factors produced by bone marrow stromal cells include the chemokine CXCL12, which despite its original designation as stroma-cell derived factor is shown in *Fig. 2* as a micro-environmental factor occurring in peripheral blood, owing to its alternate origin from nurse-like cells. Stimulation by purified recombinant CXCL12 induced the raf-dependent mitogen activated protein (MAP) kinase cascades in CLL cells, which augmented their survival and was targeted by the raf inhibitor sorafenib (Messmer et al., 2011).

In vivo, inhibition of apoptosis may occur preferentially in pseudofollicles containing CLL and accessory cells, due to cell contact and mutual paracrine and autocrine stimulation. *In vitro*, co-culture with bone-marrow-derived stromal cells, e.g. the cell line HS-5, may provide stimuli for long-term survival of CLL cells. In co-cultures of primary CLL cells with HS-5 cells, various chemokines attracting T lymphocytes, most prominently CCL4 and CCL3, were detected, which are not produced by HS-5 control cultures (Seiffert et al., 2010). The proteins found in the supernatant of HS-5 co-cultures included factors, which are commonly secreted by monocytes, e.g. soluble CD14. Among the soluble factors provided to CLL cells by co-culture with the bone marrow stromal cell line HS5, vascular endothelial growth factor (VEGF) is partly responsible for the increase in viability of co-cultivated CLL cells (Gehrke et al., 2011).

3.4 Oligonucleotides containing CpG dinucleotides

Toll like receptor 9 (TLR9) has been identified as a part of the innate immune response recognizing unmethylated foreign DNA that can be mimicked by phosphothioate oligodeoxynucleotides containing CpG dinucleotides (CpG-ODN) (Krieg, 2006). Survival and proliferation of CLL cells can be considerably enhanced by class B CpG-ODN, e.g. DSPN-30 (Decker et al., 2000). Like CD40 ligation, activation of CLL cells through TLR9 occupation by CpG-ODN was exploited as a mitogenic signal in order to obtain metaphase chromosomes for cytogenetic analysis by fluorescent in situ hybridization (Mayr et al., 2006). The importance of activated CLL cells in drug assessment is demonstrated by the example of mTOR inhibitors. In untreated CLL cells rapamycin showed an IC_{50} of 10 µM for apoptosis induction (Aleskog et al., 2008). In contrast less than one thousandth of this concentration of RAD001 or 10 nM rapamycin was sufficient for complete inhibition of the cell proliferation induced by CpG-ODN (Decker et al., 2003).

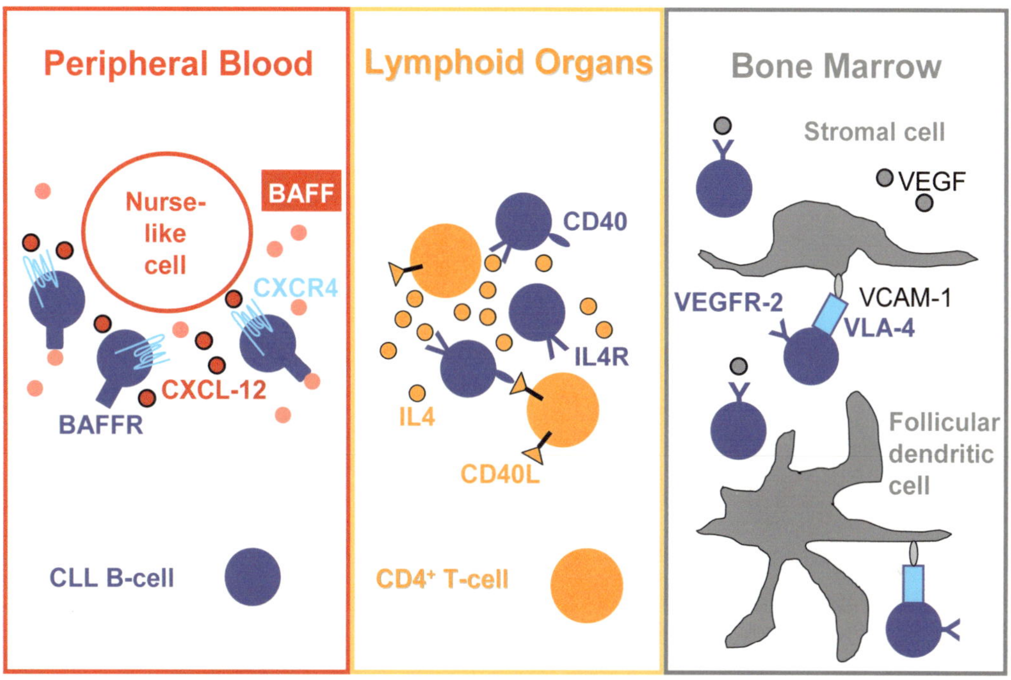

Fig. 2. Microenvironment interactions of CLL cells. The survival of CLL lymphocytes can be prolonged by contact with different accessory cells in the peripheral blood, lymphoid system and bone marrow. Some prominent interactions of CLL cells with soluble factors and cell surface molecules supplied by accessory cells are shown. On the surface of CLL cells receptors for various soluble factors are expressed, e.g. for the chemokine CXCL12, formerly designated as stroma-derived factor 1 (SDF-1), for the cytokine interleukin-4 (IL-4), and for vascular endothelial growth factor (VEGF). CD40 or the integrin VAL-4 on the surface of CLL cells interact with CD40 ligand (CD40L) on T cells or VCAM-1 on follicular dendritic cells and other stromal cells, respectively. Adapted from Munk Pedersen *et al.*, 2004.

In addition to activating CLL cells CpG-ODN were found to increase surface expression levels of co-stimulatory molecules including CD20 (Jahrsdorfer et al., 2001). Consequently, the same CpG-ODN DSPN-30 that is commonly used for activating CLL cells, increased CD20 expression on freshly isolated CLL cells, which in turn led to higher B cell depletion by the type II CD20 antibody GA101 (Patz et al., 2011).

3.5 B cell depletion from whole blood samples

Monoclonal antibodies (MABs) induce direct cell death (DCD) of tumor cells via signal transduction and additional Fc-mediated cytotoxic effects, namely antibody-dependent cell-mediated cytotoxicity (ADCC) and complement-dependent cytotoxicity (CDC) (*Fig. 3*). In order to include ADCC and CDC in measurements of overall MAB effects, the extent of tumor cell depletion by MABs from individual blood samples can be determined by multi-color flow cytometry comparing treated and untreated whole blood cultures.

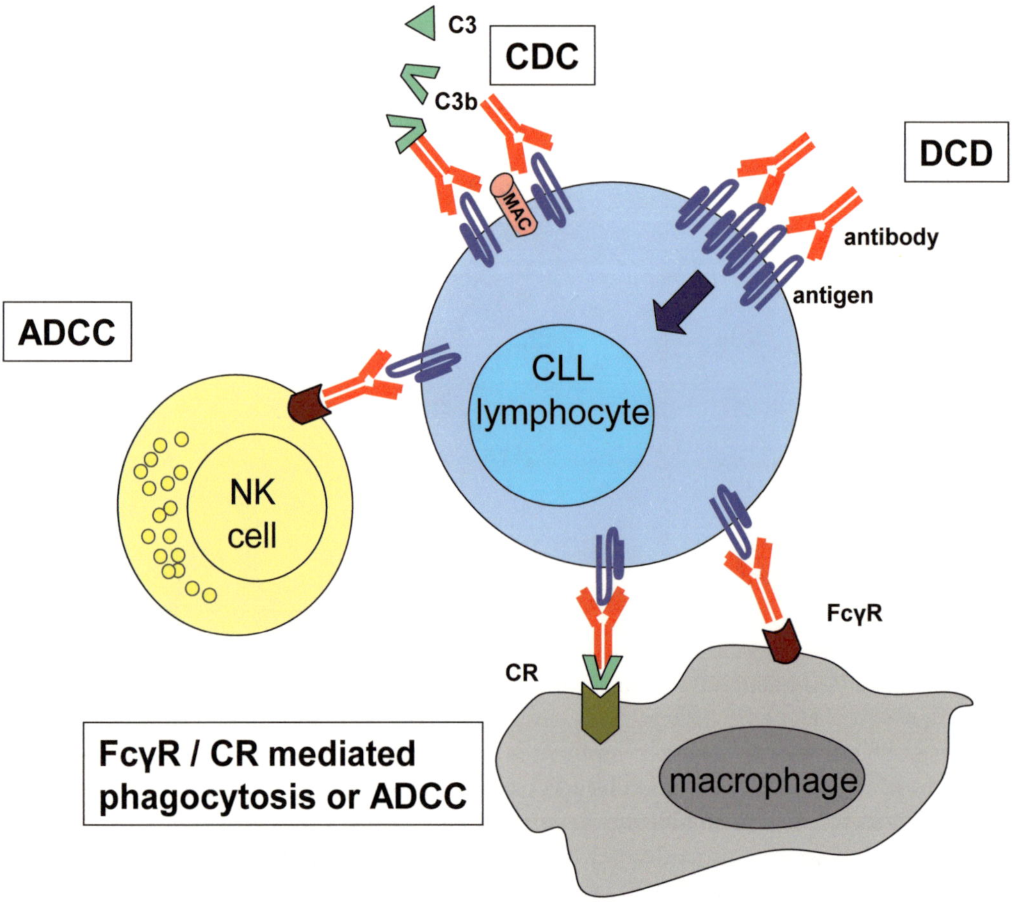

Fig. 3. Killing mechanisms of monoclonal antibodies and their assessment. Apart from direct cell death (DCD) induction in tumor cells, monoclonal antibodies exert their action via Fc-mediated functions, namely complement-mediated cytotoxicity (CDC) and antibody-dependent cell-mediated cytotoxicity (ADCC) and phagocytosis. Due to the importance of CD20 antibodies in CLL therapy, a structure crossing the cell membrane four times is shown as the surface antigen on CLL cells. This overall structural organization is shared by another emerging target for immunotherapy, the tetraspanin CD37. Ways to examine the above mechanisms on isolated CLL cells and whole blood samples are compiled in *Table* 2 and described in the text. Adapted from Olszewski & Grossbard, 2004 and Jaglowski et al., 2010.

4. Pre-clinical assessment of kinase inhibitors

Prototypic targeted therapy by the tyrosine kinase inhibitor imatinib was developed for Bcr-Abl positive leukemias, in which deregulated Abl activity is a predominant driving force (Druker et al., 2001). In contrast, the pathogenesis of CLL appears to be multi-factorial. The second generation of Abl inhibitors for treatment of imatinib-resistant Bcr-Abl positive leukemias achieves greater efficacy against mutant forms of the Abl kinase (Weisberg et al., 2007). Some of these inhibitors, e.g. dasatinib (Shah et al., 2004) and bosutinib (Puttini et al., 2006) are dual-specific and target Abl and additionally Src kinases. Since members of the latter tyrosine kinase family, e.g. Lyn (Contri et al., 2005) and Lck (Majolini et al., 1999) have been suggested to be involved in CLL pathogenesis, we conducted an assessment of dasatinib on CLL cells (Veldurthy et al., 2008). This pre-clinical investigation indicated an influence of Src kinase inhibition on the cellular survival of CLL cells with preference for the subgroups with unmutated immunoglobulin heavy chain genes or with high ZAP70 expression and thus indicated patient groups that might profit most from Src kinase inhibition. Since the fate of CLL B lymphocytes critically depends on BCR signaling (Stevenson & Caligaris-Cappio, 2004), inhibition by kinase inhibitors of survival pathways emanating from the BCR or from micro-environmental stimuli (Burger et al., 2009) represents a promising strategy for treating CLL (Gandhi, 2010).

Drug assessment on primary CLL cells serves as preparation for clinical trials and to some degree enables comparison of the efficacies of different agents and the prediction of the response of molecularly defined subgroups of CLL patients. The clearly higher dasatinib sensitivity of CLL samples with unmutated IgV_H genes as compared to mutated ones is an example for this type of correlation (Veldurthy et al., 2008). Signaling analysis revealed that treatment of primary CLL cells with dasatinib drastically reduces the level of activated SFK in CLL cells, but inhibits downstream BCR signaling pathways and induces apoptosis more strongly in the patient subgroup with aggressive disease. The extent of dasatinib-induced apoptosis in CLL cells corresponds to the concomitant decrease in the phosphorylation of the direct SFK substrates Syk and phospholipase C-γ (Song et al., 2010). Signaling analysis during SFK inhibition thus contributed to the rationale for pre-clinical assessment of Syk inhibitors on CLL cells (Baudot et al., 2009; Buchner et al., 2009). For another second generation dual Abl/Src inhibitor, bosutinib, inhibition of the receptor tyrosine kinase Axl was found to be partially responsible for its apoptosis induction in CLL cells (Ghosh et al., 2010).

Inhibition of Abl does not reduce viability of CLL cells on its own, but can sensitize CLL cells for chemotherapeutic agents, e.g. chlorambucil, by interfering with DNA repair (Aloyz et al., 2004). Inhibitors of the delta isoform of the catalytic p110 subunit of phosphatidylinositol-3-kinase (PI3K) show moderate efficiencies on primary CLL lymphocytes without activation that contrast the promising effects in clinical trials. The observed pre-clinical efficiency of the PI3K-delta inhibitor CAL-101 is not abrogated by micro-environmental stimulation and other cell types, while other cell types, e.g. natural killer cells are not influenced by CAL-101 (Herman et al., 2010).

5. Pre-clinical assessment of monoclonal antibodies

Apart from small molecules, monoclonal antibodies constitute another group of targeted therapeutics for the treatment of CLL. This group includes the first biological anti-tumor agent, namely the CD20 antibody rituximab. As a common cell surface antigen of all B cells except stem or plasma cells, CD20 has become a very effective antibody target for the treatment of B cell malignancies (Molina, 2008) including CLL despite variable surface expression on CLL cells. Together with the monoclonal anti-CD52 antibody alemtuzumab, rituximab thus may be counted among the most efficient targeted treatment options for CLL achieved so far. In a recent phase III trial inclusion of rituximab was shown to substantially improve the established fludarabine / cyclophosphamide chemotherapy regimen (Hallek et al., 2010).

Apart from DCD induction in tumor cells, monoclonal antibodies exert their action via Fc-mediated functions, namely CDC, ADCC and phagocytosis (Jaglowski et al., 2010; Olszewski & Grossbard, 2004) (*Fig. 3*). Therefore an assessment of antibody effects on CLL cells *ex vivo* can either be performed on freshly isolated CLL cells in separate dedicated assays for each mentioned mechanisms, or in a comprehensive assay from whole (*Table 2*). For assessing antibody effects on isolated CLL cells, the same procedures as for other anti-CLL agents can only be applied for the determination of DCD. For instance DCD induction by rituximab in freshly isolated CLL cells was assessed according to viable cell counts, metabolic activity and phosphatidylserine exposure and was found variable among individual samples and considerably smaller than in lymphoma cell lines (Patz et al., 2011; Stanglmaier et al., 2004). Since DCD induction in primary CLL cells may constitute only a minor fraction of overall B cell depletion as in the case of rituximab (Voso et al., 2002), it is indispensable to additionally assess Fc-mediated mechanisms. For performing ADCC assays on isolated CLL lymphocytes, effector cells need to be externally added, e.g. autologous or heterologous peripheral blood mononuclear cells or a natural killer cell line (Weitzman et al., 2009). Similarly, CDC can be assessed by monitoring changes in the membrane integrity of CLL cells after incubation in medium containing high concentrations of complete as compared to heat-inactivated serum (Golay et al., 2000; Patz et al., 2011).

Mechanism	**Isolated CLL cells**	**Whole blood**
DCD	Cytotoxicity or viability assays	Requires distinction of CLL lymphocytes from other cell populations
CDC	Comparison of effects with complete or heat-inactivated serum	Complement inhibition by cobra venom factor
ADCC	Externally added effector cells	Blocking antibodies for Fc receptors

Table 2. Determination and dissection of different mechanisms of antibody-induced cytotoxicity.

As an alternative to these separate assays, we applied a B cell depletion assay from whole blood encompassing Fc-mediated antibody-induced cytotoxicity. This assay is based on the enumeration of B lymphocytes in differentially treated whole blood samples after staining the general, B- and T- lymphocyte antigens CD45, CD19 and CD3 using three color flow cytometry and commercially available fluorescently labeled immunoreagents. B cell depletion can be calculated from the B cell counts in antibody-treated versus untreated control samples. B/T cell ratios with the T cell population as an internal standard can be used for this calculation, if T cell counts are proven to be unaffected by the antibody treatment. Alternatively absolute B cell counts can be determined using externally added fluorescent counting beads. In part the contributions of DCD, CDC and ADCC to the observed B cell depletion from whole blood samples can be dissected. Thus, we were able to show a substantial contribution of ADCC to the B cell depletion by the novel type II CD20 antibody GA101 (Moessner et al., 2010) by blocking the interaction of FcγIIIa on NK cells and macrophages and the Fc exposed on antibody-coated target cells by incubation with anti-CD16 antibody in whole blood from healthy donors but not CLL patients (Patz et al., 2011). In summary, flow cytometric determination of B cell depletion from whole blood has the potential of comparing antibody effects on individual CLL samples and of predicting clinical responses.

Resistance mechanisms to anti-CLL antibodies have been unraveled by pre-clinical models and some of the influences interfering with antibody efficacy may be recapitulated in the the present B cell depletion from whole blood samples (*Table 3*) (Reslan et al., 2009). Thus the shape of the dose response curves of GA101 or mAb37.1 observed in the B cell depletion assay (Krause et al., 2011; Patz et al., 2011) is of saturation type and suggests an influence on antibody effects of individually different levels of endogenous human IgG in the assay matrix (Preithner et al., 2006). Similarly, varying ratios of effector to target cells, the Phe158Val polymorphism of FcγIIIa (Cartron et al., 2002) as well as complement depletion (Kennedy et al., 2004) will influence B cell depletion from whole blood samples. Thus, the assay described here has the advantage of reflecting both, the efficiency of antibody-induced B cell depletion and the potential to supply host-dependent immune functions and thus should be able to predict at the individual level the clinical efficiency of therapeutics assayed *in vitro*.

Influence	**References**
Antigen density on target cells	Golay et al., 2001, Patz et al., 2011
Complement depletion	Kennedy et al., 2004
Complement inhihibitors CD59 and CD55	Golay et al., 2001
Ratio of effector to target cells	
Plasma levels of IgG	Preithner et al., 2006
Fc receptor polymorphisms	Cartron et al., 2002

Table 3. Influences on antibody efficacy in a whole blood matrix.

6. Conclusions

Due to the dependence of CLL lymphocytes on their micro-environment, the predictive value of simple cytotoxicity assays on freshly isolated CLL cells can be enhanced by activating CLL cells using procedures that mimic certain micro-environmental stimuli. In the case of monoclonal antibodies, effector cells and complement system need to be included in order to comprise indirect antibody-mediated mechanisms. For arriving at valid predictions, results of the individualized *in vitro* sensitivity testing should be linked to mechanistic and biochemical target validation studies, ideally involving genetically defined systems. Remarkably three major topics addressed in this chapter, namely the importance of accompanying signaling analysis, consideration of the micro-environment of CLL cells and combination with chemotherapeutic agents conceptually strongly overlap with general targeting strategies in contemporary pre-clinical anticancer drug discovery (Caponigro & Sellers, 2011).

7. Acknowledgements

Work in our laboratory has been supported by grants from the German Cancer Aid, German José Carreras Leukemia Foundation and CLL Global Research Foundation.

8. References

Aleskog, A., Norberg, M., Nygren, P., Rickardson, L., Kanduri, M., Tobin, G., Aberg, M., Gustafsson, M.G., Rosenquist, R. & Lindhagen, E. (2008). Rapamycin shows anticancer activity in primary chronic lymphocytic leukemia cells in vitro, as single agent and in drug combination *Leuk Lymphoma* , 49, 2333-43.

Aloyz, R., Grzywacz, K., Xu, Z.Y., Loignon, M., Alaoui-Jamali, M.A. & Panasci, L. (2004). Imatinib sensitizes CLL lymphocytes to chlorambucil *Leukemia* , 18, 409-14.

Baudot, A.D., Jeandel, P.Y., Mouska, X., Maurer, U., Tartare-Deckert, S., Raynaud, S.D., Cassuto, J.P., Ticchioni, M. & Deckert, M. (2009). The tyrosine kinase Syk regulates the survival of chronic lymphocytic leukemia B cells through PKCdelta and proteasome-dependent regulation of Mcl-1 expression *Oncogene* , 28, 3261-73.

Bosanquet, A.G., Richards, S.M., Wade, R., Else, M., Matutes, E., Dyer, M.J., Rassam, S.M., Durant, J., Scadding, S.M., Raper, S.L., Dearden, C.E. & Catovsky, D. (2009). Drug cross-resistance and therapy-induced resistance in chronic lymphocytic leukaemia by an enhanced method of individualised tumour response testing *Br J Haematol* , 146, 384-95.

Buchner, M., Fuchs, S., Prinz, G., Pfeifer, D., Bartholome, K., Burger, M., Chevalier, N., Vallat, L., Timmer, J., Gribben, J.G., Jumaa, H., Veelken, H., Dierks, C. & Zirlik, K. (2009). Spleen tyrosine kinase is overexpressed and represents a potential therapeutic target in chronic lymphocytic leukemia *Cancer Res* , 69, 5424-32.

Burger, J.A., Ghia, P., Rosenwald, A. & Caligaris-Cappio, F. (2009). The microenvironment in mature B-cell malignancies: a target for new treatment strategies *Blood* , 114, 3367-75.

Burger, J.A. & Kipps, T.J. (2006). CXCR4: a key receptor in the crosstalk between tumor cells and their microenvironment *Blood* , 107, 1761-7.

Caponigro, G. & Sellers, W.R. (2011). Advances in the preclinical testing of cancer therapeutic hypotheses *Nat Rev Drug Discov* , 10, 179-87.

Cartron, G., Dacheux, L., Salles, G., Solal-Celigny, P., Bardos, P., Colombat, P. & Watier, H. (2002). Therapeutic activity of humanized anti-CD20 monoclonal antibody and polymorphism in IgG Fc receptor FcgammaRIIIa gene *Blood* , 99, 754-8.

Collins, I. & Workman, P. (2006). New approaches to molecular cancer therapeutics *Nat Chem Biol* , 2, 689-700.

Contri, A., Brunati, A.M., Trentin, L., Cabrelle, A., Miorin, M., Cesaro, L., Pinna, L.A., Zambello, R., Semenzato, G. & Donella-Deana, A. (2005). Chronic lymphocytic leukemia B cells contain anomalous Lyn tyrosine kinase, a putative contribution to defective apoptosis *J Clin Invest* , 115, 369-78.

Crespo, M., Bosch, F., Villamor, N., Bellosillo, B., Colomer, D., Rozman, M., Marce, S., Lopez-Guillermo, A., Campo, E. & Montserrat, E. (2003). ZAP-70 expression as a surrogate for immunoglobulin-variable-region mutations in chronic lymphocytic leukemia *N Engl J Med*, 348, 1764-75.

Decker, T., Hipp, S., Ringshausen, I., Bogner, C., Oelsner, M., Schneller, F. & Peschel, C. (2003). Rapamycin-induced G1 arrest in cycling B-CLL cells is associated with reduced expression of cyclin D3, cyclin E, cyclin A, and survivin *Blood*, 101, 278-85.

Decker, T., Schneller, F., Sparwasser, T., Tretter, T., Lipford, G.B., Wagner, H. & Peschel, C. (2000). Immunostimulatory CpG-oligonucleotides cause proliferation, cytokine production, and an immunogenic phenotype in chronic lymphocytic leukemia B cells *Blood*, 95, 999-1006.

Deglesne, P.A., Chevallier, N., Letestu, R., Baran-Marszak, F., Beitar, T., Salanoubat, C., Sanhes, L., Nataf, J., Roger, C., Varin-Blank, N. & Ajchenbaum-Cymbalista, F. (2006). Survival response to B-cell receptor ligation is restricted to progressive chronic lymphocytic leukemia cells irrespective of Zap70 expression *Cancer Res*, 66, 7158-66.

Druker, B.J., Talpaz, M., Resta, D.J., Peng, B., Buchdunger, E., Ford, J.M., Lydon, N.B., Kantarjian, H., Capdeville, R., Ohno-Jones, S. & Sawyers, C.L. (2001). Efficacy and safety of a specific inhibitor of the BCR-ABL tyrosine kinase in chronic myeloid leukemia *N Engl J Med*, 344, 1031-7.

Eichhorst, B., Goede, V. & Hallek, M. (2009). Treatment of elderly patients with chronic lymphocytic leukemia *Leuk Lymphoma*, 50, 171-8.

Gandhi, V. (2010). Targeting kinases in CML CLL *Blood*, 116, 1999-2000.

Gehrke, I., Gandhirajan, R.K., Poll-Wolbeck, S.J., Hallek, M. & Kreuzer, K.A. (2011). Bone marrow stromal cell-derived VEGF rather than CLL cell-derived VEGF is essential for the apoptotic resistance of cultured CLL cells *Mol Med*.

Ghosh, A.K., Secreto, C., Boysen, J., Sassoon, T., Shanafelt, T.D., Mukhopadhyay, D. & Kay, N.E. (2010). The novel receptor tyrosine kinase Axl is constitutively active in B-cell chronic lymphocytic leukemia and acts as a docking site of nonreceptor kinases: implications for therapy *Blood*, 117, 1928-37.

Golay, J., Bologna, L., Andre, P.A., Buchegger, F., Mach, J.P., Boumsell, L. & Introna, M. (2010). Possible misinterpretation of the mode of action of therapeutic antibodies in vitro: homotypic adhesion and flow cytometry result in artefactual direct cell death *Blood*, 116, 3372-3; author reply 3373-4.

Golay, J., Zaffaroni, L., Vaccari, T., Lazzari, M., Borleri, G.M., Bernasconi, S., Tedesco, F., Rambaldi, A. & Introna, M. (2000). Biologic response of B lymphoma cells to anti-CD20 monoclonal antibody rituximab in vitro: CD55 and CD59 regulate complement-mediated cell lysis *Blood*, 95, 3900-8.

Groves, M.J., Maccallum, S., Boylan, M.T., Coates, P.J. & Tauro, S. (2009). The annexin-V assay reflects susceptibility to in vitro membrane damage in chronic lymphocytic leukemia and may overestimate cell death *Am J Hematol*, 84, 196-7.

Hallaert, D.Y., Jaspers, A., van Noesel, C.J., van Oers, M.H., Kater, A.P. & Eldering, E. (2008). c-Abl kinase inhibitors overcome CD40-mediated drug resistance in CLL: implications for therapeutic targeting of chemoresistant niches *Blood*, 112, 5141-9.

Hallek, M., Cheson, B.D., Catovsky, D., Caligaris-Cappio, F., Dighiero, G., Dohner, H., Hillmen, P., Keating, M.J., Montserrat, E., Rai, K.R. & Kipps, T.J. (2008). Guidelines for the diagnosis and treatment of chronic lymphocytic leukemia: a report from the International Workshop on Chronic Lymphocytic Leukemia updating the National Cancer Institute-Working Group 1996 guidelines *Blood* , 111, 5446-56.

Hallek, M., Fischer, K., Fingerle-Rowson, G., Fink, A.M., Busch, R., Mayer, J., Hensel, M., Hopfinger, G., Hess, G., von Grunhagen, U., Bergmann, M., Catalano, J., Zinzani, P.L., Caligaris-Cappio, F., Seymour, J.F., Berrebi, A., Jager, U., Cazin, B., Trneny, M., Westermann, A., Wendtner, C.M., Eichhorst, B.F., Staib, P., Buhler, A., Winkler, D., Zenz, T., Bottcher, S., Ritgen, M., Mendila, M., Kneba, M., Dohner, H. & Stilgenbauer, S. (2010). Addition of rituximab to fludarabine and cyclophosphamide in patients with chronic lymphocytic leukaemia: a randomised, open-label, phase 3 trial *Lancet* , 376, 1164-74.

Hamblin, T.J. (2009). Just exactly how common is CLL? *Leuk Res* , 33, 1452-3.

Hamblin, T.J., Davis, Z., Gardiner, A., Oscier, D.G. & Stevenson, F.K. (1999). Unmutated Ig V(H) genes are associated with a more aggressive form of chronic lymphocytic leukemia *Blood* , 94, 1848-54.

Hamblin, T.J., Orchard, J.A., Ibbotson, R.E., Davis, Z., Thomas, P.W., Stevenson, F.K. & Oscier, D.G. (2002). CD38 expression and immunoglobulin variable region mutations are independent prognostic variables in chronic lymphocytic leukemia, but CD38 expression may vary during the course of the disease *Blood* , 99, 1023-9.

Herman, S.E., Gordon, A.L., Wagner, A.J., Heerema, N.A., Zhao, W., Flynn, J.M., Jones, J., Andritsos, L., Puri, K.D., Lannutti, B.J., Giese, N.A., Zhang, X., Wei, L., Byrd, J.C. & Johnson, A.J. (2010). Phosphatidylinositol 3-kinase-delta inhibitor CAL-101 shows promising preclinical activity in chronic lymphocytic leukemia by antagonizing intrinsic and extrinsic cellular survival signals *Blood* , 116, 2078-88.

Jaglowski, S.M., Alinari, L., Lapalombella, R., Muthusamy, N. & Byrd, J.C. (2010). The clinical application of monoclonal antibodies in chronic lymphocytic leukemia *Blood* , 116, 3705-14.

Jahrsdorfer, B., Hartmann, G., Racila, E., Jackson, W., Muhlenhoff, L., Meinhardt, G., Endres, S., Link, B.K., Krieg, A.M. & Weiner, G.J. (2001). CpG DNA increases primary malignant B cell expression of costimulatory molecules and target antigens *J Leukoc Biol* , 69, 81-8.

Kennedy, A.D., Beum, P.V., Solga, M.D., DiLillo, D.J., Lindorfer, M.A., Hess, C.E., Densmore, J.J., Williams, M.E. & Taylor, R.P. (2004). Rituximab infusion promotes rapid complement depletion and acute CD20 loss in chronic lymphocytic leukemia *J Immunol* , 172, 3280-8.

Kepp, O., Galluzzi, L., Lipinski, M., Yuan, J. & Kroemer, G. (2011). Cell death assays for drug discovery *Nat Rev Drug Discov* , 10, 221-37.

Koopman, G., Reutelingsperger, C.P., Kuijten, G.A., Keehnen, R.M., Pals, S.T. & van Oers, M.H. (1994). Annexin V for flow cytometric detection of phosphatidylserine expression on B cells undergoing apoptosis *Blood* , 84, 1415-20.

Krause, G. & Hallek, M. (2011). On the assessment of dasatinib-induced autophagy in CLL *Leuk Res* , 35, 137-8.

Krause, G., Patz, M., Isaeva, P., Wigger, M., Baki, I., Vondey, V., Kerwien, S., Kuckertz, M., Brinker, R., Claasen, J., Frenzel, L.P., Wendtner, C.M., Heider, K.H. & Hallek, M. (2011). Action of novel CD37 antibodies on chronic lymphocytic leukemia cells *Leukemia* , in press.

Krieg, A.M. (2006). Therapeutic potential of Toll-like receptor 9 activation *Nat Rev Drug Discov* , 5, 471-84.

Lindhagen E, Nygren P, Larsson R (2008) The fluorometric microculture cyto-toxicity assay. *Nat Protoc* , 3 (8): 1364–9.

Lilienthal, N., Prinz, C., Peer-Zada, A.A., Doering, M., Ba, L.A., Hallek, M., Jacob, C. & Herling, M. (2011). Targeting the disturbed redox equilibrium in chronic lymphocytic leukemia by novel reactive oxygen species-catalytic 'sensor/effector' compounds *Leuk Lymphoma* , 52, 1407-11.

Majolini, M.B., Boncristiano, M. & Baldari, C.T. (1999). Dysregulation of the protein tyrosine kinase LCK in lymphoproliferative disorders and in other neoplasias. *Leuk Lymphoma* , 35, 245-54.

Mayr, C., Speicher, M.R., Kofler, D.M., Buhmann, R., Strehl, J., Busch, R., Hallek, M. & Wendtner, C.M. (2006). Chromosomal translocations are associated with poor prognosis in chronic lymphocytic leukemia *Blood* , 107, 742-51.

Messmer, D., Fecteau, J.F., O'Hayre, M., Bharati, I.S., Handel, T.M. & Kipps, T.J. (2011). Chronic lymphocytic leukemia cells receive RAF-dependent survival signals in response to CXCL12 that are sensitive to inhibition by sorafenib *Blood* , 117, 882-9.

Moessner, E., Brunker, P., Moser, S., Puntener, U., Schmidt, C., Herter, S., Grau, R., Gerdes, C., Nopora, A., van Puijenbroek, E., Ferrara, C., Sondermann, P., Jäger, C., Strein, P., Fertig, G., Friess, T., Schuell, C., Bauer, S., Dal Porto, J., Del Nagro, C., Dabbagh, K., Dyer, M.J.S., Poppema, S., Klein, C. & Umana, P. (2010). Increasing the efficacy of CD20 antibody therapy through the engineering of a new type II anti-CD20 antibody with enhanced direct and immune effector cell-mediated B-cell cytotoxicity *Blood* , 115, 4393-4402.

Molina, A. (2008). A decade of rituximab: improving survival outcomes in non-Hodgkin's lymphoma *Annu Rev Med* , 59, 237-50.

Munk Pedersen, I. & Reed, J. (2004). Microenvironmental interactions and survival of CLL B-cells *Leuk Lymphoma* , 45, 2365-72.

Olszewski, A.J. & Grossbard, M.L. (2004). Empowering targeted therapy: lessons from rituximab *Sci STKE* , 2004, pe30.

Patz, M., Isaeva, P., Forcob, N., Muller, B., Frenzel, L.P., Wendtner, C.M., Klein, C., Umana, P., Hallek, M. & Krause, G. (2011). Comparison of the in vitro effects of the anti-CD20 antibodies rituximab and GA101 on chronic lymphocytic leukaemia cells *Br J Haematol* , 152, 295-306.

Pharmingen. (1998). Apoptosis. Applied reagents and technologies. 2nd edition.

Pleyer, L., Egle, A., Hartmann, T.N. & Greil, R. (2009). Molecular and cellular mechanisms of CLL: novel therapeutic approaches *Nat Rev Clin Oncol* , 6, 405-18.

Preithner, S., Elm, S., Lippold, S., Locher, M., Wolf, A., da Silva, A.J., Baeuerle, P.A. & Prang, N.S. (2006). High concentrations of therapeutic IgG1 antibodies are needed to compensate for inhibition of antibody-dependent cellular cytotoxicity by excess endogenous immunoglobulin G *Mol Immunol* , 43, 1183-93.

Puttini, M., Coluccia, A.M., Boschelli, F., Cleris, L., Marchesi, E., Donella-Deana, A., Ahmed, S., Redaelli, S., Piazza, R., Magistroni, V., Andreoni, F., Scapozza, L., Formelli, F. & Gambacorti-Passerini, C. (2006). In vitro and in vivo activity of SKI-606, a novel Src-Abl inhibitor, against imatinib-resistant Bcr-Abl+ neoplastic cells *Cancer Res* , 66, 11314-22.

Reslan, L., Dalle, S. & Dumontet, C. (2009). Understanding and circumventing resistance to anticancer monoclonal antibodies *MAbs* , 1, 222-9.

Seiffert, M., Schulz, A., Ohl, S., Dohner, H., Stilgenbauer, S. & Lichter, P. (2010). Soluble CD14 is a novel monocyte-derived survival factor for chronic lymphocytic leukemia cells, which is induced by CLL cells in vitro and present at abnormally high levels in vivo *Blood* , 116, 4223-30.

Shah, N.P., Tran, C., Lee, F.Y., Chen, P., Norris, D. & Sawyers, C.L. (2004). Overriding imatinib resistance with a novel ABL kinase inhibitor *Science* , 305, 399-401.

Song, Z., Lu, P., Furman, R.R., Leonard, J.P., Martin, P., Tyrell, L., Lee, F.Y., Knowles, D.M., Coleman, M. & Wang, Y.L. (2010). Activities of SYK and PLCgamma2 predict apoptotic response of CLL cells to SRC tyrosine kinase inhibitor dasatinib *Clin Cancer Res* , 16, 587-99.

Stanglmaier, M., Reis, S. & Hallek, M. (2004). Rituximab and alemtuzumab induce a nonclassic, caspase-independent apoptotic pathway in B-lymphoid cell lines and in chronic lymphocytic leukemia cells *Ann Hematol* , 83, 634-45.

Stevenson, F.K. & Caligaris-Cappio, F. (2004). Chronic lymphocytic leukemia: revelations from the B-cell receptor *Blood* , 103, 4389-95.

Veldurthy, A., Patz, M., Hagist, S., Pallasch, C.P., Wendtner, C.M., Hallek, M. & Krause, G. (2008). The kinase inhibitor dasatinib induces apoptosis in chronic lymphocytic leukemia cells in vitro with preference for a subgroup of patients with unmutated IgVH genes *Blood* , 112, 1443-52.

Vogler, M., Butterworth, M., Majid, A., Walewska, R.J., Sun, X.M., Dyer, M.J. & Cohen, G.M. (2009). Concurrent up-regulation of BCL-XL and BCL2A1 induces approximately 1000-fold resistance to ABT-737 in chronic lymphocytic leukemia *Blood* , 113, 4403-13.

Voso, M.T., Pantel, G., Rutella, S., Weis, M., D'Alo, F., Urbano, R., Leone, G., Haas, R. & Hohaus, S. (2002). Rituximab reduces the number of peripheral blood B-cells in vitro mainly by effector cell-mediated mechanisms *Haematologica* , 87, 918-25.

Weisberg, E., Manley, P.W., Cowan-Jacob, S.W., Hochhaus, A. & Griffin, J.D. (2007). Second generation inhibitors of BCR-ABL for the treatment of imatinib-resistant chronic myeloid leukaemia *Nat Rev Cancer* , 7, 345-56.

Weitzman, J., Betancur, M., Boissel, L., Rabinowitz, A.P., Klein, A. & Klingemann, H. (2009). Variable Contribution of Monoclonal Antibodies to ADCC in patients with chronic lymphocytic leukemia *Leuk Lymphoma,* 1-8.

Wickremasinghe, R.G., Prentice, A.G. & Steele, A.J. (2011). Aberrantly activated anti-apoptotic signalling mechanisms in chronic lymphocytic leukaemia cells: clues to the identification of novel therapeutic targets *Br J Haematol* , 153, 545-56.

Zenz, T., Mertens, D., Kuppers, R., Dohner, H. & Stilgenbauer, S. (2010). From pathogenesis to treatment of chronic lymphocytic leukaemia *Nat Rev Cancer* , 10, 37-50.

Zhang G, Gurtu V, Kain SR& Yan G. (1997) Early detection of apoptosis using a fluorescent conjugate of annexin V. *Biotechniques* , 23, 525-31.

16

Interactions of the Platinum(II) Complexes with Nitrogen- and Sulfur-Bonding Bio-Molecules in Chronic Lymphocytic Leukemia

Jovana Bogojeski, Biljana Petrović and Živadin D. Bugarčić*
University of Kragujevac, Faculty of Science, Department of Chemistry
Serbia

1. Introduction

Transition metals and their reactions are in general important in the environment, in technical processes (catalysis, extraction and purification of metal complexes) and in biology and medicine (biological electron transfer, toxicology and use of metal complexes as drugs). Moreover, nonessential metal ions are very often used in biological systems either for therapeutic application or as diagnostic aids. For instance, metal complexes have been used for the treatment of many diseases (cancer, arthritis, diabetes, Alzheimer, *etc.*), but with little understanding of their mechanism of action in biological systems.(Ronconi & Sadler, 2007; Bruijnincx & Sadler, 2009) Biochemical studies have not clearly established the molecular basis for the activity and mechanism of action. The growing field of bioinorganic chemistry is presently dealing with the clarification of the mechanisms of action of metal complexes in biological systems.(Ronconi & Sadler,2007; Bruijnincx & Sadler, 2009; Jakupec et al., 2008)

Research in the area of application of metal complex compounds in medicine began with the discovery of antitumor properties of cisplatin. (Rosenberg, 1965, 1967, 1969, 1970) Today cisplatin is in routine use as therapeutics worldwide. Following the success of cisplatin a large number of analogous compounds were synthesized. All these compounds have a several common characteristics:

1. bifunctional complex compounds with *cis*-geometry
2. $PtX_2(amin)_2$ is general formula of this compounds, where X_2 are two labile monodentate or one labile bidentate ligand, and $(amine)_2$ are inert nitrogen-donor ligands
3. nitrogen-donor ligands have to containe at least one NH bond.

Despite the large number of synthesized compounds only a few of them entered the medicinal use and most are still in preclinical investigation. (Jakupec et al., 2003; Reedijk, 2009) At the Fig. 1. are presented some of platinum complexes that are in the medicinal use worldwide.

Chronic lymphocytic leukemia is the most frequent type of leukemia and it accounts for approximately 25% of all leukemias. (Chiorazzi et al., 2005) Although at the present there is no curative treatment, combinations of cytotoxic agents and of immunotherapies that generate high complete remission rates hold promise for altering the natural history of this disease. (Wierda et al., 2005) Fludarabine (9-beta-D-arabinofuranosyl-2-fluoroadenine 5′-phosphate) is the most effective purine nucleoside analogue for the treatment of indolent lymphoproliferative disorders, including Chronic lymphocytic leukemia, low-grade lymphoma, and prolymphocytic leukemia. (Eichhorst et al., 2005)

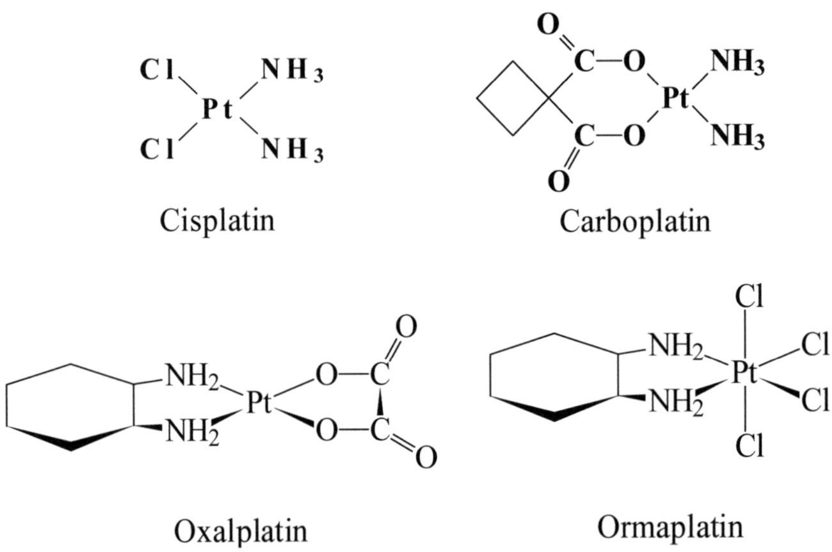

Fig. 1. The structures of some platinum complexes which are in clinical use worldwide.

The studies show that among the best drugs in the treatment of Chronic lymphocytic leukemia are the combination of Pt(II) complexes (cisplatin and oxaliplatin) and alkylating agents and nucleoside analogues such as fluradabine. (Zecevic et al., 2011) The nonoverlapping side effect profiles of oxaliplatin and fludarabine and their different but potentially complementary mechanisms of action provide a basis for investigation of the activity of the drugs in combination. The rationale for combining oxaliplatin with fludarabine is based on preclinical data showing synergistic cytotoxicity between cisplatin in combination with the nucleoside. (Wang et al., 1991; Yamauchi et al., 2001)

Consequently, knowledge of the interaction of the different Pt(II) complexes and nitrogen- and sulfur-bonding bio-molecules, and the results obtained from *in vitro* studies of this type of interactions will help in finding of good antitumor drug for the treatment of many tumors including the Chronic lymphocytic leukemia. The main topic of this chapter will be to show the results obtained in numerous studies of the interactions of the potential antitumor Pt(II) complexes and different biomolecules.

Platinum(II) has a high affinity for sulphur, so after administrating Pt(II) complex in the human body there is a strong possibility for binding with sulphur-donor bio-molecules. Sulphur-donor bio-molecules are present in large amounts in the form of peptides, proteins and enzymes. Binding of platinum complexes with sulphur-donor bio-molecules are responsible for the occurrence of toxic effects. (Lippert, 1999; Reedijk, 1999) However, a certain amount of platinum complexes being bound to nitrogen-donor bio-molecules (amino acids or DNA). Today it is generally accepted that the anti-tumor activity of platinum drugs can be ascribed to interactions between the metal complex and DNA, primarily with the genetic DNA, which is located in the nucleus. The interactions with mitochondrial DNA are less responsible for the antitumor activity of the platinum complexes. (Fuertes et al., 2003) When the Pt(II) complexe reach the DNA, the possibilities for coordination are different. Binding of Pt(II) complexes to DNA primarily occurs through the N7 atoms of guanine, while a binding to N7 and N1 of adenine and N3 of cytosine occurs in small amount. (Lippert, 1999; Reedijk, 1999) Since the DNA molecule containing a different sequence of purine and pyrimidine bases, it was found that with 60% represented the coordination of the type 1,2-(GPG), i.e., the coordination realizes *via* two molecules of guanosine-5'-monophosphate (5'-GMP), which are located on opposite strands of DNA. About 25% is represented by coordination of the type 1,2-(APG), i.e. coordination with adenosine-5'-monophosphate (5'-AMP) and 5'-GMP placed on opposite DNA strands. Other ways of coordinations (monofunctional binding of the type 1,3-(GPG), coordination *via* guanosine located on the same chain of DNA, etc.) are less frequent. On the Fig. 2. is shown the different ways of coordination of cisplatin to DNA. (Jakupec et al., 2003; Kozelka et al., 1999)

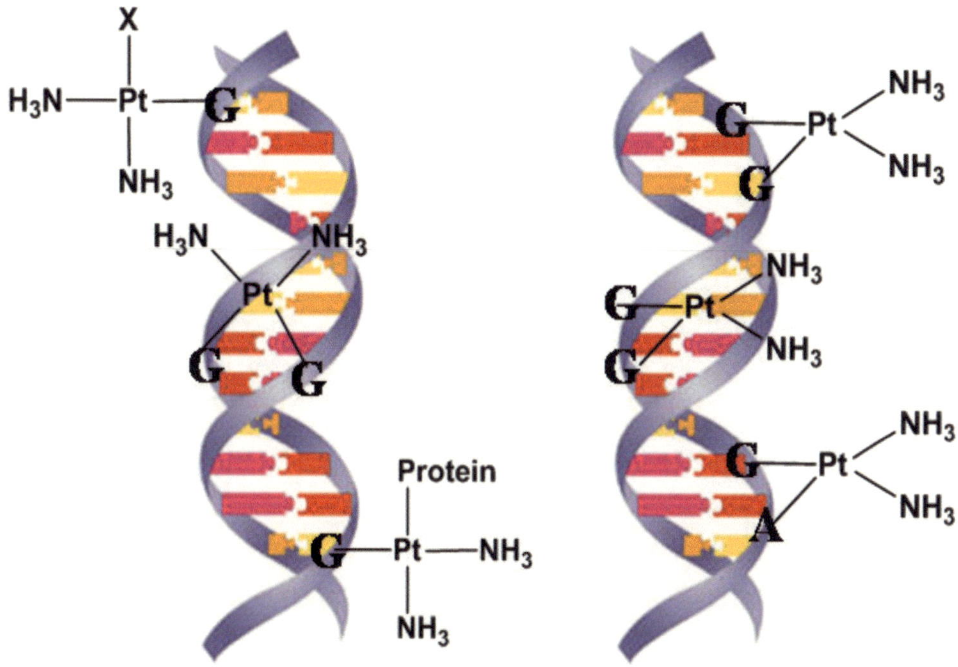

Fig. 2. The different ways of coordinations of cisplatin to DNA.

However, as noted above, the cells contain other bio-molecules which can also react with platinum complexes. High affinities for the platinum complexes show the bio-molecules that contain sulphur, as the thiols and the thioethars. Namely, Pt(II) as "soft" acid forms very stable compounds with sulphur donor ("soft" bases). The resulting compounds are responsible for the occurrence of toxicity (nephrotoxicity, neurotoxicity, resistance, etc.). Since the concentration of thiols, including glutathione (GSH) and L-cysteine, in intracellular liquid is about 10 mM, it is assumed that most of the platinum complex bound to sulphur before it comes to the molecules of DNA. (Jakupec et al., 2003; Reedijk, 2009; Lippert, 1999; Reedijk, 1999) Binding of platinum complexes to sulphur from thioethars are the kinetically favored process. The resulting Pt-S(thioethar) bond may be terminated in the presence of DNA, i.e. N7 atom of 5′-GMP can substitute the molecule of thioethar. (Reedijk, 1999; Soldatović & Bugarčić, 2005) For these reasons the compounds of the type Pt-S(thioethers) are believe to be the reservoirs of "platinum complexes" in the body, i.e. they are suitable intermediates in the reaction of Pt(II) complexes and DNA. Pt-S(thioethers) bond can be terminated in the presence of thiol molecules. The product of this substitution is thermodynamically stable. Also, Pt(II) complex can direct bind to sulphur from thiol molecules and the resulting Pt-S(thiol) bond is very stable and can not be easy broken. It is believed that compounds of the type Pt-S(thiol) are responsible for the occurrence of toxic effects during the use of Pt(II) complexes as anticancer reagents. The Pt-S(thiol) bond can be terminated in the presents of compounds known as "rescue agents", which are compounds with sulphur and they are very strong nucleophiles (diethyldithiocarbamate, thiourea, thiosulfate, GSH, cysteine, biotin, etc.). (Jakupec et al., 2003; Fuertes et al., 2003; Soldatović & Bugarčić, 2005)

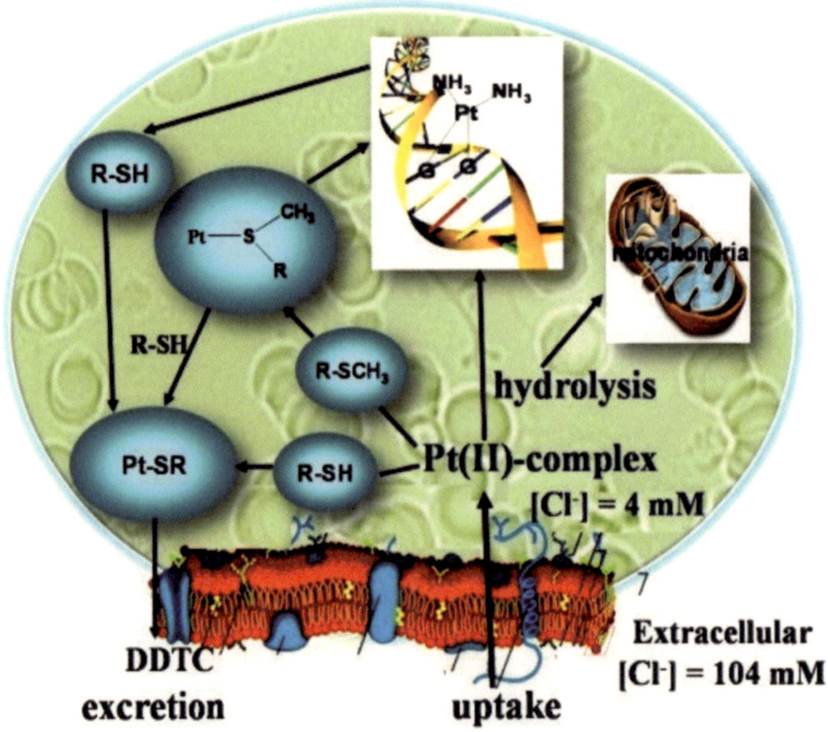

Scheme 1. Schematic presentation of the levels of action of cisplatin in the cell and possible biological consequences.

In recent years a much attention has given to studies of the antitumor activity of polynuclear Pt(II) complexes structurally similar to cisplatin.(Harris et al., 2005) The bridge ligand can be diamine ligands of the type $NH_2(CH_2)nNH_2$ (n = 6). (Mambanda et al., 2010) In the reaction with DNA primarily is obtained compound in which complex is bound simultaneously to both spirale. (Mambanda et al., 2010; Berners-Price et al., 2003) It was found that the presence of the hydrophobic part of the molecule enhances the absorption of these compounds on the cell membrane, where their activity decrease. Also, the polynuclear Pt(II) complexes with heterocyclic nitrogen compounds as bridge ligands were synthesized. (Lakomska et al., 2009)

Pt(IV) complexes are also very interesting. They react more slowly than the corresponding Pt(II) complexes.(Ali et al., 2005) It assumed that first Pt(IV) complexes by reduction translate to Pt(II) complexes and then the mechanism of action is the same as in the case of Pt(II) complexes. (Talman et al., 1997) For the reduction of Pt(IV) complexes can serve GSH, L-cysteine, L-methionine, DL-penicilamin (Lemma et al., 2000a) or ascorbic acid. (Lemma et al., 2000b)

Besides the already mentioned complexes of Pt(II), there are other platinum compounds such as *trans*-$[PtCl_2(NH_3)_2]$ which does not show antitumor activity. (Jolley et al., 2001) These complexes were also intensively studied, (Natile & Coluccia, 2001) as well as some dinuclear complexes of *trans*-geometry. (Jansen et al., 2002) Special attention in recent years were given to the investigation of dinuclear complexes of platinum and paladium. (Mock et al., 2001)

2. Interaction of monofunctional Pt(II) complexes with sulphur- and nitrogen-donor bio-molecules

Monofunctional complexes of Pt(II) are a complexes which in structure contains a stable tridentate ligand, while the fourth coordination place is occupied with labile ligand, mostly chloride ligand. Because of this structure these complexes are not able to bind bifunctionaly to the DNA molecule. Accordingly to this monofunctional complexes of Pt(II) do not exhibit antitumor properties. However, one place for coordination greatly simplifies testing of substitution reactions of these complexes. For these reasons monofunctional complexes present model molecules for the study of interactions of Pt(II) complexes and bio-molecules which contain sulphur- and nitrogen-donor ligands.

Probably the greatest interest in examining substitution reactions of the monofunctional complexes are for complexes of general formula [Pt(NNN)X], where NNN represents a tridentate ligand coordinated *via* three nitrogen donor atoms, while X is a labile ligand, usually chlorido ion. Most intensively studied compounds from this group are $[Pt(dien)Cl]^+$, where *dien* is diethylentriamine or 1,5-diamino-3-azapentane, $[Pt(bpma)Cl]^+$, where *bpma* is bis-(2-pyridylmethyl)amine, and $[Pt(terpy)Cl]^+$, where *terpy* is (2,2':6',2''-terpyridine).

2.1 Interaction of $[Pt(dien)Cl]^+$ complex with sulphur- and nitrogen-donor bio- molecules

There are a large number of studies of substitution reactions of the $[Pt(dien)Cl]^+$ complex and his aqua analog, with different ligands and in different experimental conditions. This studies including investigations of the substitution reactions of the $[Pt(dien)Cl]^+$ complex with sulphur-donor ligands, especially with thiols and thioethers and nitrogen-donor ligands.

In the substitution reactions of $[Pt(dien)Cl]^+$ with GSH it was observed that substitution process depends on the pH value at which the reaction is studied. (Đuran et al. 1991; Bose et al., 1995; Tauben et al. , 2000; Petrović B. & Bugarčić, 2001) At $pH > 7$ as the only reaction product are obtained mononuclear complexes $[Pt(dien)GS]^+$, while at $pH < 7$ a binuclear complex $[\{Pt(dien)_2GS\}]^{3+}$ with GSH as the bridging ligand forms. Also, the process of substitution is followed by deprotonation of GSH, which is observed in the reactions of other Pt(II) complexes with thiols. (Bugarčić & Đorđević, 1998) When the ligand is thioetar, S-methyl-glutathione, reactions are much faster, but the product with thiol is thermodynamically more stable. (Tauben et al., 2002) Comparing the values of rate constants of substitution reactions of $[Pt(dien)Cl]^+$ complexes with different thiols and thioethers, (Tauben et al. , 2000; Petrović B. & Bugarčić, 2001; Bugarčić & Đorđević, 1998; Lampers & Reedijk, 1990) it was noted a discrepancy of GSH compared to other thiols. GSH is a tripeptide that contains an unusual peptide linkage between the amine group of L-cysteine (which is attached by normal peptide linkage to a L-glycine) and the carboxyl group of the glutamate side-chain, with a L-cysteine molecule at the center. It was assumed that the substitution process was much slower compared to L-cysteine. However, the experimentally obtained values showed a much higher reactivity of GSH. This is explained by a suitable geometrical structure of molecules, which cause the formation of intramolecular hydrogen bond involving the proton from the thiol groups, resulting in significantly increased nucleophelicity of the sulphur atoms and therefore higher reactivity. (Bugarčić et al., 2004a;, Petrović B. & Bugarčić, 2001; Bugarčić & Đorđević, 1998)

During the substitution reaction of the $[Pt(dien)Cl]^+$ complexes with L-methionine (Petrović B. & Bugarčić, 2001; Lampers & Reedijk, 1990; Barnham et al. , 1994) as a reaction product primarily has been formed complex $[Pt(dien)(L\text{-methionine})]^{2+}$. It was noted that only in very acidic solutions ($pH < 1$) there is a possibility for protonation of the terminal amino groups of *dien* ligand, which leads to the opening of one chelate ring and the creation of *S,N*-chelat. (Chen et al., 1998) Reaction between $[Pt(dien)Cl]^+$ complexes and L-methionine was studied in the presence of 5'-GMP, assuming the existence of competition of this two ligands.(Lampers & Reedijk, 1990; Soldatović & Bugarčić, 2005) The $[Pt(dien)Cl]^+$ first reacts with L-methionine and form $[Pt(dien)(L\text{-methionine})]^{2+}$ product. Then 5'-GMP molecule coordinated to Pt(II) by substitution of coordinated L-methionine forming thermodynamically more stable $[Pt(dien)(N7\text{-}GMP)]^{2+}$ complex.

INO, 5′-IMP and 5′-GMP can coordinate to metal ions *via* N1 and N7. (Arpalahti & Lehikoinen, 1990; Arpalahti & Lippert, 1990; Caradonna & Lippard, 1988; Bose et al., 1986; Martin, 1999) Under pH = 2.5 only the N7 position of INO, 5′-IMP and 5′-GMP will be free for coordination to the central metal atom, since at this pH the N1 position is protonated. (Sigel et al., 1994) Binding through the N7 position in a neutral or weakly acidic medium has been verified. (Bugarčić et al., 2004a) 5′-GMP is more reactive toward Pt(II) complexes than either INO or 5′-IMP. Furthermore, the pH at which anti-tumor complexes bind to DNA is significantly higher than this one. It is expected that at neutral pH the phosphate residue on the nucleotide will also bind to the central metal atom as a result of its deprotonation. (Jacobs et al., 1992)

From a comparison of the reactivity of GSH or L-methionine with INO, 5′-IMP and 5′-GMP in the reaction with $[Pt(dien)(H_2O)]^{2+}$, $[Pt(dien)Cl]^+$ and $[Pt(dien)Br]^+$ (Soldatović & Bugarčić, 2005) can be concluded that these N-bonding ligands are good nucleophiles. This small difference in the reactivity of N-bondining (INO, 5′-IMP and 5′-GMP) and S-bonding nucleophiles (GSH and L-methionine) is not usually. The complex formation reactions have been studied at pH 2.5 were GSH and L-methionine are protonated. On the other hand, at pH 2.5, N7 sites of N-bonding ligands are not protonated. However, at neutral pH, although less than 10% of thiols are deprotonated, the N-bonding ligand cannot compete with the thiols. The second-order rate constant for GSH is 10^2 times higher than for the 5′-GMP. (Bugarčić et al., 2004b) Also, from obtained results, (Soldatović & Bugarčić, 2005) could be concluded that L-methionine is the best nucleophile for the Pt(II) complexes. This could be explaining by positive inductive effect of the methyl group on the sulphur. However, this is in agreement with the previous results. (Petrović B. & Bugarčić, 2001)

Competitive reactions of $[Pt(dien)Cl]^+$ with L-methionine and 5′-GMP demonstrated initially rapid formation of $[Pt(dien)(L\text{-methionine})]^{2+}$ followed by displacement of L-methionine by 5′-GMP. In the later stages the concentration of $[Pt(dien)(N7\text{-GMP})]^{2+}$ is predominant. (Soldatović & Bugarčić, 2005)

The reactions of $[Pt(dien)Cl]^+$ (10 mM) with L-methionine and 5′-GMP in a molar ratio: $[Pt(dien)Cl]^+$: L-methionine : 5′-GMP = 1:1:3 were also studied. (Soldatović & Bugarčić, 2005)

In the initial stage of the reactions (< 40 h) ^{1}H NMR peak for the free L-methionine (d 2.142 ppm) decrease in the intensity and new peak of the $[Pt(dien)(L\text{-methionine})]^{2+}$ appeared in the spectrum (d 2.544 ppm), whereas a little of the 5′-GMP reacted. In the later stages (72 h), the peaks for the bounded L-methionine and free 5′-GMP (d 8.208 ppm) decreased in intensity, whereas those for free L-methionine increased in intensity, as did those assignable to bound 5′-GMP in $[Pt(dien)(N7\text{-GMP})]^{2+}$ (d 8.624 ppm) as shown in Fig. 3

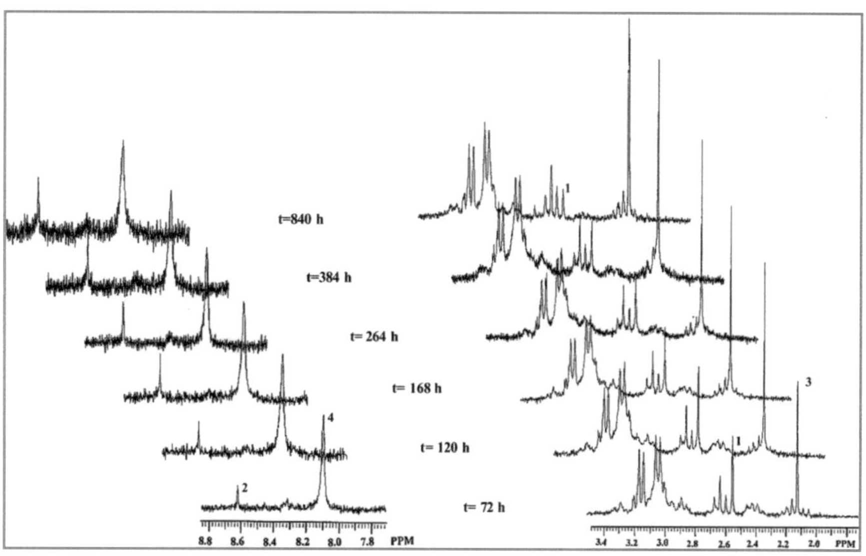

Fig. 3. ^{1}H NMR spectra of the reactions of $[Pt(dien)Cl]^+$ (10 mM) with mixture of L-methionine and 5′-GMP in the ratio 1:1:3 (where 1 is the signal for the $[Pt(dien)(L\text{-methionineh})]^{2+}$, 2 is the signal for the $[Pt(dien)(N7\text{-GMP})]^{2+}$, 3 is the signal for the free L-methionine and 4 is the signal for the free 5′-GMP. (Soldatović & Bugarčić, 2005)

Moreover, Pt–thioether adducts are more easily converted into Pt–thiolate adduct than Pt–N7–GMP adduct. (Teuben et al., 2000) On the other hand, it has been known that 5′-GMP cannot substitute thiols from Pt–thiolate adduct. (Bugarčić et al., 2004a) These findings could have implications for the mechanism of action of platinum anticancer drugs. Sulphur-bonding ligands have a much higher affinity for Pt(II) complexes than nitrogen-bonding ligands. (Bugarčić et al., 2004a; Bugarčić et al., 2002a) Moreover, nephrotoxicity has been explained by the formation of Pt–S(GSH) aduct.

Product in reactions of the $[Pt(dien)Cl]^{+}$ complexes with thioethers or nucleotides in the presence of glutathione is a very stable complexes of the type $[Pt(dien)SG]^{+}$, which confirms the fact that the Pt-S(thiol) bond is the most stable. (Bose et al., 1995) The Pt-S(thiol) bond can be terminated only in the presence of certain nucleophiles with sulphur, such as diethyldithiocarbamate, thiosulphate, thiourea. (Bugarčić et al., 2004a) Interesting is attempt to hydrolysed Pt-S(GSH) bond in the presence of transition metal ions Cu(II) and Zn(II). (Cheng & Pai, 1998)

2.2 Interaction of $[Pt(terpy)Cl]^{+}$ complex with sulphur- and nitrogen-donor bio-molecules

In addition, $[Pt(terpy)Cl]^{+}$ complex was also extensively studied. $[Pt(terpy)Cl]^{+}$ complex has some biological activity. (Becker et al., 2001) In square-planar planes it contains tridentate-coordinated terpyridine system (terpy = 2,2':6',2''-terpyridine), while the fourth coordination site occupies chloro ligand.

Tridentate-coordinated terpyridine system, because of the presence of the aromatic pyridine unit and because of their bulkiness, strongly affects on the characteristics of this complex. In fact, $[Pt(terpy)Cl]^{+}$ complex is much more reactive than complex with *dien* ligand. (Hofmann et al., 2003) The obtained values for lengths of chemical bonds between the platinum(II) and three nitrogen donor atoms of terpyridine system show that the shortest connection is to the secondary nitrogen atom. This feature is certainly reflected on its reactivity in the processes of substitution. In addition, the presence of electrostatic interactions between the pyridine units and metal ions has been observed in crystal structures of various Pt-terpy complexes. (Bailey et al., 1995)

Although the high reactivity of the complex depend on the electronic interactions between the terpyridine system and Pt(II), (Hofmann et al., 2003) bulkiness of the *terpy* ligand has great influence on the characteristics of this complex. The substitution reactions of the $[Pt(terpy)Cl]^{+}$ complexes with different thioethers has been confirmed that there is no reaction, (Petrović B. et al., 1999; Bugarčić et al., 1997) which can be attributed to the strong steric effect. Although, the reactions of $[Pt(terpy)Cl]^{+}$ complexes with some S-methyl-thioethers and thiones may occur, but in this case as the product of reactions appear dinuclear platinum complexes in which the bridge ligand is S-methyl-group. (Annibale et al., 1999) High reactivity of the $[Pt(terpy)Cl]^{+}$ complex in substitution reactions with thiols is explained by formation of intramolecular hydrogen bonds between protons from the thiol-group and outgoing chloro ligand, which further stabilizes the transition state. (Annibale et al., 1998; Petrović B. et al., 1999; Bugarčić et al., 1997)

In the reaction between biologically relevant ligands and Pt(II) complexes, DNA fragments usually coordinated through the N7 atom to Pt(II). (Bugarčić et al., 2004b) Several products of the reaction between $[Pt(terpy)Cl]^{+}$ complex and DNA fragments were synthesized and characterized by X-ray analysis, in which the presence of strong intramolecular hydrogen bonds are observed. The role of these bonds are to further stabilizes the products of the reaction. (Wong & Lippard, 1977)

The kinetics of the complex-formation reactions between $[Pt(terpy)H_2O]^{2+}$, with thiols: L-cysteine, DL-penicillamine, GSH, and with thiourea were studied. (Bugarčić et al., 2002a) Rate constants and activation parameters derived from these experiments are summarized in Table 1.

L	k_1^{298}/M^{-1} s^{-1}	ΔH$^{\neq}$/kJ mol^{-1}	ΔS$^{\neq}$/J K^{-1} mol^{-1}	ΔV$^{\neq}$/cm^3 mol^{-1}
L-Cysteine	37.8 ± 0.1	25 ± 0.5	-132 ± 2	-9.3 ± 0.4
L-Glutathione	(5.8 ± 0.1)×10^2	23 ± 1	-116 ± 3	-12.4 ± 0.6
DL-Penicillamine	12.8 ± 0.1	38 ± 1	-98 ± 3	-20.6 ± 1.0
Thiourea	(1.72 ± 0.02)×10^5	22 ± 1[b]	-73 ± 1[b]	-6.0 ± 0.3[b]

[a]All values refer to 0.10 M $HClO_4$(Bugarčić et al., 2002a) [b] Data from Jaganyi et al., 2001

Table 1. Rate constants and activation parameters for the reaction of $[Pt(terpy)H_2O]^{2+}$ with thiols and thiourea.

From Table 1. can be seen that although the thiol ligands are good entering groups for the Pt(II) complex, thiourea is the best nucleophile. From a comparison of the thiols used, it can be concluded that the variation in size, bulkiness and salvation of the entering ligands reflect in their properties as nucleophiles. The difference in nucleophilicity of the selected ligands is obvious and their reactivity follows the order; DL-penicillamine < L-cysteine < GSH < thiourea. The sensitivity of the reaction rate towards the σ-donor properties of the entering ligands is in line with that expected for an associative mode of activation. In addition, steric effects are very important as well. For example, DL-penicillamine has the lowest reactivity of the thiols used. This can be attributed to the steric effects involving the two methyl groups on carbon near the sulphur atom. At the same time, GSH is considerably more reactive than expected. This anomaly seems to suggest an appreciable anchimeric effect capable of reducing the activation energy of the substitution reaction, arising from hydrogen bonding interactions between the acidic group located in a suitable position of the nucleophile. The anchimeric effect has been reported for other reactions at Pt(II) complexes and is well known for organic reactions. (Wilkins, 1991) This clearly demonstrates that the versatile kinetic behaviour is controlled by steric hindrance on the tridentate ligand and the nucleophilicity of the entering nucleophiles. Increasing steric hindrance is expected to slow down the ligand substitution reactions, whereas increasing nucleophilicity is expected to speed up this process in terms of an associative mechanism.

A trigonal bipyramidal transition state for reaction of $[Pt(terpy)H_2O]^{2+}$ with thiols, is probably stabilized by hydrogen bonding between the entering thiol and the leaving water ligand as already proposed for the reaction of $[Pd(H_2O)_4]^{2+}$ with monodentate acetate, propionate, glycolate, and carboxylic acids (Shi & Elding, 1996, 1997) and for $[Pt(H_2O)_4]^{2+}$ with thioglycolic acid. (Bugarčić & Đorđević, 1998) These findings indicate that bond-making with the entering thiol is important in the activation process and that water is still tightly bound to the metal centre in the transition state.

Also, the reactions between $[Pt(terpy)Cl]^+$ and thiols, such as GSH, L-cysteine, DL-penicillamine and thioglycolic acid have been studied. (Petrović B. et al., 1999) These thiols are very good entering groups for Pt(II) complex. The reaction of the Pt(II) complex and DL-pencillamine is also the slowest one (Table 2.).

The complex $[Pt(terpy)Cl]^+$ appears to be more reactive than $[Pt(dien)Cl]^+$ (Table 2.) in accordance with the greater possibility of π-interaction and π-*trans* effect probably operating as well. The Pt-N distance to the middle nitrogen atom of the terpyridine ligand, 1.930(4) A is slightly shorter than the distances of Pt to the other two nitrogen atoms, N1, 2.018(5) and N3 2.030(5). (Hofmann et al., 2003)

	$k_2/M^{-1}s^{-1}$ $[Pt(dien)Cl]^+$	$k2/M^{-1}s^{-1}$ [Pt(terpy)Cl]+
Thiglycolic acid	7.86×10^{-3}	5.62×10^{-2}
L-Cysteine	1.43×10^{-3}	1.06×10^{-2}
D-penicillamine	8.04×10^{-4}	6.02×10^{-3}
Glutathione	3.85×10^{-3}	7.77×10^{-2}

Table 2. The second-order rate constants for the reactions between thiols and Pt(II) complexes at T = 295 K. (Petrović B. et al., 1999)

As in the case of $[Pt(dien)H_2O]^{2+}$, the kinetic data clearly show that 5′-GMP is more reactive to $[Pt(terpy)H_2O]^{2+}$ than either INO and 5′-IMP in 0.1 M $NaClO_4$ and at pH = 2.5. (Bugarčić et al., 2004a) On the contrary, in the reactions of $[Pd(SMC)(H_2O)_2]^{2+}$ with the same nucleophiles, (Bugarčić et al., 2002b) the most reactive one was INO, which can be attributed to a primary process that involves partial preassociation of the metal complex with the phosphate group in 5′-GMP and 5′-IMP. Furthermore, the pH at which antitumour complexes bind to DNA is significantly higher than used in this study. It is expected that at neutral pH the phosphate residue on the nucleotide will also bind to the central metal atom as a result of its deprotonation. (Jacobs et al., 1992) From a comparison of the reactivity of thiols (L-cysteine, DL-penicillamine and GSH) (Bugarčić et al., 2002a), with INO, 5′-IMP and 5′-GMP in the reaction with $[Pt(terpy)H_2O]^{2+}$, it can be concluded that these N-bonding ligands are even better nucleophiles than the mentioned thiols. The preference of these N-bonding nucleophiles over thiols in acidic solutions needs to be addressed. It must be kept in mind that the reactions with thiols have been investigated at pH 1, where all thiols were protonated. On the other hand, at pH 2.5 the N7 sites of INO, 5′-IMP and 5′-GMP are not protonated. However, at or near neutral pH, although less than 10% of thiols are deprotonated, the N-bonding bases cannot compete with the thiol containing amino acids and peptides. (Bose et al., 1995;, Volckova et al., 2002) Therefore, binding primarily takes place through the sulphur donor sites. However, for the GSMe system, rapid coordination to the sulphur atom followed by migration to the N7 site of the purine was observed. (Teuben et al., 1977) Similar competition experiments of the bifunctional platinum complex, *cis*-dichloro-(ethylendiamine)platinum(II) and its hydrolysed forms with a mixture of 5′-GMP or dGpG and thioether containing di- and tri-peptides, also afforded sulphur bound intermediates, followed by the formation of N7 coordinated guanine products. (Barnhham et al., 1996)

Several sulphur donor ligands are usually co-administered with platinum drugs to reduce the toxicity. (Chen et al., 1998; Berners-Price et al., 1996) Some of them, such as GSH, DEDTC, thiosulfate and thiourea, were used in the study with $[Pt(terpy)(cyst\text{-}S)]^{2+}$ and $[Pt(terpy)(gua\text{-}N7)]^{2+}$ complexes. (Bugarčić et al., 2004a) The X-ray structure of the $[Pt(terpy)(cyst\text{-}S)]^{2+}$ and $[Pt(terpy)(gua\text{-}N7)]^{2+}$ complexes were determinated. (Bugarčić et al., 2004a)

The $[Pt(terpy)(cyst\text{-}S)]^{2+}$ complex is unreactive toward nitrogen binding ligands and cysteine cannot be replaced by N7 from INO, 5′-IMP and 5′-GMP. However, very strong sulphur-donor nucleophiles, such as DEDTC, thiosulfate and thiourea, could reverse the Pt–cysteine bond under pH *ca.* 6. (Bugarčić et al., 2004a) This results clearly show that therapeutic nucleophilic agents for platinum drugs, such as DEDTC, thiosulfate and thiourea, may help to displace Pt from Pt–cysteine adducts and in that way could reduce nephrotoxicity.

It is widely accepted that, once formed, the Pt–nucleobase complexes are inert under mild conditions and in the absence of strong *trans*-labilising ligands. (Lippert, 1999) In contrast, the presence of strong nucleophiles, for instance sulphur-containing bio-molecules, could facilitate the dissociation of N-coordinated nucleobases from the Pt(II) complex. In particular, various sulphur-containing molecules have aroused considerable interest owing to their important roles in the biological processing of anticancer platinum drugs. (Reedijk,1999) The substitution reactions of monofunctional $[Pt(dien)(L\text{-}N7)]^{2+}$ (L = adenosine or guanosine) with thiourea have been studied in acidic aqueous solution. (Mikola et al., 1999) The substitution of guanosine from $[Pt(terpy)(guo\text{-}N7)]^{2+}$ by some sulphur-donor nucleophiles which have been used as protecting agents were studied. (Bugarčić et al., 2004a) This result strongly indicate that all studied sulphur-donor nucleophiles could substitute guanosine from the Pt(II) complex. Also it is noticed that DEDTC and thiosulfate are the strongest nucleophiles and that these nucleophiles can very easily substitute guanosine from $[Pt(terpy)(guo\text{-}N7)]^{2+}$. However, the tripeptide GSH is a very efficient nucleophile as well. This observation could be very important since it is already known that GSH has numerous cellular functions, including the detoxification of chemotherapeutic agents. However, GSH has been used as protecting agent and administered before or after cisplatin. (Reedijk, 1999) Cisplatin readily reacts with GSH and as much as 67% of the administered platinum has been found to coordinate to GSH. However, the role of GSH appears to be dual: GSH deactivates and activates cisplatin. (Volckova et al., 2002) The higher effectiveness of cisplatin has also been demonstrated by co-administering cisplatin and GSH in patients. However, it is not clear whether this increase in effectiveness is due to the reduced toxicity or due to the modification of the platinum drug by binding to the metal. Currently there is much interest in the mechanisms responsible for the development of resistance. Such resistance is often associated with increased cellular GSH, consistent with the view that GSH protects cells against foreign compounds and the effects of radiation. (Jaganyi & Tiba, 2003) From our results we can conclude that the employed rescue or protecting agents such as thiourea, thiosulfate and DEDTC can much easier substitute guanosine than L-cysteine form the $[Pt(terpy)X]^{2+}$ complex (X is guo-*N7* or cyst-*S*). This is in excellent agreement with previous investigations, where has been shown that the Pt–S (cysteine) bond is very stable. (van Boom et al., 1999; Teuben et al., 2000; Pitteri et al., 2001) The thiolate ion is capable of providing a stronger binding affinity owing to its better σ-donating ability. Such a Pt–S bond is considered relatively inert may cause the inhibition of the anticancer activity of platinum drugs.

The kinetics for the complex formation of the $[Pt(terpy)Cl]^+$ with 5′-GMP in the presence and absence of GSH at pH *ca.* 6, with a concentration ratio $[Pt(terpy)Cl]^+$: GSH : 5′-GMP = 1 : 2 : 10 were studied. (Bugarčić et al., 2004b) The second order rate constants, obtained from linear least-squares analysis of the kinetic data (Bugarčić et al., 2004b) clearly point to a kinetic preference of $[Pt(terpy)Cl]^+$ toward the GSH at pH *ca.* 6. 5′-GMP is also a very good nucleophile for Pt(II) complexes, but at neutral pH cannot compete with GSH. The second-order rate constant for GSH is 10^2 times higher than for 5′-GMP. This is also reflected in the competition reactions utilizing mixtures of GSH and GMP. Also, proton and ^{195}Pt NMR data did not show any N7 coordination of GMP, in spite of its excess, in the presence of thiols. (Teuben et al., 2000) However, at or near neutral pH, although less than 10% of thiols are deprotonated, the N-bonding bases cannot compete with the thiol containing amino acids and peptides. (Bugarčić et al., 2004a; Teuben et al., 2000) Therefore, binding primarily takes place through the sulphur donor sites. However, for the GSMe system, rapid coordination to the sulphur atom followed by migration to the N7 site of the purine was observed. (van Boom et al., 1999; Barnham et al., 1994)

The progress of the reaction of $[Pt(terpy)Cl]^+$ with other compounds over extended periods of time can be monitored with techniques such as HPLC which allows aliquots separated from the reaction mixture at programmed times to be analyzed. The studied reactions were carried out in water, without any buffer, since buffer ions (*e.g.* phosphate) are potential ligands for Pt(II). The pH of each solution was regularly checked over the reaction time, and was shown to be kept between 4.5 and 5.5. The products formed were isolated by reversed-phase HPLC and characterized by MALDI-TOF mass spectrometry. As expected, the products obtained corresponded to the adducts $[Pt(terpy)(GS)]^+$ and $[Pt(terpy)(5'\text{-}GMP)]^+$ (m/z 734,2 and 789,8, respectively). The reaction between $[Pt(terpy)Cl]^+$, GSH and 5′-GMP was then followed by HPLC. The ratio of the three compounds in the repeated assays was 1:1:12, respectively. It was observed that $[Pt(terpy)Cl]^+$ reacted much faster with GSH than with 5′-GMP, but this did not prevent a small amount (< 16%) of $[Pt(terpy)(5'\text{-}GMP)]^+$ from being formed at the very beginning of the process. The relative proportion of this adduct remained virtually constant throughout the reaction process, which indicates that once formed it remains unaltered. The possibility that $[Pt(terpy)(GS)]^+$ reactes with the excess of 5′-GMP present in the reaction mixture to give $[Pt(terpy)(5'\text{-}GMP)]^+$ can be ruled out, unless GSH can replace 5′-GMP from $[Pt(terpy)(5'\text{-}GMP)]^+$ at the same reaction rate. The identity of the formed adducts was confirmed by mass spectrometric analysis of the products isolated from the reaction mixture by HPLC (Fig. 4.). (Bugarčić et al., 2004b)

2.3 Interaction of $[Pt(bpma)Cl]^+$ complex with sulphur- and nitrogen-donor bio-molecules

In recent years, an intensive investigation of the substitution reactions of Pt(II) complexes which containing an inert tridentate nitrogen donor ligand with two or three pyridine units was performed. The role of these studies is to explain the effect of present pyridine on the reactivity of these compounds. For example, the complex $[Pt(bpma)Cl]^+$, containes tridentate nitrogen donor ligand consisting of two pyridines connected *via* amide.

This complex in substitution reactions react faster than the $[Pt(dien)Cl]^+$ complex, but slower compared to $[Pt(terpy)Cl]^+$ complex. The substitution reactions of this complex with thiols. (Jaganyi & Tiba, 2003) pyridine, derivatives of pyridine (Pitteri et al., 2001), 5′-GMP, azoles and diazines (Bogojeski and Bugarčić, 2011) were studied. It is interesting that the aqua complex, $[Pt(bpma)(H_2O)]^{2+}$, which crystallizes with perchlorate as external ions, acts as a double base acid, because in the process of deprotonation the second stage involved coordinated amido group. (Pitteri et al., 2002)

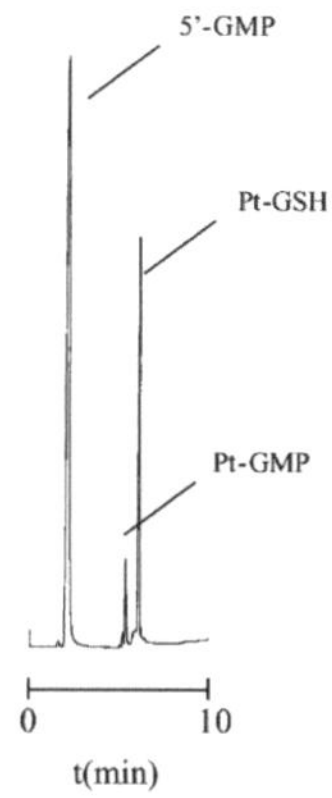

Fig. 4. HPLC profile of an aliquot of the reaction mixture [Pt(terpy)Cl]+/glutathione/5′-GMP = 1:1:12 after 1 week reaction time.

The substitution reactions of $[Pt(bpma)Cl]^+$ and $[Pt(bpma)(H_2O)]^{2+}$ with L-methionine, GSH and 5′-GMP were studied. (Bugarčić et al., 2007) The reactions of the chloro complexes were followed in the presence of 10 mM NaCl and at pH ≈ 5, whereas the reactions of the aqua complexes were studied at pH 2.5.The nucleophilic attack of these ligands occurs *via* the sulphur donor of the thioether group in the case of L-methionine and of the thiol group in the case of GSH. L-methionine appears to be a better nucleophile than GSH under these experimental conditions. This could be explained by the positive inductive effect of the methyl group on the sulphur donor. (Bugarčić et al., 2007)

Transformation from Pt–S(thioether) to Pt–N7(GMP) coordination seems to be common. (Reedijk, 1999; Soldatović & Bugarčić, 2005) To obtain more quantitative data for the stability differences between Pt-DNA and Pt–S(thioether) adducts, it was performed DFT calculations applying the model reaction (Eq. 1.) (L_3 is terpy, bpma, dien, gly-met-S,N,N), where guanine approximates the guanosine-based interactions and SR_2 represents a generic thioether:

$$[L_3Pt\text{-}(N7\text{-}guanine)]^{2+} + S(CH_3)_2 \longrightarrow [L_3Pt\text{-}S(CH_3)_2]^{2+} + guanine \quad (1)$$

In all cases guanine coordination to the L_3Pt fragment is much more favored than thioether coordination. As shown in Table 3.

The $[Pt(bpma)Cl]^+$ and $[Pt(bpma)(H_2O)]^{2+}$ complexes are more reactive than [PtCl(gly-met-S,N,N)] and $[Pt(glymet\text{-}S,N,N)(H_2O])^+$. This can be explained by the steric effect of the coordinated $S\text{–}CH_3$ group in the *cis* position in $[Pt(gly\text{-}met\text{-}S,N,N)(H_2O)]^+$ and [PtCl(gly-met-S,N,N)]. Moreover, another reason for the higher reactivity of the $[Pt(bpma)(H_2O])^{2+}$ and $[Pt(bpma)Cl]^+$ complexes is the presence of two pyridine rings in the coordination sphere. This has been studied in detail for a set of monofunctional Pt(II) complexes with tridentate ligands in which the number and position of the amine and pyridine groups were systematically varied. (Hofmann et al., 2003) The presence of π-acceptor ligands promotes the electrophilicity of the metal center and thereby the nucleophilic attack. (Hofmann et al., 2003; Jaganyi et al., 2001) This behavior distinguishes these complexes from classic platinum drugs where such effects are not present.

L_3	B3LYP/LANL2DZp	B3LYP(CPCM)/LANL2DZp// B3LYP/LANL2DZp
terpy	running (ca. 27 kcal/mol)	Still running kcal/mol
bpma	+28.7 kcal/mol	+12.8 kcal/mol
dien	+34.1 kcal/mol	+11.0 kcal/mol
Gly-Met-N,N,S	+21.5 kcal/mol	+9.5 kcal/mol
Gly-Met-N,N,S (without H-bond)	+17.5 kcal/mol	+8.5 kcal/mol

Table 3. DFT results for model eq. (1)

^{1}H NMR spectroscopy was used to investigate the substitution reactions of the chloro complexes $[Pt(bpma)Cl]^+$ and [PtCl(gly-met-S,N,N)] with 5'-GMP. The substitution reactions were studied in D_2O at 298 K. (Bugarčić et al., 2007)

The reaction of [PtCl(gly-met-S,N,N)] with 5'-GMP is approximately 50 times slower than the reactions of this complex with L-methionine or GSH. This could be accounted for in terms of steric effects of the incoming 5'-GMP and the complex as well. On the other hand, for the reactions with $[Pt(bpma)Cl]^+$ the rate constants are of the same order of magnitude, but L-methionine is the best nucleophile and 5'-GMP is the poorest one. However, the $[Pt(bpma)Cl]^+$ complex is much more reactive towards 5'-GMP than [PtCl(gly-met-S,N,N)]. (Bugarčić et al., 2007) This is in agreement with earlier published findings. (Volckova et al., 2002; Tauben et al., 2000)

Substitution reactions of the complex $[Pt(bpma)(H_2O)]^{2+}$ with TU, DMTU and TMTU Cl^-, Br^-, I^- and SCN^-, were studied in aqueous 0.10 M $NaClO_4$ at pH 2.5. (Jaganyi et al., 2006) Based on the second order rate constants, k_2, it can be concluded that the reactivity of the nucleophiles towards the complex follows the order: TMTU < TU < DMTU. The observed trend for the platinum complex was also reported earlier in the literature for the substitution reactions of the coordinated water molecule from $[Pt(dien)(H_2O)]^{2+}$, $[Pt(terpy)(H_2O)]^{2+}$ and $[Pt(bpma)(H_2O)]^{2+}$ complexes. (Shoukry et al., 1998; Bugarčić et al., 2004c)

The observed trends can be attributed to the different structures (in terms of steric and inductive effects) of these three nucleophiles. The order of increasing steric hindrance for these nucleophiles is: TMTU < DMTU < TU. Theoretically, it would be expected that TU would react much faster than the other two nucleophiles. Instead, it turns out that DMTU is a much better nucleophile than TMTU and TU. This enhanced reactivity is due to the inductive effect introduced by the two methyl groups in the case of the DMTU, which over compensate the steric effect. (Jaganyi et al., 2006)

3. Interaction of bifunctional Pt(II) complexes with sulphur- and nitrogen-donor bio-molecules

In order to achieve the best possible strategy in the designing of antitumor platinum complexes, it is necessary to know how mentioned compounds react with various sulfur- and nitrogen-donor bio-molecules. Significant information about these interactions were obtained from a number of studies implemented in *vitro*, among which are investigation of the substitution reactions of bifunctional platinum complexes with various bio-molecules at different conditions.

Cisplatin is most investigated bifunctional Pt(II) complex. (Redijk, 1999, 2009; Lippert, 1999) In details has been described how cisplatin coordinate to a molecule of DNA. (Redijk, 1999, Lippert, 1999) In addition to investigate the interaction with the classical nucleoside (Barry et al., 2005; Anzellotti et al., 2005) The interactions with AMP, ADP and ATP were investigated, and the best reactivity toward Pt(II) complexes showed to be ATP. (Arpalahti & Lehikoinen, 1990; Arpalahti & Lippert, 1990; Caradonna & Lippard, 1988; Bose et al., 1986; Martin, 1999) Also, the interactions of cisplatin with sulfur-donor bio-molecules, L-cysteine, GSH, L-methionine were studied. GSH is more reactive than L-cysteine. (Bugarčić et al., 2004a) In reactions with L-methionine, amino acid coordinates bidentate to platinum building *S,N*-chelate. If the amino acids is presented in excess the reaction may lead to the bidentate coordination of two molecules of amino acid for Pt(II)-ion. (Norman et al., 1992) The competitive reaction between cisplatin, L-methionine and 5'-GMP in the mixture were also examined. A predominant product is complex $[Pt(NH_3)_2(N7\text{-}GMP)_2]$, while compounds $[Pt(N,L\text{-methionine})(N7\text{-}GMP)(NH_3)]$ and $[Pt(N,L\text{-methionine})_2]$ are formed in a very small concentrations. (Kung et al., 2001) The competitive reactions between 5′-GMP and thiols were also studied, but only found product where is platinum coordinated to sulphur from thiols. (Volckova et al., 2002) The reactions of cisplatin with 5′-GMP and GSH were studied spectrophotometricaly at 37 ^{o}C. NMR technique was also applied to study the reactions of cisplatin with guanosine-5′-monophosphate. (Petrović D. et al., 2007) The rate constants for the reactions of cisplatin with 5′-GMP, obtained by ^{1}H NMR experiments and obtained by Uv–Vis experiments, are in a good agreement. However, these results are in a good agreement with the published results. (Barnham et al., 1994)

Fig. 5. show ^{1}H NMR spectra of the reaction between cisplatin and 5′-GMP. The peak for the free 5′-GMP is at d 8.22 ppm, and for the product the peaks are at d 8.69 and at 8.71 ppm. The peak at 8.69 ppm is smaller than the peak at 8.71 ppm at the later stage of the reaction. (Petrović D. et al., 2007)

During the reaction the peak at 8.71 ppm, which corresponds to the product, $[Pt(NH_3)_2Cl(N7\text{-}GMP)]^+$, increased in intensity, while the peak for the free 5′-GMP (d 8.22 ppm) decreased in intensity. At the end of the reaction all 5′-GMP is coordinated to Pt(II), and the peak for the free 5′-GMP disappears as shown in Fig. 5.

The reactions of cisplatin with GSH were studied spectrophotometricaly, and it has been found that GSH is better nucleophile for cisplatin than 5′-GMP, (Petrović D. et al., 2007) what is also in agreement with previously published results. (Soldatović & Bugarčić, 2005; Hagrman et al., 2004)

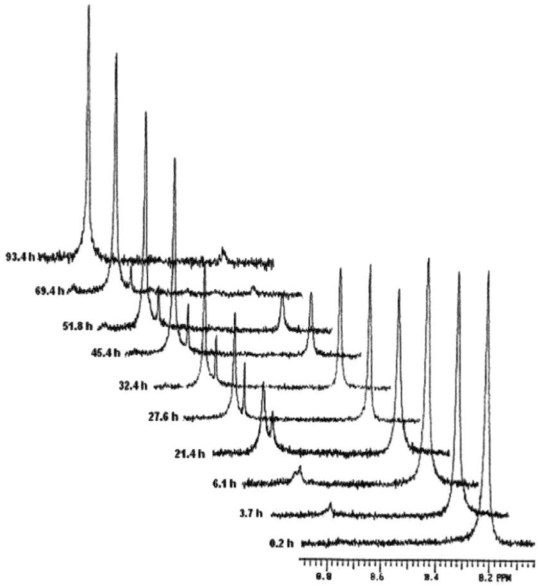

Fig. 5. ^{1}H HMR spectra of a solution of cisplatin (7.5 mM) and 5′-GMP (7.5 mM) in D_2O at pH 7.4 and 298 K recorded as a function of time.

Substitution reactions of the complexes *cis*-$[Pt(NH_3)_2Cl_2]$, $[Pt(SMC)Cl_2]^-$, $[Pt(en)Cl_2]$, and $[Pt(dach)Cl_2]$, with selected biologically important ligands, *viz.* 5′-GMP, L-histidine and 1,2,4-triazole, were studied. (Bogojeski et al., 2010) All reactions were studied in aqueous 25 mM Hepes buffer in the presence of 5 mM NaCl at pH = 7.2 under *pseudo*-first-order conditions as a function of concentration at 310 K by using Uv/Vis spectrophotometry. The substitution reactions were studied in the presence of 5 mM chloride to be close to the conditions in the cell where the concentration is ca. 4 mM. Two consecutive reaction steps, which both depend on the nucleophile concentration, were observed in all cases.

The most reactive N-donor nucleophile is 1,2,4 triazole. L-Histidine has the same order of reactivity as 5′-GMP and it is only slightly faster than 5′-GMP. The difference in the reactivity of these nucleophiles can be accounted in terms of electronic and steric effects. 5′-GMP is sterically more crowded than L-histidine and that can be the reason why the reactions with 5′-GMP are a bit slower. From a comparison of the values of the second-order rate constants for the first reaction step, k_2, it can be concluded that the order of reactivity of the complexes is: $[Pt(SMC)Cl_2]^-$ > *cis*-$[Pt(NH_3)_2Cl_2]$ > $[Pt(en)Cl_2]$ > $[Pt(dach)Cl_2]$. The high reactivity of $[Pt(SMC)Cl_2]^-$ can be attributed to the strong *trans*-labilization effect of the coordinated sulfur atom from the S-methyl-L-cysteine chelate. Such labilization has clearly been illustrated by an earlier study. (Bugarčić et al., 2004b) The reactivity of the complexes *cis*-$[Pt(NH_3)_2Cl_2]$, $[Pt(en)Cl_2]$ and $[Pt(dach)Cl_2]$ depends on steric effects. The $[Pt(dach)Cl_2]$ complex is the sterically most crowded one and the reactions are found to be slower than those with $[Pt(en)Cl_2]$ and *cis*-$[Pt(NH_3)_2Cl_2]$. The reactions with $[Pt(dach)Cl_2]$ were expected to be slower than those with $[Pt(en)Cl_2]$, because the Pt(II) center should be less electrophilic due to the positive inductive effect of the cyclohexane ring. (Summa et al., 2006) The second step of the reaction are significantly slower than the reactions of the first step in all cases.

Transformation from Pt-S(thioether) to Pt-N7(GMP) coordination seems to be common in biological processes. (Reedijk, 1999; Soldatović & Bugarčić, 2005; Jansen et al., 2002; van Boom et al., 1999; Tauben et al., 2000; Barnham et al., 1996) We performed quantum chemical calculations to gain more insight into this process. To obtain more quantitative data for the difference in stability between Pt-DNA and Pt-S(thioether) adducts, DFT calculations were performed.

In all cases guanine coordination to the fragments $Pt(NH_3)_2$, Pt(en) and Pt(dach) is much more favored than thioether coordination. For the first step in the gas phase Pt-N7(Gua) is more stable than Pt-S(thioether) by *ca.* 31-33 kcal/mol, and for the second step by 32-34 kcal/mol.

Finally, this result could be the first to clearly show how much the Pt-N7(Gua) adduct is more stable than the Pt-S(thioether) adduct. This is important since Pt-S(thioether) adducts have been postulated to be a drug reservoir for the binding of platinum to DNA, which may act as intermediates and then be transformed into Pt-N7(Gua) adduct. (Lippert, 1999; Reedijk, 1999; Jansen et al., 2002; van Boom et al., 1999;, Jung & Lippard, 2007)

The kinetics and mechanism of ligand substitution reactions of $[Pt(SMC)Cl_2]$ with biologically relevant ligands were studied as a function of chloride and nucleophile concentrations at pH 2.5 and 7.2. (Soldatović et al., 2009) It was observed that the slope and intercept obtained from the linear dependence of the observed rate constant on the nucleophile concentration strongly depend on the $[Cl^-]$ for all the studied substitution reactions. At high $[Cl^-]$, the rate constant for the forward reaction is almost zero and that for the back reaction follows the order: L-methionine > GSH ~ INO > 5'-GMP. Ion-pair formation between the positively charged Pt(II) complex and the chloride ion is suggested to account for the saturation kinetics observed for the back reaction.

At the highest $[Cl^-]$ of 0.1 M the binding of the nucleophiles is drastically slowed down and almost completely suppressed. This will be the case during the transport of such anti-tumour complexes in blood. At low chloride concentrations as found in cells, effective binding of the studied nucleophiles will occur. The order of reactivity L-met > GSH ~ INO > 5'-GMP clearly shows the high affinity of the Pt(II) complex for thioether. These interactions are more favourable because the transformation from Pt-S(thioether) to Pt-N7 coordination was observed. (Soldatović & Bugarčić, 2005) In our earlier work we did not observe any measurable transformation from Pt-S(thiol) to Pt-N7 coordination. (Bugarčić et al., 2004b) The lower reactivity of 5'-GMP compared to INO can be explained by the fact that at pH 2.5 the N7 position of inosine is almost fully deprotonated whereas in 5'-GMP it is still partially protonated (N7 p*Ka* = 2.33). (Bugarčić et al., 2004b) At pH = 7.2, it is possible that the 5'-monophosphate residue of the nucleotide (p*Ka* a 6) binds to the metal center, which can lead to additional complications in the complex-formation at higher pH and slower second-order rate constants are obtained.

A set of three oxaliplatin derivatives containing 1,2-*trans*-R,R-diaminocyclohexane (dach) as a spectator ligand and different chelating leaving groups X-Y, *viz.*, [Pt(dach)(O,O-cyclobutane-1,1-dicarboxylate)], or Pt(dach)(CBDCA), $[Pt(dach)(N,O\text{-glycine})]^+$, or Pt(dach)(gly), and $[Pt(dach)(N,L\text{-methioninehionine})]^+$, or Pt(dach)(L-Met), where L-Met is L-methionine, were synthesized and the crystal structure of Pt(dach)(gly) was determined by X-ray diffraction. (Summa et al., 2007) The effect of the leaving group on the reactivity of the resulting Pt(II) complexes was studied for the nucleophiles thiourea, GSH and L-Met under *pseudo*-first-order conditions as a function of nucleophile concentration and temperature, using Uv–Vis spectrophotometric techniques. ^{1}H NMR spectroscopy was used to follow the substitution of the leaving group by guanosine 5′-monophosphate (5′-GMP^{2-}). The rate constants for all reactions of direct substitution of the X–Y chelate by the selected nucleophiles, showing that the nature of the chelate, viz., O–O (CBDCA^{2-}), N–O (glycine) or S–N(L-Met), respectively, plays an important role in the kinetic and mechanistic behavior of the Pt(II) complex.

The nature of the chelate, being O–O(CBDCA^{2-}), N–O(glycine) or S–N(L-Met) was shown to play an important role in the kinetic and mechanistic behavior of the Pt(II) complexes. Pt(dach)(CBDCA) exhibits a higher reactivity towards the sulfur donor L-Met than Pt(dach)(gly), whereas the order is the opposite for the nitrogen donor 5′-GMP^{2-} and the sulfur donors thiourea and GSH in the first reaction step. The Pt–N bond was always found to be very strong, especially for the reaction with 5′-GMP^{2-}, in which the 1:1 reaction product [Pt(N-gly)(N7-GMP)] is very stable and hardly (7%) reacts with another molecule of 5′-GMP^{2-} to form the 1:2 product. By contrast, the liberation of H_2CBDCA in Pt(dach)(CBDCA) in the second reaction step was faster than the rate-determining first reaction step and could not be analyzed under the selected experimental conditions. The mechanism of the substitution reactions is associative as supported by the large and negative values of $\Delta S^{\#}$.

Multinuclear complexes of platinum(II) represent a third generation of antitumor drugs as and platinum(IV) complexes. (Esposito & Najjar, 2002) The reason for the increasing interest in multinuclear complexes is their ability to form DNA adducts that differ significantly from those formed cisplatin and related complexes, (McGregor et al., 1999) which results in a completely different anti tumor behaviour. The biological activity of polynuclear platinum complexes maybe modulated by the geometry and number of leaving groups in the coordination sphere of platinum atoms as well as by the nature of linkers connecting the platinum centers. In contrast with the mononuclear complexes, such as antitumor cisplatin and clinically ineffective transplatin, in the dinuclear case both geometries are antitumor active. (Farrell, 2004)

We compared the cytotoxic capacity of platinum complexes (Fig. 6.) towards TOV21G, HCT 116 tumour human cell lines and human MSC, normal rapidly dividing cells (Fig. 7.). (Jovanović et al., 2011)

All complexes displayed a dose-dependent and time-dependent cytotoxicity towards the tested cell lines but the most cytotoxic effect showed towards TOV21G cells (Fig. 7). The complex [$PtCl_4$(dach)] at the lower concentrations induced significantly higher cytotoxic effect towards TOV21G cells then other four complexes.

HCT116 cells were more resistant to the cytotoxic effects of selected complexes (Fig. 7). Again, [$PtCl_4$(dach)] was the most efficient and exerted very similar activity towards HCT116 cells as cisplatin.

The complexes **Pt2** and **Pt3** displayed cytotoxicity towards MSC similar as cisplatin, but the other three complexes **Pt1**, [$PtCl_4$(dach)] and [$PtCl_4$(bipy)] were more toxic. (Jovanović et al., 2011)

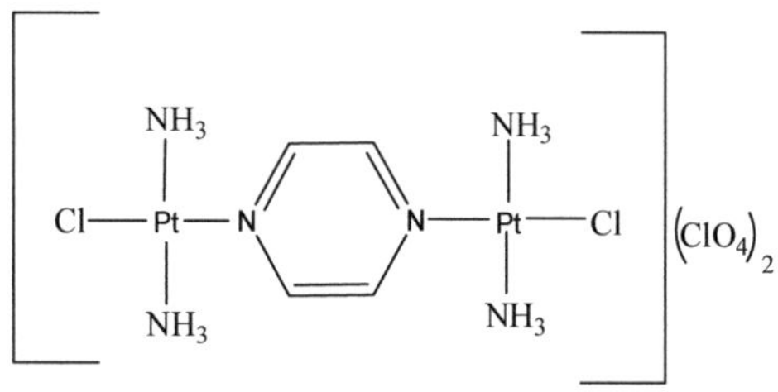

[{*trans*-Pt(NH_3)$_2$Cl}$_2$(μ-pyrazine)](ClO_4)$_2$, **Pt1**

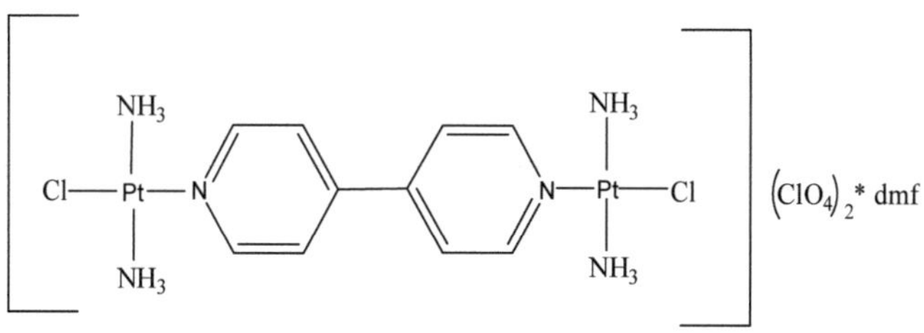

[{*trans*-Pt(NH_3)$_2$Cl}$_2$(μ-4,4'-bipyridyl)](ClO_4)$_2$·DMF, **Pt2**

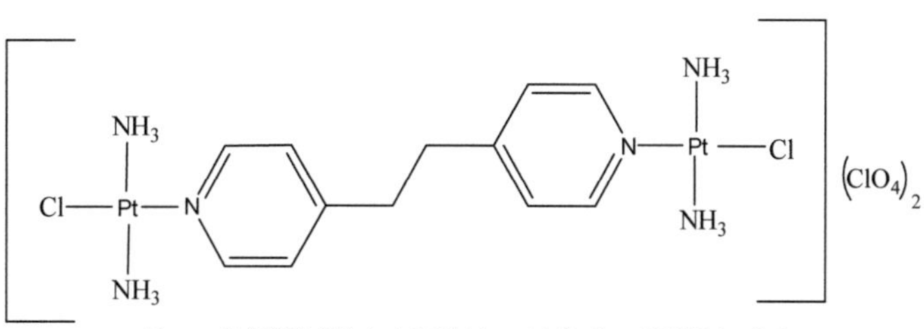

[{*trans*-Pt(NH_3)$_2$Cl}$_2$(μ-1,2-bis(4-pyridyl)ethane)](ClO_4)$_2$, **Pt3**

Fig. 6. Structures of investigated dinuclear platinum(II) complexes.

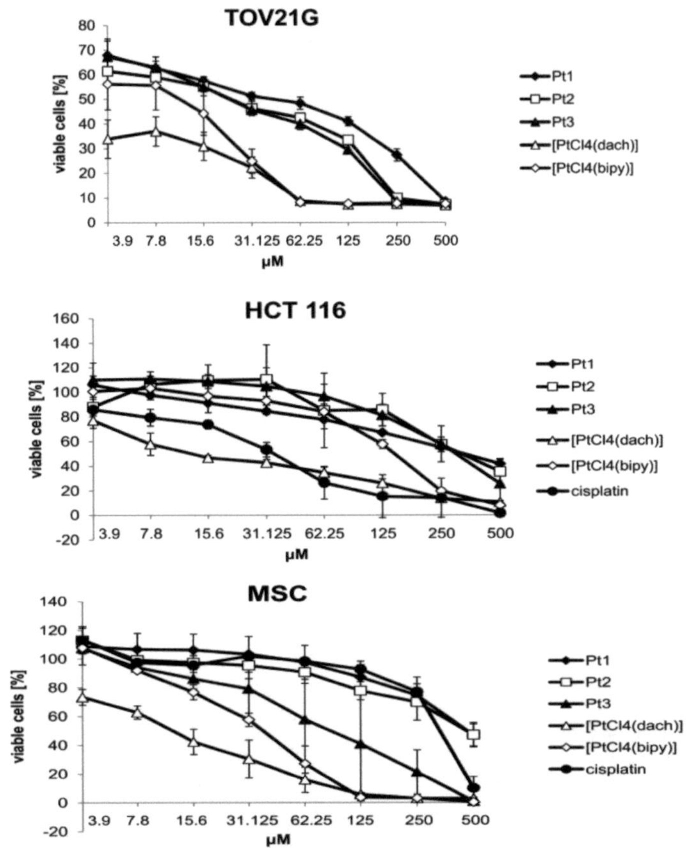

Fig. 7. Cytotoxic activity of tested complexes measured by MTT test (Mean+/-SE).

4. Conclusion

Results presented here, could contribute to a better understanding of the precise biochemical mechanism of some Pt(II) complexes. Moreover, the results of the substitution reactions with biologically relevant ligands could help to get more information on the possible interaction modes of Pt(II) complexes with *in vivo* targets and their representative application in the study of their anti-tumour properties. Detailed knowledge of the interactions between transition metal ions complexes with biomolecules and stability of final products under varying experimental conditions is fundamental for future investigations of new pharmacological agents and discovery of the alternative tumor treatment. Connecting theoretical calculations, chemistry, biochemistry and cellular biology and establishement of the structure-activity relationship Pt(II) complexes will help to solve some of the questions and will finally result in more tailored drug design. Numerous data imply that interactions of Pt(II) complexes and investigation of the mechanism of their reaction with DNA fragments (purine and pyrimidine bases, as well as oligonucleotides) are important for antitumor activity of Pt(II) complexes and the results of studies presented above contribute to that. Investigations of the interaction of Pt(II) complexes with other S-donor biomolecules can help us to get better insights in the destiny of anti-tumor drugs in the cells after their uptake, as well as to obtain more information about the inner cellular processes, which are affected by therapy.

Further research in this area will be based on the synthesis and investigation of the substitution reactions of the transition metals complexes especially Pt(II), Pt(IV), Au(III) and Ru(II/III) complexes. This complexes are investigated in order to find compounds that would demonstrate greater anti-tumour activity and less toxicity and resistance compared to cisplatin. It turned out that some complexes of Pt(IV) are toxic to cancers where cisplatin developed resistance. A good feature of the complexes of Pt(IV) is that some of them can be taken orally. When the complex of Pt(IV) enters the cell, it leads to the reduction of Pt(IV) to Pt(II) and binding to DNA. Au(III) is isoelectronic with Pt(II) and forms square planar complexes, and is therefore a good candidate for the synthesis of new complexes that could show better properties than the complexes of Pt(II). Also, complexes of Ru(II/III) are potential anti-cancer agents and consequently the study of these complexes is of great importance.

5. Acknowledgements

The authors gratefully acknowledge financial support from the Ministry of Education and Science of the Republic of Serbia, project No. 172011.

6. References

Ali M. S.; Khan S. R. A.; Ojima H.; Guzman I. Y.; Whitmire K. H.; Siddik Z. H. & Khokhar A. R. (2005). Model platinum nucleobase and nucleoside complexes and antitumor activity: X-ray crystal structure of [PtIV(trans-1R,2R-diaminocyclohexane)trans(acetate)2(9-ethylguanine)Cl]NO_3H_2O. *Journal of Inorganic Biochemistry*, Vol. 99, pp. 795-804, ISSN:0162-0134.

Annibale G.; Bergamini P.; Bertolasi V.; Cattabriga M.; Lazzaro A.; Marchi A. & Vertuani G. (1999). Platinum assisted cyclization of S-methyl 3-acyl-2-methyldithiocarbazates under mild conditions. Crystal structure of $[Pt_2(\mu\text{-SMe})(terpy)_2][ClO_4]_3$. *Journal of the Chemical Society, Dalton Transactions: Inorganic Chemistry*, No. 21, pp. 3877-3882, ISSN:0300-9246.

Annibale G.; Brandolisio M.; Bugarčić Ž. D. & Cattalini L. (1998). Nucleophilicity of thiols towards planar tetracoordinated platinum(II) complexes. *Transition Metal Chemistry*, Vol. 23, pp. 715-719, ISSN:0340-4285.

Anzellotti A. I.; Ma E. S. & Farell N. (2005). Platination of Nucleobases To Enhance Noncovalent Recognition in Protein-DNA/RNA Complexes. *Inorganic Chemistry*, Vol. 44, pp. 483-485, ISSN:0020-1669.

Arpalahti J. & Lehikoinen P. (1990). Kinetics of complexation of aquated (diethylenetriamine)platinum(II) with inosine and 1-methylinosine as a function of pH. *Inorganic Chemistry*, Vol. 29, pp. 2564-2567, ISSN:0020- 1669.

Arpalahti J. & Lippert B. (1990) Coordination of aquated cis-platinum(II) diamines to purine nucleosides. Kinetics of complex formation. *Inorganic Chemistry*, Vol. 29, pp. 104-110, ISSN:0020-1669.

Bailey J. A.; Hill M. G.; Marsh R. E.; Miskowski V. M.; Schaeefer W. P. & Gray H. B. (1995). Electronic Spectroscopy of Chloro(terpyridine)platinum(II). *Inorganic Chemistry,* Vol. 34, pp. 4591-4599, ISSN:0020-1669.

Barnham K. J.; Djuran M.I.; del Socorro P. & Sadler P.J. (1994). Intermolecular displacement of S-bound L-methionine on platinum(II) by guanosine 5'-monophosphate: implications for the mechanism of action of anticancer drugs. *Journal of the Chemical Society, Chemical Communications,* No. 6, pp. 721–722, ISSN:0022-4936.

Barnham K. J.; Guo Z. J. & Sadler P. J. (1996). Stabilization of monofunctional platinum-nucleotide adducts: reactions of N-acetyl-L-methionine complexes with guanosine 5'-monophosphate and guanylyl(3'-5')guanosine. *Journal of the Chemical Society, Dalton Transactions,* No. 13, pp. 2867-2876, ISSN:0300-9246.

Barnham K. J.; Djuran M. I.; Murdoch P. d. S.; Ranford J. D. & Sadler P. J. (1996). Ring-Opened Adducts of the Anticancer Drug Carboplatin with Sulfur Amino Acids. *Inorganic Chemistry,* Vol. 35, pp. 1065-1072, ISSN:0020-1669.

Barry C. G.; Day C. S. & Bierbach U. (2005). Duplex-Promoted Platination of Adenine-N3 in the Minor Groove of DNA: Challenging a Longstanding Bioinorganic Paradigm. *Journal of the American Chemical Society,* Vol. 127, pp. 1160-1169, ISSN:0002-7863.

Becker K.; Herold-Mende C.; Park J. J.; Lowe G. & Shirmer R. H. (2001). Human thioredoxin reductase is efficiently inhibited by (2,2':6',2''-terpyridine)platinum(II) complexes. Possible implications for a novel antitumor strategy. *Journal of medicinal chemistry,* Vol. 44, pp. 2784-2792, ISSN:0022-2623.

Berners-Price S. J.; Barnham K. J.; Frey U. & Sadler P. J. (1996). Kinetic analysis of the stepwise platination of single- and double-stranded GG oligonucleotides with cisplatin and cis-$[PtCl(H_2O)(NH_3)_2]^+$. *Chemistry--A European Journal,* Vol. 2, pp. 1283-1291, ISSN:0947-6539.

Berners-Price S. J.; Davies M. S.; Cox J. W.; Thomas D. S. & Farrell N. (2003) Competitive reactions of interstrand and intrastrand DNA-Pt adducts: A dinuclear-platinum complex preferentially forms a 1,4-interstrand cross-link rather than a 1,2 intrastrand cross-link on binding to a GG 14-mer duplex. *Chemistry--A European Journal,* Vol. 9, pp. 713-725, ISSN:0947-6539.

Bogojeski J.; Bugarčić Ž. D.; Puchta R. & van Eldik R. (2010). Kinetic studies on the reactions of different bifunctional platinum(II) complexes with selected nucleophiles. *European Journal of Inorganic Chemistry,* No. 34, 5439-5445, ISSN:1434-1948.

Bogojeski J. & Bugarčić Ž. D. (2011). Kinetic and thermodznamic studies on reactions of $[Pt(bpma)Cl]^+$ and $[Pt(bpma)H_2O]^{2+}$ (bpma = bis-(2-pyridylmethyl)amine) with some azoles and diazines. *Transaction Metal Chemistry,* Vol. 36, pp. 73-78, ISSN:0340-4285.

Bose N.; Cornelius R. D. & Viola R. E. (1986). Multinuclear NMR studies and the kinetics of formation of platinum(II)-adenine nucleotide complexes. *Journal of the American Chemical Society,* Vol. 108, pp. 4403-4408, ISSN:0002- 7863.

Bose N.; Moghaddas S.; Weaver E. L. & Cox E. H. (1995). Reactivity of Glutathione and Cysteine toward Platinum(II) in the Presence and Absence of Guanosine 5'-Monophosphate. *Inorganic Chemistry,* Vol. 34, pp. 5878-5883, ISSN:0020-1669.

Bruijnincx P. C. A. & Sadler P. J. (2009). Controlling platinum, ruthenium, and osmium reactivity for anticancer drug design. *Advances in Inorganic Chemistry,* Vol. 61, pp. 1-62, ISSN:0898-8838.

Bugarčić Ž. D.; Đorđević B. V. & Đuran M. I. (1997). Mechanism of the reactions between chloro(2,2':6',2''-terpyridine)platinum(II) and ligands containing a thiol group. *Journal of the Serbian Chemical Society*, Vol. 62, pp. 1031-1036, ISSN:0352-5139.

Bugarčić Ž. D. & Đorđević B. V. (1998). Kinetics and mechanism of the reaction of platinum(II) complexes with thioglycolic acid. *Monatshefte fuer Chemie*, Vol. 129, pp. 1267-1274, ISSN:0026-9247.

Bugarčić Ž. D.; Liehr G. & van Eldik R. (2002). Kinetics and mechanism of the reactions of $[Pt(terpy)H_2O]^{2+}$ with thiols in acidic aqueous solution. Synthesis and crystal structure of $[Pt(terpy)(tu)](ClO_4)^2$ (tu = thiourea). *Journal of the Chemical Society, Dalton Transactions*, No. 14, pp. 2825-2830, SSN:1472-7773.

Bugarčić Ž. D.; Shoukry M. M. & van Eldik R. (2002). Equilibrium and kinetic data for the interaction of diaqua-(S- methyl-l-cysteine)palladium(II) with biologically relevant ligands. *Journal of the Chemical Society, Dalton Transactions*, No. 21, pp. 3945-3951, SSN:1472-7773.

Bugarčić Ž. D.; Heinemann F. W. & van Eldik R. (2004). Substitution reactions of $[Pt(terpy)X]^{2+}$ with some biologically relevant ligands. Synthesis and crystal structure of $[Pt(terpy)(cyst\text{-}S)](ClO_4)_2$□$0.5H_2O$ and $[Pt(terpy)(guo\text{-}N7)](ClO_4)_2$□0.5guo□$1.5H_2O$. *Dalton Transactions*, No. 2, pp. 279-286, ISSN:1477-9226.

Bugarčić Ž. D.; Soldatović T.; Jelić R.; Alguero B. & Grandas A. (2004). Equilibrium, kinetic and HPLC study of the reactions between platinum(II) complexes and DNA constituents in the presence and absence of glutathione. *Dalton Transactions*, No. 22, pp. 3869-3877, ISSN:1477-9226.

Bugarčić Ž. D.; Petrović B. & Zangrando E.(2004). Kinetics and mechanism of the complex formation of $[Pd(NNN)Cl]^+$ with pyridines in methanol: synthesis and crystal structure of $[Pd(terpy)(py)](ClO_4)_2$. *Inorganica Chimica Acta*, Vol. 357, pp. 2650-2656, ISSN:0020-1693.

Bugarčić Ž. D.; Rosić J.; Petrović B. V.; Summa N.; Puchta R. & van Eldik R. (2007). Kinetics and mechanism of the substitution reactions of $[Pt(bpma)Cl]^+$, [PtCl(gly-met-S,N,N)] and their aqua analogs with L-methionine, glutathione and 5'-GMP. *Journal of Biological Inorganic Chemistry*, Vol. 12., pp. 1141-1150, ISSN:0949-8257.

Caradonna J. P. & Lippard S. J. (1988). Synthesis and characterization of [d(ApGpGpCpCpT)]2 and its adduct with the anticancer drug cis-diamminedichloroplatinum(II). *Inorganic Chemistry*, Vol. 27, pp. 1454-1466.

Chen Y.; Guo Z.; Murdoch P. S.; Zang E. & Sadler P. J. (1998). Interconversion between S- and N-bound L-methionine adducts of $Pt(dien)^{2+}$ (dien = diethylenetriamine) via dien ring-opened intermediates. *Journal of the Chemical Society, Dalton Transactions: Inorganic Chemistry*, No. 9, pp. 1503-1508.

Cheng C. C. & Pai C. H. (1998). Specific displacement of glutathione from the Pt(II)-glutathione adduct by Cu(II) in neutral phosphate buffer. *Journal of Inorganic Biochemistry*, Vol. 71, pp. 109-113.

Chiorazzi N.; Rai K. R. & Ferrarini M. (2005). Chronic lymphocytic leukemia. *New England Journal of Medicine*, Vol. 352, pp. 804-815, ISSN:0028-4793.

Eichhorst B. F.; Busch R. Hopfinger G. et al. (2005) Fludarabine plus cyclophosphamide versus fludarabine alone in first line therapy of younger patients with chronic lymphocytic leukemia. *Blood*, Vol. 107, pp. 885-891.

Esposito B.P. & Najjar R. (2002). Interactions of antitumoral platinum- group metallodrugs with albumin, *Coordination Chemistry Reviews,* Vol. 232, pp. 137-149, ISSN 0010-8545.

Farrell N. (2004). Polynuclear platinum drugs in: A. Sigel, H. Sigel (Eds.), Metal ions in biological systems, New York and Basel Marcel Dekker Inc., New York, pp. 251–296.

Frey U.; Ranford J.D. & Sadler P.J. (1993). Ring-opening reactions of the anticancer drug carboplatin: NMR characterization of cis-[Pt(NH_3)$_2$(CBDCA-O)(5'-GMP-N7)] in solution. *Inorganic Chemistry,* Vol. 32, pp. 1333-1340, ISSN:0020-1669.

Fuertes M. A.; Alonso C. & Perez J. M. (2003). Biochemical modulation of cisplatin mechanisms of action: enhancement of antitumor activity and circumvention of drug resistance. *Chemical Reviews,* Vol. 103, pp. 645-662, ISSN:0009-2665.

Hagrman D.; Goodisman J. & Soud A-K. (2004). Kinetic study on the reactions of platinum drugs with glutathione. *Journal of Pharmacology and Experimental Therapeutics,* Vol. 308, pp. 658-666, ISSN:0022-3565.

Harris A.; Qu Y. & Farell N. (2005). Unique Cooperative Binding Interaction Observed between a Minor Groove Binding Pt Antitumor Agent and Hoeschst Dye 33258. *Inorganic Chemistry,* Vol. 44, pp. 1196-1198, ISSN:0020-1669.

Hofmann A.; Jaganyi D.; Munro O. Q.; Liehr G. & van Eldik R. (2003). Electronic Tuning of the Lability of Pt(II) Complexes through □ -Acceptor Effects. Correlations between Thermodynamic, Kinetic, and Theoretical Parameters. *Inorganic Chemistry,* Vol. 42, pp. 1688-1700, ISSN:0020-1669.

Jacobs R.; Prinsloo F. & Breet E. (1992). Kinetics of binding of DNA nucleotides to antitumor type complexes. *Journal of the Chemical Society, Chemical Communications,* No. 3, pp. 212-213, ISSN:0022-4936.

Jaganyi D.; Hofmann A. & van Eldik R. (2001). Controlling the lability of square-planar PtII complexes through electronic communication between □ -acceptor ligands. *Angewandte Chemie, International Edition,* Vol. 40, pp. 1680-1683, ISSN:1433-7851.

Jaganyi D. & Tiba F. (2003). Substitution of [Pt(terpy)H_2O]$^{2+}$ and [Pt(bpma)H_2O]$^{2+}$ with thiols in acidic aqueous solution. terpy = 2,2':6'2''-terpyridine; bpma = bis(2-pyridylmethyl)amine. *Transition Metal Chemistry,* Vol. 28, pp. 803-807, SSN:0340-4285.

Jaganyi D.; Tiba F.; Munro O. Q.; Petrović B. & Bugarčić Ž. D. (2006). Kinetic and mechanistic study on the reactions of [Pt(bpma)(H_2O)]$^{2+}$ and [Pd(bpma)(H_2O)]$^{2+}$ with some nucleophiles. Crystal structure of [Pd(bpma)(py)](ClO_4)$_2$. *Dalton Transactions,* No. 24, pp. 2943-2949, ISSN:1477-9226.

Jakupec M. A.; Galanski M. & Keppler B. K. (2003). Tumour-inhibiting platinum complexes-state of the art and future perspectives. *Reviews of Physiology, Biochemistry and Pharmacology,* Vol. 146, pp. 1-53, ISSN:0303-4240.

Jakupec M. A.; Galanski M.; Arion V. B.; Hartinger C. G. & Keppler B. K. (2008). Antitumor metal compounds: more than theme and variations. *Dalton Transactions,* No. 2, pp. 183-194, ISSN:1477-9226.

Jansen B. A. J.; Brouwer J. & Reedijk J. (2002). Glutathione induces cellular resistance against cationic dinuclear platinum anticancer drugs. *Journal of Inorganic Biochemistry,* Vol. 89, pp. 197-202, ISSN:0162-0134.

Jolley J. N.; Yanovsky A. I.; Kelland L. R. & Nolan K. B. (2001). Synthesis and antitumour activity of platinum(II) and platinum(IV) complexes containing ethylenediamine-derived ligands having alcohol, carboxylic acid and acetate substituents. Crystal and molecular structure of $[PtL_4Cl_2]$ H_2O where L_4 is ethylenediamine-N,N'-diacetate. *Journal of Inorganic Biochemistry*, Vol. 83, pp. 91-100, ISSN:0162-0134.

Jovanović S.; Soldatović T.; Milovanović M.; Volarević V.; Čanović D.; Arsenijević N. & Bugarčić Ž. D. (2011). Ligand substitution reactions of Pt(IV) and dinuclear Pt(II) complexes with 5′-GMP and their cytotoxic properties. Submitted in European Journal of Medicinal Chemistry

Jung Y. & S. J. Lippard (2007). Direct Cellular Responses to Platinum-Induced DNA Damage. *Chemical Reviews*, Vol. 107, pp. 1387-1407, ISSN:0009-2665.

Kozelka J.; Legendre F.; Reeder F. & Chottard J. C. (1999). Kinetic aspects of interactions between DNA and platinum complexes. *Coordination Chemistry Reviews*, Vol. 190-192.

Kung A.; Strickman D. B.; Galanski M. & Keppler B. K. (2001). Comparison of the binding behavior of oxaliplatin, cisplatin and analogues to 5'-GMP in the presence of sulfur-containing molecules by means of capillary electrophoresis and electrospray mass spectrometry. *Journal of Inorganic Biochemistry*, Vol. 86, pp. 691-698, ISSN:0162-0134.

Lakomska I.; Kooijman H.; Spek A. L.; Shen W. & Reedijk J. (2009). Mono- and dinuclear platinum(II) compounds with 5,7-dimethyl-1,2,4-triazolo[1,5-a]pyrimidine. Structure, cytotoxic activity and reaction with 5'-GMP. *Dalton Transactions*, Vol. 48, pp. 10736-10741, ISSN:1477-9226.

Lampers L. M. & Reedijk J. (1990). Reversibility of binding of cisplatin-methionine in proteins by diethyldithiocarbamate or thiourea: a study with model adducts. *Inorganic Chemistry*, Vol. 29, pp. 217-222, ISSN:0020-1669.

Lemma K.; Shi T. & Elding L. I. (2000). Kinetics and mechanism for reduction of the anticancer prodrug trans,trans,trans-$[PtCl_2(OH)_2(c\text{-}C_6H_{11}NH_2)(NH_3)]$ (JM335) by thiols. *Inorganic chemistry*, Vol. 39, pp. 1728-1734, ISSN:0020-1669.

Lemma K.; Sargeson A. M. & Elding L. I. (2000). Kinetics and mechanism for reduction of oral anticancer platinum(IV) dicarboxylate compounds by L-ascorbate ions. *Dalton Transaction*, No. 7, pp. 1167-1172, ISSN:1470-479X.

Lippert B. (1999). Cisplatin, Chemistry and Biochemistry of Leading Antitumor Drugs ,Wiley-VCH, Zuruch.

Lippert B. (1999). Impact of Cisplatin on the recent development of Pt coordination chemistry: a case study. *Coordination Chemistry Reviews*, Vol. 182, pp. 263-295, ISSN:0010-8545.

Mambanda A.; Jaganyi D.; Hochreuther S. & van Eldik R. (2010). Tuning the reactivity of chelated dinuclear Pt(II) complexes through a flexible diamine linker. A detailed kinetic and mechanistic study. *Dalton Transactions*, Vol. 39, 3595-3608, ISSN:1477-9226.

Martin R. B. , *Cisplatin, Chemistry and Biochemistry of Leading Antitumor Drugs*, ed. B. Lippert, Wiley-VCH, Zurich, 1999, p. 193-200.

McGregor T.D.; Balcarova Z.; Qu Y.; Tran M.-C.; Zaludova R.; Brabec V. & Farrell N. (1999). Sequence-dependent conformational changes in DNA induces by polinuclear platinum complexes. *Journal of Inorganic Biochemistry*, Vol. 77, pp. 43-46, ISSN:0162-0134.

Mikola M.; Klika K. D.; Hakala A. & Arpalahti J. (1999). Substitution Reactions of Platinum(II)-Nucleobase Complexes by Associative Mechanism Involving Pseudorotation of the Five-Coordinate Intermediate. *Inorganic Chemistry*, Vol. 38, pp. 571-578, ISSN:0020-1669.

Mock C.; Puscasu I.; Rauterkus M. J.; Tallen G.; Wolff J. E. A. & Krebs B. (2001). Novel Pt(II) anticancer agents and their Pd(II) analogues: syntheses, crystal structures, reactions with nucleobases and cytotoxicities. *Inorganica Chimica Acta*, Vol. 319, pp. 109-116, ISSN:0020-1693.

Natile G. & Coluccia M. (2001). Current status of trans-platinum compounds in cancer therapy. *Coordination Chemistry Reviews*, Vol. 216-217, pp. 383-410, ISSN:0010-8545.

Norman R. E.; Ranford J. D. & Sadler P. J. (1992). Studies of platinum(II) methionine complexes: metabolites of cisplatin. *Inorganic Chemistry*, Vol. 31, pp. 877-888,ISSN:0020-1669.

Petrović B. & Bugarčić Ž. D. (2001). Kinetics and mechanism of complex formation between $[Pt(dien)Cl]^+$ and thiols and thioethers. *Journal of Coordination Chemistry*, Vol. 53, pp. 35-45, ISSN:0095-8972.

Petrović B. V.; Đuran M. I. & Bugarčić Ž. D. (1999). Binding of platinum(II) to some biologically important thiols. Metal-Based Drugs, Vol. 6, pp. 355-360, ISSN:0793-0291.

Petrović D.; Stojimirović B.; Petrović B.; Bugarčić Z. M. & Bugarčić Ž. D. (2007). Studies of interactions between platinum(II) complexes and some biologically relevant molecules. Bioorganic & Medicinal Chemistry, Vol. 15, pp. 4203-4211, ISSN:0968-0896.

Pitteri B.; Marangoni G.; Cattalini L.; Visentin F.; Bertolasi V. & Gilli P. (2001). The role of the non-participating groups in substitution reactions at cationic Pt(II) complexes containing tridentate chelating nitrogen donors. Crystal structure of {Pt[bis(2-pyridylmethyl)amine](py)}$(CF_3SO_3)_2$. *Polyhedron*, Vol. 20, pp. 869-880, ISSN:0277-5387.

Pitteri B.; Annibale G.; Marangoni G.; Bertolasi V. & Ferretti V. (2002). Base hydrolysis kinetics and equilibria of [bis(2-pyridylmethyl)amine]chloroplatinum(II) and crystal and molecular structures of [Pt(bpma)Cl]Cl H_2O and $[Pt(bpma)(OH_2)](ClO_4)_2$ $2H_2O$. *Polyhedron*, 2002, Vol. 21, pp. 2283-2291, ISSN:0277-5387.

Reedijk J. (1999). Why does cisplatin reach guanine-N7 with competing S-donor ligands available in the cell? *Chemical Reviews*, Vol. 99, pp. 2499-2510, ISSN:0009-2665.

Reedijk J. (2009). Platinum anticancer coordination compounds: study of DNA binding inspires new drug design. *European Journal of Inorganic Chemistry*, No. 10, pp. 1303-1312, ISSN:1434-1948.

Ronconi L. & Sadler P. J. (2007). Using coordination chemistry to design new medicines. *Coordination Chemistry Reviews*, Vol. 251, pp. 1633-1648, ISSN:0010-8545.

Rosenberg B. & Camp L. V. (1965). INHIBITION OF CELL DIVISION IN ESCHERICHIA COLI BY ELECTROLYSIS PRODUCTS FROM A PLATINUM ELECTRODE, *Nature, Vol. 205, pp.* 698-699, ISSN:0028-0836.

Rosenberg B.; Camp L. V.; Trosko J. E. & Mansour V. H. (1969). Platinum compounds: a new class of potent antitumor agents. *Nature*, Vol. 222, pp. 385-386, ISSN:0028-0836.

Rosenberg B. & Camp L. V. (1970). Successful regression of large solid sarcoma 180 tumors by platinum compounds. *Cancer Research*, Vol. 30, pp. 1799-1802, ISSN:0008-5472.

Rosenberg B.; Camp L. V.; Grimley E. B. & Thomson A. J. (1967). Inhibition of growth or cell division in Escherichia coli by different ionic species of platinum(IV) complexes. *Journal of Biological Chemistry*, Vol. 242, pp. 1347-1352, ISSN:0021-9258.

Shi T. & Elding L. I. (1996). Equilibrium and High-Pressure Kinetic Study of Formation and Proton-Assisted Aquation of Monodentate Acetate, Propionate, and Glycolate Complexes of Palladium(II) in Aqueous Solution. *Inorganic Chemistry*, Vol. 35, pp. 735-740, ISSN:0020-1669.

Shi T. & Elding L. I. (1997). Linear Free Energy Relationships for Complex Formation Reactions between Carboxylic Acids and Palladium(II). Equilibrium and High-Pressure Kinetics Study. *Inorganic Chemistry*, Vol. 34, pp. 528-536, ISSN:0020-1669.

Shoukry A.; Rau T.; Shoukry M. & van Eldik R. (1998). Kinetics and mechanisms of the ligand substitution reactions of bis(amine)(cyclobutane-1,1-dicarboxylato)palladium(II). *Journal of the Chemical Society, Dalton Transactions*, No. 18, pp. 3105-3112.

Sigel H.; Massoud S. S.; Corfu N. A. (1994). Comparison of the Extent of Macrochelate Formation in Complexes of Divalent Metal Ions with Guanosine (GMP^{2-}), Inosine (IMP^{2-}), and Adenosine 5'-Monophosphate (AMP^{2-}). The Crucial Role of N-7 Basicity in Metal Ion-Nucleic Base Recognition. *Journal of the American Chemical Society*, Vol. 116, pp. 2958-2971, ISSN:0002-7863.

Soldatović T. & Bugarčić Ž. D. (2005). Study of the reactions between platinum(II) complexes and -methionine in the presence and absence of 5'-GMP. *Journal of Inorganic Biochemistry*, Vol. 99, pp. 1472-1479, ISSN:0162-0134.

Soldatović T.; Bugarčić Ž. D. & van Eldik R. (2009). Influence of the chloride concentration on ligand substitution reactions of $[Pt(SMC)Cl_2]$ with biologically relevant nucleophiles. *Dalton Transactions*, No. 23, pp. 4526-4531, ISSN:1477-9226.

Summa N.; Schiessl W.; Puchta R.; van Eikema Hommes N. & van Eldik R. (2006). Thermodynamic and Kinetic Studies on Reactions of Pt(II) Complexes with Biologically Relevant Nucleophiles. *Inorganic Chemistry*, Vol. 45, pp. 2948-2959, ISSN:0020-1669.

Summa N.; Soldatović T.; Dahlenburg L.; Bugarčić Ž. D. & van Eldik R. (2007). Kinetics and mechanism of the substitution reactions of $[Pt(bpma)Cl]^{+}$, [PtCl(gly-met-S,N,N)] and their aqua analogs with L-methionine, glutathione and 5'-GMP. *Journal of Biological Inorganic Chemistry*, Vol. 12, pp. 1141-1150, ISSN:0949-8257.

Talman E. G.; Bruning W.; Reedijk J.; Spek A. L. & Veldman N. (1997). Crystal and Molecular Structures of Asymmetric cis- and trans-Platinum(II/IV) Compounds and Their Reactions with DNA Fragments. *Inorganic Chemistry*, Vol. 36, pp. 854-861, ISSN:0020-1669.

Tauben J. M.; Rodrugez M.; Zubiri & Reedijk J. (2000). Glutathione readily replaces the thioether on platinum in the reaction with $[Pt(dien)(GSMe)]^{2+}$ (GSMe = S-methylated glutathione); a model study for cisplatin-protein interactions. *Dalton*, No. 3, pp. 369-372, ISSN:1470-479X.

Teuben J. M.; van Boom S. S. G. E. & Reedijk J. (1997). Intramolecular migration of coordinated platinum from a sulfur to N7 in the nucleopeptide Met-d(TpG) (5'-Omethioninate-N-ylcarbonylthymidine 2'-deoxyguanosine monophosphate). *Journal of the Chemical Society, Dalton Transactions*, No. 21, pp. 3979-3980, ISSN:0300-9246.

van Boom S.S.G.E.; Chen B.W; Tauben J.M. & Reedijk J. (1999). Platinum-Thioether Bonds Can Be Reverted by Guanine-N7 Bonds in Pt(dien)2+ Model Adducts. *Inorganic Chemistry*, Vol. 38, pp. 1450-1455.

Volckova E.; Dudones L. P. & Bose R. N. (2002). HPLC determination of binding of cisplatin to DNA in the presence of biological thiols: implications of dominant platinum-thiol binding to its anticancer action. *Pharmaceutical research*, Vol. 19, pp. 124-131, ISSN:0724-8741.

Wierda W.; O'Brien S.; Wen S.; Faderl S.; Garcia-Manero G.; Thomas D.; Do K-A.; Cortes J.; Koller C.; Beran M.; Ferrajoli A.; Giles F.; Lerner S.; Albitar M.; Kantarijan H. & Keating M. (2005) Chemoimmunotherapy with fludarabine, cyclophosphamide, and rituximab for relapsed and refractory chronic lymphocytic leukemia. *Journal of Clinical Oncology*, Vol. 23, pp. 4070-4078 ISSN:0732-183X.

Wang Y. F.; Curtis J. E.; Lipton J.; Minkin S. & McCulloch E. A. (1991) Cytosine arabinoside (ara-C) and cisdichlorodiammineplatinumII (cisplatin) alone and in combination: effects on acute myeloblastic leukemia blast cells in culture and in vivo. *Leukemia*, Vol. 5, pp. 522-527.

Wilkins R. G. (1991) *Kinetics and Mechanism of Reactions of Transition metal Complexes*, 2nd edn., Verlag, Berlin, p. 300.

Wong Y. S. & Lippard S. J. (1977). X-ray crystal structure of a 2:2 chloroterpyridineplatinum(II)-adenosine-5'-monophosphate intercalation complex. *Journal of the Chemical Society, Chemical Communications*, No. 22, pp. 824-825, ISSN:0022-4936.

Yamauchi T.; Nowak B. J.; Keating M. J. & Plunkett W. (2001). DNA repair initiated in chronic lymphocytic leukemia lymphocytes by 4-hydroperoxycyclophosphamide is inhibited by fludarabine and clofarabine. *Clinical Cancer Research*, Vol. 7, pp. 3580-3589.

Zecevic A.; Sampath D.; Ewald B.; Chen R.; Wierda W. & Plunkett W.. (2011) Killing of Chronic Lymphocytic Leukemia by the Combination of Fludarabine and Oxaliplatin Is Dependent on the Activity of XPF Endonuclease. *Clinical Cancer Research*, Vol. 17, pp. 4731-4741, ISSN:1078-0432.

17

Infectious Diseases and Clinical Complications During Treatment in CLL

Farhad Abbasi
Bushehr University of Medical Sciences
Iran

1. Introduction

Infectious complications continue to be one of the major causes of morbidity and mortality in patients with chronic lymphocytic leukemia (CLL). The pathogenesis of infections in these patients is multifactorial (Wadhwa & Morrison, 2006). Predisposition to infection in CLL is mediated through various abnormalities including both the immune defects inherent in the primary disease (impairment in humoral and cellular immunity) and in the further immunosuppression related to management of CLL (Morra et al., 1999). Increased infectious events may arise from the multiple courses of immunosuppressive therapy and progressive deterioration of a patient's immune system over the course of disease (Elter et al., 2009). Hypogammaglobulinemia is an important predisposing factor for infection in patients with early-stage disease and for those treated with conventional alkylating agents (Wadhwa & Morrison, 2006). It is probably the most important immune defect increases the risk of severe bacterial infections and its frequency and severity has direct relationship with the duration of the disease (Morra, et al., 1999). The majority of disease-specific complications in CLL, notably infection and autoimmunity, relate to the underlying alterations in immune function. Both cellular and humoral immunity are impaired with qualitative and quantitative defects in B cells, T cells, NK cells, neutrophils and the monocyte/macrophage lineage. Virtually all patients have reduced immunoglobulin levels, even in early stages, and this is associated with an increased frequency and severity of infection (Dearden, 2008). The immunodeficiency chiefly manifests as hypogammaglobulinaemia but involves all elements of the immune system. It is caused by the interpolation of tumor cells among immunological cells and mediated by bi-directional cell contact and secretion of cytokines, which both sustain and invigorate the tumor and suppress immunity. CLL treatment generally makes the immunodeficiency worse (Hamblin & Hamblin, 2008). The proportion of patients treated with purine analogs and monoclonal antibodies such as rituximab and alemtuzumab is increasing. As a result of this therapy, these patients often experience profound and sustained T-cell immunodeficiency. Consequently, the spectrum of organisms causing infections in these patients is changing from common bacterial organisms to less common opportunistic pathogens such as Pneumocystis, Listeria, mycobacteria, herpesviruses and Candida (Wadhwa & Morrison, 2006). The early recognition of infections as well as prophylactic administration of appropriate antibiotics has been the mainstay of managing infections in patients with CLL. Hopefully, increasing understanding of the molecular events underlying the neoplastic change in CLL will lead to more targeted and less immunosuppressive therapeutic modalities (Ravandi & O'Brien S, 2006).

2. Infectious diseases in chronic lymphocytic leukemia

Patients with lymphoid malignancies such as chronic lymphocytic leukemia are at increased risk for infectious morbidity and mortality. Defects in cell-mediated immunity appear to be a major predisposing factor in these patients. An expanding spectrum of pathogens associated with lymphocytopenia and depletion of CD4 has been described in the setting of therapy with purine analogs. Infectious diseases in chronic lymphocytic leukemia are categorized as bacterial, viral, fungal and parasitic infection. CLL is characterized by progressive defects in humoral- and cell-mediated immunity. These defects are manifested as a propensity to develop infections with encapsulated, and less frequently, with gram-negative enteric bacteria. In addition, reactivation of viruses such as herpesvirus is not uncommon. Treatment of the disease exacerbates immunosuppression by depleting immune effectors and broadening the spectrum of potentially offending pathogens (Wierda, 2003). Neutrophil count, serum immunoglobulin G level and granulocyte chemotaxis are predicting factors of susceptibility to infections. Phagocytosis and intracellular killing of granulocytes are intact in patients with CLL (Itälä et al, 1996, 1998). Over the past decade, the introduction of nucleoside analogs and monoclonal antibodies into the treatment of patients with CLL has resulted in higher rates and longer duration of response. This is a significant step towards achieving the ultimate goal of disease-eradication and improved survival. A continuing problem, however, is the susceptibility of these patients to infections. Profound dysregulation of the host immune system in patients with CLL and its impact on the clinical course of the disease are well established. A number of investigators have sought to identify the mechanisms underlying this innate immune dysfunction, which is further exacerbated by the actions of the potent therapeutic agents (Ravandi & O'Brien S, 2006). A characteristic spectrum of infectious complications has been described for specific treatment agents. With chlorambucil, most infections are bacterial in origin, caused by common Gram-positive and -negative organisms. Recurrent infections are a hallmark, with the respiratory tract being the most common site of infection. The pathogenesis of infection with the purine analogues is related to the quantitative and qualitative T-cell abnormalities induced by these agents. Risk factors for infection identified in patients treated with fludarabine include advanced-stage disease, prior CLL therapy, response to therapy, elevated serum creatinine, hemoglobin < 12 g/dl, and decreased serum IgG. As compared with patients receiving chlorambucil, patients receiving fludarabine have more major infections and herpes virus infections. However, Pneumocystis, Aspergillus, and cytomegalovirus (CMV) infections are uncommon. The use of alemtuzumab is complicated by frequent opportunistic infections. CMV reactivation is especially problematic, occurring in 10%-25% of patients (Morrison, 2009). The humanized, anti-CD52 monoclonal antibody alemtuzumab has shown notable activity for both untreated and fludarabine-refractory CLL. The antibody not only targets malignant cells but also affects normal, healthy immune cells. The cumulative effects of the malignancy and successive courses of treatments adversely impinge on a patient's defense response to certain bacterial, fungal, and viral infections (Elter et al., 2009). Severe lymphopenia is one of the most profound hematologic effects of alemtuzumab, often predisposing patients to infectious complications such as herpes simplex virus, cytomegalovirus, and Pneumocystis jirovecii pneumonia. Opportunistic infections secondary to mycobacterial sources have been documented less frequently (Saadeh & Srkalovic, 2008).

2.1 Bacterial infection

Patients with chronic lymphocytic leukemia are at an increased risk for infections with bacteria which require complement for osponization (Heath & Cheson, 1985). Patients with chronic leukemias typically are affected by infections due to the underlying hematologic condition, particularly hypogammaglobulinemia in CLL patients. With active treatment, particularly those agents that cause defects in cell-mediated immunity, the incidence of opportunistic infections increases although endogenous bacterial, mycobacterial, and fungal infections also occur (Young, 2011). These defects are manifested as a propensity to develop infections with encapsulated bacteria, and less frequently, with gram-negative enteric bacteria. Bacterial pneumonia, urinary tract infection, sepsis, meningitis, typhlitis or neutropenic enterocolitis and soft tissue infections are common infections occur in CLL patients with bacterial source (Perkins et al., 2002). Staphylococcus spp., Streptococcus spp. (especially Streptoccoccus pneumonia) Enterococcus spp., Enterobacteriaceae, Hemophillus influenza, Pseudomonas spp. (especially Pseudomonas aeruginosa), Listeria monocytogenes, Nocardia, Vibrio vulnificus etc. are bacteria that cause infection in CLL patients (Travade et al, 1986; Barton & Ratard, 2006). Infections are one of the most important causes of mortality in CLL patients, and Streptococcus pneumoniae has been considered the most important single pathogen in this group (Sinisalo et al., 2007). In a survey on CLL patients with pneumonia, Pneumococcus was the most frequent agent followed by Pseudomonas aeruginosa, Pneumocystis carinii and Aspergillus fumigates. (Batlle et al., 2001).

2.2 Epstein-Bar virus infection

Epstein-Barr virus (EBV) is a gammaherpesvirus which infects greater than 90% of the world population. Infection is nonsymptomatic in healthy individuals, but has been associated with a number of lymphoproliferative disorders when accompanied by immunosuppression. Like all herpesviruses, EBV has both latent and lytic replication programs, which allows it to evade immune clearance and persist for the lifetime of the host (Bajaj et al., 2001). The most common primary symptoms of EBV infection are fever, skin eruption, lymphadenopathy, hepatosplenomegaly, eyelid edema, pharyngitis, cardiac arrhythmia and arthralgia (Li et al. 2004; C. Berger 2003). EBV can cause meningoencephalitis or central nervous system tumor-like lesion in immunocompromised patient (Khalil et al., 2008; Turkulov et al., 1999). This virus plays an important role in the etiology of nasopharyngeal carcinoma, adenocarcinoma of the parotid glands, gastric carcinoma, Burkitt's lymphoma and lymphoproliferative syndromes (Zahorodnia, 2011). EBV is pathogenically associated with a well defined group of lymphoid and epithelial tumors in which the virus directly drives transformation of infected cells. Recent evidence however indicates that this virus may infect a subpopulation of tumor cells in patients with chronic lymphocytic leukemia (Dordević, 2006). As one the most important clinical presentation of EBV and other herpesviruses is central nervous system (CNS) involvement; Rapid, sensitive and economical detection and identification of human herpesviruses as causative agents of CNS infections is clinically important. The traditional methods for the detection of herpesviruses in CNS infections all suffer from limitations. Polymerase chain reaction (PCR) is the best laboratory test. Multiplex nested consensus PCR provide a rapid, sensitive and economical method for detection of viral infections and is applicable to small volumes of CSF samples (Tafreshi, 2005). The spectrum of drugs active against EBV remains very limited. Gancyclovir and acyclovir are used in medical practice. The search of new compounds active against EBV remains necessary (Zahorodnia, 2011).

2.3 Cytomegalovirus infection

Human cytomegalovirus (CMV) is one of herpesviruses that commonly infect humans. Advances in molecular virology coupled with improvements in diagnostic methods and treatment options have vastly improved ability to manage CMV infection, but many uncertainties remain, including the mechanisms of persistence and pathogenesis and its hypothesized roles in a variety of human illnesses (Boeckh & Geballe, 2011). It is a recognized cause of morbidity and mortality in immunocompromised individuals (Emery, 2001). Primary infection with CMV is followed by persistence of the virus in a latent form. During life, the virus can reactivate, resulting in renewed shedding of the virus or development of disease. Significant progress has been made in detecting CMV, but in the immunocompromised patients, establishing the diagnosis of CMV infection can still be problematic (Vancíková & Dvorák, 2001).

Cellular immune responses are important against virus infections (Sester et al, 2002). CMV infection causes significant morbidity and mortality in the setting of immunodeficiency (Ozdemir et al, 2002). It can cause serious clinical complications in eye (retinitis), lung, central nervous system and other organs in immunocompromised individuals (Bronke et al, 2005; Reeves et al, 2005). For diagnosis the most sensitive molecular amplification methods such as PCR should be used. Treatment of infection depends mainly on the immune status of the host (Vancíková & Dvorák, 2001). The availability of sensitive diagnostic tests such as pp65 antigenemia has made the early diagnosis of CMV possible (Kusne et al, 1999). CMV should be suspected as a cause of pneumonia in immunocompromised patients and diagnosis may require invasive procedures bronchoalveolar lavage (BAL) and transbronchial lung biopsy (TBLB) may be required for diagnosis of CMV pneumonitis. (Yadegarynia et al, 2009). In immunocompetent patients only symptomatic treatment is recommended, while in immunocompromised patients antiviral therapy should be used. The most commonly used antiviral agents are: ganciclovir, foscarnet, cidofovir, valganciclovir and valaciclovir (Vancíková & Dvorák, 2001). Although it remains rare, ganciclovir-resistant CMV disease is increasingly seen in clinical practice, potentially fostered by the prolonged use of antiviral agents in high-risk patients. Treatment of drug-resistant CMV is currently non-standardized and may include foscarnet, cidofovir, CMV hyperimmune globulins or leflunomide (Eid & Razonable, 2010).

2.4 Herpes simplex virus infection

Herpes simplex viruses type 1 and 2 (HSV-1 and HSV-2) are alpha herpes viruses. Humans are the only natural host and they can be transmitted through oral or genital secretions. These viruses are ubiquitous all over the world, with different percentage rates (Dordević,

2006). They can infect both skin and nerves and develop latent infection within the dorsal root and trigeminal ganglia. Infection with these viruses is common and causes a wide range of clinical syndromes (Midak-Siewirska et al, 2010). HSV infections range in severity from common cutaneous outbreaks to life-threatening central nervous system and deep organ involvement (Higgins et al 1999). Atypical clinical manifestations of HSV may occur in immunocompromised patients. HSV-2 infection is responsible for significant neurological morbidity, perhaps more than any other virus (JR. Berger et al, 2008). Herpes esophagitis is common in immunosuppressed patients, but has rarely been reported in immunocompetent individuals, in whom it appears to be a self-limited illness (Canalejo Castrillero et al, 2010). Pneumonia, hepatitis, gasterointestinal involvement and disseminated infection may occur in immunocompromised patients (Longerich et al, 2005; Medlicott et al, 2005; Massler et al, 2011). Multiple herpes virus co-infection (HSV and EBV) may occur in patients with chronic lymphocytic leukemia (Mercadal et al, 2006). HSV infections have a severe and rapidly progressive course especially in immunocompromised patients, leading to significant morbidity and mortality. Therefore, rapid and reliable laboratory diagnosis of HSV infections is important for initiation of early antiviral therapy. PCR, direct fluorescein antibody (DFA) methods and cell culture are used for diagnosis (Cordes et al, 2011). There is evidence that acyclovir is effective for preventing and treating HSV infections. There is no evidence that valaciclovir is more effective than acyclovir, or that a high dose of valaciclovir is better than a low dose (Nolan, 2009). Antiviral-resistant herpes virus infection has become a great concern for immunocompromised patients (Shiota et al, 2011).

2.5 Hepatitis B virus infection

Recent studies emphasize the risk of hepatitis B virus (HBV) reactivation among patients with hematologic malignancies of B lineage, in which HBV has been recently hypothesized to play a pathogenetic role. Occult HBV infection is significantly more prevalent among patients with CLL and may contribute to the susceptibility of patients with CLL to HBV reactivation, whether exposed or not to biological agents (Rossi et al, 2009). Chemotherapy-induced HBV reactivation is a serious problem in chronic HBV carriers with hematologic malignancies. In Yağci's study all patients with chronic lymphocytic leukemia experienced chemotherapy-induced HBV reactivation regardless of the chemotherapy regimen. CLL patients who are HBV carriers are at significant risk of chemotherapy-induced HBV reactivation (Yağci et al, 2006). Reactivation of HBV in HBsAg-positive patients is a well-documented complication of cytotoxic or immunosuppressive therapy and has also been observed after treatment with rituximab (Heider et al, 2004). Patients may be treated with lamivudine or lamivudine plus adefovir dipivoxil combination therapy to control viral replication and allow for long-term anti-cancer chemotherapy (Cortelezzi et al, 2006). lamivudine is highly effective in inhibiting HBV proliferation and can be used to prevent HBV flare-up during chemotherapy in patients with positive HBs antigen (Heider et al, 2004).

2.6 Fungal infection

Opportunistic fungal infection may occur in patient with CLL. Candida and Aspergillus are common fungi. Invasive Candida infections are important causes of morbidity and mortality in immunocompromised patients. The cornerstone of diagnosis remains the detection of the organism by culture with identification of the isolate at the species level; in vitro susceptibility testing is mandatory for invasive isolates. Options for initial therapy of candidaemia and other invasive Candida infections in non-granulocytopenic patients include fluconazole or one of the three approved echinocandin compounds; liposomal amphotericin B. Voriconazole are secondary alternatives. In granulocytopenic patients, an echinocandin or liposomal amphotericin B is recommended as initial therapy. Indwelling central venous catheters serve as a main source of infection independent of the pathogenesis of candidaemia and should be removed whenever feasible. Dose reduction or discontinuation of pre-existing immunosuppressive treatment (particularly glucocorticosteroids) should be performed. Ophthalmoscopy is recommended prior to the discontinuation of antifungal chemotherapy to rule out endophthalmitis or chorioretinitis (Ruhnke et al, 2011).

Morbidity and mortality caused by invasive Aspergillus infections are increasing. This is because of the higher number of patients with malignancies treated with intensive immunosuppressive therapy regimens as well as their improved survival from formerly fatal bacterial infections. Clinical diagnosis is based on radiologic findings and non-culture based diagnostic techniques such as galactomannan or DNA detection in blood or bronchoalveolar lavage samples. Most promising outcomes can be expected in patients at high risk for aspergillosis in whom antifungal treatment has been started pre-emptively, backed up by laboratory and imaging findings. The gold standard of systemic antifungal treatment is voriconazole, which has been proved to be significantly superior to conventional amphotericin B and has led to a profound improvement of survival rates in patients with cerebral aspergillosis. Liposomal amphotericin B at standard dosages appears to be a suitable alternative for primary treatment, while caspofungin, amphotericin B lipid complex or posaconazole have shown partial or complete response in patients who had been refractory to or intolerant of primary antifungal therapy. Combination therapy with two antifungal compounds may be a promising future strategy for first-line treatment (Maschmeyer et al, 2007).

Cryptococcus neoformans is an important fungal pathogen of immunocompromised individuals. Lung and CNS are two important organs involved by Cryptococcus neoformans (Price et al, 2011). Diagnosis is based on direct microscopic examination of India ink preparations and PCR (Ndiaye et al, 2011; Sidrim et al, 2010; Mseddi et al, 2011). Amphotericin B and flucytosine is used for treatment (Thalla et al, 2009). Histoplasmosis (Van Koeveringe & Brouwer, 2010), fusariosis (Campo et al, 2010) and other uncommon fungal infection may be seen in immunocomromised patients.

2.7 Pnemocystis jirovecii infection

Pneumocystis jiroveci pneumonia (formerly Pneumocystis carinii pneumonia) occurs frequently in patients with immunodeficiency (Otahbachi et al, 2007). Pneumocystis carinii pneumonia (PCP) in patients with chronic lymphocytic leukaemia (CLL) who have not been treated with fludarabin are rare, although clinically relevant CD4 T-cell depletion can occur in longstanding CLL without prior treatment with purine analogues (Vavricka et al, 2004). It is associated with a wide spectrum of clinical presentations (Gal et al, 2002). The most frequent symptoms are: fever, dyspnea, non-productive cough, thoracic pain, chills and severe hypoxaemia (Pagano et al, 2002). For diagnosis of PCP bronchoalveolar lavage (BAL) cytology and transbronchial lung biopsy (TBLB) may be required (Bijur et al, 1996). Because Pneumocystis cannot be cultured, diagnosis relies on detection of the organism by colorimetric or immunofluorescent stains or by polymerase chain reaction. Trimethoprim-sulfamethoxazole is the preferred drug regimen for both treatment and prevention of PCP, although a number of alternatives are also available. Corticosteroids are an important adjunct for hypoxemic patients (Kovacs et al, 1994).

2.8 Mycobacterium avium complex infection

Mycobacterium avium complex (MAC) primarily causes respiratory infection in patients with underlying lung disease or disseminated disease in immunocompromised patients (Azzam et al, 2009). MAC is clinically important since it can cause severe infections in immunocompromised individuals (Rodrigues et al, 2009). Severe lymphopenia is one of the most profound hematologic effects of alemtuzumab, often predisposing patients to infectious complications such as herpes simplex virus, cytomegalovirus, and Pneumocystis jirovecii pneumonia. Opportunistic infections secondary to mycobacterial sources like mycobacterium avium complex have been documented less frequently (Saadeh & Srkalovic, 2008). A diagnosis requires a high index of suspicion in patients with immunocompromised status who present with prolonged fever, with or without organ-specific symptoms and signs. Therefore, clinical specimens must be sent for mycobacterial cultures for a definite diagnosis (Saritsiri et al, 2006). Microscopic evaluation, culture and PCR may be necessary for diagnosis (Haas et al, 1998). Combination of clarithromycin, rifabutin and ethambutol has proven to be the most efficacious therapy and therefore it is considered as standard therapy for disseminated MAC infection. Clarithromycin, rifabutin and azithromycin given as primary prophylaxis can diminish the risk of disseminated MAC infection (Fätkenheuer et al, 1998).

2.9 Adenovirus infection

Adenovirus infections are widespread in society and are occasionally associated with severe, but rarely with life-threatening, disease in otherwise healthy individuals. In contrast, adenovirus infections present a real threat to immunocompromised individuals and can result in disseminated and fatal disease (Andersson et al, 2010). It is an important cause of morbidity and mortality in the immunocompromised host (Gavin & Katz, 2002). Adenovirus infection has been reported following alemtuzumab treatment in CLL patients (Martin et al, 2006). There is no formally approved treatment of adenovirus infections today, and existing antiviral agents evaluated for their antiadenoviral effect give inconsistent results (Andersson et al, 2010). ribavirin and cidofovir are used for treatment of adenovirus infection (Gavin & Katz, 2002).

2.10 Other microorganism infection

Other opportunistic and non-opportunistic organisms like toxoplamosis, tuberculosis, non tuberculosis mycobacteria, herpes zoster infection, etc may infect CLL patients (Herrero et al, 1995; Mehta et al, 1997; Juliusson & Liliemark, 1996; Krebs et al, 2000)

3. Management

3.1 Diagnosis

Appropriate diagnosis is important for treatment. Different diagnostic methods may be needed to achieve diagnosis. Culture (blood, urine, sputum, etc.), search for antigens

(Legionella pneumophila serogroup 1, galactomannan, and Streptococcus pneumonia), CSF analysis, radiologic modality (x-ray, CT scan, MRI, etc.), broncoscopy, endoscopy, tissue biopsy and other diagnostic test may be used to find the etiologic agents (Batlle et al., 2001; Krebs et al, 2000).

3.2 Treatment

Appropriate antibacterial, antiviral and anti fungal treatment can be life saving (for specific treatment of each microorganism see above). Immunoglobulins are an important component of host defense against infections. They also play a central role in immune regulation. A wide spectrum of human diseases is associated with decreased or abnormal regulation of immunoglobulin levels. Recently intravenous (IV) preparations of immunoglobulin have become available for clinical studies. There are already substantial data indicating a useful role for IV immunoglobulin in patients with primary hypogammaglobulinemia, neonates predisposed to group B streptococcal infections, individuals with ITP, children with Kawasaki disease, bone marrow transplant patients predisposed to CMV infections and in individuals with CLL (Berkman et al, 1988). Intravenous immunoglobulin (IVIG) replacement therapy reduces the number of bacterial infections in CLL patients. However, due to the complexity of immunodeficiency in CLL and the cost-effectiveness of replacement therapy, it is important to identify patients who are likely to benefit from the treatment and to investigate which dose should be used. Low dose of gammaglobulin intravenously can restore normal serum IgG levels in hypogammaglobulinaemic B-CLL patients, and leads to a decreased number of febrile episodes and admissions to hospital due infections (Jurlander et al, 1994, 1995). IVIG has been shown to be a useful prophylactic therapy against infections (Gamm et al, 1994). Granulocyte colony stimulating factor (G-CSF) supplementation may improve the rate of infectious complications by reducing the duration of drug-induced neutropenia (Südhoff et al, 1997). It can be used safely and effectively in CLL-patients with severe bacterial infections to restore neutropenia (Hollander et al, 1991). Granulocyte macrophage colony stimulating factor (GM-CSF) is also effective in improving CLL associated chronic neutropenia and also enhances impaired granulocyte chemiluminescence. Thus, GM-CSF could be helpful for giving chemotherapy without neutropenic delays and for prophylaxis of infectious complications in CLL patients (Itälä et al, 1996, 1998).

3.3 Prophylaxis

Patients with advanced disease who receive cytotoxic therapy may benefit from antibacterial prophylaxis. Risk of infection can potentially be reduced by administration of intravenous immunoglobulin and use of prophylactic antibiotics for individuals who are at high risk (5). Treatments of CLL enhance the risk of myelosuppression and infection, so these patients may need antibiotic, antiviral, and antimycotic prophylaxis during and after their administration (Todisco, 2009). Antimicrobial prophylaxis, particularly anti-Pneumocystis prophylaxis, may be indicated in selected patients (Young, 2011). Consideration of primary prophylaxis against M. avium complex infections in aggressively treated patients with advanced B-CLL or other clinical indications may be warranted (Saadeh & Srkalovic, 2008). Some investigators recommend routine antibacterial and antiviral prophylaxis during and after purine nucleoside analogues treatment (Perkins et al.,

2002). An understanding of the patients at highest risk and duration of risk are important in developing recommendations for empirical management, antimicrobial prophylaxis and targeted surveillance (Thursky et al, 2006).

3.4 Vaccination

Routine vaccination should be maintained in CLL patients and vaccination early in the course of treatment may result in improve protection (Young, 2011). Antibody response rates to vaccine antigens are lower in patients with CLL compared to normal host. However, if the vaccine has been administered at an early stage of the disease and before starting chemotherapy and the development of hypogammaglobulinaemia, a significant vaccination response to antigens will be obtained in almost 40% of the CLL patients. Early administration of vaccine may be beneficial in CLL patients (Sinisalo et al., 2007). Bacterial polysaccharide vaccines would seem to be ineffective in antibody formation in patients with CLL. However, protein and conjugate vaccines appear to be more immunogenic and their responses may be further enhanced with ranitidine adjuvant treatment (Sinisalo et al, 2003). Response rate to Haemophilus influenzae type b (Hib) conjugate vaccine among adult and elderly patients with chronic lymphocytic leukaemia was 43% in Sinsalo's study (Sinsalo et al, 2002). It is recommended to vaccinate CLL patients with S. pneumoniae and Haemophilus influenzae type b (Hib) vaccines as soon as the diagnosis of CLL is made, early in the course of the disease with determination of post-vaccination antibody levels (Hartkamp et al, 2001). Antibody production after vaccination against common pathogen in CLL patients may improve by treatment histamine type-2 receptor blockade such as ranitidine (Jurlander et al, 1994, 1995). Influenza vaccination is recommended for patients with B-cell CLL however immune response to influenza vaccination appears to be poor (Van der Velden et al, 1995). New well-designed investigations are needed to develop appropriate vaccination strategies and evaluate vaccination efficacy in infection morbidity and mortality in CLL (Sinisalo et al, 2003).

4. Conclusion

Infectious complications are leading causes of morbidity and mortality in CLL patients. High index of suspicious and using appropriate diagnostic methods, treatment and prophylaxis can enhance survival of patients.

5. Acknowledgment

With special thanks to Dr Soolmaz Korooni.

6. References

Andersson EK, Strand M, Edlund K, Lindman K, Enquist PA, Spjut S, Allard A, Elofsson M, Mei YF, Wadell G. (2010). Small-molecule screening using a whole-cell viral replication reporter gene assay identifies 2-{[2-(benzoylamino)benzoyl]amino}-benzoic acid as a novel antiadenoviral compound. *Antimicrob Agents Chemother.* Vol.54, No.9, (September 2010), pp.3871-7, ISSN 0066-4804

Azzam HC, Gahunia MK, Sae-Tia S, Santoro J. (2009). Mycobacterium avium-avium-associated typhlitis mimicking appendicitis in an immunocompetent host. *Am J Med Sci.* Vol.337, No.3, (March 2009), pp. 218-20, ISSN 0002-9629

Bajaj BG, Murakami M, Robertson ES. (2001). Molecular biology of EBV in relationship to AIDS-associated oncogenesis. *Cancer Treat Res.* Vol.133, (2001), pp. 141-62, ISSN 0927-3042

Barton JC, Ratard RC. (2006).Vibrio vulnificus bacteremia associated with chronic lymphocytic leukemia, hypogammaglobulinemia, and hepatic cirrhosis: relation to host and exposure factors in 252 V. vulnificus infections reported in Louisiana. *Am J Med Sci.* Vol.332, No.4, (October 2006), pp. 216-20, ISSN 0002-9629

Batlle M, Ribera JM, Oriol A, Rodríguez L, Cirauqui B, Xicoy B, Grau J, Feliu J, Flores A, Millá F. (2001). Pneumonia in patients with chronic lymphocytic leukemia. Study of 30 episodes. *Med Clin (Barc).* Vol.116, No.19, (May 2001), pp. 738-40, ISSN 0025-7753

Berger C. Infectious mononucleosis. *Ther Umsch.* Vol.60, No.10, (October 2003), pp. 625-30, ISSN 0040-5930

Berger JR, Houff S. (2008). Neurological complications of herpes simplex virus type 2 infection. *Arch Neurol.* Vol.65, No.5, (May 2008), pp. 596-600. ISSN 0003-9942

Berkman SA, Lee ML, Gale RP. (1988). Clinical uses of intravenous immunoglobulins. *Semin Hematol.* Vol.25, No. 2, (April 1988), pp. 140-58, 0037-1963

Bijur S, Menon L, Iyer E, Deshpande J, Sivaraman A, Vaideeswar P, Mahashur AA. (1996). Pneumocystis carinii pneumonia in human immunodeficiency virus infected patients in Bombay: diagnosed by bronchoalveolar lavage cytology and transbronchial lung biopsy. *Indian J Chest Dis Allied Sci.* Vol.38, No.4, (October-December 1996), pp. 227-33, ISSN 0377-9343

Boeckh M, Geballe AP. (2011). Cytomegalovirus: pathogen, paradigm, and puzzle. *J Clin Invest.* Vol.121, No.5, (May 2011), pp. 1673-80, ISSN 0021-9738

Bronke C, Palmer NM, Jansen CA, Westerlaken GH, Polstra AM, Reiss P, Bakker M, Miedema F, Tesselaar K, van Baarle D. (2005). Dynamics of cytomegalovirus (CMV)-specific T cells in HIV-1-infected individuals progressing to AIDS with CMV end-organ disease. *J Infect Dis.* Vol.191, No.6, (March 2005), pp. 873-80, ISSN 1553-6203

Campo M, Lewis RE, Kontoyiannis DP. (2010). Invasive fusariosis in patients with hematologic malignancies at a cancer center: 1998-2009. *J Infect.* Vol.60, No.5, (May 2010), pp. 331-7, ISSN 1553-6203

Canalejo Castrillero E, García Durán F, Cabello N, García Martínez J. (2010). Herpes esophagitis in healthy adults and adolescents: report of 3 cases and review of the literature. *Medicine (Baltimore).* Vol.89, No.4, (July 2010), pp. 204-10, ISSN 0025-7974

Cordes C, Tiemann M, Tiemann K, Knappe D, Hoffmann M, Gottschlich S. (2011). Epstein-Barr virus-associated diffuse large B-cell lymphoma of the hypopharynx. *B-ENT.* Vol.7, No.1, (2011), pp. 43-6, ISSN 1781-782X

Cortelezzi A, Viganò M, Zilioli VR, Fantini NN, Pasquini MC, Deliliers GL, Colombo M, Lampertico P. (2006). Adefovir added to lamivudine for hepatitis B recurrent infection in refractory B-cell chronic lymphocytic leukemia on prolonged therapy with Campath-1H. *J Clin Virol.*Vol.35, No.4, (April 2006), pp. 467-9, ISSN 1386-6532

Dearden C. (2008). Disease-specific complications of chronic lymphocytic leukemia. *Hematology Am Soc Hematol Educ Program.* (2008), pp.450-6, ISSN 1520-4391

Dordević H. (2006). Serological response to herpes simplex virus type 1 and 2 infection among women of reproductive age. *Med Pregl.* Vol.59, No.11-12, (November-December 2006), pp. 591-7, ISSN 0025-8105

Eid AJ, Razonable RR. (2010). New developments in the management of cytomegalovirus infection after solid organ transplantation. *Drugs.* Vol.70, No.8, (Fall 2009), pp. 965-81, ISSN 0012-6667

Elter T, Vehreschild JJ, Gribben J, Cornely OA, Engert A & Hallek M. (2009). Management of infections in patients with chronic lymphocytic leukemia treated with alemtuzumab. *Ann Hematol.* Vol.88, No.2, (February 2009), pp.121-32, ISSN 0939-5555

Emery VC.(2001). Investigation of CMV disease in immunocompromised patients. *J Clin Pathol.* Vol.54, No.2, (February 2001), pp. 84-8, ISSN 0021-9746

Fätkenheuer G, Salzberger B, Diehl V. (1998). Disseminated infection with Mycobacterium avium complex (MAC) in HIV infection. *Med Klin (Munich).* Vol.93, No.6, (Jun 1998), pp. 360-4, ISSN 0723-5003

Gal AA, Plummer AL, Langston AA, Mansour KA. Gal AA, Plummer AL, Langston AA, Mansour KA. *Pathol Res Pract.* Vol.198, No.8, (2002), pp. 553-8, ISSN 0344-0338

Gamm H, Huber C, Chapel H, Lee M, Ries F, Dicato MA. (19994). Intravenous immune globulin in chronic lymphocytic leukaemia. *Clin Exp Immunol.* Vol.97, No. Suppl 1, (July 1994), pp. 17-20, ISSN 0009-9104

Gavin PJ, Katz BZ. (2002). Intravenous ribavirin treatment for severe adenovirus disease in immunocompromised children. *Pediatrics.* Vol.110, No.1, (July 2002), pp.9, ISSN 0031-4005

Haas WH, Amthor B, Engelmann G, Rimek D, Bremer HJ. (1998). Preoperative diagnosis of Mycobacterium avium lymphadenitis in two immunocompetent children by polymerase chain reaction of gastric aspirates. *Pediatr Infect Dis J.* Vol.17, No.11, (November 1998), pp. 1016-20, ISSN 0891-3668

Hamblin AD & Hamblin TJ. (2008). The immunodeficiency of chronic lymphocytic leukaemia. *Br Med Bull.* Vol.47, No.1, (2008), pp. 49-62, ISSN 0007-1420

Hartkamp A, Mulder AH, Rijkers GT, van Velzen-Blad H, Biesma DH. (2001). Antibody responses to pneumococcal and haemophilus vaccinations in patients with B-cell chronic lymphocytic leukaemia. *Vaccine.* Vol.19, No. (13-14), (February 2001), pp. 1671-7, ISSN 0264-410X

Heath ME, Cheson BD. (1985). Defective complement activity in chronic lymphocytic leukemia. *Am J Hematol.* Vol.19, No.*1*, (May 1985), pp. 63-73, ISSN 0361-8609.

Heider U, Fleissner C, Zavrski I, Jakob C, Dietzel T, Eucker J, Ockenga J, Possinger K, Sezer O. (2004). Treatment of refractory chronic lymphocytic leukemia with Campath-1H in combination with lamivudine in chronic hepatitis B infection. *Eur J Haematol.* Vol.72, No.1, (January 2004), pp. 64-6, ISSN 0902-4441

Herrero M, Cabrera JR, Briz M, Forés R, Díez JL, Regidor C, Sanjuán I, Fernández MN. (1995). Treatment with fludarabine of chronic refractory lymphoid leukemia. *Sangre (Barc).* Vol.40, No.2, (April 1995), pp. 115-9, ISSN 0036-3634

Higgins JP, Warnke RA. (1999). Herpes lymphadenitis in association with chronic lymphocytic leukemia. *Cancer.* Vol.86, No.7, (October 1999), pp. 1210-5. ISSN 0008-5472.

Hollander AA, Kluin-Nelemans HC, Haak HR, Stern AC, Willemze R, Fibbe WE. (1991). Correction of neutropenia associated with chronic lymphocytic leukaemia following treatment with granulocyte-macrophage colony-stimulating factor. Ann Hematol. Vol.62, No. 1, (February 1991), pp. 32-4, ISSN 0939-5555

Itälä M, Vainio O, Remes K.(1996). Functional abnormalities in granulocytes predict susceptibility to bacterial infections in chronic lymphocytic leukaemia. *Eur J Haematol.* Vol.57, No.*1*, (July 1996), pp. 46-53, ISSN 0902-4441

Itälä M, Pelliniemi TT, Remes K, Vanhatalo S, Vainio O. (1998). Long-term treatment with GM-CSF in patients with chronic lymphocytic leukemia and recurrent neutropenic infections. *Leuk Lymphoma.* Vol.32, No. (1-2), (December 1998), pp. 165-74. ISSN 1042-8194

Juliusson G, Liliemark J. (1996). Long-term survival following cladribine (2-chlorodeoxyadenosine) therapy in previously treated patients with chronic lymphocytic leukemia. *Ann Oncol.* Vol.7, No. 4, (April 1996), pp. 373-9, ISSN 0923-7534

Jurlander J, Geisler CH, Hansen MM. (1994). Treatment of hypogammaglobulinaemia in chronic lymphocytic leukaemia by low-dose intravenous gammaglobulin. *Eur J Haematol.* Vol.53, No. 2, (August 1994), pp. 114-8, ISSN 0902-4441

Jurlander J, de Nully Brown P, Skov PS, Henrichsen J, Heron I, Obel N, Mortensen BT, Hansen MM, Geisler CH, Nielsen HJ. (1995). Improved vaccination response during ranitidine treatment, and increased plasma histamine concentrations, in patients with B cell chronic lymphocytic leukemia. *Leukemia.* Vol.9, No. 11, (November 1995), pp. 1902-9, ISSN 0887-6924

Khalil M, Enzinger C, Wallner-Blazek M, Scarpatetti M, Barth A, Horn S, Reiter G. (2008). Epstein-Barr virus encephalitis presenting with a tumor-like lesion in an immunosuppressed transplant recipient. *J Neurovirol.* Vol.14, No.6, (October 2008), pp. 574-8, ISSN 1355-0284

Kovacs JA, Masur H. Evolving health effects of Pneumocystis: one hundred years of progress in diagnosis and treatment. *Schweiz Med Wochenschr.* Vol.124, No.(1-2), (Jun 1994), pp. 73-8, ISSN 0036-7672

Krebs T, Zimmerli S, Bodmer T, Lämmle B. (2000). Mycobacterium genavense infection in a patient with long-standing chronic lymphocytic leukaemia. *J Intern Med.* Vol.248, No. 4, (October 2000), pp. 343-8, ISSN 0954-6820

Kusne S, Shapiro R, Fung J. (1999). Prevention and treatment of cytomegalovirus infection in organ transplant recipients. *Transpl Infect Dis.* Vol.1, No.*3*, (September 1999), pp. 187-203, ISSN 1398-2273

Li ZY, Lou JG, Chen J. (2004). Analysis of primary symptoms and disease spectrum in Epstein-Barr virus infected children. *Zhonghua Er Ke Za Zhi.* Vol.42, No.1, (Jane 2004), pp. 20-2, ISSN 0578-1310

Longerich T, Eisenbach C, Penzel R, Kremer T, Flechtenmacher C, Helmke B, Encke J, Kraus T, Schirmacher P. (2005).Recurrent herpes simplex virus hepatitis after liver retransplantation despite acyclovir therapy. *Liver Transpl.* Vol.11, No.*10*, (October 2005), pp. 1289-94. ISSN 1527-6465

Martin SI, Marty FM, Fiumara K, Treon SP, Gribben JG, Baden LR. (2006). Infectious complications associated with alemtuzumab use for lymphoproliferative disorders. *Clin Infect Dis.* Vol.43, No.1, (July 2006), pp. 16-24, ISSN 1058-4838

Maschmeyer G, Haas A, Cornely OA. (2007). Invasive aspergillosis: epidemiology, diagnosis and management in immunocompromised patients. *Drugs.* Vol.67, No.11, (2007), pp. 1567-601, ISSN 0012-6667

Massler A, Kolodkin-Gal D, Meir K, Khalaileh A, Falk H, Izhar U, Shufaro Y, Panet A. (2011). Infant lungs are preferentially infected by adenovirus and herpes simplex virus type 1 vectors: role of the tissue mesenchymal cells. *J Gene Med.* Vol.13, No.2, (February 2011), pp.101-13, ISSN 1099-498X

Medlicott SA, Falck VG, Laupland KB, Akbari M, Beck PL. (2005). Herpes simplex virus type II infection of ileum mesothelium: a case report and review of the literature. *Can J Gastroenterol.* Vol.19, No.6, (Jun 2005), pp. 367-71. ISSN 0835-7900

Mehta J, Powles R, Singhal S, Riley U, Treleaven J, Catovsky D. (1997). Antimicrobial prophylaxis to prevent opportunistic infections in patients with chronic lymphocytic leukemia after allogeneic blood or marrow transplantation. *Leuk Lymphoma.* Vol.26, No. (1-2), (June 1997), pp. 83-8. ISSN 1042-8194

Mercadal S, Martinez A, Nomdedeu B, Rozman M, Gaya A, Salamero O, Campo E. (2011). Herpes simplex and Epstein-Barr virus lymphadenitis in a patient with chronic lymphocytic leukemia treated with fludarabine. *Eur J Haematol.* Vol.77, No.5, (November 2006), pp. 442-4, ISSN 0902-4441

Midak-Siewirska A, Karabin K, Chudzik E, Dzieciatkowski T, Przybylski M, Majewska A, Łuczak M, Młynarczyk G. (2010).Application of real-time PCR assay for investigating the presence of herpes simplex virus type 1 DNA. *Med Dosw Mikrobiol.* Vol.62, No.1, (2010), pp. 85-92, ISSN 0025-8601

Morra E, Nosari A& Montillo M. (2006). Infectious complications of chronic lymphocytic leukemia. *Hematol Cell Ther.* Vol.41, No.4, (Agust 2006), pp.145-51, ISSN 1269-3286

Morrison VA. (2009). Infectious complications in patients with chronic lymphocytic leukemia: pathogenesis, spectrum of infection, and approaches to prophylaxis. *Clin Lymphoma Myeloma.* Vol.9, No.5, (October 2009), pp. 365-70, ISSN 1938-0712

Mseddi F, Sellami A, Sellami H, Cheikhrouhou F, Makni F, Ayadi A. (2011). Two new media Pinus halepensis seed agar and blackberry agar for rapid identification of Cryptococcus neoformans. *Mycoses.* Vol.54, No.4, (July 2011), pp. 350-3, ISSN 0933-7407

Ndiaye M, Diagne NR, Seck LB, Sow AD, Sène MS, Diop AG, Sow HD, Ndiaye MM.(2011). Cryptococcal meningitis in children: description of 3 cases. *Med Trop (Mars).* Vol.71, No.2, (April 2011), pp. 176-8, ISSN 0025-682X

Nolan A. (209). Interventions for prevention and treatment of herpes simplex virus in cancer patients. *Evid Based Dent.* Vol.10, No.4, (2009), pp. 116-7, ISSN 1462-0049

Otahbachi M, Nugent K, Buscemi D. (2007). Granulomatous Pneumocystis jiroveci Pneumonia in a patient with chronic lymphocytic leukemia: a literature review and hypothesis on pathogenesis. *Am J Med Sci.* Vol.333, No.2, (February 2007), pp. 131-5. ISSN 0002-9629

Ozdemir E, St John LS, Gillespie G, Rowland-Jones S, Champlin RE, Molldrem JJ, Komanduri KV. (2002). Cytomegalovirus reactivation following allogeneic stem cell transplantation is associated with the presence of dysfunctional antigen-specific CD8+ T cells. *Blood.* Vol.100, No.1, (November 2002), pp. 3690-7, ISSN *0006-4971*

Pagano L, Fianchi L, Mele L, Girmenia C, Offidani M, Ricci P, Mitra ME, Picardi M, Caramatti C, Piccaluga P, Nosari A, Buelli M, Allione B, Cortelezzi A, Fabbiano F, Milone G, Invernizzi R, Martino B, Masini L, Todeschini G, Cappucci MA, Russo D, Corvatta L, Martino P, Del Favero A. (2002). Pneumocystis carinii pneumonia in patients with malignant haematological diseases: 10 years' experience of infection in GIMEMA centres. *Br J Haematol.* Vol.117, No.2, (May 2002), pp. 379-86, ISSN 1365-2141

Perkins JG, Flynn JM, Howard RS, Byrd JC. (2002). Frequency and type of serious infections in fludarabine-refractory B-cell chronic lymphocytic leukemia and small lymphocytic lymphoma: implications for clinical trials in this patient population. *Cancer.* Vol.94, No.7, (April 2002), pp. 2033-9, ISSN 0008-5472.

Price MS, Betancourt-Quiroz M, Price JL, Toffaletti DL, Vora H, Hu G, Kronstad JW, Perfect JR. (2007) . Cryptococcus neoformans Requires a Functional Glycolytic Pathway for Disease but Not Persistence in the Host. *MBio.* Vol.2, No.3, (Jun 2011), pp. 103-11, ISSN 2150-7511

Ravandi F & O'Brien S. (2006). Immune defects in patients with chronic lymphocytic leukemia. *Cancer Immunol Immunother.* Vol.55, No.2, (February 2006), pp. 197-209, ISSN 0340-7004

Reeves M, Sissons P, Sinclair J. (2005). Reactivation of human cytomegalovirus in dendritic cells. *Discov Med.* Vol.5, No.26, (April 2005), pp. 170-4, ISSN 1539-6509

Rodrigues L, Sampaio D, Couto I, Machado D, Kern WV, Amaral L, Viveiros M. (2009). The role of efflux pumps in macrolide resistance in Mycobacterium avium complex. *Int J Antimicrob Agents.* Vol.34, No.6, (December 2009), pp. 529-33, ISSN 0924-8579

Rossi D, Sala L, Minisini R, Fabris C, Falleti E, Cerri M, Burlone ME, Toniutto P, Gaidano G, Pirisi M. (2009). Occult hepatitis B virus infection of peripheral blood mononuclear cells among treatment-naive patients with chronic lymphocytic leukemia. *Leuk Lymphoma.* Vol.50, No.4, (April 2009), pp.604-11, ISSN 1042-8194

Ruhnke M, Rickerts V, Cornely OA, Buchheidt D, Glöckner A, Heinz W, Höhl R, Horré R, Karthaus M, Kujath P, Willinger B, Presterl E, Rath P, Ritter J, Glasmacher A, Lass-Flörl C, Groll AH. (2011). Diagnosis and therapy of Candida infections: joint recommendations of the German Speaking Mycological Society and the Paul-Ehrlich-Society for Chemotherapy. *Mycoses.* Vol.54, No.4, (July 2011), pp. 279-310, ISSN 0933-7407

Saadeh CE, Srkalovic G. (2008). Mycobacterium avium complex infection after alemtuzumab therapy for chronic lymphocytic leukemia. *Pharmacotherapy.* Vol.28, No.2, (February 2008), pp. 281-4, ISSN 0277-0008

Saritsiri S, Udomsantisook N, Suankratay C. (2006). Nontuberculous mycobacterial infections in King Chulalongkorn Memorial Hospital. J Med Assoc Thai. Vol.89, No.12, (December 2006), pp. 2035-46, ISSN 0125-2208

Sester M, Sester U, Gärtner BC, Girndt M, Meyerhans A, Köhler H.(2002). Dominance of virus-specific CD8 T cells in human primary cytomegalovirus infection. *J Am Soc Nephrol.* Vol.13, No.10, (October 2002), pp. 2577-84, ISSN 1046-6673

Shiota T, Lixin W, Takayama-Ito M, Iizuka I, Ogata M, Tsuji M, Nishimura H, Taniguchi S, Morikawa S, Kurane I, Mizuguchi M, Saijo M. (2011). Expression of herpes simplex virus type 1 recombinant thymidine kinase and its application to a rapid antiviral sensitivity assay. *Antiviral Res.* Vol.91, No.2, (Jun 2011), pp. 142-149, ISSN 0166-3542

Sidrim JJ, Costa AK, Cordeiro RA, Brilhante RS, Moura FE, Castelo-Branco DS, Neto MP, Rocha MF. (2010). Molecular methods for the diagnosis and characterization of Cryptococcus: a review. *Can J Microbiol.* Vol.56, No.6, (Jun 2010), pp. 445-58, ISSN 0008-4166

Sinisalo M, Aittoniemi J, Käyhty H, Vilpo J. (2003). Vaccination against infections in chronic lymphocytic leukemia. *Leuk Lymphoma.* Vol.44, No. 4, (April 2003), pp. 649-52. ISSN 1042-8194

Sinsalo M, Aittoniemi J, Käyhty H, Vilpo J. (2002). Haemophilus influenzae type b (Hib) antibody concentrations and vaccination responses in patients with chronic lymphocytic leukaemia: predicting factors for response. *Leuk Lymphoma.* Vol.43, No. 10, (October 2002), pp. 1967-9. ISSN 1042-8194

Sinisalo M, Vilpo J, Taurio J, Aittoniemi J. (2007). Antibody response to 7-valent conjugated pneumococcal vaccine in patients with chronic lymphocytic leukaemia. *Vaccine.* Vol.26, No.1, (December 2007), pp. 82-7, ISSN **0264-410X**

Südhoff T, Arning M, Schneider W. (1997). Prophylactic strategies to meet infectious complications in fludarabine-treated CLL. *Leukemia.* Vol.11, No. Suppl 2, (April 1997), pp. 38-41, ISSN 0887-6924

Tafreshi NK, Sadeghizadeh M, Amini-Bavil-Olyaee S, Ahadi AM, Jahanzad I, Roostaee MH. (2005). Development of a multiplex nested consensus PCR for detection and identification of major human herpesviruses in CNS infections. *J Clin Virol.* Vol.32, No.4, (April 2005), pp. 318-24, ISSN1386-6532

Thalla R, Kim D, Venkat KK, Parasuraman R. (2009). Sequestration of active Cryptococcus neoformans infection in the parathyroid gland despite prolonged therapy in a renal transplant recipient. *Transpl Infect Dis.* Vol.11, No.4, (August 2009), pp. 349-52, ISSN 1398-2273

Thursky KA, Worth LJ, Seymour JF, Miles Prince H, Slavin MA. (2006). Spectrum of infection, risk and recommendations for prophylaxis and screening among patients with lymphoproliferative disorders treated with alemtuzumab. *Br J Haematol.* Vol.132, No. 1, (January 2006), pp. 3-12, ISSN 0902-4441

Todisco M. (2009). Chronic lymphocytic leukemia: long-lasting remission with combination of cyclophosphamide, somatostatin, bromocriptine, retinoids, melatonin, and ACTH. *Cancer Biother Radiopharm.* Vol.24, No. 3, (June 2009), pp. 353-5, ISSN 1084-9785

Travade P, Dusart JD, Cavaroc M, Beytout J, Rey M. (1986). Severe infections associated with chronic lymphoid leukemia. 159 infectious episodes in 60 patients. *Presse Med.* Vol.15, No.34, (October 1986), pp. 1715-8, ISSN **0755-4982**

Turkulov V, Madle-Samardzija N, Brkić S. (1999). Meningoencephalitis as the only manifestation of Epstein-Barr virus infection. *Med Pregl.* Vol.52, No.(9-10), (September 1999), pp. 391-3, ISSN 0025-8105

Vancíková Z, Dvorák P.(2001). Cytomegalovirus infection in immunocompetent and immunocompromised individuals-a review. *Curr Drug Targets Immune Endocr Metabol Disord. 2001* Vol.1, No.2, (February 2001), pp. 179-87, ISSN 1568-0088

Van der Velden AM, Mulder AH, Hartkamp A, Diepersloot RJ, van Velzen-Blad H, Biesma DH. (1995). Influenza virus vaccination and booster in B-cell chronic lymphocytic leukaemia patients. *Eur J Intern Med.* Vol.12, No. 5, (September 1995), pp. 420-424, ISSN 0953-6205

Van Koeveringe MP, Brouwer RE. (2010). Histoplasma capsulatum reactivation with haemophagocytic syndrome in a patient with chronic lymphocytic leukaemia. *Neth J Med.* Vol.*68*, No.12, (December *2010*), pp. 418-21, ISSN 0300-2977

Vavricka SR, Halter J, Hechelhammer L, Himmelmann A. (2004). Pneumocystis carinii pneumonia in chronic lymphocytic leukaemia. *Postgrad Med J.* Vol.80, No.942, (April 2004), pp. 236-8, ISSN 0022-3859

Wadhwa PD & Morrison VA. (2006). Infectious complications of chronic lymphocytic leukemia. *Semin Oncol.* Vol.33, No.2, (April 2006), pp. 240-9, ISSN 0093-7754

Wierda WG.(2003). Immunologic monitoring in chronic lymphocytic leukemia. *Curr Oncol Rep.* Vol.5, No.5, (September 2003), pp. 419-25, ISSN 1523-3790

Yadegarynia D, Abbasi F, Haghighi M, Korooni Fardkhani S, Yadegarynia S. Pneumonitis due to cytomegalovirus in an immunocompromised patient. *Iranian Journal of Clinical Infectious Disease* Vol.4, No.4, (Fall 2009), pp. 238-240, ISSN 1735-5109

Yağci M, Acar K, Sucak GT, Aki Z, Bozdayi G, Haznedar R. (2006). A prospective study on chemotherapy-induced hepatitis B virus reactivation in chronic HBs Ag carriers with hematologic malignancies and pre-emptive therapy with nucleoside analogues. *Leuk Lymphoma.* Vol.47, No.8, (August 2006), pp. 1608-12, ISSN 1042-8194

Young JA. (2011). Epidemiology and management of infectious complications of contemporary management of chronic leukemias. (2011). *Infect Disord Drug Targets.* Vol.11, No.1, (February 2011), pp. 3-10, ISSN 1871-5265

Zahorodnia SD, Nesterova NV, Danylenko VP, Bukhtiarova TA, Baranova HV, Holovan' AV. (2011). Effect of isonicotinic acid derivates on reproduction of Epstein-Barr virus. *Mikrobiol Z.* Vol.73, No.2, (March-April 2011), pp. 65-72, ISSN 1028-0987

18

Emerging Therapies in Chronic Lymphocytic Leukemia

Reslan Lina and Dumontet Charles
Université Lyon 1, Lyon,
France

1. Introduction

The introduction of new therapies has opened new therapeutic hopes in the field of treating Chronic Lymphocytic Leukemia (CLL). CLL is extremely heterogeneous in its clinical course; some patients live for decades with no need for treatment, whereas others develop aggressive clinical course with a survival of less than 2-3 years. The decision to treat CLL patients should be guided by clinical staging, the presence of symptoms and disease activity (Diehl et al. 1999).

Once the diagnosis of CLL has been made, the treating physician is faced with the decision of not only how to treat the patient, but when to initiate therapy. In general practice, newly diagnosed patients with asymptomatic early-stage disease (Rai 0, Binet A) are monitored without therapy until they have evidence of disease progression. Studies from the French Cooperative Group on CLL, (Dighiero et al. 1998) the Cancer and Leukemia Group B,(Shustik et al. 1988) the Spanish Group PETHEMA, (Montserrat et al. 1996) and the Medical Research Council (Catovsky et al. 1988) confirm that the use of alkylating agents in patients with early-stage disease does not prolong survival (Group. 1999). Patients at intermediate (I and II) or high-risk (III and IV) according to the modified Rai classification or Binet stage B or C usually require the initiation of treatment at presentation. Some of these patients (in particular Rai intermediate risk or Binet stage B) can still be monitored without therapy until they exhibit evidence of progressive or symptomatic disease.

During the past decade there have been major advances in understanding the pathogenesis of the disease and more efficient treatments have been developed. CLL treatments have seen the transition from single-agent alkyator-based therapies to nucleoside analogs, combination chemotherapy, and recently to monoclonal antibodies (MAbs) and chemoimmunotherapy.

The use of immunotherapy is emerging as an exciting modality with significant potential to advance the treatment of B-cell malignancies. In the field of lymphoproliferative diseases rituximab, followed by the anti-CD52 antibody alemtuzumab, has changed the therapeutic landscape of B-cell cancers, particularly in patients with non-Hodgkin's lymphoma (NHL) with more recent indications in the setting of CLL (Cheson 2006).

Novel therapies are being evaluated both in pre-clinical studies and in clinical trials. These treatments include new MAbs such as ofatumumab, GA101, veltuzumab, epratuzumab, lumiliximab, TRU-016 as well as agents targeting the anti-apoptotic Bcl-2 family of proteins, antisense oligonucleotides and other agents. This review attempts to summarize the current knowledge of these treatments and point to potential opportunities in the future with other targeted therapies currently being explored.

2. Best compounds of alkylating agents and purine analogs used in CLL

Chlorambucil, an alkylating agent, has been considered the "gold standard" for several decades. Due to its low toxicity and its oral administration, this drug remains the appropriate option for non-fit, elderly patients as well as for younger fit patients. Chlorambucil achieved higher remission rates (Overall response rates (ORR) 89%, Complete responses (CR) 59%) when administered at a fixed dose of 15 mg daily up to achievement of a CR or occurrence of grade 3 toxicity, for a maximum of six months (Jaksic et al. 1997). However, chlorambucil is no longer considered an appropriate option for younger or physically fit patients because of its low to non-existent CR rate (Catovsky et al. 2007).

Besides chlorambucil, cyclophosphamide (C) is another alkylating agent with activity in CLL patients. It is generally utilized in combination regimen. (Hansen et al. 1988; Raphael et al. 1991).

Fludarabine is the best purine analog studied in CLL. When used as single agent, it achieves superior ORR and longer progression-free survival (PFS) rates compared with other treatment regimens containing alkylating agents or corticosteroids (Anaissie et al. 1998; Plunkett et al. 1993; Rai et al. 2000). In phase III studies in naive CLL patients, fludarabine induced more CRs (7–40%) as well as longer duration of remission than other chemotherapies or chlorambucil. However, overall survival (OS) was not improved by this drug when used as a single agent (Johnson et al. 1996; Leporrier et al. 2001; Rai et al. 2000; Steurer et al. 2006).

Bendamustine, a hybrid of an alkylating nitrogen mustard group and a purine-like benzimidazole, has been used for more than 30 years in Germany. Results of a recent randomized trial, comparing bendamustine to chlorambucil, showed that more patients achieved CRs with bendamustine than with chlorambucil (31% vs. 2%). Moreover, the median PFS was 21.6 months and 8.3 months for bendamustine and chlorambucil, respectively (Knauf et al. 2009).

3. Rituximab: The first anti-CD20 MAb

Rituximab has revolutionized the therapeutic approach for patients with a wide variety of B-cell malignancies, including CLL. Rituximab is a chimeric human-mouse MAb with a high affinity for the CD20 surface antigen, a transmembrane protein that is expressed on pre-B cells and normal differentiated B lymphocytes. The predominant mechanism of action of rituximab-induced cell death is proposed to be primarily the result of antibody-dependent cell-mediated cytotoxicity (ADCC), complement-dependent cytotoxicity (CDC) and direct cell death (Di Gaetano et al. 2003; Golay et al. 2000; Manches et al. 2003).

Rituximab was first approved in the United States for the treatment of relapsed or refractory, low grade or follicular, B-cell NHL (Grillo-Lopez et al. 1999) then approved in Europe, for the treatment of relapsed stage III/IV follicular NHL (Gopal & Press 1999;

McLaughlin et al. 1998). In CLL, rituximab is less active as single agent than in other lymphomas, unless very high doses or denser dosing regimen are used. The objective response rates observed in CLL patients are ranged between 25% and 35% (Huhn et al. 2001; Itala et al. 2002).

In contrast, the greatest benefit of rituximab is demonstrated when used in combination with chemotherapy. Multiple combinations are currently in use and others are in investigational phases. Here, we will present some of these combinations to highlight the synergistic effect of rituximab with other agents.

The combination of fludarabine with rituximab prolonged the PFS and OS of CLL patients compared to fludarabine alone (Byrd et al. 2005).

A phase II study performed by the German CLL Study Group (GCLLSG) of fludarabine and rituximab in both refractory and previously untreated patients resulted in an ORR of 87% with a subset achieving CR (Schulz et al. 2002).

CALGB 9712 evaluated fludarabine in combination with rituximab given either concurrently or sequentially. Patients in the concurrent arm experienced more severe hematologic and infusion-related toxicity, but the ORR was 90% with a CR of 47% compared with an ORR of 78% and CR of 28% in the sequential arm (Byrd et al. 2003).

Likewise, rituximab induced a high ORR and complete remission rates when combined either with fludarabine/cyclophosphamide in refractory/relapsed CLL patients (73% and 25%, respectively) (Wierda et al. 2005) or in those with previously untreated CLL (95% and 72%, respectively) (Tam et al. 2008). The superiority of fludarabine, cyclophosphamide plus rituximab (FCR) compared to fludarabine and cyclophosphamide, alone was also confirmed in randomized phase III trials (Hallek 2008; Robak 2008; Tam et al. 2008).

In the CLL8 protocol of the German CLL Study Group (GCLLSG), 817 treatment-naive, physically fit patients (aged 30–81 years) were randomly assigned to receive either fludarabine, cyclophosphamide, and rituximab (FCR group) or fludarabine and cyclophosphamide (FC group). At 3 years after randomization, 65% of patients in the FCR group were free of progression compared with 45% in the FC group ($P < 0.0001$); The three-year survival rates were 87% and 83% for FCR-treatment and FC-treatment ($p=0.012$), respectively. FCR treatment was more frequently associated with hematologic adverse events, particularly neutropenia; these results suggest that the choice of FCR as first-line treatment prolongs OS of CLL patients (Hallek et al., 2010).

Furthermore, when combined with pentostatin and cyclophosphamide in previously untreated CLL patients, rituximab achieved a significant clinical activity despite poor risk-based prognoses, including achievement of minimal residual disease in some patients (Kay et al. 2007; Keating et al. 2005; Tam et al. 2006).

The German CLL Study Group initiated two studies to explore the combination of bendamustine plus rituximab in patients with relapsed CLL (Fischer 2008) and in previously untreated CLL patients (Fischer 2009). Results showed an ORR of 77%, CR rate of 15% for relapsed patients and an OR of 91%, CR of 33% for untreated ones. A retrospective Italian study was conducted in 109 relapsed/refractory CLL patients. Results showed that the combination of rituxmab plus bendamustine was an effective and well-tolerated treatment for these patients, producing a remarkable high CR rate and mild toxicity (Iannitto et al. 2011).

Investigations of the mechanism underlying the anti-tumor activity of rituximab as a single agent and in combination with chemotherapy are ongoing. By understanding these mechanisms, it might be possible to further enhance current cell killing strategies or develop novel agents and strategies.

4. Newer anti-CD20 antibodies for CLL

4.1 Ofatumumab

Ofatumumab is a fully humanized MAb targeting a small-loop CD20 epitope distinct from that of rituximab (Teeling et al. 2004). Compared to rituximab, it demonstrates an increased target-binding affinity to CD20 and slower dissociation rates. It exhibits stronger complement-mediated toxicity and shows potent lysis of rituximab-resistant cells.

In phase I/II study in relapsed/refractory CLL patients, ofatumumab achieved an ORR of 44%; however, these were almost exclusively partial responses (Coiffier et al. 2008). In a phase I/II dose-escalation trial, the efficacy and safety of single-agent ofatumumab (300-1000 mg) have been evaluated in 40 patients with relapsed or refractory Follicular Lymphoma (FL). Rapid, efficient and sustained peripheral B-cell depletion was observed in all dose groups. The ORR in evaluable patients (n=36) was 43% (Hagenbeek et al. 2008).

This antibody was recently approved by the Food and Drug Administration (FDA) for fludarabine and alemtuzumab refractory CLL patients and for fludarabine refractory patients with bulky disease. Ofatumumab was administered in these two groups with an ORR of 58% and 47%, respectively (Wierda G 2009). It is currently being combined with other agents in CLL, including bendamustine.

A recently completed phase II trial of ofatumumab in combination with fludarabine and cyclophosphamide demonstrated CRs in up to 50% of patients with previously untreated CLL, despite poor prognostic factors (Wierda G 2009). The median PFS has not been reached with the short median follow-up of 8 months.

Moreover, a randomized phase II study was conducted using two dose schedules of ofatumumab (500 mg and 1000 mg) in combination with fludarabine 25 mg/m2 and cyclophosphamide 250 mg/m2. The CR rate was 32% for the 500-mg and 50% for the 1000-mg cohort; the ORR was 77% and 73%, respectively (Wierda et al. 2010).

4.2 GA101

GA101 is the first humanized type II anti-CD20 MAb with glycolengineered Fc portion and a modified elbow hinge (Bello & Sotomayor 2007). The adapted Fc region gives GA101 a 50-fold higher binding affinity to FCγRIII (CD16) compared to a non-glycoengineered antibody, resulting in 10- to 100-fold increase in ADCC against $CD20^+$ NHL cell lines via the activation of effector cells (Umana 2006). Moreover, the modified elbow hinge area also results in strong induction of direct cell death of several NHL cell lines and primary malignant B cells *in vitro* (Alduaij W & S. 2009; Bello & Sotomayor 2007; Umana 2006). However, these modifications result in reduced CDC activity (Umana 2007). In vitro B-cell depletion assays with whole blood from healthy and leukemic patients showed that the combined activity of ADCC, CDC, and apoptosis for GA101 was significantly superior to rituximab (Alduaij W & S. 2009; Patz M 2009; Umana 2006; Zenzl 2009).

The enhanced efficacy of GA101 has been also shown *in vivo*. In xenograft models of Diffuse large B-cell lymphoma (DLBCL) and mantle cell lymphoma, treatment with GA101 resulted in CR and long-term survival compared with tumor stasis achieved with rituximab (Umana 2006). In cynomolgus monkeys, GA101 (10 and 30 mg/kg infused on days 0 and 7) showed significantly superior depletion of B cells compared to rituximab (10 mg/kg) from day 9 to day 35 and was more efficacious at clearing B cells from lymph nodes and the spleen (Umana 2007).

Initial phase I study of patients with relapsed/refractory CD20+ disease (n=21), including CLL, DLBCL, and other NHLs, for whom no therapy of higher priority was available (95% of patients had previously received rituximab), GA101 demonstrated a favorable safety profile with no dose-limiting toxicities (Salles 2009). The depletion of B-cell was rapid and sustained in the majority of patients. Nine of the evaluable patients responded to therapy (ORR, 43%; five CR/unconfirmed CR and four partial responses), with responses observed at all dose levels and across all FcγRIIIA genotypes.

The pharmacokinetics of GA101 are generally similar to those of rituximab and dose-dependent. However, significant inter- and intra-patient variabilities have been observed, the clinical relevance of which will need further investigation [86]. Results from a phase I study in patients with previously treated B-CLL (n=13) who were given single-agent GA101 (400–2000 mg; nine infusions) showed similar safety and pharmacokinetic profiles to those observed in the previously described patients with NHL, except for an increased incidence of neutropenia (Morschhauser 2009).

GA101 is currently being explored as a single agent in phase II studies in relapsed/refractory B-CLL and indolent/aggressive NHL, and in combination with chemotherapy in a phase Ib study.

4.3 Veltuzumab (IMMU-106)

Veltuzumab is a humanized CD20 MAb (type I) constructed recombinantly on the framework regions of epratuzumab, with complementarity-determining regions (CDRs) identical to rituximab, except for a single amino acid in CDR3 of the variable heavy chain. It showed anti-proliferative, apoptotic, and ADCC effects *in vitro* similar to rituximab, but with significantly slower off-rates and increased CDC in several human lymphoma cell lines. In addition, at very low doses, given either intravenously or subcutaneously, veltuzumab showed a potent anti-B cell activity in cynomolgus monkeys and controlled tumor growth in mice bearing human lymphomas (Goldenberg et al. 2009).

In a phase I/II dose-escalating clinical trial in patients with recurrent NHL, the ORR for veltuzumab-treatement was 41% (33/81), including 17 patients (21%) with CR or unconfirmed CR (Morschhauser et al. 2009). Veltuzumab caused B-cell depletion after the first infusion even at the lowest dose of 80 mg/m^2, which persisted after the fourth infusion, and was well tolerated, with no evidence of immunogenicity.

Veltuzumab is additionally being developed for subcutaneous administration, which may provide advantages for this agent versus other MAbs (Goldenberg et al. 2010). Veltuzumab is undergoing clinical trials using a low-dose subcutaneous formulation in patients with NHL and CLL.

5. Other MAbs for CLL

5.1 Alemtuzumab

Alemtuzumab is a recombinant, fully humanized, MAb targeting the CD52 antigen. CD52 is expressed on virtually all lymphocytes at various stages of differentiation, as well as monocytes, macrophages and eosinophils, whereas hematopoeitic stem cells, erythrocytes and platelets do not express it (Hale et al. 1990). A high level of CD52 is found on T-prolymphocytic leukemia, followed by B-CLL, with the lowest levels expressed on normal B cells. The mechanisms of action of alemtuzumab include CDC, ADCC and induction of apoptosis (Mone et al. 2006).

The use of alemtuzumab monotherapy is approved in the United States in the first-line treatment of patients with CLL. In a pivotal phase II study in 93 patients with fludarabine-refractory disease, alemtuzumab yielded an ORR of 33% with a median OS of 16 months (Keating et al. 2005).

Alemtuzumab has been approved for the initial treatment of CLL based on randomized trial conducted including 297 patients who received either alemtuzumab or chlorambucil. The antibody induced an ORR rate of 83.2% with 24.2% CRs compared with 55.4% and 2%, for alemtuzumab and chlorambucil, respectively (Hillmen et al. 2007). In addition, alemtuzumab has proven efficacy even in patients with poor prognostic factors, including high-risk genetic markers such as deletions of chromosome 11 or 17 and p53 mutations (Lozanski et al. 2004; Stilgenbauer & Dohner 2002). The combination of alemtuzumab with fludarabine was investigated in a phase II trial with relapsed CLL patients. The ORR was 83% including 30% CR (Elter et al. 2005). The combination of both alemtuzumab with rituximab has been also studied in patients with lymphoid malignancies including patients with refractory/relapsed CLL, producing an ORR of 52% with 8% CR (Faderl et al. 2003).

The combination of fludarabine, cyclophosphamide plus alemtuzumab (FCA) was recently compared to fludarabine, cyclophosphamide plus rituximab (FCR) in a phase III study by "the french Cooperative Group On CLL and WM" (FCGCLL/MW) and "the Groupe Ouest-est d'Etudes des Leucemies Aigues et Autres Maladies du Sang" (GOELAMS). Response rates of the first 100 patients were reported in a preliminary analysis with safety data presented for the entire cohort of 178 patients. The ORR in the first 100 patients was 96% for FCR compared to 85% in the FCA arm (p=0.086) with a CR rate of 78% in the FCR arm versus 58% in the FCA arm (p=0.072). Increased toxicity of FCA compared with FCR was found, preventing the use of the FCA combination outside of clinical trials (Lepretre 2009).

5.2 Lumiliximab

Lumiliximab is an anti-CD23 macque-human chimeric MAb with a strong similarity to the human antibody. The CD23 antigen is a low-affinity IgE receptor that is found in high levels in CLL patients (Fournier et al. 1992). Lumiliximab inhibits the IgE secretion *in vitro,* binds complement and mediates ADCC by binding FcγRI and RII receptors.

A phase I pilot study reported a limited single-agent activity in patients with refractory/relapsed CLL (Byrd et al. 2007b). Based on preclinical evidences of synergistic improvement of survival when lumiliximab was combined with fludarabine or rituximab, a phase I/II trial evaluated the safety and efficacy of lumiliximab in combination with FCR in 31 patients of relapsed CLL patients (Byrd J 2008). This combination regimen yielded an ORR of 65%, which was comparable to the results seen with FCR in the pivotal phase II study conducted by the M.D. Anderson Cancer Center (Byrd J 2008; Wierda et al. 2005). Lumiliximab/FCR appeared to double the CR rate compared to FCR alone (52% vs. 25%) without increasing the rate of toxicities.

5.3 Epratuzumab

Epratuzumab is a humanized anti-CD22 MAb currently in clinical trials for treatment of NHL and autoimmune disorders (Leonard & Goldenberg 2007). Epratuzumab is selectively active against normal and neoplastic B-cells. This MAb acts as an immunomodulatory agent in contrast to rituximab which is an actually cytotoxic therapeutic antibody. *In vitro*, epratuzumab has demonstrated the ability to elicit ADCC and induce CD22 phosphorylation and signaling, both of which may contribute as potential mechanisms of action (Carnahan et al. 2007; Carnahan et al. 2003).

Phase I/II studies demonstrated objective responses across various dose levels in both relapsed/refractory FL (24%) (Leonard et al. 2003) and DLBCL (15%) (Leonard et al. 2004).

Epratuzumab has also been combined with rituximab in phase II studies showing at least an additive benefit while toxicities of the combination were comparable with those of single-agent rituximab (Leonard et al. 2005). In a recent international, multicenter trial evaluating rituximab plus epratuzumab in patients with post-chemotherapy relapsed/refractory, indolent NHL, an objective response was seen in 54% FL patients including 24% with CR/unconfirmed CR (CRu) whereas 57% of Small Lymphocytic Lymphoma patients had ORs including 43% with CR/Cru (Leonard et al. 2008). Rituximab-naive patients had an ORR of 50%, whereas patients who previously responded to rituximab had an ORR of 64%.

Thus, the combination of epratuzumab and rituximab induced durable responses in patients with recurrent, indolent NHL. Epratuzumab is also being evaluated in combination with rituximab plus cyclophosphamide, doxorubicin, vincristine, and prednisone (CHOP) and as a therapy in other B-cell neoplasms (Micallef et al. 2006).

5.4 TRU-016

TRU-016 is a CD37-directed small modular immunopharmaceutical protein composed of IgG1 variable regions (VL and VH) and a small, engineered constant region. CD37 is expressed at high concentrations on the surface of B cells and mature B-cell lymphomas and leukemias. *In vitro* studies demonstrated that the chimeric version of TRU-016 induced apoptosis and ADCC-dependent cytotoxicity in CLL cells (Zhao, Lapalombella et al. 2007).

Interim results of a phase I study of TRU-016 reported a favorable toxicity profile and partial responses at higher doses (Andritsos 2009).

6. Emerging drugs

6.1 Bcl-2 inhibitors

The expression of high levels of anti-apoptotic Bcl-2 protein is characteristic of CLL cells (Hanada et al. 1993). Many studies have suggested that an increased ratio of anti- to pro-apoptotic proteins such as Bcl-2/Bax is correlated with poor response to chemotherapy, disease progression and shorter survival (Pepper et al. 1997; Robertson et al. 1996).

Modulation of anti-apoptotic proteins is a promising strategy to sensitize cells to antileukemic agents. Preclinical data have shown that inhibition of Bcl-2, inhibition of the interaction between Bcl-2 or Bcl-xL and partner proteins with compounds such as ABT-737 (Mason et al. 2009) or inhibition of Mcl-1 were associated with increased sensitivity to antileukemic agents (Hallaert et al. 2007).

Numerous novel agents have shown *in vitro* promise in overcoming the pro-apoptotic defects in CLL cells. These do not, however, always translate into a therapeutic *in vivo* effect.

6.2 Oblimersen sodium (G3139)

Oblimersen sodium is a phosphorothioate antisense oligodeoxynucleotide composed of 18 nucleotides targeting the first six codons of the open reading frame of the bcl-2 mRNA. Preclinical evaluation has demonstrated good antineoplastic effect in B-cell cancers; several clinical trials have confirmed its safety and efficacy both alone and in combination with other therapeutics.

A phase I/II clinical trial was conducted in patients with relapsed or refractory CLL to determine the maximum tolerated dose (MTD), efficacy, safety, and pharmacokinetics of oblimersen sodium. A total of 40 patients (who had received at least one prior chemotherapy regimen containing a purine analogue) were treated (14 in Phase I and 26 in Phase II) with single-agent oblimersen sodium in doses ranging from 3 to 7 mg/kg/day in the phase I portion of the study. The MTD for the phase II part of the study was determined to be 3 mg/kg/day with higher doses of oblimersen sodium being associated with a cytokine release reaction characterized by fever, rigors and hypotension. This was attributed to the release of large amounts of cytokines. Thus, oblimersen sodium has shown a modest single-agent activity in heavily pretreated patients with advanced CLL (O'Brien et al. 2005).

A phase II trial was conducted to evaluate the safety and efficacy of the combination of fludarabine, rituximab and oblimersen in previously untreated or relapsed/previously treated CLL patients. Preliminary results have been encouraging especially in the setting of CLL with poor prognostic markers (Marvromatis 2006; Mavromatis 2005).

A randomized phase III trial of fludarabine and cyclophosphamide (FC) with or without oblimersen sodium in 241 patients with relapsed or refractory CLL who had received at least one prior fludarabine-containing regimen has been conducted. The rate of CR/nodular PR was significantly higher for patients treated with FC plus oblimersen, 17% versus 7%, respectively. The oblimersen treated group was associated with a significant survival benefit (O'Brien et al. 2007).

Overall, oblimersen has shown new hope and potential in the management of CLL, enhancing the efficacy of other commonly used agents. Further studies with oblimersen should have a special focus on correlating response and survival outcomes with Bcl-2 overexpression and subsequent decrease in Bcl-2 protein.

6.3 Navitoclax (ABT-263)

Navitoclax (ABT-263), a novel, orally bioavailable, small molecule, binds with high affinity to anti-apoptotic proteins Bcl-2, Bcl-xL, and Bcl-w, promoting apoptosis. *In vitro*, navitoclax shows potent targeted cytotoxicity against T and B lymphoid malignancies that over-express Bcl-2. A phase I trial demonstrated oral navitoclax monotherapy to be well-tolerated and to have anti-tumor activity in CLL patients.

Phase II study was conducted in patients with heavily pretreated CLL, the drug attained an objective response rate of 33% (currently confirmed in 19% of patients); 58% of patients with baseline nodal enlargement showed shrinkage of greater than 50%.

The combination of navitoclax with bendamustine/rituximab was effective for patients with relapsed or refractory CLL and presented encouraging results in a phase II trial. Moreover, phase III studies showed that the combination of navitoclax with fludarabine/cyclophosphamide/rituximab combination improved outcomes in CLL patients (Kipps 2010).

6.4 Obatoclax (GX15-070)

Obatoclax is a hydrophobic molecule, developed as a Bcl-2 family antagonist. This agent inhibits several anti-apoptotic Bcl-2 family proteins including Bcl-x_L, Bcl-2, Bcl-w, BCL-B, A-1 and Mcl-1. It induces the release of Bak from Mcl-1, the liberation of Bim from both Bcl-2 and Mcl-1 as well as the formation of an active Bak/Bax complex. Moreover, it can promote the release of cytochrome c from mitochondria leading to apoptosis (Konopleva et al. 2008).

A phase I trial of obatoclax was conducted in heavily pretreated patients with advanced CLL. Obatoclax was administered at doses ranging from 3.5 to 14 mg/m^2 as a 1-hour infusion and from 20 to 40 mg/m^2 as a 3-hour infusion every 3 weeks. Obatoclax demonstrated biologic as well as modest clinical activity in these patients with one (4%) of 26 patients achieving a partial response (O'Brien et al. 2009).

7. Newer treatment options

7.1 Lenalidomide

The immunomodulatory agent lenalidomide has shown activity in CLL in the relapsed/refractory as well as in the untreated setting.

Activity in CLL was first demonstrated by Chanan-Khan *et al.* in a phase II study. 25 mg of lenalidomide was administered in this trial daily on days 1 through 21 of a 28-day cycle in 45 pretreated CLL patients (Chanan-Khan et al. 2006). This regimen was associated with a 47% ORR and a 9% CR rate.

Ferrajoli *et al.* adopted this dose escalation scheme in 45 patients with relapsed CLL. The dosing started at 10 mg daily for 28 days, with dose escalation to a maximum of 25 mg/day as tolerated. The ORR was 32% with 7% of patients achieving a CR (Ferrajoli et al. 2008). Moreover, lenalidomide therapy was well tolerated and induced durable remissions in elderly patients with CLL (Badoux et al. 2011).

The combination of lenalidomide plus rituximab is currently being investigated in 60 patients with relapsed CLL patients. 37 patients are to date evaluable for response. The ORR was 68%, no CR was achieved. The results obtained suggest that the combination of rituximab and lenalidomide is superior to the single agent lenalidomide.

Currently, a study is recruiting participants to evaluate the combination of fludarabine plus rituximab with or without lenalidomide or cyclophosphamide in treating patients with symptomatic CLL.

7.2 Flavopiridol (Alvocidib)

Flavopiridol, a synthetic flavon, induces apoptosis in CLL cell lines by targeting cyclin-dependent kinases.

It shows high activity in CLL patients with relapsed high-risk CLL (Byrd et al. 2007a; Phelps et al. 2009). A phase II trial on relapsed CLL patients with genetically high risk features achieved an ORR of 53%, including one CR (Lin et al. 2009). Currently, a registration trial for flavopiridol in relapsed CLL is conducted in the United States and Europe.

8. Conclusion

A refreshing change is taking place in CLL research. There is an increasing interest to fully understand all subsets of CLL patients in order to develop novel and specific agents which cater to individualized needs of each subset. Currently available therapies are only partially efficient in CLL; thus, obvious clinical and scientific needs to develop new therapeutic options are under investigation to circumvent the limitations of currently used therapies in CLL.

Further studies should elucidate the role of these new agents and their combinations in the management of CLL.

9. References

Alduaij W, P.S., Ivanov A, Honeychurch J, Beers & S. 2009, 'New-generation anti-CD20 monoclonal antibody (GA101) evokes homotypic adhesion and actin-dependent, lysosome-mediated cell death in B-cell lymphom [abstract]', *ASH Annual Meeting Abstracts*, vol. 114:725.

Anaissie, E.J. et al. 1998, 'Infections in patients with chronic lymphocytic leukemia treated with fludarabine', *Ann Intern Med*, vol. 129, no. 7, pp. 559-66.

Andritsos, L., Furman, R., Flinn, I.W., Foreno-Torres, A. , Flynn, J. M., Stromatt, S. C., Byrd, J. C. 2009, 'A Phase 1 Trial of TRU-016, An Anti-CD37 Small Modular Immunopharmaceutical (SMIPTM) Protein in Relapsed and Refractory CLL: Early Promising Clinical Activity [abstract 3017].', *J Clin Oncol.*, vol. 27.

Badoux, X.C. et al. 2011, 'Lenalidomide as initial therapy of elderly patients with chronic lymphocytic leukemia', *Blood.*

Bello, C. & Sotomayor, E.M. 2007, 'Monoclonal antibodies for B-cell lymphomas: rituximab and beyond', *Hematology Am Soc Hematol Educ Program*, pp. 233-42.

Byrd J, C.J., Flinn I, et al. 2008, ' Lumiliximab in combination with FCR for the treatment of relapsed chronic lymphocytic leukemia (CLL): results from a phase I/II multicenter study', *Ann Oncol* vol. 19(suppl 4):iv130 (Abstract 145).

Byrd, J.C. et al. 2007a, 'Flavopiridol administered using a pharmacologically derived schedule is associated with marked clinical efficacy in refractory, genetically high-risk chronic lymphocytic leukemia', *Blood*, vol. 109, no. 2, pp. 399-404.

Byrd, J.C. et al. 2007b, 'Phase 1 study of lumiliximab with detailed pharmacokinetic and pharmacodynamic measurements in patients with relapsed or refractory chronic lymphocytic leukemia', *Clin Cancer Res*, vol. 13, no. 15 Pt 1, pp. 4448-55.

Byrd, J.C. et al. 2003, 'Randomized phase 2 study of fludarabine with concurrent versus sequential treatment with rituximab in symptomatic, untreated patients with B-cell chronic lymphocytic leukemia: results from Cancer and Leukemia Group B 9712 (CALGB 9712)', *Blood*, vol. 101, no. 1, pp. 6-14.

Byrd, J.C. et al. 2005, 'Addition of rituximab to fludarabine may prolong progression-free survival and overall survival in patients with previously untreated chronic lymphocytic leukemia: an updated retrospective comparative analysis of CALGB 9712 and CALGB 9011', *Blood*, vol. 105, no. 1, pp. 49-53.

Carnahan, J. et al. 2007, 'Epratuzumab, a CD22-targeting recombinant humanized antibody with a different mode of action from rituximab', *Mol Immunol*, vol. 44, no. 6, pp. 1331-41.

Carnahan, J. et al. 2003, 'Epratuzumab, a humanized monoclonal antibody targeting CD22: characterization of in vitro properties', *Clin Cancer Res*, vol. 9, no. 10 Pt 2, pp. 3982S-90S.

Catovsky, D. et al. 1988, 'The UK Medical Research Council CLL trials 1 and 2', *Nouv Rev Fr Hematol*, vol. 30, no. 5-6, pp. 423-7.

Catovsky, D. et al. 2007, 'Assessment of fludarabine plus cyclophosphamide for patients with chronic lymphocytic leukaemia (the LRF CLL4 Trial): a randomised controlled trial', *Lancet*, vol. 370, no. 9583, pp. 230-9.

Chanan-Khan, A. et al. 2006, 'Clinical efficacy of lenalidomide in patients with relapsed or refractory chronic lymphocytic leukemia: results of a phase II study', *J Clin Oncol*, vol. 24, no. 34, pp. 5343-9.

Cheson, B.D. 2006, 'Monoclonal antibody therapy of chronic lymphocytic leukemia', *Cancer Immunol Immunother*, vol. 55, no. 2, pp. 188-96.

Coiffier, B. et al. 2008, 'Safety and efficacy of ofatumumab, a fully human monoclonal anti-CD20 antibody, in patients with relapsed or refractory B-cell chronic lymphocytic leukemia: a phase 1-2 study', *Blood*, vol. 111, no. 3, pp. 1094-100.

Di Gaetano, N. et al. 2003, 'Complement activation determines the therapeutic activity of rituximab in vivo', *J Immunol*, vol. 171, no. 3, pp. 1581-7.

Diehl, L.F. et al. 1999, 'The American College of Surgeons Commission on Cancer and the American Cancer Society. The National Cancer Data Base report on age, gender, treatment, and outcomes of patients with chronic lymphocytic leukemia', *Cancer*, vol. 86, no. 12, pp. 2684-92.

Dighiero, G. et al. 1998, 'Chlorambucil in indolent chronic lymphocytic leukemia. French Cooperative Group on Chronic Lymphocytic Leukemia', *N Engl J Med*, vol. 338, no. 21, pp. 1506-14.

Elter, T. et al. 2005, 'Fludarabine in combination with alemtuzumab is effective and feasible in patients with relapsed or refractory B-cell chronic lymphocytic leukemia: results of a phase II trial', *J Clin Oncol*, vol. 23, no. 28, pp. 7024-31.

Faderl, S. et al. 2003, 'Experience with alemtuzumab plus rituximab in patients with relapsed and refractory lymphoid malignancies', *Blood*, vol. 101, no. 9, pp. 3413-5.

Ferrajoli, A. et al. 2008, 'Lenalidomide induces complete and partial remissions in patients with relapsed and refractory chronic lymphocytic leukemia', *Blood*, vol. 111, no. 11, pp. 5291-7.

Fischer, K., Cramer, P., Stilgenbauer, S., Busch, R., Balleisen, L., Kilp, J., Fink, A-M., Boettcher, S., Ritgen, M., Kneba,M.,Staib, P., Döhner, H., Schulte, S., Eichhorst, B.F., Hallek, M., Wendtner, C-M., and the German CLL Study Group (GCLLSG) 2009, ' Bendamustine Combined with Rituximab (BR) in First-Line Therapy of Advanced CLL: A Multicenter Phase II Trial of the German CLL Study Group (GCLLSG)', *Blood*, vol. (ASH Annual Meeting Abstracts) 114: 205.

Fischer, K., Stilgenbauer, S., Schweighofer, C.D. , Busch, R., Renschler, J., Kiehl, M., Balleisen, L., Eckart, M.J., Fink, A-M., Kilp,J., Ritgen, M., Böttcher, S., Kneba, M., Döhner, H., Eichhorst, B.F., Hallek, M., Wendtner, C-M., and The German CLL Study Group 2008, 'Bendamustine in combination with rituximab (BR) for patients with relapsed chronic lymphocytic leukemia (CLL): A multicentre phase II trial of the German CLL Study Group (GCLLSG).', *Blood*, vol. 112, p. 128.

Fournier, S. et al. 1992, 'CD23 antigen regulation and signaling in chronic lymphocytic leukemia', *J Clin Invest*, vol. 89, no. 4, pp. 1312-21.

Golay, J. et al. 2000, 'Biologic response of B lymphoma cells to anti-CD20 monoclonal antibody rituximab in vitro: CD55 and CD59 regulate complement-mediated cell lysis', *Blood*, vol. 95, no. 12, pp. 3900-8.

Goldenberg, D.M. et al. 2010, 'Veltuzumab (humanized anti-CD20 monoclonal antibody): characterization, current clinical results, and future prospects', *Leuk Lymphoma*, vol. 51, no. 5, pp. 747-55.

Goldenberg, D.M. et al. 2009, 'Properties and structure-function relationships of veltuzumab (hA20), a humanized anti-CD20 monoclonal antibody', *Blood*, vol. 113, no. 5, pp. 1062-70.

Gopal, A.K. & Press, O.W. 1999, 'Clinical applications of anti-CD20 antibodies', *J Lab Clin Med*, vol. 134, no. 5, pp. 445-50.

Grillo-Lopez, A.J. et al. 1999, 'Overview of the clinical development of rituximab: first monoclonal antibody approved for the treatment of lymphoma', *Semin Oncol*, vol. 26, no. 5 Suppl 14, pp. 66-73.

Group., C.T.C. 1999, 'Chemotherapeutic options in chronic lymphocytic leukemia: a meta-analysis of the randomized trials', *J Natl Cancer Inst.*, vol. 91:861-868.

Hagenbeek, A. et al. 2008, 'First clinical use of ofatumumab, a novel fully human anti-CD20 monoclonal antibody in relapsed or refractory follicular lymphoma: results of a phase 1/2 trial', *Blood*, vol. 111, no. 12, pp. 5486-95.

Hale, G. et al. 1990, 'The CAMPATH-1 antigen (CDw52)', *Tissue Antigens*, vol. 35, no. 3, pp. 118-27.

Hallaert, D.Y. et al. 2007, 'Crosstalk among Bcl-2 family members in B-CLL: seliciclib acts via the Mcl-1/Noxa axis and gradual exhaustion of Bcl-2 protection', *Cell Death Differ*, vol. 14, no. 11, pp. 1958-67.

Hallek, M., Fingerle-Rowson, G., Fink, A.M., et al. 2008, ' Immunochemotherapy with fludarabine (F), cyclophosphamide (C), and rituximab (R) (FCR) versus fludarabine and cyclophosphamide (FC) improves response rates and progression-free survival (PFS) of previously untreated patients (pts) with advanced chronic lymphocytic leukemia (CLL) [abstract]', *Blood*, vol. 112(11):125 Abstract 325.

Hallek, M. et al., 'Addition of rituximab to fludarabine and cyclophosphamide in patients with chronic lymphocytic leukaemia: a randomised, open-label, phase 3 trial', *Lancet*, vol. 376, no. 9747, pp. 1164-74.

Hanada, M. et al. 1993, 'bcl-2 gene hypomethylation and high-level expression in B-cell chronic lymphocytic leukemia', *Blood*, vol. 82, no. 6, pp. 1820-8.

Hansen, M.M. et al. 1988, 'CHOP versus prednisolone + chlorambucil in chronic lymphocytic leukemia (CLL): preliminary results of a randomized multicenter study', *Nouv Rev Fr Hematol*, vol. 30, no. 5-6, pp. 433-6.

Hillmen, P. et al. 2007, 'Alemtuzumab compared with chlorambucil as first-line therapy for chronic lymphocytic leukemia', *J Clin Oncol*, vol. 25, no. 35, pp. 5616-23.

Huhn, D. et al. 2001, 'Rituximab therapy of patients with B-cell chronic lymphocytic leukemia', *Blood*, vol. 98, no. 5, pp. 1326-31.

Iannitto, E. et al. 2011, 'Bendamustine with or without rituximab in the treatment of relapsed chronic lymphocytic leukaemia: an Italian retrospective study', *Br J Haematol*, vol. 153, no. 3, pp. 351-7.

Itala, M. et al. 2002, 'Standard-dose anti-CD20 antibody rituximab has efficacy in chronic lymphocytic leukaemia: results from a Nordic multicentre study', *Eur J Haematol*, vol. 69, no. 3, pp. 129-34.

Jaksic, B. et al. 1997, 'High dose chlorambucil versus Binet's modified cyclophosphamide, doxorubicin, vincristine, and prednisone regimen in the treatment of patients with advanced B-cell chronic lymphocytic leukemia. Results of an international multicenter randomized trial. International Society for Chemo-Immunotherapy, Vienna', *Cancer*, vol. 79, no. 11, pp. 2107-14.

Johnson, S. et al. 1996, 'Multicentre prospective randomised trial of fludarabine versus cyclophosphamide, doxorubicin, and prednisone (CAP) for treatment of advanced-stage chronic lymphocytic leukaemia. The French Cooperative Group on CLL', *Lancet*, vol. 347, no. 9013, pp. 1432-8.

Kay, N.E. et al. 2007, 'Combination chemoimmunotherapy with pentostatin, cyclophosphamide, and rituximab shows significant clinical activity with low accompanying toxicity in previously untreated B chronic lymphocytic leukemia', *Blood*, vol. 109, no. 2, pp. 405-11.

Keating, M.J. et al. 2005, 'Early results of a chemoimmunotherapy regimen of fludarabine, cyclophosphamide, and rituximab as initial therapy for chronic lymphocytic leukemia', *J Clin Oncol*, vol. 23, no. 18, pp. 4079-88.

Kipps, T.J., Wierda, W.G., Jones, J.A., Swinnen, L.J., Yang, J., Cui, Y., Busman, T., Krivoshik, A., Enschede, S., and Humerickhouse, R. 2010, 'Navitoclax (ABT-263) Plus Fludarabine/Cyclophosphamide/Rituximab (FCR) or Bendamustine/Rituximab (BR): A Phase 1 Study In Patients with Relapsed/Refractory Chronic Lymphocytic Leukemia (CLL) ', vol. ASH Annual Meeting Abstracts 2010; Abstract 2455.

Knauf, W.U. et al. 2009, 'Phase III randomized study of bendamustine compared with chlorambucil in previously untreated patients with chronic lymphocytic leukemia', *J Clin Oncol*, vol. 27, no. 26, pp. 4378-84.

Konopleva, M. et al. 2008, 'Mechanisms of antileukemic activity of the novel Bcl-2 homology domain-3 mimetic GX15-070 (obatoclax)', *Cancer Res*, vol. 68, no. 9, pp. 3413-20.

Leonard, J.P. et al. 2005, 'Combination antibody therapy with epratuzumab and rituximab in relapsed or refractory non-Hodgkin's lymphoma', *J Clin Oncol*, vol. 23, no. 22, pp. 5044-51.

Leonard, J.P. et al. 2003, 'Phase I/II trial of epratuzumab (humanized anti-CD22 antibody) in indolent non-Hodgkin's lymphoma', *J Clin Oncol*, vol. 21, no. 16, pp. 3051-9.

Leonard, J.P. et al. 2004, 'Epratuzumab, a humanized anti-CD22 antibody, in aggressive non-Hodgkin's lymphoma: phase I/II clinical trial results', *Clin Cancer Res*, vol. 10, no. 16, pp. 5327-34.

Leonard, J.P. & Goldenberg, D.M. 2007, 'Preclinical and clinical evaluation of epratuzumab (anti-CD22 IgG) in B-cell malignancies', *Oncogene*, vol. 26, no. 25, pp. 3704-13.

Leonard, J.P. et al. 2008, 'Durable complete responses from therapy with combined epratuzumab and rituximab: final results from an international multicenter, phase 2 study in recurrent, indolent, non-Hodgkin lymphoma', *Cancer*, vol. 113, no. 10, pp. 2714-23.

Leporrier, M. et al. 2001, 'Randomized comparison of fludarabine, CAP, and ChOP in 938 previously untreated stage B and C chronic lymphocytic leukemia patients', *Blood*, vol. 98, no. 8, pp. 2319-25.

Lepretre, S., Aurran, T., Mahe, B., et al. 2009, ' Immunochemotherapy with Fludarabine (F), Cyclophosphamide (C), and Rituximab (R) (FCR) Versus Fludarabine (F), Cyclophosphamide (C) and MabCampath (Cam) (FCCam) in Previously Untreated Patients (pts) with Advanced B-Chronic Lymphocytic Leukemia (BCLL): Experience On Safety and Efficacy within a Randomised Multicenter Phase III Trial of the french Cooperative Group On CLL and WM (FCGCLL/MW) and the "Groupe Ouest-Est d'Etudes Des Leucemies Aigues Et Autres Maladies Du sang" (GOELAMS) : CLL2007FMP (for fit medically patients).', *ASH Annual Meeting Abstracts. 2009;114(22):538-.*

Lin, T.S. et al. 2009, 'Phase II study of flavopiridol in relapsed chronic lymphocytic leukemia demonstrating high response rates in genetically high-risk disease', *J Clin Oncol*, vol. 27, no. 35, pp. 6012-8.

Lozanski, G. et al. 2004, 'Alemtuzumab is an effective therapy for chronic lymphocytic leukemia with p53 mutations and deletions', *Blood*, vol. 103, no. 9, pp. 3278-81.

Manches, O. et al. 2003, 'In vitro mechanisms of action of rituximab on primary non-Hodgkin lymphomas', *Blood*, vol. 101, no. 3, pp. 949-54.

Marvromatis, B., Rai, K., Wallace, P.K., et al. 2006, 'Impact of prognostic markers on outcomes in patients with advanced chronic lymphocytic leukemia treated with the regimen of fludarabine/rituximab plus oblimersen (Bcl-2 Antisense) ', *[abstract 6609] ASCO Annual Meeting Proceedings; 2006. p.24.*

Mason, K.D. et al. 2009, 'The BH3 mimetic compound, ABT-737, synergizes with a range of cytotoxic chemotherapy agents in chronic lymphocytic leukemia', *Leukemia*, vol. 23, no. 11, pp. 2034-41.

Mavromatis, B., Rai, K.R., Wallace, P.K., et al. 2005, 'Efficacy and Safety of the Combination of Genasense™ (Oblimersen Sodium, Bcl-2 Antisense Oligonucleotide), Fludarabine and Rituximab in Previously Treated and Untreated Subjects with Chronic Lymphocytic Leukemia', *ASH Annual Meeting Abstracts 2005;106:2129.*

McLaughlin, P. et al. 1998, 'Rituximab chimeric anti-CD20 monoclonal antibody therapy for relapsed indolent lymphoma: half of patients respond to a four-dose treatment program', *J Clin Oncol*, vol. 16, no. 8, pp. 2825-33.

Micallef, I.N. et al. 2006, 'A pilot study of epratuzumab and rituximab in combination with cyclophosphamide, doxorubicin, vincristine, and prednisone chemotherapy in patients with previously untreated, diffuse large B-cell lymphoma', *Cancer*, vol. 107, no. 12, pp. 2826-32.

Mone, A.P. et al. 2006, 'Alemtuzumab induces caspase-independent cell death in human chronic lymphocytic leukemia cells through a lipid raft-dependent mechanism', *Leukemia*, vol. 20, no. 2, pp. 272-9.

Montserrat, E. et al. 1996, 'Fludarabine in resistant or relapsing B-cell chronic lymphocytic leukemia: the Spanish Group experience', *Leuk Lymphoma*, vol. 21, no. 5-6, pp. 467-72.

Morschhauser, F., Cartron, G., Lamy, T., et al. 2009, 'Phase I study of RO5072759 (GA101) in relapsed/refractory chronic lymphocytic leukemia [abstract]. ASH Annual Meeting Abstracts. 2009;114:884.'.

Morschhauser, F. et al. 2009, 'Humanized anti-CD20 antibody, veltuzumab, in refractory/recurrent non-Hodgkin's lymphoma: phase I/II results', *J Clin Oncol*, vol. 27, no. 20, pp. 3346-53.

O'Brien, S. et al. 2007, 'Randomized phase III trial of fludarabine plus cyclophosphamide with or without oblimersen sodium (Bcl-2 antisense) in patients with relapsed or refractory chronic lymphocytic leukemia', *J Clin Oncol*, vol. 25, no. 9, pp. 1114-20.

O'Brien, S.M. et al. 2009, 'Phase I study of obatoclax mesylate (GX15-070), a small molecule pan-Bcl-2 family antagonist, in patients with advanced chronic lymphocytic leukemia', *Blood*, vol. 113, no. 2, pp. 299-305.

O'Brien, S.M. et al. 2005, 'Phase I to II multicenter study of oblimersen sodium, a Bcl-2 antisense oligonucleotide, in patients with advanced chronic lymphocytic leukemia', *J Clin Oncol*, vol. 23, no. 30, pp. 7697-702.

Patz M, F.N., Muller B, et al. 2009, 'Depletion of chronic lymphocytic leukemia cells from whole blood. Samples mediated by the anti-CD20 antibodies rituximab and GA101 [abstract]', vol. ASH Annual Meeting Abstracts 114, p. 2365.

Pepper, C. et al. 1997, 'Bcl-2/Bax ratios in chronic lymphocytic leukaemia and their correlation with in vitro apoptosis and clinical resistance', *Br J Cancer*, vol. 76, no. 7, pp. 935-8.

Phelps, M.A. et al. 2009, 'Clinical response and pharmacokinetics from a phase 1 study of an active dosing schedule of flavopiridol in relapsed chronic lymphocytic leukemia', *Blood*, vol. 113, no. 12, pp. 2637-45.

Plunkett, W. et al. 1993, 'Fludarabine: pharmacokinetics, mechanisms of action, and rationales for combination therapies', *Semin Oncol*, vol. 20, no. 5 Suppl 7, pp. 2-12.

Rai, K.R. et al. 2000, 'Fludarabine compared with chlorambucil as primary therapy for chronic lymphocytic leukemia', *N Engl J Med*, vol. 343, no. 24, pp. 1750-7.

Raphael, B. et al. 1991, 'Comparison of chlorambucil and prednisone versus cyclophosphamide, vincristine, and prednisone as initial treatment for chronic lymphocytic leukemia: long-term follow-up of an Eastern Cooperative Oncology Group randomized clinical trial', *J Clin Oncol*, vol. 9, no. 5, pp. 770-6.

Robak, T., Moiseev, S., Dmoszynska, A., et al. 2008, 'Rituximab, fludarabine, and cyclophosphamide (R-FC) prolongs progression free survival in relapsed or refractory chronic lymphocytic leukemia (CLL) compared with FC alone: final results from the international randomized phase III REACH trial', *Blood*, vol. 112(11):LBA-1 Abstract 157420.

Robertson, L.E. et al. 1996, 'Bcl-2 expression in chronic lymphocytic leukemia and its correlation with the induction of apoptosis and clinical outcome', *Leukemia,* vol. 10, no. 3, pp. 456-9.

Salles, G., Morschhauser, F., Lamy, T., et al. 2009, 'Phase I study of RO5072759 (GA101) in patients with relapsed/refractory CD20 non-Hodgkin lymphoma (NHL) [abstract] ASH Annual Meeting Abstracts. 2009;114:1704.'.

Schulz, H. et al. 2002, 'Phase 2 study of a combined immunochemotherapy using rituximab and fludarabine in patients with chronic lymphocytic leukemia', *Blood,* vol. 100, no. 9, pp. 3115-20.

Shustik, C. et al. 1988, 'Treatment of early chronic lymphocytic leukemia: intermittent chlorambucil versus observation', *Hematol Oncol,* vol. 6, no. 1, pp. 7-12.

Steurer, M. et al. 2006, 'Single-agent purine analogues for the treatment of chronic lymphocytic leukaemia: a systematic review and meta-analysis', *Cancer Treat Rev,* vol. 32, no. 5, pp. 377-89.

Stilgenbauer, S. & Dohner, H. 2002, 'Campath-1H-induced complete remission of chronic lymphocytic leukemia despite p53 gene mutation and resistance to chemotherapy', *N Engl J Med,* vol. 347, no. 6, pp. 452-3.

Tam, C.S. et al. 2008, 'Long-term results of the fludarabine, cyclophosphamide, and rituximab regimen as initial therapy of chronic lymphocytic leukemia', *Blood,* vol. 112, no. 4, pp. 975-80.

Tam, C.S. et al. 2006, 'Fludarabine, cyclophosphamide, and rituximab for the treatment of patients with chronic lymphocytic leukemia or indolent non-Hodgkin lymphoma', *Cancer,* vol. 106, no. 11, pp. 2412-20.

Teeling, J.L. et al. 2004, 'Characterization of new human CD20 monoclonal antibodies with potent cytolytic activity against non-Hodgkin lymphomas', *Blood,* vol. 104, no. 6, pp. 1793-800.

Umana, P., Moessner, E., Bruenker, P., et al. 2007, ' GA101, a novel humanized type II CD20 antibody with glycoengineered Fc and anhanced cell death induction, exhibits superior anti-tumor efficacy and superior tissue B cell depletion in vivo. Blood 2007;110: 694a (Abstract 2348). '.

Umana, P., Moessner, E., Bruenker, P., Unsin, G., Puentener, U., Suter, T., et al. 2006, 'Novel third-generation humanized Type II CD20 antibody with glycoengineered Fc and modified elbow hinge for enhanced ADCC and superior apoptosis induction', *Blood,* vol. 108 ; (abstract #229).

Wierda G, K.T., Mayer J, et al. 2009, 'High activity of single-agent ofatumumab, a novel CD20 monoclonal antibody in fludarabine- and alemtuzumab-refractory or bulky fludarabine - refractory chronic lymphocytic leukemia, regardless of prior rituximab exposure [abstract].EHA Annual Meeting 2009;0919.'.

Wierda, W. et al. 2005, 'Chemoimmunotherapy with fludarabine, cyclophosphamide, and rituximab for relapsed and refractory chronic lymphocytic leukemia', *J Clin Oncol,* vol. 23, no. 18, pp. 4070-8.

Wierda, W.G. et al. 2010, 'Chemoimmunotherapy with O-FC in previously untreated patients with chronic lymphocytic leukemia', *Blood,* vol. 117, no. 24, pp. 6450-8.

Zenzl, T., Volden, M., Mast, T., et al. 2009, 'In vitro activity of the type II anti-CD20 antibody GA101 in refractory, genetic high-risk CLL [abstract]', vol. ASH Annual Meeting Abstracts 2009;114:2379.

19

Heat Shock Proteins in Chronic Lymphocytic Leukaemia

Nina C. Dempsey-Hibbert, Christine Hoyle and John H.H. Williams
Chester Centre for Stress Research, University of Chester
United Kingdom

1. Introduction

Over the last decade, research has implicated a group of molecular chaperones termed Heat Shock Proteins (HSPs) as major contributors to cancer progression and the development of chemo-resistance. HSPs were initially discovered as a group of proteins that were strongly induced in response to heat shock and other cellular stresses. Under non-stress conditions, they have a wide variety of roles within many sub-cellular compartments where they facilitate protein folding, prevent protein unfolding and assist protein transport across membranes. Due to their roles in maintaining protein conformation, HSPs are vital when other cellular proteins start to unfold due to cellular stress such as high temperature, exposure to cytotoxic chemicals or oxidative stress and are up-regulated rapidly in these situations (Ciocca and Calderwood, 2005). Under these stressful conditions, HSPs prevent protein aggregation, stabilise cell membranes and inhibit many of the key steps in cell death pathways (Beere & Green, 2001), thereby enabling cell survival in conditions that would otherwise be lethal. Importantly, in normal cells, once the stress has passed, HSP levels return to baseline and these proteins return to their regular house-keeping duties. However, a growing body of research shows that in tumour cells, including Chronic Lymphocytic Leukaemia (CLL) cells, HSPs remain elevated and may contribute to prolonged tumour cell survival via several mechanisms that remain to be fully revealed.

Human HSPs were originally identified as stress-induced proteins and were traditionally split into five families based on their molecular weight. These five families were the HSP27, HSP60, HSP90, HSP70 and HSP110 families. However, the sequencing of the human genome led to the identification of additional members of well established HSP families. Furthermore, the expansion of these HSP families resulted in many HSPs being referred to by several different names. Therefore, attempts to draw comparisons between studies examining specific HSPs has proved challenging. Consequently, Kampinga et al. (2009) recently introduced guidelines for the nomenclature of human HSPs which ensures that the genes and proteins are named in a consistent manner (Table 1). Readers are referred to Kampinga et al. (2009) for a complete listing of human HSP nomenclature. This chapter will focus on the involvement of the major HSPs, HSPB1 (Hsp27) HSPA1A (Hsp72) and HSPC1 (Hsp90) in the development and progression of CLL.

Gene Name	New Protein Name	Old Names
HSPB1	HSPB1	Hsp27, Hsp28; Hsp25
DNAJB1	DNAJB1	Hsp40
HSPD1	HSPD1	Hsp60
HSPA8	HSPA8	HSC70, Hsp71, Hsp73
HSPA9	HSPA9	Mortalin, mtHsp70, GRP75
HSPA1A	HSPA1A	Hsp72, Hsp70-1, HSPA1
HSPC1	HSPC1	Hsp90, HSP90A, Hsp89, HSP90AA
HSPH2	HSPH2	Hsp110

(Adapted from Kampinga et al. 2009)

Table 1. New nomenclature for human HSPs referred to in this chapter

The up-regulation of a number of HSPs in response to stress stimuli is regulated by the transcription factor Heat Shock Factor-1 (HSF1) (Wu, 1995). Under non-stress conditions, members of the DNAJ and HSPA families along with HSPC1 are bound to monomeric HSF1 within the cytosol. However, under stress conditions these HSPs dissociate from HSF1 and bind misfolded proteins, suggesting that these HSPs have a higher affinity for misfolded proteins compared to HSF1. As a consequence HSF1 trimerises and migrates to the nucleus where, in this state, it has a high binding affinity for cis-acting DNA sequence elements known as Heat Shock Elements (HSEs) in the promoter region of the HSP genes resulting in transcription of HSP genes (Sorger , 1991). Once the stress is discontinued, the trimeric forms of HSF1 dissociate from the HSEs and are converted back to HSF1 monomers with the inability to bind DNA. It is believed that the increase in HSPs within the cell following the heat shock response are themselves negative regulators of HSF, binding to HSF and preventing further trimerisation (Wu, 1995). HSPC1 has been shown to be a negative regulator of HSF1, as immunodepletion of HSPC1 results in enhanced HSF1 activity (Zou et al. 1998).

2. HSPs in cancer

The potential importance of HSPs in tumour biology is clear when considering their activities in light of the Hanahan & Weinberg concept of the hallmarks of cancer (Hanahan & Weinberg 2000; Hanahan & Weinberg 2011), where the development of a malignant phenotype requires six modifications:

- self-sufficiency with respect to growth signals
- limitless replicative potential
- insensitivity to anti-growth signals
- sustained angiogenesis
- capacity for tissue invasion and metastasis
- evasion of apoptosis

HSPs have the potential to contribute to each of these modifications, and three HSPs (HSPB1, HSPA1A and HSPC1) can be shown to influence at least two of these modifications. Not surprisingly it is these three HSPs that feature most in tumour studies.

HSPB1 belongs to the family of small heat shock proteins. Besides its role as an ATP-independent molecular chaperone, it is involved in the regulation of cell differentiation, the acquisition of thermotolerance and the inhibition of apoptosis and cell senescence. HSPB1 is up-regulated in response to a wide variety of stress stimuli such as oxidative stress, exposure to anti-cancer agents and radiation (Lanneau et al. 2008). As a molecular chaperone, HSPB1 prevents protein aggregation and stabilises partially denatured proteins ensuring refolding by other chaperones such as HSPA1A and HSPC1.

HSPA1A is the main inducible member of the HSPA family and is not normally present in significant concentrations in non-stressed normal cells. HSPA1A mainly exists as a dimer, and similarly to HSPB1 is up-regulated in response to a wide variety of stress stimuli and promotes cell survival. HSPA1A has a high affinity for hydrophobic amino acids and will rapidly bind to partially denatured proteins in preparation for refolding or disposal.

HSPC1 is the most abundant member of the HSPC family, and is constitutively expressed in all eukaryotic cells where it binds a specific set of 'client proteins' including steroid receptors, non-receptor tyrosine kinases and cyclin-dependent kinases (McLaughlin et al. 2002). HSPC1 operates as part of a multimeric chaperone complex which includes members of the HSPA and DNAJ families, along with many other 'co-chaperones' and immunophillins (Holzbeierlein et al. 2010). It exists as a dimer, consisting of three major domains per monomer; A C-terminal homodimerisation domain, a middle ATP-hydrolysis-regulating domain, and an N-terminal, ATP binding domain (Krukenberg et al. 2011).

At one time HSPs were thought to be solely intracellular proteins (iHSPs). However certain HSPs have been found to be released from viable cells into the extracellular milieu (eHSPs) (Hightower & Guidon, 1989; Hunter-Lavin et al. 2004) and have also been found expressed on the tumour cell surface (sHSPs). The exact mechanism involved in the transport of these HSPs from the cytosol to the cell surface and extracellular environment have not been fully determined, but evidence suggests that HSPs may employ a number of methods including lipid-raft transport (Hunter-Lavin et al. 2004; Gastpar et al 2005; Vega et al. 2008), exosomal transport (Clayton et al. 2005) and ABC transporters (Mambula & Calderwood 2006). Regardless of their route of exit, sHSPs and eHSPs have critical roles in a variety of processes ranging from cell invasion and metastasis to immunomodulation.

3. Intracellular HSPs

3.1 Intracellular HSPs and prognosis

The up-regulation of HSPs inside cancer cells compared to normal cells has been well documented and has led to numerous studies investigating their prognostic and therapeutic potential (Calderwood et al. 2006; Ciocca et al. 2005; Sherman & Multhoff. 2007). In many cases high levels of HSPs have been found to be advantageous to the cancer cell, which is hardly surprising when considering that HSPB1, HSPA1A and HSPC1 are all anti-apoptotic factors, and would suggest that these proteins should have prognostic potential. However, although elevated HSPA1A, HSPB1, and HSPC1 are associated with poor prognosis in leukaemia, this pattern is not repeated in other cancers (Table 2) (Jaattela, 1999; Ciocca & Calderwood, 2005). In a minority of cancer types, the over-expression of HSPs appears to correlate with a positive prognosis for the patient (Kawanishi et al. 1999; Sagol et al. 2002; Santarosa et al. 1997) and at present it is still unclear as to how HSP expression may influence cancer progression.

Increased levels of HSPB1 have been documented in various cancers including breast, liver and prostate (Cornford et al. 2000; Romani et al. 2007; Vargas-Roig et al. 1997) and high levels have been found to correlate with poor prognosis (Duval et al. 2006; Thomas et al. 2005). However, there are contradictions within the literature; In breast cancer, for example, increased levels of HSPB1 have been associated with prolonged survival in oestrogen receptor-negative cases (Love & King, 1994). Low levels of HSPB1 in ovarian cancer have also been found to correlate with decreased survival (Geisler et al. 2004). However, these contradictions may be attributed to HSPB1, (synonymous with p24 and p29), being an oestrogen-regulated protein (Adams & McGuire, 1985; Ciocca & Luque, 1991).

Increases in HSPA1A have been observed in breast cancer (Tauchi et al. 1991), colorectal cancer (Milicevic et al. 2007; Shotar, 2005), kidney cancer (Ramp et al. 2007) and leukaemia (Chant et al. 1995; Thomas et al. 2005). Additionally, elevated HSPA1A has been associated with resistance to cancer therapy and/or poor prognosis for the patient (Thomas et al. 2005; Vargas-Roig et al. 1998). However, the relationship between the presence of HSPs and prognosis cannot be extrapolated to all cancers, as high intracellular HSPA1A expression has been correlated with a positive prognosis in oesophageal (Kawanishi et al. 1999), pancreatic (Sagol et al. 2002) and renal cancer (Santarosa et al. 1997).

HSPC1 levels are elevated in a number of cancer types including oesophageal squamous cell carcinoma (Wu et al. 2009), invasive breast carcinoma (Zagouri et al. 2010) and leukaemia (Thomas et al. 2005). Furthermore, in some cases, elevated HSPC1 levels have been associated with decreased survival and adverse karyotypes (Pick et al. 2007; Thomas et al. 2005).

Cancer type	HSPA1A	HSPB1	HSPC1
Breast	Poor	Variable	n/d
Endometrial	Poor	n/d	Good
Kidney	Good	n/d	n/d
Leukaemia	Poor	Poor	Poor
Lung	n/d	n/d	n/d
Osteosarcoma	Good	Poor	Variable
Ovary	n/d	Poor	n/d

(Adapted from Jaattela, (1999) and Ciocca & Calderwood, (2005))

Table 2. Association of HSP over-expression with prognosis

It is clear that different HSPs have distinct roles in normal cells and therefore it is not inconceivable that they may also have a variety of roles in tumour development. Indeed, the over-expression of one particular HSP within a tumour cell does not necessarily signify elevated levels of other HSPs within the same patient; In CLL particularly, HSPB1, HSPA1A and HSPC1 increases have been observed amongst patients but not necessarily simultaneously (Dempsey et al. 2010a). Similarly there is little correlation between the expression of HSPB1, HSPA1A and HSPC1 in prostate cancer (Cornford et al. 2000) or AML (Thomas et al. 2005). It is therefore imperative to understand the individual roles of these proteins in cancer development by studying them together within a specific sample but also considering them as distinct entities.

3.2 Intracellular HSPs and resistance to apoptosis

Mechanistic investigations have shown that HSPB1 interferes with the apoptotic pathway in several ways including the prevention of cytochrome c and Smac/DIABLO release from the mitochondria (Chauhan et al. 2003a; Paul et al. 2002) and direct interaction with cytochrome c (Garrido et al. 2001; LeBlanc, 2003; Samali et al. 2001) and Daxx (Charrette et al. 2000) thereby inhibiting their function. There is clear evidence that HSPB1 levels correlate with chemo-resistance (Schepers et al. 2005; Vargas-Roig et al. 1998). Studies designed to explore the role of HSPB1 in the development of chemo-resistance have utilised various techniques including siRNA and gene transfection. Depletion of HSPB1 has been shown to overcome resistance to drug-induced apoptosis (Chauhan et al. 2003b) while transfection of full-length HSPB1 into cancer cells confers resistance to Cisplatin and Doxorubicin (Richards et al. 1996).

HSPA1A is involved in carcinogenesis at many different stages from the enhancement of activity of many different oncogenes and inhibition of tumour suppressor genes such as p53 (Yaglom et al. 2007), to promoting the survival of tumour cells through inhibition of apoptosis (Khaleque et al. 2005; Nylandsted et al. 2000). Similarly to HSPB1, HSPA1A interacts with several key proteins in cell death pathways (Beere & Green, 2001). Direct interaction with APAF-1 and mutated p53 (Iwaya et al. 1995; Lehman et al. 1991) has been documented as well as direct inhibition of procaspases. Several studies have shown that depletion of HSPA1A results in increased sensitivity to chemotherapeutic drugs (Zhao & Shen, 2005) and ultimately apoptosis of various cell lines including breast, colon and prostate (Nylandsted et al. 2000), highlighting the importance of this protein for cell survival.

A wide variety of client proteins are held by HSPC1 in both tumour and non-tumour cells, and as a result it is involved in several vital signalling pathways including PI3K/Akt, Erk1/2, JNK and NFκB pathways. It is the chaperoning of a variety of oncoproteins such as mutant B-Raf (Grbovic et al. 2006), Bcr/Abl (An et al. 2000) and mutant p53 (Lin et al. 2008), as well as the signalling pathway components, that has sparked interest into HSPC1's potential role in tumour development and progression. HSPC1 also cooperates with HSPA1A in inhibiting apoptosome formation. Furthermore, HSPC1 interferes with death receptor mediated apoptosis by stabilising the anti-apoptotic protein Receptor Interacting Protein (RIP) thereby promoting cell survival.

Clearly HSPB1, HSPA1A and HSPC1 interfere with apoptotic signalling at multiple points (Figure 1).

4. Extracellular HSPs

4.1 Extracellular HSPs in immunomodulation

As a consequence of their molecular chaperoning role, HSPs exit the cell bound to a wide variety of antigenic peptides. These extracellular HSP-peptide complexes bind to surface receptors on Antigen Presenting Cells (APCs) in a process termed cross-presentation (Bolhassani & Rafati, 2008). During the process of necrosis, when cell stress is highest and the cellular components leak out of the cell, these HSP-peptide complexes are abundant and can signal stress to local APCs, which in-turn can induce a Cytotoxic T-Lymphocyte (CTL)

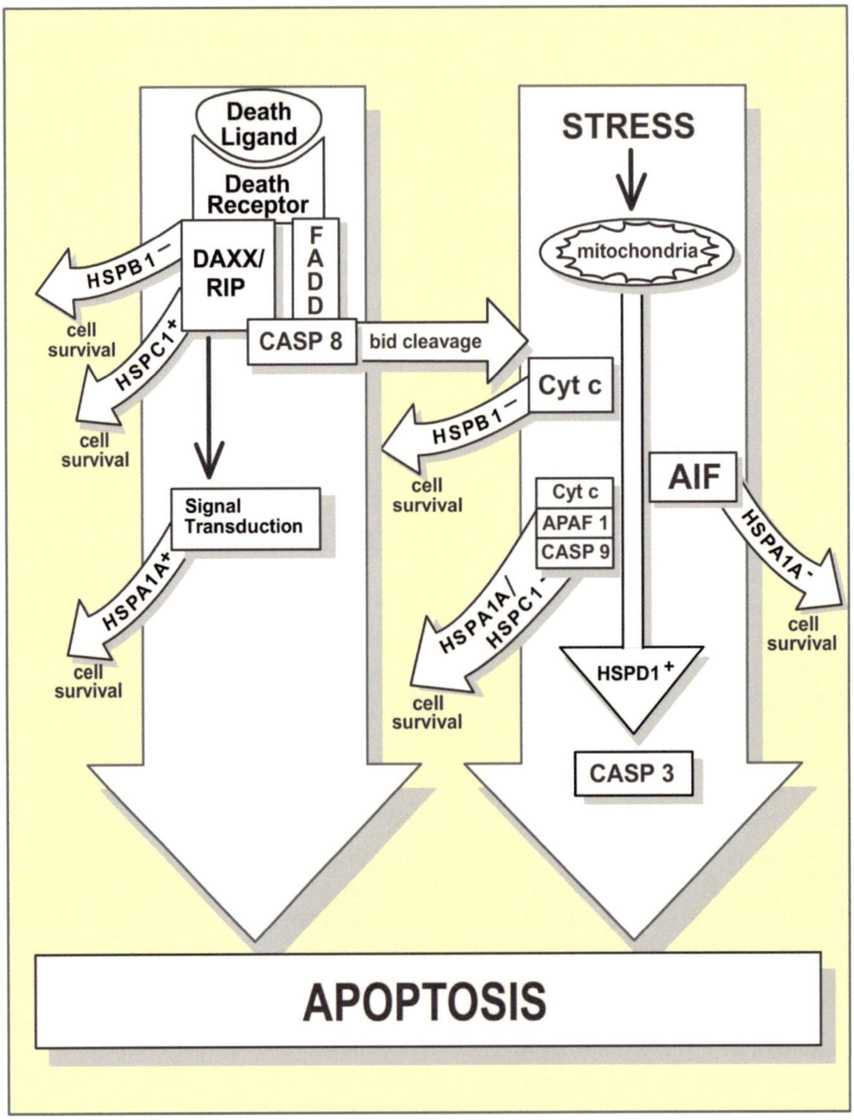

Fig. 1. Regulation of the Death Receptor and Mitochondrial Apoptosis Pathways by HSPs (Taken from Dempsey, 2009). Two main arrows represent the Death Receptor-mediated- and mitochondrial- apoptosis pathways. HSPB1 inhibits apoptosis by directly interacting with Daxx, and sequestering cytochrome c released from the mitochondria. HSPD1 has been shown to directly promote the proteolytic maturation of caspase-3, thereby displaying a pro-apoptotic role. HSPA1A inhibits apoptosis by inhibiting the activation of protein kinases involved in signal transduction pathways (e.g. JNK), binding to AIF thereby neutralising its effects and binding to Apaf-1 resulting in inhibition of apoptosome formation. HSPC1 has been shown to stabilise the anti-apoptotic protein, RIP and has also been shown to work synergistically with HSPA1A to inhibit apoptosome formation. Apoptosis induced by Death Receptors also results in activation of the mitochondrial pathway via cleavage of the pro-apoptotic protein Bid. A minus sign indicates negative regulation while a positive sign indicates positive regulation.

response. Similarly, viable tumour cells with high HSP levels may also actively release HSP-peptide complexes into the surrounding environment. Research investigating the HSP-APC interactions has revealed a number of APC receptors capable of binding HSPs; Scavenger receptors (SRs), Toll-like receptors (TLRs), CD40, CD14 and CD91 (Calderwood et al. 2007; Basu et al. 2001) allow HSP-peptide complexes to interact with a number of different immune cell types including Dendritic cells, Macrophages, Monocytes and NK-cells (Murshid et al. 2008).

The binding of HSPA1A-peptide complexes to the SR LOX-1 on Dendritic cells, for example, results in the internalisation of the HSP-peptide complex (Arnold-Schild et al. 1999) via the phagocytic pathway, and re-presentation of the antigenic peptide on MHC-I on the Dendritic cell surface. Work by Kurotaki et al. (2007) has revealed the significance of HSPs in this antigen cross presentation process; Dendritic cells were found to bind and internalise HSPC1-peptide complexes and generate a T-cell response, while unconjugated peptide was unable to stimulate this same response. In order for APCs to effectively activate a T-cell response, they must undergo maturation to express appropriate co-stimulatory molecules. Indeed, HSPA1A has been shown to stimulate the expression of CD40, CD83 and CD86 on Dendritic cells (Bausero et al. 2005; Kuppner et al. 2001). Additionally, the expression and release of pro-inflammatory cytokines such as IL-1β, IL-6, IL-12 and TNF-α is stimulated by HSPs (Asea et al. 2000; Baretto et al. 2003; Todryk et al. 1999). There appears to be a positive feedback system in which APC-released pro-inflammatory cytokines augment transcription and release of HSPA1A from tumour cells (Baretto et al. 2003). The immunomodulatory properties of extracellular HSPs have identified them as a potential 'danger signal', released by cells in order to signal stress to the immune system (Todryk et al. 2000; Williams & Ireland 2008). Furthermore, as HSP-peptide complexes can induce both innate and adaptive immunity, they have become attractive candidates for immunotherapy protocols. Clinical trials have investigated the use of HSP-based vaccines on solid tumours and lymphomas but results have been inconclusive (Murshid et al. 2008). The technique involves isolating and purifying HSP from the patient's tumour cells and re-applying this as a vaccine in order to stimulate an immune response. A critical advantage of using such treatments is that, by exploiting the chaperoning ability of HSPs, a broad range of tumour-specific peptides, unique to that specific tumour will be targeted.

4.2 Distinct roles of membrane bound HSPs

A number of HSPs are also present on the tumour cell surface, and have distinct roles dependent on the specific HSP. HSPA1A in particular has been found embedded in the cell membrane of a variety of tumour cell types (Kleinjung et al. 2003; Pfister et al. 2007) and work from our lab has shown sHSPA1A on CD5+/CD19+ cells from CLL patients (Dempsey et al. 2010a). To date, it appears that the membrane localisation of HSPA1A is specific to tumour cells and has attracted much attention as a potential therapeutic target (Gehrmann et al. 2008; Krause et al. 2004), the implications of which will be discussed later in this chapter.

sHSPA1A acts a recognition structure for activated NK-cells (Gehrmann et al. 2003; Gross et al. 2003; Multhoff et al. 1999) and is therefore detrimental for the tumour cell. The region of the HSPA1A molecule exposed to the extracellular milieu of tumours has been identified as the 14-mer peptide TKDNNLLGRFELSG (TKD peptide) (Multhoff et al. 2001). The stimulation of NK cells using the TKD peptide and low dose IL-2 results in up-regulation of CD94/CD56 on NK cells and initiates NK-cell killing of sHSPA1A+ tumour cells (Gross et al. 2003; Gross et al. 2008; Multhoff et al. 1999). Interestingly, purified (perforin-free) granzyme B from NK-cells was shown to bind to HSPA1A and result in granzyme B internalisation into sHSPA1A+ tumour cells (Gross et al. 2003). Stimulation of NK-cells was also observed following incubation with sHSPA1A+ tumour-cell derived exosomes (Gastpar et al. 2005). Wei et al. (1996) demonstrated that sHSPA1A is also a target for δγT-cells. Furthermore, the induced *in-vivo* expression of sHSPA1A on tumour cells increases their immunogenicity, resulting in both a CTL-mediated and NK-cell mediated response and rejection of the tumour (Chen et al. 2002a). The expression of sHSPA1A, therefore, overcomes many of the characteristics that tumour cells develop to evade immune recognition, including down-regulation of MHC molecules, and down-regulation of co-stimulatory and adhesion molecules (Bausero et al, 2005; Chen et al. 2002a). The literature to date, suggests that the cellular location of HSPA1A is crucial in determining disease outcome as iHSPA1A is advantageous to the tumour, while sHSPA1A appears to be detrimental.

In contrast to this theory, the small number of studies to date, investigating the presence of sHSPA1A in primary cells from leukaemic patients suggest that its presence may in fact be detrimental for the patient. The study by Gehrmann et al. (2003) demonstrated that although sHSPA1A acted as a recognition structure for NK cells, sHSPA1A expression could be correlated with unfavourable or intermediate cytogenetics. Similarly, sHSPA1A levels were found to be higher in AML patients with treatment-refractory disease and active disease than patients in complete remission, suggesting a correlation with poor prognosis (Steiner et al. 2006). Furthermore, AML patients continuing to express moderately high levels of sHSPA1A after achieving remission were shown to have a shorter relapse-free survival time than remission patients with lower levels of sHSPA1A (Steiner et al. 2006). No correlation between sHSPA1A expression and stage of AML or resistance to chemotherapy could be determined by Steiner et al. (2006), suggesting that surface localisation of HSPA1A cannot be investigated in isolation. Schilling et al. (2007) demonstrated co-expression of HSPA1A with phosphatidylserine (PS) on the surface of hypoxic tumour cell lines. Additionally, exogenously added HSPA1A was shown to bind to PS on the cell surface and enhance the response to radiation. The results indicate that the radiotherapy-resistance observed in many hypoxic tumours may be overcome by prior treatment with HSPA1A.

In addition to HSPA1A, cell surface expression of HSPC1 and HSPB1 on tumour cells has been reported (Becker et al. 2004; Brameshuber et al. 2010; Ferrarini et al. 1992; Shin et al. 2003). sHSPC1 has been shown to be involved in tissue invasion and metastasis (Eustace et al. 2004), while the role of sHSPB1 is still unclear. Indeed, inhibiting cell surface expression of HSPC1, both *in-vitro* and *in-vivo*, reduces cell motility and invasiveness (Eustace et al. 2004; Tsutsumi et al. 2008). Work by Sidera et al. (2008) proposes that in some cancer cell types, sHSPC1 interacts with and activates HER-2, resulting in homodimerisation with ErbB-3, signal transduction pathway activation and ultimately actin rearrangement. Secretion of HSPC1 in exosomes has also been discovered, and has been shown to contribute to cancer cell invasiveness (McCready et al. 2010).

It is clear that extracellular HSPs have critical roles in tumour development and immune responses and we therefore suggest that mechanistic investigations of tumour biology should include analysis of extracellular, as well as intracellular, HSPs.

5. HSPs in leukaemia

Although a large amount of data exists regarding the expression of HSPs in cancer, the majority of studies have focused on solid tumours. Cells within a solid tumour mass are subjected to high levels of stress; the tumour microenvironment is often hypoxic and nutrient deficient and there may be infiltration by large numbers of immune cells. Therefore it is not surprising that HSP levels are elevated in many solid tumour types. Leukaemia cells however, are not subjected to these same stresses and as a result may not necessarily show elevated levels of HSPs.

Of the limited number of studies investigating HSP expression in leukaemia, a number have focused on correlating HSP expression with prognosis and clinical outcome, while others have directed research towards HSP expression and susceptibility to apoptosis. One study by Thomas et al. (2005) explored the expression of intracellular HSPB1, HSPD1, HSPA1A, HSPC1 and HSPH2 in both peripheral blood and bone marrow from patients with Acute Myeloid Leukaemia (AML). It was noted that complete remission rates were higher in patients with lower HSP expression and that overall survival was also significantly longer in these patients. Similarly, overall survival was found to be significantly greater in Myelodysplastic Syndrome (MDS) patients with lower HSPB1, HSPD1, HSPC1 and HSPH2 expression (Duval et al. 2006). A study exploring the expression of surface HSPA1A (sHSPA1A) in bone marrow aspirates from AML patients demonstrated that patients in complete remission express significantly lower levels of sHSPA1A when compared to patients with active AML (Steiner et al. 2006). Taken together these results suggest that higher levels of HSP expression both internally and on the surface of the leukaemic cell are advantageous to the cancer cell and therefore an adverse factor for the patient. This is in contrast to studies that have demonstrated the involvement of sHSPA1A in immune recognition and tumour regression (Chen et al. 2002; Multhoff et al. 1999; Gross et al. 2003; Gross et al. 2008).

HSP expression in AML and MDS has also been found to correlate with expression of the myeloblast surface antigen CD34, a well established poor prognostic factor (Duval et al. 2006; Thomas et al. 2005). Moreover, AML and MDS patients with intermediate or unfavourable karyotypes display a higher level of HSP expression than patients with favourable karyotypes. In contrast, Steiner et al. (2006) did not establish a correlation between sHSPA1A expression and cytogenetic risk group or FAB subtype. A study into expression of HSPD1, HSPA1A, HSPA8 (constitutive and heat-inducible forms) and HSPC1 in AML cells showed a heterogeneous expression of all three HSPs and no correlation was found between this extensive range of HSP expression and clinical outcome (Chant et al. 1995). However, a more recent study by the same group demonstrated that although AML cells show a broad range of HSPA1A expression, this expression correlates with susceptibility to apoptosis (Chant et al. 1996). Surprisingly, the correlation between HSPA1A expression and apoptosis was positive, indicating that cells with higher levels of the protein are more susceptible to apoptosis. This finding is contradictory to the theory that HSPA1A protects cells from apoptosis. In spite of this correlation between HSPA1A and apoptosis, none was found between expression of HSPC1 and susceptibility to apoptosis. In contrast, levels of HSPA1A in MDS did not correlate with either pro- or anti-apoptotic protein levels (Duval et al. 2006). However, levels of HSPB1, HSPD1, HSPC1 and HSPH2 negatively correlated with the expression of the pro-apoptotic proteins Bad and Bak, while correlating positively with the anti-apoptotic proteins Bcl-2 and Bcl-Xl.

Research into acute lymphoblastic leukaemia (ALL) has shown decreased expression of HSPA1A and HSPB1 in bone marrow aspirates from patients who achieved complete remission when compared to those patients who did not achieve complete remission (Campos et al. 1999). Additionally, ALL cells displaying the Bcr/Abl fusion protein contained high levels of HSPA1A (Nimmanapalli et al. 2002). Further studies have demonstrated that HSPA1A contributes to the Bcr-Abl–mediated resistance to apoptosis by chemotherapeutic agents such as etoposide. Moreover, down-regulation of HSPA1A can sensitise these Bcr/Abl ALL cells to cytotoxic drugs (Guo et al. 2005). The Bcr/Abl fusion protein was shown to be a client protein of HSPC1. Furthermore, inhibition of HSPC1, but not HSPA1A, in myeloid cells was found to result in degradation of Bcr/Abl (Peng et al. 2007).

6. HSPs in chronic lymphocytic leukaemia

An extensive study by our group analysed the levels of HSPB1, HSPA1A and HSPC1 in CD5+/CD19+ and CD5-/CD19+ cells from CLL patients and normal lymphocytes from control subjects (Dempsey et al. 2010a). At first glance, it would appear that levels of both iHSPC1 and iHSPB1 are significantly higher in CLL patients overall than normal age-matched control subjects. An initial analysis of our data would also support the hypothesis that elevated intracellular HSP leads to tumour cells being resistant to apoptosis (Khaleque et al. 2005; Nylandsted et al. 2000; Thomas et al. 2005; Vargas-Roig et al. 1998); Caspase-3, a marker of apoptosis, was found to be lower in CLL patients compared to age-matched control subjects, while levels of iHSPB1 and iHSPC1 were higher in CLL patients. We also observed a negative correlation between levels of caspase-3 and iHSPB1. An observed difference in caspase-3 levels between CLL and control subjects is not surprising since the underlying basis of CLL is an inability for B-lymphocytes to commit to apoptosis. There was, however, no difference in caspase-3 levels between patients at different stages of the disease which suggests that the progression of CLL is more likely to be a result of an increased cellular clonal replication rather than an increased resistance to apoptosis from the same cells. A more detailed analysis of the data has demonstrated that CLL patients in different Binet stages express distinct levels of iHSPC1; Levels of iHSPC1 in Binet stage A patients are significantly higher than levels observed in Binet stage B and C patients. This is surprising, as the anti-apoptotic nature of these proteins would suggest they may be elevated in patients with a more advanced disease. However, the elevated levels of HSPC1 in patients with a less severe disease could be interpreted as a stress response in the early stages of the disease, which aids CLL cells in surviving immune destruction. As the disease progresses and CLL cells replicate uncontrollably, these very high HSPC1 levels are no longer required for cell survival and therefore begin to decrease.

Our data has also revealed that CLL patients can be divided into two groups based on their expression of iHSPA1A in CD5+/CD19+ cells; one group of patients presents very low levels of iHSPA1A while the other group expresses levels up to 1000-fold higher. This is also the case for sHSPA1A, although the difference is less pronounced. It should be noted that patients expressing very low levels of iHSPA1A are not necessarily the same patients that express low levels of sHSPA1A as no correlation between sHSPA1A and iHSPA1A could be found. Interestingly these CLL patients classified into the 'low sHSPA1A or iHSPA1A expressing' groups display HSPA1A levels similar to levels in non-malignant CD5-/CD19+ cells from the same patients and also lymphocytes from control subjects. In spite of this differential expression of HSPA1A amongst CLL patients, neither sHSPA1A nor iHSPA1A can be correlated with stage of disease or cytogenetic abnormality. Our data supports the work by Chant et al. (1995) who have demonstrated a wide range of HSP expression amongst AML patients. We have also determined that CLL patients with stable disease (not requiring treatment) possess significantly higher levels of iHSPA1A than patients with progressive disease (requiring treatment), which is in line with the decrease in HSPC1 seen as the disease progresses.

There is also considerable variation in the levels of extracellular HSPA1A (eHSPA1A) present in the serum of CLL patients. When considered as a group, levels of eHSPA1A in CLL patients are not significantly different from levels in control subjects. However, a more detailed analysis of the data reveals a correlation between the levels of extracellular and intracellular HSPA1A in CLL patients. Interestingly patients receiving corticosteroid treatment display significantly lower levels of HSPA1A in serum when compared to patients not receiving corticosteroid treatment, with some steroid-treated patients showing near-undetectable levels of eHSPA1A. This suggests that steroid treatment may totally inhibit the secretion of HSPA1A, although this remains to be confirmed. However, in addition to their negative effects on lymphocyte proliferation, T-cell activation and NK-cell function, corticosteroids have been shown to regulate transcription factors. As eHSPA1A and iHSPA1A levels correlate and eHSPA1A levels are lower in steroid-treated patients, it could be deduced that the transcription of HSPA1A has been inhibited. This conclusion is supported by the decrease in HSPA1A release observed following commencement of glucocorticoid treatment in CLL patients.

CLL patients often display resistance to corticosteroid therapy which is attributed to the imbalanced expression of glucocorticoid receptor (GR) isoforms. Indeed, higher expression of the transcriptionally inactive glucocorticoid receptor-beta (GR-beta) in relation to the hormone-activated transcription factor GR-alpha has been observed in CLL cells (Shahidi et al. 1999). However, as the GR is a client protein of HSPC1, variation in HSPC1 concentration may result in defective ligand binding, which may also contribute to resistance (Bailey et al. 2001). Indeed it has been demonstrated that the ratio of HSPC1 to GR expression is significantly higher in steroid-resistant compared to steroid-sensitive multiple sclerosis patients (Matysiak et al. 2008). This suggests that CLL patients in Binet stage A, whose HSPC1 expression is high, may have a reduced sensitivity for the steroid.

In summary although HSPs appear to be elevated in CLL patients compared to control subjects, closer examination of the data reveals that this is not the case in all CLL patients and in fact, there is a large variability in HSPB1, HSPA1A and HSPC1 amongst patients which can be associated with disease stage and also treatment regime. The results indicate that the concept of HSPs being over-expressed in cancer may in fact be oversimplified. Indeed, it is now becoming apparent that there is also great variability in HSP expression in solid tumours such as breast cancer (Zagouri et al. 2010). These findings are crucial in helping to determine whether future treatments targeting HSPs maybe considered as a universal option.

7. Heat shock proteins as therapeutic targets

Many of the most recently developed anti-cancer treatments are targeted towards a single specific oncoprotein. Although in many cases, this has been largely successful (Flaherty et al. 2010; Kantarjian et al. 2003) cancer cells may acquire resistance to these treatments via a number of mechanisms including secondary mutations in the target binding domain and activation of alternative signalling pathways (Nazarian et al. 2010; Shah et al. 2002). Indeed, by their very nature, cancers accumulate oncogenic mutations as they progress and therefore a treatment strategy that involves the selective targeting of a specific protein kinase, for example, is unlikely to show continued success. As stated earlier, HSPs contribute to each of the six hallmarks of cancer and as a result have multiple molecular targets. In particular, HSPC1 appears to play a fundamental role in the development and maintenance of several tumour characteristics (Neckers, 2007). HSPC1 binds and stabilises a broad array of mutated oncoproteins (An et al. 2000; Minami et al. 2002; Pashtan et al. 2008), so the targeting of this single chaperone, should in theory, destabilise and degrade a wide variety of signalling kinases, therefore simultaneously targeting a number of cell signalling pathways. Furthermore, by selectively inhibiting HSPC1, all six 'hallmarks of cancer' (Hanahan & Weinberg, 2001; Hanahan & Weinberg, 2011) can be targeted in parallel, thereby dramatically reducing the probability that a resistant clone will develop. Since the identification of the first HSPC1 inhibitors 25 years ago, interest into these novel therapies has expanded considerably and the development of newer inhibitors has focussed on increasing efficacy and reducing side effects. Indeed a large body of data now exists documenting their anti-cancer effects on a wide variety of tumour cell types (Kim et al. 2009) both in isolation and in combination with common chemotherapeutic agents. HSPC1 inhibitors are currently grouped according to their site of action; N-terminal inhibitors and C-terminal inhibitors.

7.1 N-terminal HSPC1 inhibitors

The original N-terminal inhibitors, geldanamycin (GA) and radicicol were naturally occurring antibacterial products discovered in *Streptomyces hygroscopicus*. Initial experiments using these compounds revealed binding to HSPC1 and consequent degradation of the HSPC1 client protein v-src (Whitesell et al. 1994). Although subsequent experiments proved that these natural HSPC1 inhibitors were able to cause the degradation of a wide range of client proteins, the non-specific toxicity of these compounds prevented their clinical use. However, these experiments led to the development of the first clinically applicable HSPC1 inhibitor, 17-AAG (17-allylamino-17-demethoxygeldanamycin, also known as tanespimycin) (Holzbeierlein et al. 2010). As a derivative of GA, 17-AAG resulted in the degradation of a variety of oncogenic proteins in a number of tumour cell types, while displaying reduced toxicity. This compound was entered into clinical trials and tested on a broad array of cancers including a large variety of haematological malignancies such as AML, ALL, CML and CLL. Detailed reviews of clinical trial data can be found in Kim et al. (2009), Taldone et al. (2008) and Holzbeierlein et al. (2010). In addition to showing initial promise as a novel therapy in isolation, 17-AAG also demonstrated synergism with a number of chemotherapeutic agents such as Bortezomib (Richardson et al. 2010), Trastuzumab (Modi et al. 2007) and Paclitaxel (Ramalingam et al. 2008). An alternative derivative of GA, 17-DMAG (17-dimethylaminoethylamino-17-demethoxygeldanamycin, also known as alvespimycin) was subsequently produced, with greater solubility and showed similar initial success in phase I and II clinical trials. Based on the results using 17-AAG and 17-DMAG, interest into the development of alternative HSPC1 inhibitors has increased greatly and has produced a number of N-terminal inhibitors including IPI-504 (Retaspimycin hydrochloride), AUY922, BIIB021 and SNX-2112 (Eccles et al. 2009; Hanson & Vesole, 2009; Lundgren et al. 2009; Okawa et al. 2008). In spite of these promising results and continuous research and development, clinical trials involving N-terminal inhibitors have not been without limitations. Hepatotoxicity and poor solubility of the drugs have been frequently reported. Furthermore, despite the idea of targeting the six 'hallmarks of cancer' through the inhibition of HSPC1, drug resistance has become an issue. This has been attributed to the increase in HSPB1 and HSPA1A following HSPC1 inhibition (Dakappagari et al. 2010; Ravagnan et al. 2001) due to enhanced activity of HSF-1, thereby increasing cellular resistance to apoptosis. This increase in HSPB1 and HSPA1A appears to be a complication related to the use of all N-terminal inhibitors (Taldone et al. 2008). A review by Holzbeierlein et al. (2010) highlights three significant clinical trials involving 17-AAG in which no anti-cancer response was observed and recruitment into the trials was terminated prematurely. Similarly, unexpected problems have been encountered using 17-DMAG. Another issue with HSPC1 inhibition is that, in addition to chaperoning many oncogenic proteins, HSPC1 also chaperones many other proteins with anti-tumour activities. The tumour suppressor proteins LKB1 (Boudeau et al. 2003), LATS1, LATS2 (Huntoon et al. 2010) and wild-type p53 (Walerych et al. 2004) are all down-regulated following treatment with HSPC1 inhibitors. These results highlight the potential disadvantages of HSPC1 inhibitor therapies.

7.2 C-terminal HSPC1 inhibitors

Research into HSPC1 inhibitors has primarily focused on N-terminal inhibition, however a small number of C-terminal inhibitors have been identified. Novobiocin was the first C-terminal HSPC1 inhibitor to be identified, and similarly to GA, is a naturally occurring antibiotic produced in *Streptomyces niveu*. However, novobiocin was found to have a weak affinity for its target and as a result was not therapeutically applicable. Subsequently, research has focused on the synthesis of novobiocin analogues with a stronger affinity for HSPC1. According to a review by Holzbeierlein et al. (2010), over 300 analogues have been screened resulting in the identification of compounds with improved activity and selectivity of tumour over non-tumour cells. It has also been noted that the anti-cancer agent cisplatin and the polyphenolic flavanoid Epigallocatechin-3-gallate (EGCG) can inhibit HSPC1 activity via C-terminal inhibition (Soti et al. 2002; Yin et al. 2009). Cisplatin has been used as a conventional chemotherapy for decades due to its ability to form DNA adducts and therefore prevent DNA transcription. By binding to the C-terminal, cisplatin hinders nucleotide binding. Treatment of a human ovarian cell line with EGCG was found to inhibit HSPC1 activity and therefore result in the degradation of several client proteins including ErbB2, Raf-1, and phosphorylated Akt (Yin et al. 2009).

C-terminal inhibitors appear to have many non-specific effects and as a result have not been entered into clinical trials (Sreedhar et al. 2004). However, recent research has revealed that C-terminal inhibition, unlike N-terminal inhibition, does not result in the enhanced activity of HSF-1 (Conde et al. 2009; Holzbeierlein et al. 2010). Indeed, treatment of Xenopus oocytes with heat shock in the presence of novobiocin results in a dose dependent decrease in HSF-1 transcriptional activity (Conde et al. 2009). In contrast similar treatment of these cells in the presence of GA resulted in a dose-dependent increase in HSF-1 activity. This lack of HSF-1 induction is a very attractive attribute of C-terminal inhibitors and therefore research and development into synthetic C-terminal inhibitors continues.

7.3 Important HSPC1 client proteins in CLL

Research into the involvement of HSPC1 in cancer progression has identified a wide variety of client proteins that may contribute to the progression of both solid tumours and haematological malignancies. There are a number of HSPC1 clients that have been implicated in the development and progression of CLL in particular (Johnson et al. 2007) and therefore the use of HSPC1 inhibitors as a treatment option appears attractive. The list of HSPC1 client proteins is continually expanding suggesting that novel therapeutic targets in CLL may present themselves in the future.

The tyrosine kinase Zeta-associated Protein-70 (ZAP-70) is a well established poor prognostic factor and an HSPC1 client (Bartis et al. 2007). In normal T-cells, ZAP-70 is associated with the TCR where it functions in downstream TCR signalling (Cruse et al. 2007). However, although ZAP-70 is present in normal pre-B-cells, its expression should be lost on maturation of the cell. Hence, the presence of ZAP-70 in CLL cells is indicative of an immature clone. A study by Crespo et al. (2003) found that ZAP-70 expression in CLL correlates with disease progression and survival, and also correlates with another well established CLL prognostic factor, IgV_H mutational status. Castro et al. (2005) demonstrated that ZAP-70 in CLL cells co-immunoprecipitates with HSPC1, while ZAP-70 from normal T-cells does not. In addition, treatment of ZAP-70$^+$ CLL cells with HSPC1 inhibitors resulted in degradation of ZAP-70, while treatment of T-cells from CLL and control patients with HSPC1 inhibitors did not affect the expression of ZAP-70. Manipulation of ZAP-70$^-$ CLL cells to express ZAP-70 was shown to activate HSPC1 and induce sensitivity to 17-AAG.

The tumour suppressor protein p53, encoded by the *TP53* gene is frequently mutated in CLL, and other cancer types. Mutant p53$^+$ CLL patients show increased resistance to a wide range of chemotherapeutic agents (Sturm et al. 2003) and therefore are often treated as a distinct sub-group of patients. Indeed agents that act independently of the p53 pathway, such as the monoclonal antibodies rituximab and alemtuzumab and other agents such as lenalidomide, are often used as alternative first-line treatments for patients with a 17p deletion (mutated p53 status). HSPC1 inhibitor treatment of CLL cells results in a dose-dependent reduction in mutant p53 levels, a simultaneous up-regulation of wild type p53 and consequent cytotoxicity (Lin et al. 2007). This treatment also results in an increase in p21, an inducer of cell cycle arrest.

It should be noted that this same study showed that CLL cells without a p53 mutation were also sensitive to HSPC1 inhibitor treatment. However, this could be due to activation of wild-type p53 and consequent p53-dependent apoptosis. Further research has shown a synergistic effect between 17-DMAG and Doxorubicin, demonstrating a sensitisation of p53 mutated cells to Doxorubicin-induced cell death (Robles et al. 2006).

HSPC1 chaperones a broad array of protein kinases involved in signal transduction pathways including phosphorylated Akt, Lyn, B-Raf and IκK (Broemer et al. 2004; da Rocha Dias et al. 2005; Sato et al. 2000; Trentin et al. 2011). The interaction of HSPC1 with these phosphorylated kinases prevents dephosphorylation of the kinase and its subsequent inactivation, therefore maintaining its activity. The over-activity of Akt (Ringshausen et al. 2002), Lyn (Contri et al. 2005), and implied elevation of IκK (Hertlein et al. 2010) in CLL cells has been previously observed and thought to contribute to cell survival and activation of downstream kinases. Indeed, as IκK regulates the activation of the NF-κB family of transcription factors, its over-activity has implications for a large number of NF-κB target genes including Bcl-2, X-IAP, c-FLIP and Mcl-1 (Hertlein et al. 2010). In fact, a number of these proteins have been implicated in the progression of CLL and have been found to correlate with poor prognosis (Pepper et al. 2008; Pepper et al. 2009) which may suggest a clear link to over-activity of NF-κB. Nevertheless, HSPC1 inhibitor treatment has been shown to destabilise Akt, Lyn and IκK (Hertlein et al. 2010; Johnson et al. 2007; Jones et al. 2004; Lin et al. 2007; Trentin et al. 2008), in CLL cells resulting in proteosomal degradation of these HSPC1 clients and ultimately apoptosis. A study by McCraig et al. (2011) showed that CD40 stimulation of CLL cells *in-vitro* increased the expression of the anti-apoptotic protein Mcl-1 and enhanced cell survival, suggesting that Mcl-1 may be responsible for *in-vivo* survival of CLL cells following CD40 stimulation by T-cells. 17-DMAG treatment of CLL cells was found to result in down-regulation of Mcl-1 even in the presence of CD40 stimulation and inhibit *in-vitro* survival (Hertlein et al. 2010; McCraig et al. 2011) suggesting that *in-vivo* treatment with 17-DMAG may prevent CLL survival associated with T-cell stimulation in lymph nodes.

The B-cell restricted enzyme, Activation-Induced Cytidine Deaminase (AID) has been shown to have prognostic significance in CLL (Heintel et al. 2004; Palacios et al. 2010). This enzyme is required in normal B-cells for somatic hypermutation and class switch recombination (CSR) and is induced following interaction of CD40 with CD40L on T-cells in germinal centres. However, AID expression has been found in CLL cells circulating in peripheral blood and has been found to correlate with unmutated IgV_H status and unfavourable cytogenetics (Heintel et al. 2004). AID expressing CLL cells were also shown to expresses high levels of anti-apoptotic proteins and proliferation factors (Palacios et al. 2010). It was proposed that these high levels of AID and ongoing CSR are a consequence of recent contact with the proliferation centres and provides further evidence that the microenvironment plays a critical role in CLL cell survival and disease progression. Interestingly, AID is an HSPC1 client and chemical inhibition of HSPC1 activity results in destabilisation and proteosomal degradation of AID and reduced antibody diversification (Orthwein et al. 2010).

It would appear that HSPC1 inhibitor treatment of CLL cells targets a wide variety of client proteins, many of which have been implicated in the progression of the disease.

Furthermore, HSPC1 inhibitor-induced cell death appears to be p53 independent suggesting that it may also be useful in the treatment of patients with a mutated p53 status. However, it is well established that CLL has an extremely heterogeneous clinical course and as a result patients show great variation in their responses to specific treatments. Results from our lab have shown that CLL patients also show great heterogeneity in HSP levels with some patients expressing very high levels of a particular HSP and some patients expressing extremely low levels (Dempsey et al. 2010a). These results indicate that although targeting HSPs may appear an attractive strategy, it may not be successful in all patients. Therefore, HSP analysis may prove useful in providing a personalised treatment.

7.4 Effect of HSPC1 inhibition on normal cells

As HSPC1 is abundant in non-tumour cells, the use of HSPC1 inhibitors as anti-cancer therapies may seem impractical. Indeed, the survival of normal cells following exposure to stressors such as ionising radiation or cytotoxic drugs is dependent upon activation of signal transduction pathways, the components of which are HSPC1 client proteins. This is important as in the clinical setting, both tumour and non-tumour cells may have been pre-exposed to cytotoxic drugs or ionising radiation as part of previous therapy. Little is known about the effects of HSPC1 inhibition on signal transduction pathways in stressed non-tumour cells and whether the response to HSPC1 inhibitors depends upon the pre-existing levels of HSPA1A and HSPB1 in target cells. Although HSPC1 inhibitors have been shown to be highly tumour-specific, this has recently been questioned (Gooljarsingh et al. 2006). If correct, introduction of these inhibitors into the systemic circulation, where they will have access to both tumour and non-tumour cells, may introduce complications and this issue warrants further investigation.

7.5 Targeting HSPA1A

At present, the modulation of HSPA1A activity using chemical inhibitors does not appear to be achievable in the clinical setting. Although, several compounds are able to inhibit the activity of HSF-1 and therefore regulate HSPA1A, the associated toxicity with HSF-1 and HSPA1A inhibitors is too severe. Furthermore, the inhibition of HSF-1 appears to have a number of associated effects such as the up-regulation of Hsp32, which itself is anti-apoptotic (Lin et al. 2004; Yao et al. 2007). The flavanoid quercetin and the benzylidene lactam KNK-437 have both been shown to inhibit HSPA1A and HSPB1 and sensitise cells to chemotherapeutic drugs or hyperthermia (Taba et al. 2011; Sahin et al. 2011; Zanini et al. 2007). Furthermore, the ability of KNK-437 to enhance the anti-tumour activity of HSPC1 inhibitors has been demonstrated (Guo et al. 2005), although as yet, this has not been tested on primary cells. These data suggest that if the solubility issues and non-specific effects of these inhibitors can be resolved, HSF-1 and/or HSPA1A may prove effective therapeutic targets. Recent work by Zaarur et al. (2006) used a high throughput screening programme to identify chemicals with the capacity to inhibit the heat shock response. Although a number of compounds were identified, one in particular, Emunin, showed very low levels of toxicity while sensitising cells to HSPC1 inhibitors and proteosome inhibitors. Interestingly, this compound appeared to have a novel mode of action as it did not affect HSF-1 activity. Although its exact mechanism remains to be determined, it appears to possess a specific regulatory affect on HSP protein translation. A further benefit of using this type of compound is that if, as in some cases, the over-expression of HSPs in a tumour is HSF-1 independent (Zaarur et al. 2006), manipulating the stress response in this way may still prove advantageous.

The surface expression of HSPA1A on tumour cells provides a novel focus for anti-cancer therapies. The ability of membrane embedded HSPA1A to bind and stimulate NK-cells and induce killing of sHSPA1A+ tumour cells (Gross et al. 2003; Gross et al. 2008; Multhoff et al. 1999) has led to trials involving *ex-vivo* stimulation of autologous NK-cells with TKD peptide and low dose IL-2. This patient-specific technique involves obtaining leukocyte concentrates from the patient by leukapheresis, purifying PBMCs and stimulating them with TKD peptide/low dose IL-2 for four days. Following stimulation, the activated PBMC preparation is re-infused into the patient. Re-infusion is repeated every fortnight for a maximum of five doses (Krause et al. 2004). This technique has been shown to eliminate the primary tumour, prevent metastasis and significantly increase life expectancy in tumour mouse models (Mutlhoff et al. 2000; Stangl et al. 2006). Furthermore, use of this technique in patients with lower rectal carcinoma and non-small cell lung carcinoma was found to increase NK-cell cytotoxicity against sHSPA1A+ tumour cells (Krause et al. 2004) and was found to be well tolerated. However, it should be noted that patients included in this study did not show complete remission following treatment but these were patients with advanced disease and were refractory to standard chemotherapy. A subsequent case study using another advanced disease patient was unsuccessful in attaining remission, but did demonstrate the maintenance of NK-cell cytolytic activity following TKD-IL-2 stimulation (Milani et al. 2009). These data suggest that *ex-vivo* TKD/IL-2 stimulation of autologous NK-cells may have therapeutic potential.

As an alternative strategy to inhibiting the activity of HSPs, recent work from our lab attempted to manipulate the cellular location of HSPs in order to sensitise CLL cells to chemotherapeutic agents (Dempsey et al. 2010b). As mentioned earlier, a number of HSPs associate with lipid rafts and incorporate into the plasma membrane (Gastpar et al. 2005; Nagy et al. 2007; Vega et al. 2008) where they may remain or may be released into the extracellular environment. Vigh et al. (2007b) have proposed a 'membrane sensor model' in which cell stress may be detected at the membrane level and the cell is able to produce a stress response. It is proposed that stress signals originating from the cell membrane result in activation of specific HSP genes and movement of these newly synthesised HSPs to the membrane where they facilitate in stabilising the cell membrane (Vigh et al. 2007a) and therefore facilitating cell survival (Figure 2). It is proposed that a change in membrane fluidity and microdomain organisation (Torok et al. 2003; Vigh et al. 2007a) may be sufficient to result in such membrane stress signals. Our group used several membrane fluidising treatments including aliphatic alcohol, local anaesthetic or mild hyperthermia to fluidise the cell membrane and induce movement of HSPs to the cell surface (Dempsey et al. 2010b). The result was a change in the cellular localisation of HSPA1A, HSPD1, and to a lesser extent, HSPB1 and HSPC1. We found that this movement to the cell surface resulted in a transient decrease in internal levels of HSPs. This temporary decrease in anti-apoptotic HSPs allowed a number of chemotherapeutic agents including Doxorubicin, Cyclophosphamide and TRAIL to act on the cells resulting in significant cytotoxicity of CLL cells. Interestingly, by combining membrane fluidising treatments with chemotherapeutic agents, low doses of drugs were able to cause considerable apoptosis. These low doses were unable to cause cytotoxicity in isolation. We found that inhibiting the movement of HSPs using methyl-β-cyclodextrin (mβcd), a cholesterol sequestering agent, and inhibitor of lipid raft transport, prior to combination treatment, prevented the synergistic effect of fluidising treatment and chemotherapeutic drug. The results suggest that manipulation of HSP cellular location may be an attractive strategy for enhancing the chemotherapeutic treatment of CLL. Furthermore, this method does not rely on CLL patients expressing similar levels of internal HSPs and therefore is an attractive therapeutic approach for a heterogeneous disease. Furthermore, the data may point to a revival of targeted hyperthermia to induce HSP translocation in combination with other therapeutic agents.

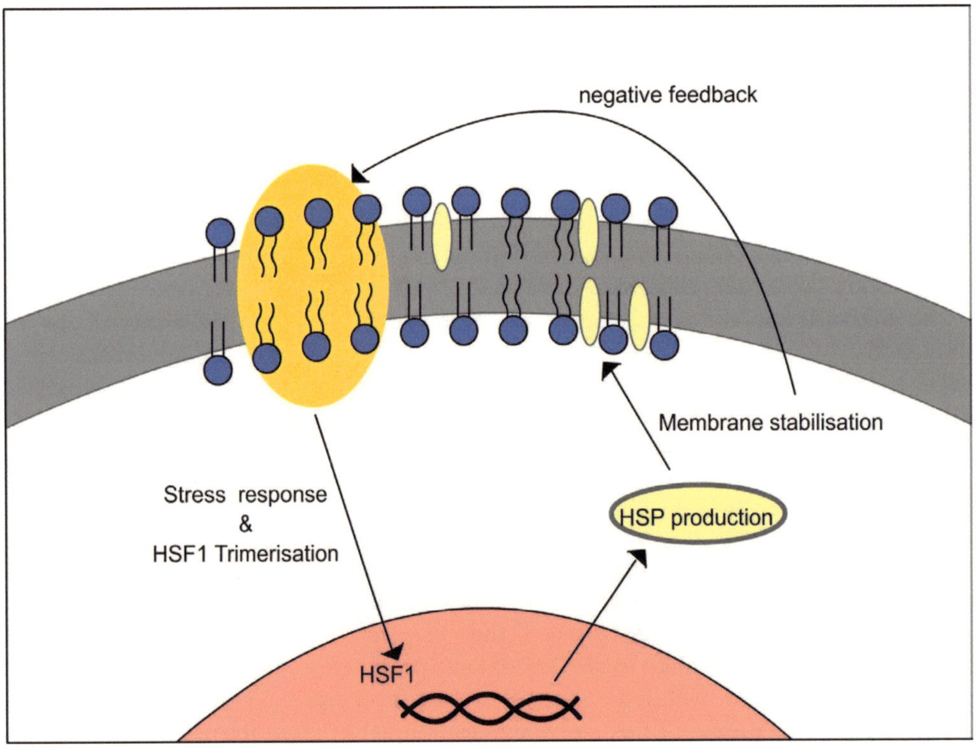

Fig. 2. Induction of an HSP Response via Alteration in Membrane Fluidity (Taken from Dempsey, 2009). Change in membrane fluidity is detected at the membrane, activating a membrane signal which results in the transcription of HSP genes. Newly synthesised HSPs then move to the membrane resulting in membrane stabilisation and re-established membrane-lipid order. This stabilisation effect may itself be a negative feedback regulator to turn off HSP transcription.

8. Conclusion

The up-regulation of HSPs in cancer has led to a large variety of studies investigating their prognostic and therapeutic potential. Due to the stressful nature of tumour development, it is not surprising that these anti-apoptotic proteins remain elevated in cancer cells. The anti-apoptotic characteristics of these proteins enable tumour cells to survive in otherwise lethal conditions and hence have been associated with a poor prognosis and resistance to therapy.

These elements alone suggest HSPs may be suitable targets for therapy. However after considering that a number of HSPs are involved in the modifications required for cancer development (the six 'hallmarks of cancer'), they become particularly attractive. Further work on inhibiting HSP activity is required before such compounds can be considered as routine therapies. Extracellular HSPs have been shown to have critical roles in cancer progression with surface-bound HSPC1 in particular contributing to cell invasion and metastasis. Conversely, sHSPA1A has been shown to be detrimental to the tumour, stimulating NK-cell responses and resulting in tumour regression, while a number of extracellular HSPs present tumour-derived peptides to APCs resulting in antigen cross-presentation and T-cell responses. The beneficial effects of these extracellular HSPs have also formed the basis of research into HSP-based therapies focusing on increasing the immune response against tumours. Increasing HSP translocation via cell membrane fluidisation may therefore have the double benefit of increasing the susceptibility of tumours to chemotherapeutic agents and stimulating the immune response. Our work on CLL has found that HSPA1A, HSPB1 and HSPC1 are located inside CLL cells, on the cell surface and also in the serum of CLL patients. However, the pattern of patient variability within and between specific HSPs suggests that analysis of patient HSP profile would be beneficial in directing therapy.

9. References

Adams, D.J. & McGuire, W.L. (1983). Quantitative Enzyme-linked Immunosorbent Assay for the Estrogen-regulated Mr 24,000 Protein in Human Breast Tumors: Correlation with Estrogen and Progesterone Receptors. *Cancer Research*. 45(6):2445-2449

An, W.G., Schulte, T.W. & Neckers, L.M. (2000). The heat shock protein 90 antagonist geldanamycin alters chaperone association with p210(bcr-abl) and v-src proteins before their degradation by the proteasome. *Cell Growth & Differentiation*. 11(7):355-360

Arnold-Schild, D., Hanau, D., Spehner, D., Schmid, C., Rammensee, H.G., de la Salle, H. & Schild, H. (1999). Cutting Edge: Receptor-Mediated Endocytosis of Heat Shock Proteins by Professional Antigen-Presenting Cells. *The American Association of Immunologists*. 162(7):3757-3760

Asea, A., Kraeft, S.K., Kurt-Jones, E.A., Stevenson, M.A., Chen, L.B., Finberg, R.W., Koo, G.C. & Calderwood, S.K. (2000). HSP70 stimulates cytokine production through a CD14-dependant pathway, demonstrating its dual role as a chaperone and cytokine. *Nature Medicine*. 6(4):435-442

Bailey, S., A. G. Hall, A. D. J. Pearson and C. P. F. Redfern (2001). The role of AP-1 in glucocorticoid resistance in leukaemia. *Leukaemia Research*. 15(3):391-397.

Barreto, A., Gonzalez, J.M., Kabingu, E.K., Asea, A. & Fiorentino, S. (2003). Stress-induced release of HSC70 from human tumors. *Cellular Immunology*. 222(2):97–104

Bartis, D., Boldizsar, F., Kvell, K., Szabo, M., Palinkas, L., Nemeth, P., Monostori, E. & Berki, T. (2007). Intermolecular relations between the glucocorticoid receptor, ZAP-70 kinase, and Hsp-90. *Biochemical and Biophysical Research Communications*. 354(1):253-258

Basu, S., Binder, R., Ramalingam, T. & Srivastava, P. (2001). CD91 is a common receptor for Heat Shock Proteins gp96, hsp90, hsp70, and calreticulin. *Immunity*. 14(3):303-313

Bausero,M.A., Gastpar, R., Multhoff, G. & Asea, A. (2005). Alternative Mechanism by which IFN-γ Enhances Tumor Recognition: Active Release of Heat Shock Protein 72. *Journal of Immunology*. 175(5):2900-2912

Becker, B., Multhoff, G., Farkas, B., Wild, P.J., Landthaler, M., Stolz, W. & Vogt, T. (2004). Induction of Hsp90 protein expression in malignant melanomas and melanoma metastases. *Experimental Dermatology*.13(1):27–32.

Beere, H.M. & Green, D.R. (2001). Stress management - heat shock protein-70 and the regulation of apoptosis. *Trends in Cell Biology*. 11(1):6-10

Bolhassani, A. & Rafati, S. (2008). Heat-shock proteins as powerful weapons in vaccine development. *Expert Review Vaccines*. 7(8):1185-1189

Boudeau, J., Deak, M., Lawlor, M.A., Morrice, N.A. & Alessi, D.R. (2003). Heat-shock protein 90 and Cdc37 interact with LKB1 and regulate its stability. *Journal of Biochemistry*. 370(3):849-857

Brameshuber, M., Weghuber, J., Ruprecht, V., Gombos, I., Horvath, I., Vigh, L., Eckerstorfer, P., Kiss, E., Stockinger, H. & Schutz, G.J. (2010). Imaging of Mobile Long-lived Nanoplatforms in the Live Cell Plasma Membrane. *The Journal of Biological Chemistry*. 285(53):41765-41771

Broemer, M., Krappmann, D. & Scheidereit, C. (2004). Requirment of Hsp90 acitvity for IκB kinase (IKK) biosynthesis and for constitutive and inducible IKK and NF-κB function. *Oncogene*. 23(31):5378-5386

Calderwood, S.K., Khaleque, M. A., Sawyer, D.B. & Ciocca, D.R. (2006). Heat shock proteins in cancer: chaperones of tumorigenesis. *Trends in Biochemical Sciences*. 31(3):164-172

Calderwood, S.K., Mambula, S.S., Gray Jr., P.J. & Theriault, J.R. (2007). Extracellular heat shock proteins in cell signalling. *FEBS Letters*. 581(19):3689-3694

Campos, L., Chautard, S., Viallet, A. & Guyotat, D. (1999). Expression of heat-shock proteins in acute leukaemia cells. *Haematologica*. 84:13.

Castro, J.E., Prada, C.E., Loria, O., Kamal, A., Chen, L., Burrows, F.J. & Kipps, T.J. (2005). ZAP-70 is a novel conditional heat shock protein 90 (Hsp90) client: inhibition of Hsp90 leads to ZAP-70 degradation, apoptosis, and impaired signaling in chronic lymphocytic leukemia. *Blood*. 106(7):2506-2512

Chant, I. D., Rose, P. E., & Morris, A. G. (1995). Analysis of Heat-Shock Protein Expression in Myeloid-Leukemia Cells by Flow-Cytometry. *British Journal of Haematology*. 90(1):163-168.

Chant, I. D., Rose, P. E., & Morris, A. G. (1996). Susceptability of AML cells to in vitro apoptosis correlates with heat shock protein 70 (hsp70) expression. *British Journal of Haematology*. 93(4):898-902.

Charette, S.J., Lavoie, J.N., Lambert, H. & Landry, J. (2000). Inhibition of Daxx-mediated apoptosis by heat shock protein 27. *Molecular and Cellular Biology*. 20(20):7602-7612

Chauhan, D., Li, G., Hideshima, T., Podar, K., Mitsiades, C., Mitsiades, N., Catley, L., Tai, Y.T., Hayashi, T., Shringarpure, R., Burger, R., Munshi, N., Ohtake, Y., Saxena, S. & Anderson, K.C. (2003a). Hsp27 inhibits release of mitochondrial protein Smac in multiple myeloma cells and confers dexamethasone resistance. *Blood*. 22(3):816-834

Chauhan D, Li GL, Shringarpure R, Podar K, Ohtake Y, Hideshima T, Anderson KC (2003b). Blockade of Hsp27 overcomes bortezomib/proteasome inhibitor PS-341 resistance in lymphoma cells. *Cancer Research.* 63(19):6174-6177

Chen, X., Tao, Q., Yu, H., Zhang, L. & Cao, X. (2002a). Tumor cell membrane-bound heat shock protein 70 elicits antitumor Immunity. *Immunology Letters.* 84(2):81-87

Chen, L.G., Widhopf, G., Huynh, L., Rassenti, L., Rai, K.R., Weiss, A. & Kipps, T.J. (2002b). Expression of ZAP-70 is associated with increased B-cell receptor signaling in chronic lymphocytic leukemia. *Blood.* 100(13):4609-4614

Ciocca, D.R. & Calderwood, S.K. (2005). Heat shock proteins in cancer: diagnostic, prognostic, predictive, and treatment implications. *Cell Stress & Chaperones.* 10(2):86-103

Ciocca, D.R. & Calderwood, S.K. (2005). Heat shock proteins in cancer: diagnostic, prognostic, predictive and treatment implications. *Cell Stress & Chaperones.* 10(2):86-103

Ciocca, D.R. & Luque, E.H. (1991). Immunological Evidence for the Identity Between the Hsp27 Estrogen-Regulated Heat-Shock Protein and the P29 Estrogen Receptor-Associated Protein in Breast and Endometrial Cancer. *Breast Cancer Research and Treatment.* 20(1):33-42

Clayton, A., Turkes, A., Navabi, H., Mason, M.D. & Tabi, Z. (2005). Induction of heat shock proteins in B-cell exosomes. *Journal of Cell Science.* 118(16):3631-3638

Conde, R., Belak, Z.R., Nair, M., O'Carroll, R.F. & Ovsenek, N. (2009). Modulation of Hsf1 activity by novobiocin and geldanamycin. *International journal of Biochemistry and Cell Biology.* 87(6):845-851

Contri, A. Brunati, A.M., Trentin, L., Cabrelle, A., Miorin, M., Cesaro, L., Pinna, L.A., Zambello, R., Semenzato, G. & Donella-Deana, A. (2005). Chronic lymphocytic leukaemia B Cells contain anomalous Lyn tyrosine kinase, a putative contribution to defective apoptosis. *The Journal of Clinical Investigation.* 115(2):369-378

Cornford, P.A., Dodson, A.R., Parsons, K.F., Desmond, A.D., Woolfenden, A., Fordham, M., Neoptolemos, J.P., Ke, Y. & Foster, C.S. (2000). Heat Shock Protein Expression Independently Predicts Clinical Outcome in Prostate Cancer. *Cancer Research.* 60(24):7099-7105

Crespo, M., Bosch, F., Villamor, N., Bellosillo, B., Colomer, D., Rozman, M., Marce, S., Lopez-Guillermo, A., Campo, E. & Montserrat, E. (2003). Zap-70 expression as a surrogate for immunoglobulin-variable-region mutations in chronic lymphocytic leukemia. *N. Engl. J. Med.* 348, 1764–1775

Cruse, J.M., Lewis, R.E., Webb, R.N., Sanders, C.M. & Suggs, J.L. (2007). Zap-70 and CD38 as predictors of IgVH mutation in CLL. *Experimental and Molecular Pathology.* 83(3):459-461

Dakappagari, N. Neely, L. Tangri, S. Lundgren, K. Hipolito, L. Estrellado, A. Burrows, F & Zhang, H. (2010). An investigation into the potential use of Hsp70 as a novel tumour biomarker for Hsp90 inhibitors. *Biomarkers.* 15(1):31-38

Dempsey, N.C. (2009). *Heat Shock Protein Localisation in Haematological Malignancies.* Doctoral Thesis. University of Liverpool. Liverpool, UK.

Dempsey, N.C., Leoni, F., Ireland, H.E., Hoyle, C., & Williams, J.H.H. (2010). Differential Heat Shock Protein Localization in Chronic Lymphocytic Leukemia. *Journal of Leukocyte Biology*. 87(2):467-476.

Dempsey, N.C., Ireland, H.E., Smith, C.M., Hoyle, C.F. & Williams, J.H.H. (2010). Heat Shock Protein translocation induced by membrane fluidization increases tumor-cell sensitivity to chemotherapeutic drugs. *Cancer Letters*. 296(2):256-267

Duval, A., Olaru, D., Campos, L., Flandrin, P., Nadal, N. & Guyotat, D. (2006). Expression and prognostic significance of heat-shock proteins in myelodysplastic Syndromes. *Haematologica*. 91(5):713-714

Eccles, S.A., Massey, A., Raynaud, F.I., Sharp, S.Y., Box, G., Valenti, M.V., et al. (2008). NVP-AUY922: A Novel Heat Shock Protein 90 Inhibitor Active against Xenograft Tumor Growth, Angiogenesis, and Metastasis. *Cancer Research*. 86(8):2850-2860

Eustace BK, Sakurai T, Stewart JK, Yimlamai D, Unger C, Zehetmeier C, Lain B, Torella C, Henning SW, Beste G, Scroggins BT, Neckers L, Ilag LL, Jay DG. (2004). Functional proteomic screens reveal an essential extracellular role for hsp90 alpha in cancer cell invasiveness. *Nature Cell Biology*. 3(9):1098-1100

Faried, A., Sohda, M., Nakajima, M., Miyazaki, T., Kato, H. & Kuwano, H. (2004). Expression of heat-shock protein Hsp60 correlated with the apoptotic index and patient prognosis in human oesophageal squamous cell carcinoma. *European Journal of Cancer*. 40(18):2804-2811

Ferrarini, M., Heltai, S., Zocchi, M.R. & Rugarli, C. (1992). Unusual Expression and Localisation of Heat-Shock Proteins in Human Tumor-Cells. *International Journal of Cancer*. 51(4):613-619

Flaherty, K.T., Puznov, I., Kim, K.B., Ribas, I., McArther, G.A., Sosman, J.A., O'Dwyer, P.J., Lee, R.J., Grippo, J.F., Nolop, K. &Chapman, P.B (2010). Inhibition of Mutated, Activated BRAF in Metastatic Melanoma. The New England Journal of Medicine. 363(9):809-819

Garrido, C., Gurbuxani, S., Ravagnan, L. & Kroemer, G. (2001). Heat Shock Proteins: Endogenous Modulators of Apoptotic Cell Death. *Biochemical & Biophysical Research Communications*. 286(3):433-442

Gastpar, R., Gehrmann, M., Bausero, M.A., Asea, A., Gross, C., Schroeder, J.A. & Multhoff, G. (2005). Heat Shock Protein 70 Surface-Positive Tumor Exosomes. *Cancer Research*. 5;65(12):5238-47.

Gehrmann, M., H. Schmetzer, G. Eissner, T. Haferlach, W. Hiddemann and G. Multhoff (2003). Membrane-bound heat shock protein 70 in acute myeloid leukemia: a tumor-specific recognition structure for the cytolytic activity of autologous natural killer cells. *Haematologica*. 88(4): 474-476.

Gehrmann, M., Radons, J., Molls, M. & Multhoff, G. (2008). The therapeutic implications of clinically applied modifiers of heat shock protein 70 (Hsp70) expression by tumor cells. *Cell Stress & Chaperones*. 13(1):1-10

Geisler, J.P., Tammela, J.E., Manahan, K.J., Geisler, H.E., Miller, G.A., Zhou, Z. & Wiemann, M.C. (2004). HSP27 in patients with ovarian carcinoma: still an independent prognostic indicator at 60 months follow-up. *European Journal of Gynaecological Oncology*. 25(2):165-168

Giaginis, C., Daskalopoulou, S.S., Vgenopoulou, S., Sfiniadakis, I., Kouraklis, G. & Theocharis, S.E. (2009). Heat Shock Protein-27, -60 and -90 expression in gastric cancer: association with clinicopathological variables and patient survival. *BMC Gastroenterology*. 9:1-10

Glaessgen, A., Jonmarker, S., Lindberg, A., Nilsson, B., Lewensohn, R., Ekman, P., Valdman, A. & Egevad, L. (2008). Heat shock proteins 27, 60 and 70 as prognostic markers of prostate cancer. *APMIS*. 116(10):888-895

Gooljarsingh, L.T. Fernandes, C. Yan, K. Zhang, H. Grooms, M. Johanson, K. Sinnamon, R.H. Kirkpatrick, R. B. Kerrigan, J. Lewis, T. Arnone, M. King, A.J. Lai, Z. Copeland, R.A. & Tummino, P.J. (2006). A Biochemical rationale for the anticancer effects of Hsp90 inhibitors: slow, tight binding inhibition by geldanamycin and its analogues. *PNAS*. 103(20):7625-7630

Gross, C., Hansch, D., Gastpar, R. & Multhoff, G. (2003). Interaction of Heat Shock Protein 70 Peptide with NK Cells Involves the NK Receptor CD94. *Biological Chemistry*. 384(2):267 - 279

Gross, C., Holler, E., Stangl, S., Dickinson, A., Pockley, A.G., Asea, A.A., Mallappa, N., & Multhoff, G. (2008). An Hsp70 peptide initiates NK cell killing of leukemic blasts after stem cell transplantation. *Leukemia Research*. 32(4):527-534

Guo, F., Sigua, C., Bali, P., George, P., Fiskus, W., Scuto, A. & Annavarapu, S. (2005). Mechanistic role of heat shock protein 70 in Bcr-Abl–mediated resistance to apoptosis in human acute leukemia cells. *Blood*. 105(3):1246-1255

Hanahan, D. & Weinberg, R.A. (2000). The Hallmarks of Cancer. *Cell*. 100(1):57–70

Hanahan, D. & Weinberg, R.A. (2011). Hallmarks of Cancer: The Next Generation. *Cell*. 144(5):646-674

Hanson, B.E. & Vesole, D.H. (2009). Retaspimycin hydrochloride (IPI-504): a novel heat shock protein inhibitor as an anti-cancer agent. *Expert Opinion on Investigational Drugs*. 18(9):1375-1383

Heintel, D., Kroemer, E., Kienle, D., Schwarzinger, I., Gleiss, a, Schwarzmeier, J., Marculescu, R., et al. (2004). High expression of activation-induced cytidine deaminase (AID) mRNA is associated with unmutated IGVH gene status and unfavourable cytogenetic aberrations in patients with chronic lymphocytic leukaemia. *Leukemia*. 18(4):756-62

Hertlein, E. Wagner, A.J. Jones, J. Lin, T.S. Maddocks, K.J. Towns, W.H. Goettl, V.M. Zhang, X. Jarjoura, D. Raymond, C.A. West, D.A. Croce, C.M. Byrd, J.C. & Johnson, A.J. (2010). 17-DMAG targets the Nuclear-Factor-{kappa}B family of proteins to induce apoptosis in Chronic Lymphocytic Leukaemia: clinical implications of Hsp90 inhibition. *Blood*. 116(1):45-53

Holzbeierlein, J.M., Windsperger, A. & Vielhauer, G. (2010). Hsp90: A Drug Target? *Current Oncology Reports*. 12:95-101

Hightower, L. E., Guidon, P. T. (1989) Selective release from cultured mammalian cells of heat-shock (stress) proteins that resemble glia-axon transfer proteins. *Journal Cellular Physiology*. 138:257–266.

Hunter-Lavin, C., Davies, E. L., Bacelar, M., Marshall, M. J., Andrew, S. M. and Williams, J. H. H. (2004). Hsp70 release from peripheral blood mononuclear cells. *Biochemical and Biophysical Research Communications*. 324(2):511-517.

Huntoon, C.J., Nye, M.D., Geng, L., Peterson, K.L., Flatten, K.S., Haluska, P., Kaufmann, S.H., Karnitz, L.M. (2010). Heat shock protein 90 inhibition depletes LATS1 and LATS2, two regulators of the mammalian hippo tumor suppressor pathway. *Cancer Research*. 70(21):8642-8650

Iwaya, K., Tsuda, H., Fujita, S., Suzuki, M. & Hirohashi, S. (1995). Natural State of Mutant P53 Protein and Heat-Shock Protein-70 in Breast-Cancer Tissues. *Laboratory Investigation*. 72(6):707-714

Jaattela, M. (1999). Escaping Cell Death: Survival Proteins in Cancer. *Experimental Cell Research*. 248:30-43

Johnson, A.J., Wagner, A.J., Cheney, C.M., Smith, L.L., Lucas, D.M., Guster, S.K., Grever, M.R., Lin, T.S. & Byrd, J.C. (2007). Rituximab and 17-allylamino-17-demethoxygeldanamycin induce synergistic apoptosis in B-cell chronic lymphocytic leukaemia. *British Journal of Haematology*. 139(5):837-844

Jones, D.T., Addison, E., North, J.M., Lowdell, M.W., Hoffbrand, A.V., Mehta, A.B., Ganeshaguru, K., Folarin, N.I. & Wickremasinghe, R.G. (2004). Geldanamycin and herbimycin A induce apoptotic killing of B chronic lymphocytic leukemia cells and augment the cells' sensitivity to cytotoxic drugs. *Blood*. 103(5):1855-1861

Kampinga, H.H., Hageman, J., Vos, M.J., Kubota, H., Tanguay, R.M., Bruford, E.A., Cheetham, M.E., Chen, B. & Hightower, L.E. (2009). Guidelines for the nomenclature of the human heat shock proteins. *Cell Stress and Chaperones*. 14(1):105-111

Kantarjian, H.M.,O'Brien, S.,Cortes, J., Giles, F.J.,Rios, M.B., Shan, J.Q., Faderl, S., Garcia-Manero, G., Ferrajoli, A., Verstovsek, S., Wierda, W., Keating, M. & Talpaz, M. (2003). Imatinib mesylate therapy improves survival in patients with newly diagnosed Philadelphia chromosome-positive chronic myelogenous leukemia in the chronic phase - Comparison with historic data. *Cancer*. 98(12):2636-2642

Kawanishi, K., Shiozaki, H., Doki, Y., Sakita, I., Inoue, M., Yano, M., Tsujinaka, T., Shamma, A. & Monden, M. (1999). Prognostic significance of heat shock proteins 27 and 70 in patients with squamous cell carcinoma of the esophagus. *Cancer*. 85(8):1649-1657

Khaleque, M.A., Bharti, A., Sawyer, D., Gong, J.L., Benjamin, I.J., Stevenson, M.A. & Calderwood, S.K. (2005). Induction of heat shock proteins by heregulin beta 1 leads to protection from apoptosis and anchorage-independent growth. *Oncogene*. 24(43): 6564-6573

Kim, Y. S. Alarcon, S. V. Lee, S. Lee, M.-J. Giaccone, G. Neckers, L. & Trepel, J. B. (2009). Update on Hsp90 inhibitors in clinical trial. *Current Topics in Medicinal Chemistry*. 9(15):1479-1492

Kleinjung, T., Arndt, O., Feldmann, H., Bockmühl, U., Gehrmann, M., Zilch, T., Pfister, K., Schönberger, J., Marienhagen, J. & Eilles, C. (2003). Heat shock protein 70 (Hsp70) membrane expression on head-and-neck cancer biopsy - a target for natural killer (NK) cells. *International Journal of Radiation Oncology Biology Physics*. 57(3):820-826

Krause, S.W., Gastpar, R., Andreesen, R., Gross, C., Ullrich, H., Thonigs, G., Pfister, K. & Multhoff, G. (2004). Treatment of colon and lung cancer patients with ex vivo heat shock protein 70-peptide-activated, autologous natural killer cells: a clinical phase I trial. *Clinical Cancer Research*. 10(11):3699-3707

Krukenberg, K.A., Street, T.O., Lavery, L.A. & Agard, D.A. (2011). Conformational dynamics of the molecular chaperone Hsp90. *Quarterly Reviews of Biophysics*. 44(2):229-255

Kuppner, M.C., Gastpar, R., Gelwer, S., Nossner, E., Ochmann, O., Scharner, A. & Issels, R.D. (2001). The role of heat shock protein (hsp70) in dendritic cell maturation: Hsp70 induces the maturation of immature dendritic cells but reduces DC differentiation from monocyte precursors. *European Journal of Immunology*. 31(5):1602-1609

Kurotaki, T., Tamura, Y., Ueda, G., Oura, J., Kutomi, G., Hirohashi, Y., Sahara, H., Torigoe, T., Hiratsuka, H., Sunakawa, H., Hirata, K. & Sato, N. (2007). Efficient cross-presentation by heat shock protein 90-peptide complex-loaded dendritic cells via an endosomal pathway. *Journal of Immunology*. 179(3):1803-1813

Lanneau, D., Brunet, M., Frisan, E., Solary, E., Fontenay, M., Garrido, C. (2008). Heat shock proteins: essential proteins for apoptosis regulation. *Journal of Cellular and Molecular Medicine*. 12(3):743-761

Le Blanc, A.C. (2003). Natural cellular inhibitors of caspases. *Progress in Neuro-Psychopharmacology & Biological Psychiatry*. 27:215-229

Lehman, T.A., Bennett, W.P., Metcalf, R.A., Welsh, J.A., Ecker, J., Modali, R.V., Ullrich, S., Romano, J.W., Appella, E., Testa, J.R., Gerwin, B.I. & Harris, C.C. (1991). P53 Mutations, Ras Mutations and P53-Heat Shock 70 Protein complexes in Human Lung-Carcinoma Cell-Lines. *Cancer Research*. 51(15):4090:4096

Li, Y., Zhang, T., Schwartz, S.J. & Sun, D. (2009). New developments in Hsp90 inhibitors as anti-cancer therapeutics: Mechanisms, clinical perspective and more potential. *Drug Resistance Updates*. 12(1-2)17-27

Lin, K., Rockliffe, N., Johnson, G.G., Sherrington, P.D. & Pettitt, A.R. (2007). Hsp90 inhibition has opposing effects on wild-type and mutant p53 and induces p21 expression and cytotoxicity irrespective of p53/ATM status in chronic lymphocytic leukaemia cells. *Oncogene*. 27(17): 2445-2455

Love, S. & King, R.J.B. (1994). A 27kDa Heat-Shock-Protein that has anomalous prognostic powers in early and advanced breast-cancer. *British Journal Of Cancer*. 69(4):743-748

Lundgren, K., Zhang, H., Brekken, J., Huser, N., Powell, R.E., Timple, N., Busch, D.J., Neely, L., Sensintaffar, J.L., Yang, Y.C., McKenzie, A., Friedman, J., Scannevin, R., Kamal, A., Hong, K., Kasibhatla, S.R., Boehm, M.F., Burrows, F.J. (2009). BIIB021, an orally available, fully synthetic small-molecule inhibitor of the heat shock protein Hsp90. *Molecular Cancer Therapeutics*. 8(4):921-929

Mambula, S.S. & Calderwood, S.K. (2006). Heat induced release of Hsp70 from prostate carcinoma cells involves both active secretion and passive release from necrotic cells. *International Journal of Hyperthermia*. 22(7):575-585

Matysiak, M., B. Makosa, A. Walczak and K. Selmaj (2008). Patients with multiple sclerosis resisted to glucocorticoid therapy: abnormal expression of heat-shock protein 90 in glucocorticoid receptor complex. *Multiple Sclerosis* 14(7): 919-926

McCraig, A.M., Cosimo, E., Leach, M.T. & Michie, A.M. (2011). Dasatinib inhibits B cell receptor signalling in chronic lymphocytic leukaemia but novel combination approaches are required to overcome additional pro-survival microenvironmental signals. *British Journal of Haematology*. 153:199-211

McCready, J., Sims, J.D., Chan, D. & Jay, D.J. (2010). Secretion of extracellular Hsp90α via exosomes increases cancer cell motility: a role for plasminogen activation. *BMC Cancer*. 10:294-304

McLaughlin, S.H., Smith, H.W. & Jackson, S.E. (2002). Stimulation of the Weak ATPase Activity of Human Hsp90 by a Client Protein. *Journal of Molecular Biology*. 315:787-798

Milicevic, Z. T., Petkovic, M. Z., Drndarevic, N. C., Pavlovic, M. D., & Todorovic, V. N. (2007). Expression of heat shock protein 70 (HSP70) in patients with colorectal adenocarcinoma - immunohistochemistry and Western blot analysis. *Neoplasma*. 54(1):37-45.

Minami, Y., Kiyoi, H., Yamamoto, Y., Ueda, R., Saito, H. & Naoe, T. (2002). Selective apoptosis of tandemly duplicated FLT3-transformed leukemia cells by Hsp90 inhibitors. *Leukemia*. 16(8): 1535-1540

Modi, S., Stopeck, A.T., Gordon, M.S., Mendelson, D., Solit, D.B., Bagatell, R., Ma, W., Wheler, J., Rosen, N., Norton, L., Cropp, G.F., Johnson, R.G., Hannah, A.L. & Hudis, C.A. (2007). Combination of Trastuzumab and Tanespimycin (17-AAG, KOS-953) Is Safe and Active in Trastuzumab-Refractory HER-2–Overexpressing Breast Cancer: A Phase I Dose-Escalation Study. *Journal of Clinical Oncology*. 25(34):5410-5417

Murshid, A., Gong, J. & Calderwood, S.K. (2008). Heat-shock proteins in cancer vaccines: agents of antigen cross presentation. *Expert Reviews in Vaccines*. 7(7):1019-1030

Nagy, E., Balogi, Z., Gombos, I., Akerfelt, M., Bjorkbom, A., Balogh, G., Torok, Z., Maslyanko, A., Fiszer-Kierzkowska, A., Lisowska, K., Slotte, P.J., Sistonen, L., Horvath, I. & Vigh, L. (2007). Hyperfluidisation-coupled membrane microdomain reorganisation is linked to activation of the heat shock response in a murine melanoma cell line. *PNAS*. 104(19):7945-7950

Nazarian, R., Shi, H., Wang, Q., Kong, X., Koya, R.C., Lee, H., Chen, Z., Lee, M.K., Attar, N., Sazegar, H., Chodon, T., Nelson, S.F., McArthur, G., Sosman, J.A., Ribas, A. & Lo, R.S. (2010). Melanomas acquire resistance to B-RAF(V600E) inhibition by RTK or N-RAS upregulation. *Nature*. 468(7326):973-977

Neckers, L. (2007). Heat shock protein 90: the cancer chaperone. *Journal of Bioscience*. 32(3):517–530

Nimmanapalli, R., O'Bryan, E., Huang, M., Bali, P., Burnette, P.K., Loughran, T., Tepperberg, J., Jove, R. & Bhalla, K. (2002). Molecular Characterization and Sensitivity of STI-571 (Imatinib Mesylate, Gleevec)- resistant, Bcr-Abl-positive, Human Acute Leukemia Cells to SRC Kinase Inhibitor PD180970 and 17-Allylamino-17-demethoxygeldanamycin. *Cancer Research*. 62:5761–5769,

Nylandsted, J., Brand, K., & Jaattela, M. (2000). Heat shock protein 70 is required for the survival of cancer cells. *Mechanisms of Cell Death*. 926:122-125.

Okawa, Y., Hideshima, T., Steed, P., Vallet, S., Hall, S., Huang, K., Rice, J., Barabasz, A., Foley, B., Ikeda, H., Raje, N., Kiziltepe, T., Yasui, H., Enatsu, S., Anderson, K.C. (2009). SNX-2112, a selective Hsp90 inhibitor, potently inhibits tumor cell growth, angiogenesis, and osteoclastogenesis in multiple myeloma and other hematologic tumors by abrogating signaling via Akt and ERK. *Blood*. 113(4):846-855

Orthwein, A., Patenaude, A.-M., Affar, E. B., Lamarre, A., Young, J. C., & Di Noia, J. M. (2010). Regulation of activation-induced deaminase stability and antibody gene diversification by Hsp90. *The Journal of experimental medicine*. 207(12):2751-65

Palacios, F., Moreno, P., Morande, P., Abreu, C., Correa, A., Porro, V., Landoni, A. I., et al. (2010). High expression of AID and active class switch recombination might account for a more aggressive disease in unmutated CLL patients: link with an activated microenvironment in CLL disease. *Blood*. 115(22):4488-96

Pashtan, I., Tsutsumi, S., Wang, S.Q., Xu, W.P., Neckers, L. (2008). Targeting Hsp90 prevents escape of breast cancer cells from tyrosine kinase inhibition. *Cell Cycle*. 7(18): 2936-2941

Paul, C., Manero, F., Gonin, S., Kretz-Remy, C., Virot, S. & Arrigo, A.P. (2002). Hsp27 as a negative regulator of cytochrome c release. *Molecular and Cellular Biology*. 22(3):816-834

Peng, C., Li, D. & Li, S. (2007). Heat Shock Protein 90. A Potential Therapeutic Target in Leukemic Progenitor and Stem Cells Harboring Mutant BCR-ABL Resistant to Kinase Inhibitors. *Cell Cycle*. 6(18):2227-2231

Pepper, C., Lin, T.T., Pratt, G., Hewamana, S., Brennan, P., Hiller, L., Hills, R., Ward, R., Starczynski, J., Austen, B., Hooper, L., Stankovic, T. & Fegan, C. (2008). Mcl-1 expression has in vitro and in vivo significance in chronic lymphocytic leukemia and is associated with other poor prognostic markers. *Blood*. 112(9):3807-3817

Pepper, C., Hewamana, S., Brennan, P. & Fegan, C. (2009). NF-kappaB as a prognostic marker and therapeutic target in chronic lymphocytic leukemia. *Future Oncology*. 5(7):1027-37

Pfister, K., Radons, J., Busch, R., Tidball, J.G., Pfeifer, M., Freitag, L., Feldmann, H.J., Milani, V., Issels, R. & Multhoff, G. (2007). Patient survival by Hsp70 membrane phenotype. *American Cancer Society*. 110(4):926-935

Pick, E., Kluger, Y., Giltnane, J.M., Moeder, C., Camp, R.L., Rimm, D.L. & Kluger, H.M. (2007). High HSP90 expression is associated with decreased survival in breast cancer. *Cancer Research*. 67(7): 2932-7.

Ramalingam, S.S., Egorin, M.J., Ramanathan, R.K., Remick, S.C., Sikorski, R.P., …Lagattuta, T.F., Chatta, G.S., Friedland, D.M., Stoller, R.G., Potter, D.M., Ivy, S.P. & Belani, C.P. (2008). A phase I study of 17-allylamino-17-demethoxygeldanamycin combined with paclitaxel in patients with advanced solid malignancies. *Clinical Cancer Research*. 14(11): 3456-3461

Ramp, U., Mahotka, C., Heikaus, S., Shibata, T., Grimm, M.O., Willers, R. & Gabbert, H.E. (2007). Expression of heat shock protein 70 in renal cell carcinoma and its relation to tumor progression and prognosis. *Histology and Histopathology*. 22:1019-1107

Ravagnan, L., Gurbuxani, S., Susin, A., Maisse, C., Daugas, E., Zamzami, N., Mak, T., Jaatella, Penninger, J.M., Garrido, C. & Kroemer, G. (2001). Heat-shock protein 70 antagonizes apoptosis-inducing factor. *Nature Cell Biology*. 3(9): 839-843

Richards, E.H., Hickey, E., Weber, L., Masters, J.R.W. (1996). Effect of overexpression of the small heat shock protein HSP27 on the heat and drug sensitivities of human testis tumor cells. *Cancer Research*. 56(10):2446-2451

Richardson, P.G., Badros, A.Z., Jagannath, S., Tarantolo, S., Wolf, J.L., Albitar, M., Berman, D., Messina, M. & Anderson, K.C. (2010). Tanespimycin with bortezomib: activity in relapsed/refractory patients with multiple myeloma. *British Journal of Haematology*. 150(4):428-437

Ringshausen, I., Schneller, F., Bogner, C., Hipp, S., Duyster, J., Peschel, C., Decker, T. (2002). Constitutively activated phosphatidylinositol-3 kinase (PI-3K) is involved in the defect of apoptosis in B-CLL: association with protein kinase Cdelta. *Blood*. 100(10):3741-3748.

Robles, A.I., Wright, M.H., Gandhi, B., Feis, S.S., Hanigan, C.L., Wiestner, A. & Varticovski, L. (2006). Schedule-dependent synergy between the heat shock protein 90 inhibitor 17-(dimethylaminoethylamino)-17-demethoxygeldanamycin and doxorubicin restores apoptosis to p53-mutant lymphoma cell lines. *Clinical Cancer Research*. 12(21): 6547-6556

Romani, A.A., Crafa, P., Desenzani, S., Graiani, G., Lagrasta, C., Sianesi, M., Soliani, P. & Borghetti, A.F. (2007). The expression of HSP27 is associated with poor clinical outcome in intrahepatic cholangiocarcinoma. *BMC Cancer*. 7(232):232

Sagol, O., Tuna, B., Coker, A., Karademir, S., Obuz, F., Astarcioglu, H., Kupelioglu, A., Astarcioglu, I. & Topalak, O. (2002). Immunohistochemical detection of PS2 protein and heat shock protein-70 in pancreatic adenocarcinomas. relationship with disease extent and patient survival. *Pathology Research & Practice*.198(2):77-84.

Sahin, E., Sahin, M., Sanlioğlu, A.D. & Gümüslü, S. (2011). KNK437, a benzylidene lactam compound, sensitises prostate cancer cells to the apoptotic effect of hyperthermia. *International Journal of Hyperthermia*. 27(1):63-73

Samali, A., Cai, J., Zhivotovsky, B., Jones, D.P. & Orrenius, S. (1999). Presence of a pre-apoptotic complex of pro-caspase-3, Hsp60 and Hsp10 in the mitochondrial fraction of Jurkat cells. *EMBO Journal*. 18(8):2040-2048

Samali, A., Robertson, J.D., Peterson, E., Manero, F., van Zeijl, L., Paul, C., Cotgreave, I.A., Arrigo, A.P. & Orrenius, S. (2001). Hsp27 protects mitochondria of thermotolerant cells against apoptotic stimuli. *Cell Stress and Chaperones*. 6(1):49-58

Santarosa, M., Favaro, D., Quaia, M. & Galligioni, E. (1997). Expression of heat shock protein 72 in renal cell carcinoma: Possible role and prognostic implications in cancer patients. *European Journal of Cancer*. 33(6):873-877

Sato, S., Fujita, N. & Tsuruo, T. (2000). Modulation of Akt kinase activity by binding to Hsp90. *PNAS*. 97(20): 10832–10837

Schepers, H., Geugien, M., van der Toorn, M., Bryantsev, A.L., Kampinga, H.H., Eggen, B.J.L. & Vellenga, E. (2005). HSP27 protects AML cells against VP-16-induced apoptosis through modulation of p38 and c-Jun. *Experimental Haematology*. 33(6):660-670

Schilling, D., Gehrmann, M., Steinem, C., De Maio, A., Pockley, A.G., Abend, M., Molls, M. Multhoff, G. (2007). Binding of heat shock protein 70 to extracellular phosphatidylserine promotes killing of normoxic and hypoxic tumor cells. *FASEB Journal*. 23(8):2467-77

Schneider, J., Jimenez, E., Marenbach, K., Romero, H., Marx, D. & Meden, H. (1999). Immunohistochemical detection of HSP60-expression in human ovarian cancer. Correlation with survival in a series of 247 patients. *Anticancer Research*. 19(3A): 2141-2146

Shah, N.P., Nicoll, J.M., Nagar, B., Gorre, M.E., Paquette, R.L., Kuriyan, J. & Sawyers, C.L. (2002). Multiple BCR-ABL kinase mutations confer polyclonal resistance to the tyrosine kinase inhibitor Imatinib (STI571) in chronic phase and blast crisis chronic myeloid leukemia. *Cancer Cell*. 2:117-125

Shahidi, H., A. Vottero, C. A. Stratakis, S. E. Taymans, M. Karl, C. A. Longui, G. P. Chrousos, W. H. Daughaday, S. A. Gregory and J. M. D. Plate (1999). Imbalanced expression of the glucocorticoid receptor isoforms in cultured lymphocytes from a patient with systemic glucocorticoid resistance and chronic lymphocytic leukemia. *Biochemical and Biophysical Research Communications*. 254(3): 559-565.

Shan, Y.X., Liu, T.J., Su, H.F., Samsamshariat, A., Mestril, R. & Wang, P.H. (2003). Hsp10 and Hsp60 modulate Bcl-2 family and mitochondria apoptosis signaling induced by doxorubicin in cardiac muscle cells. *Journal of Molecular and Cellular Cardiology*. 35(9):1135-1143

Sherman, M. & Multhoff, G. (2007). Heat Shock Proteins in Cancer. *Annals of the New York Academy of Sciences*. 1113:192-201

Shotar, A. M. (2005). P53 and heat shock protein 70 expressions in colorectal adenocarcinoma. *Saudi Medical Journal*. 26(10):1602-1606.

Sidera, K., Gaitanou. M., Stellas, D., Matsas, R. & Patsavoudi, E. (2008). A Critical Role for HSP90 in Cancer Cell Invasion Involves Interaction with the Extracellular Domain of HER-2. *The Journal of Biological Chemistry*. 283(4):2031–2041

Shin BK, Wang H, Yim AM, Le Naour F, Brichory F, Jang JH, Zhao R, Puravs E, Tra J, Michael CW, Misek DE, Hanash SM. (2003). Global profiling of the cell surface proteome of cancer cells uncovers an abundance of proteins with chaperone function. *Journal of Biological Chemistry*. 278(9):7607-1

Sorger, P.K. (1991). Heat Shock Factor and the Heat Shock Response. *Cell*. 65(3):363-366

Soti, C., Racz, A. & Csermely, P. (2002). A Nucleotide-Dependent Molecular Switch Controls ATP Binding at the C-Terminal Domain of Hsp90. *The Journal of Biological Chemistry*. 277(9):7066-7075

Sreedhar, A.S., Soti, C. & Csermely, P. (2004). Inhibition of Hsp90: a new strategy for inhibiting protein kinases. *Biochemica & Biophysica Acta*. 1697:233-242

Steiner, K., Graf, M., Hecht, K., Reif, S., Rossbacher, L., Pfister, K., Kolb, H.J., Schmetzer, H.M. & Multhoff, G. (2006). High HSP70-membrane expression on leukemic cells from patients with acute myeloid leukemia is associated with a worse prognosis. *Leukemia*. 20:2076–2079

Sturm, I., Bosanquet, AG., Hermann, S., Guner, D., Dorken, B. & Daniel, P.T. (2003). Mutation of p53 and consecutive selective drug resistance in B-CLL occurs as a consequence of prior DNA-damaging chemotherapy. *Cell Death & Differentiation.* 10:477-484

Taba, K., Kuramitsu, Y., Ryozawa, S.,Yoshida, K., Tanaka, T., Mori-Iwamoto, S., Maehara, S., Maehara, Y., Sakaida, I., Nakamura, K. (2011). KNK437 Downregulates Heat Shock Protein 27 of Pancreatic Cancer Cells and Enhances the Cytotoxic Effect of Gemcitabine. *Chemotherapy.* 57(1):12-16

Taldone, T., Gozman, A., Maharaj, R. & Chiosis, G. (2008). Targeting Hsp90: small-molecule inhibitors and their clinical development. *Current Opinion in Pharmacology.* 8(4):370-4

Tauchi, K., Tsutsumi, Y., Hori, S., Yoshimura, S., Osamura, R.Y. & Watanabe, K. (1991). Expression of Heat-Shock Protein-70 and C-Myc Protein in Human Breast-Cancer – An Immunohistochemical Study. *Japanese Journal of Clinical Oncology.* 21(4):256-263

Thomas, X., Campos, L., Mounier, C., Cornillon, J., Flandrin, P., Le, Q.H., Piselli, S. & Guyotat, D. (2005). Expression of heat-shock proteins is associated with major adverse prognostic factors in acute myeloid leukemia. *Leukaemia Research.* 29:1049-1058

Todryk, S., Melcher, A.A., Harwick, N., Linardakis, E., Bateman, A., Colombo, M.P., Stoppacciaro, A. & Vile, R.G. (1999). Heat shock protein 70 induced during tumor cell killing induces Th1 cytokines and targets immature dendritic cell precursors to enhance antigen uptake. *Journal of Immunology.* 163(3):1398-1408

Todryk, S., Melcher, A.A., Dalgleish, A.G., Vile, R.G. (2000). Heat shock proteins refine the danger theory. *Immunology.* 99:334-337

Torok, Z., Tsvetkova, N.M., Balogh, G., Horvath, I., Nagy, E., Penzes, Z., Hargitai, J., Bensaude, O., Csermely, P., Crowe, J.H., Maresca, B. & Vıgh, L. (2003). Heat shock protein coinducers with no effect on protein denaturation specifically modulate the membrane lipid phase. *PNAS.* 100(6):3131–3136

Trentin, L., Frasson, M., Donella-Deana, A., Frezzato, F., Pagano ,M.A., Tibaldi, E., Gattazzo, C., Zambello, R., Semenzato, G. & Brunati, A.M. (2008). Geldanamycin-induced Lyn dissociation from aberrant Hsp90-stabilized cytosolic complex is an early event in apoptotic mechanisms in B-chronic lymphocytic leukemia. *Blood.* 112(12):4665-74

Tsutsumi, S., Scroggins, B., Koga, F., Lee, M.J., Trepel, J., Felts, S., Carreras, C. & Neckers, L. (2008). A small molecule cell-impermeant Hsp90 antagonist inhibits tumor cell motility and invasion. *Oncogene.* 27: 2478–2487

Urushibara, M., Kageyama, Y., Akashi, T., Otsuka, Y., Takizawa, T,. Koike, M. & Kihara, K. (2007). HSP60 may predict good pathological response to neoadjuvant chemoradiotherapy in bladder cancer. *Japanese Journal of Clinical Oncology.* 37(1):56-61

Vargas-Roig, L.M., Gago, F.E., Tello, O., Anzar, J.C. & Ciocca, D.R. (1998). Heat Shock Protein Expression and Drug Resistance in breast cancer patients treated with induction chemotherapy. *International Journal of Cancer.* 79:468-475

Vega, V.L., Rodrıguez-Silva, M., Frey, T., Gehrmann, M., Diaz, J.C., Steinem, C., Multhoff, G., Arispe, N. & De Maio, A. (2008). Hsp70 Translocates into the Plasma Membrane after Stress and Is Released into the Extracellular Environment in a Membrane-

Associated Form that Activates Macrophages. *Journal of Immunology.* 180(6):4299-4307

Vigh, L., Horvath, I., Maresca, B. & Harwood, J.L. (2007a). Can the stress protein response be controlled by 'membrane-lipid therapy'? *Trends in Biochemical Sciences.* 32(8):357-363

Vigh, L., Nakamoto, H., Landry, J., Gomez-Munoz, A., Harwood, J.L. & Horvath, I. (2007b). Membrane Regulation of the Stress Response from Prokaryotic Models to Mammalian Cells. *Annals of the New York Academy of Sciences.* 1113:40–51

Walerych, D., Kudla, G., Gutkowska, M., Wawrzynow, B., Muller, L., King, F.W., Helwak, A., Boros, J., Zylicz, A., Zylicz, M. (2004). Hsp90 chaperones wild-type p53 tumor suppressor protein. *Journal of Biological Chemistry.* 279(47):48836-45

Wei, Y.Q., Zhao, X., Kariya, Y., Fukata, H., Teshigawara, K. & Uchida, A. (1996). Induction of autologous tumor killing by heat treatment of fresh human tumor cells: involvement of gamma delta T cells and heat shock protein 70. *Cancer Research.* 56(5):1104–1110.

Whitesell, L., Mimnaugh, E.G., De Costa, B., Myers, C.E. & Necker, L.M. (1994). Inhibition of heat shock protein HSP90-pp60 heteroprotein complex formation by benzoquinone ansamycins: Essential role for stress proteins in oncogenic transformation. *PNAS.* 91:8324-8328

Williams, J. H. H. and Ireland, H. E. (2008). Sensing danger - Hsp72 and HMGB1 as candidate signals. *Journal of Leukocyte Biology.* 83(3):489-492.

Wu, C. (1995). Heat Shock Treanscription Factors. Structure & Regulation. *Annual Review of Cell and Developmental Biology.* 11:441-469

Wu, X., Wanders, A., Wardega, P., Tinge, B., Gedda, L., Bergstrom, S., Sooman, L., Gullbo, J., Bergqvist, M., Hesselius, P., Lennartsson J. & kman, S. (2009). Hsp90 is expressed and represents a therapeutic target in human oesophageal cancer using the inhibitor 17-allylamino-17-demethoxygeldanamycin. *British Journal of Cancer.* 100, 334–343

Xanthoudakis, S., Roy, S., Rasper, D., Hennessey, T., Aubin, Y., Cassady, R., Tawa, P., Ruel, R., Rosen, A. & Nicholson, D.W. (1999). Hsp60 accelerates the maturation of pro-caspase-3 by upstream activator proteases during apoptosis. *EMBO Journal.* 18(8):2049-2056

Yaglom, J.A., Gabai, V.L. & Sherman, M.Y. (2007). High Levels of Heat Shock Protein Hsp72 in Cancer Cells Suppress Default Senescence Pathways. *Cancer Research.* 67(5):2373-2381

Yao, P., Nussler, A., Liu, L., Hao, L., Song, F., Schirmeier, A. & Nussler, N. (2007). Quercetin protects human hepatocytes from ethanol-derived oxidative stress by inducing heme oxygenase-1 via the MAPK/Nrf2 pathways. *Journal of Hepatology.* 47(2):253-61

Yin, Z., Henry, E.C. & Gasiewicz, T.A. (2009). (-)-Epigallocatechin-3-gallate is a novel Hsp90 inhibitor. *Biochemistry.* 48(2):336-45.

Zaarur, N., Gabai, V.L., Porco, J.A. Jr., Calderwood, S. & Sherman, M.Y. (2006). Targeting Heat Shock Response to Sensitise Cancer Cells to Proteosome and Hsp90 Inhibitors. *Cancer Research.* 66(3): 1783-1791

Zagouri, F., Sergentanis, T.N., Nonni, A., Papadimitriou, C.A., Michalopoulos, N.V., Domeyer, P., Theodoropoulos, G., Lazaris, A., Patsouris, E., Zogafos, E., Pazaiti, A. & Zografos

G.C. (2010). Hsp90 in the continuum of breast ductal carcinogenesis: Evaluation in precursors, preinvasive and ductal carcinoma lesions. *BMC Cancer*. 10:353-341

Zanini, C., Giribaldi, G., Mandili, G., Carta, F., Crescenzio, N., …Bisaro, B., Doria, A., Foglia, L., Di Montezemolo, C., Timeus, F. & Turrini, F. (2007). Inhibition of heat shock proteins (HSP) expression by quercetin and differential doxorubicin sensitization in neuroblastoma and Ewing's sarcoma cell lines. *Journal of Neurochemistry*. 103(4):1344-1354

Zhao, Z.G. & Shen, W.L. (2005). Heat shock protein 70 antisense oligonucleotide inhibits cell growth and induces apoptosis in human gastric cancer cell line SGC-7901. *World Journal of Gastroenterology*. 11(1):73-78

Zou, J.Y., Guo, Y.L., Guettouche, T., Smith, D.F., Voellmy, R. (1998). Repression of heat shock transcription factor HSF1 activation by HSP90 (HSP90 complex) that forms a stress-sensitive complex with HSF1. *Cell*. 94(4):471-480

20

Present and Future Application of Nanoparticle Based Therapies in B-Chronic Lymphocytic Leukemia (B-CLL)

Eduardo Mansilla[1,2], Gustavo H. Marin[2], Luis Núñez[3], Gustavo Larsen[4], Nelly Mezzaroba[5] and Paolo Macor[5]

[1]National University of La Rioja, UNLAR, La Rioja,
[2]CUCAIBA, Ministry of Health, La Plata, Buenos Aires
[3]University of Chicago, Chicago, Illinois, USA and Bio-Target, Chicago, Illinois,
[4]LNK Chemsolutions, Lincoln Nebraska, USA and Bio-Target, Chicago,
[5]Department of Life Science, University of Trieste,
[1,2]Argentina
[3,4]USA
[5]Italy

1. Introduction

We describe a variety of polymer biodegradable nanoparticles (BNPs) that can be created in an attempt to find an effective and durable treatment for B-Chronic Lymphocytic Leukemia (B-CLL). Many different drugs including those like Chlorambucil (CLB) that has been the gold standard B-CLL´s chemotherapeutic treatment preference for years (1), or even those not traditionally considered or used as antineoplastic agents like Hydroxychloroquine (HCQ) (2), can safely be encapsulated inside nanoparticles and specifically be targeted to the selected tumor cells by the coating of monoclonal antibodies in their surface (3,4). In this way all these drugs could be released in a steady manner exclusively into the desired neoplastic cells. This would give several advantages in relation to traditional drug delivery methods as a significant less toxicity is produced in non cancer cells while very high concentrations of the therapeutic compounds with great apoptotic effect are reached only at the targeted selected B-CLL cells level.

Therapeutic systems of this kind are relatively easy to produce in the large scale, are probably very safe, and will elicit a negligible immune response (3). BNPs like the ones we have developed, will offer a great promise as non-viral biocompatible and biodegradable vectors and carriers of drugs, peptides or other substances, with targeting capacities to specific cell sites by surface receptors of monoclonal antibodies (mAbs). Our data indicate that these nanoparticles with surface mAbs are suitable as a selective drug delivery method to treat B-CLL, other lymphomas and probably autoimmune disease such as Rheumathoid Arthritis and Lupus Erythematosus between many others. When loaded with the lysosomotropic agent HCQ alone, or combined with CLB, they elicited a strong apoptotic effect (3) (4). Additional data revealed that these BNPs were non-toxic for healthy animals, and had prolonged an outstanding survival in mice models of human lymphoma and B-CLL. There is a real need to comprehend and define all the basic processes needed in order to commercially produce viable products of this kind. This includes the present knowledge that has been acquired in the development and use of nanoparticles for the cure of B-CLL as well as all the possibilities that have been opened by their introduction, such as regulatory/safety, environmental, health and societal implications of these new treatments (5).

2. B-CLL and the need for new therapeutic approaches: An opportunity for nanoparticle systems

B-CLL is the most common form of leukemia in the western world. It results from a relentless accumulation of small mature monoclonal lymphocytes. Following a recent demonstration of a significant increase in the proliferative pool of CLL cells in vivo, the gradual accumulation of malignant B-CLL cells seems to be primarily the consequence of their selective survival advantages relative to their normal B-cell counterparts (6). As the disease is mainly caused by defective apoptosis it is thus a good candidate for treatment by pro-apoptotic agents. Even though a large amount of research has been done during the last past years, the prognosis has not changed (7). A major problem with treating patients with cancer and B-CLL by traditional chemotherapeutic regimes is that their tumors often develop a multidrug resistant (MDR) phenotype and subsequently become insensitive to a range of different chemotoxic drugs. One cause of MDR is overexpression of the drug-effluxing protein, P-glycoprotein. It is now apparent that P-glycoprotein may also possess a more generic antiapoptotic function that protects P-glycoprotein–expressing cancer cells and normal cells from death (8). B-CLL cells with unfavorable cytogenetic alterations such as deletion of chromosome 17p with loss of p53 are often resistant to fludarabine and cyclophosphamide (9,10). Similarly, CLL cells from patients with advanced disease stages or having a history of prior chemotherapy, exhibit elevated oxidative stress (11) and thus may have a greater potential to acquire additional mutations and genetic abnormalities, leading to drug resistance and disease progression.

3. The history of the first biodegradable nanoparticle system for the treatment of B-CLL and lymphomas that could also work for autoimmune disease

By the end of 2007 Dr. Luis Núñez, a biochemist that founded with Dr. Gustavo Larsen, Bio-Target, a Chicago, USA, start-up nanotechnology company, with a new interesting intellectual property in the production of biodegradable nanoparticles that could be loaded with many drugs and coated with monoclonal antibodies, contacted Dr. Eduardo Mansilla in La Plata, Argentina, and agreed to develop together ideas and products in this direction. By that time Dr. Mansilla was very involved in B-CLL research, and for many years looked for a system that could deliver HCQ in enough concentrations inside tumor B-CLL cells. In this situation the technology offered by Bio-Target seemed to him the wright one to use. In less than six months the research group in Argentina of which Dr. Gustavo H. Marin was also intensively participating, had the particles ready and the in vitro testing done with superior results, having the anti-CD20 antibody Rituximab coated in the surface of the BNPs. The nanoparticles were specifically attaching to the B-CLL cells and as they were penetrating them, an outstanding apoptotic process was seen with more than 95% killing effect in less than 48 hrs. In this way, we produced and tested in vitro in an amazing fast time the first biodegradable nanoparticle system in the history of medicine with a non-traditional antineoplastic old drug such as HCQ and a monoclonal antibody approved by the FDA, Rituximab, for the treatment of B-cell malignancies, with very good efficacy. We did some further testing with particles coated with the anti-CD19 mAb and its combination with the anti-CD20, as well as mixtures of HCQ and CLB. Then, we offered our technology to the Italian group, from Trieste, conducted by Dr. Paolo Macor in order to do more in vitro testing and a large animal study in a mouse model of Burkkit´s lymphoma. The results were reproduced in the same manner with similar results in vitro. The animal study was a great surprise, as almost all animals treated with the nanoparticle system were alive after more than 120 days, while the control group was all dead by that time. After that, we started conversations with United States and European research groups to introduce this technology into further more animal studies not only for B-CLL and Lymphoma but also for autoimmune disease, specially SLE and Reumathoid Arthritis, as well as a human clinical trial for B-CLL patients. At this time, it is clear that the developmental steps of this new technology was successful and done in just a few months, later on, the industrialization and approval by regulatory agencies, as well as the commercialization and final benefit of the patients is taking an unacceptable but predictable long time and delay. These new therapeutic strategies are really urgently needed, especially because they could easily switch on new apoptotic responses and restore sensitivity to drugs in B-CLL cells. In this way, nanoparticle-based "smart" therapeutics will generate both evolutionary as well as revolutionary products in the near future for B-CLL. There is enough evidence now, in order to think that these systems will profoundly impact the next generation of treatments for this disease and probably others. If this is to happen, there will be a few key biological requirements for such technologies to be introduced and routinely used by the onco- hematology community. All these aspects, specially related to their design, delivery capacity and their tremendous selectivity in their targeting to specific B-CLL cell sites, is urgently needed to be addressed.

4. Old drugs re-discovered to be used inside BNPs for B-CLL

CLB, which belongs to a family of drugs known as alkylating agents, has been in use for decades to treat hematological malignancies including B-CLL (12). This drug is given orally, which is normally an advantage but in this case, causes problems because the rate at which the drug is absorbed into the bloodstream can vary tremendously from patient to patient (13). Drug developers have tried a variety of techniques to offer new forms of delivery of this interesting old drug, but each of these methods has proven less than optimal (14). Now, however, we have created these BNPs that appear to could solve these issues and hold the promise of improving the utility of CLB not only in B-CLL but in many other cancer therapies. This could also be true for many other old onco-hematologic chemo-therapeutic agents with a fairly interesting efficacy and safety profile that could be re-discovered for their use in B-CLL and other leukemias and lymphomas by delivering them in nanoparticles. This could be the case of doxorubicin or tamoxifene (15,16), or even bendamustine. This last drug has been used for more than 30 years in the treatment of lymphoma, but little is known about the optimal dosing schedule in relapsed or refractory B-cell chronic lymphocytic leukemia (CLL). Various dose and treatment schedules have been used empirically, and several studies have shown impressive efficacy specially in heavily pre-treated and treatment-refractory patients (17,18).

5. Non-classical drugs for the treatment of B-CLL: HCQ, magnolol, honokiol, parthenolide, phenylethyl-isothio-cyanate (PEITC) and others delivered in BNPs

Many compounds non-traditionally used as anti-neoplastic agents have been shown to put cancer cells into pro-apoptotic programs and could be very useful for B-CLL treatment. A great diversity of still undefined compounds with anti-cancer properties can be obtained from botanical species. The pharmaceutical industry has been substantially but slowly scaling-up research efforts and partnering up with research universities for finding natural herbal and natural alternatives to fight cancer instead of the conventional expensive and tedious large scale process of screening thousands of synthetic compounds to find a final cure or solution to cancer. Scientists have given proof of the valuable anti-inflammatory, antioxidant, and cholesterol-lowering benefits of resveratrol, curcumin, and green polyphenols, natural compounds between many other that are found in red wine, curry, and green tea extracts respectively (17,18). Some of these natural products could be effective in B-CLL by activating different cell death pathways. The active principles of a group of very well known herbs like tanacetum parthenium, magnolia grandiflora, cruciferous vegetables, turmeric, and many others, have been previously described as components of different Japanese, Latin American or Chinese traditional medicine having recognized anti-angiogenic and/or anti-tumor properties (19). Many of the difficulties found in human application of these drugs have been related mainly to bioavailibility and toxicological issues. In this way and considering that these drugs are usually very cheap and can be obtained from botanical species in unlimited amounts it is very interesting to speculate in its use in B-CLL by its administration inside nanoparticles. It is an interesting issue that many of these herbs contain parthenolide (PTL) as one of their major active components (20). This last substance is a sesquiterpene lactone, a novel natural NF-kappa B inhibitor with antineoplastic properties (21). In general, parthenolide is well tolerated by humans, making it a good candidate for further clinical testing as an anti B-CLL agent. Obtained mainly from Tanacetum parthenium , Magnolia grandiflora and other plants, it has recently demonstrated an interesting anti-tumoral activity against CLL, some solid tumors and acute myeloid leukemia (21,22), but it was only tried in B-CLL in a study done by our group (23). We showed for the first time that PTL has a potent apoptotic effect on B-CLL cells without a great impact on normal PBMC (24). PTL displayed potent cytotoxic and apoptotic effects on B-CLL cells in vitro. B-CLL cells treated with PTL resulted in a dose and time dependent cytotoxicity. PTL mediated cytotoxicity occurred at a concentration of 1 μ M and above. A significant decrease in the cell viability of B-CLL cells obtained from 5 patients was seen after one day of culture (38.1± 6.37%) and at 72 h (90± 5.19%) with a PTL concentration of 8 μ M. (Fig. 1). All these responses were dose and time dependent for PTL values from 1 to 10 uM. By contrast, this compound had little apoptotic or cytotoxic effect in PBMCs of healthy donors even at higher concentrations. These results provided clues for interesting pathways involving different aspects of B-CLL cell apoptosis that could be exploited in therapies with this product. It could be speculated that parthenolide increased the amount of the NF-kappa B inhibitory protein, I kappa B-alpha, and decreased NF-kappa B DNA binding activity. All this evidence suggests that parthenolide may provide an anti-B-CLL effect and could be a potentially effective repertoire for chronic lymphocytic leukemia treatment specially if given in combination with other drugs in nanoparticle systems. Even though all our patients were Rai II and CD38-, compromising mainly a potentially less aggressive category of disease, the results obtained in this work were more than satisfactory and probably could also be transfered to patients with a poor prognosis. As this compound had little cytotoxic in vitro impact on normal human PBMCs, side effects in the clinical setting could probably be minimized, especially if given inside a nanoparticle system, and this of course, will be a very important aspect to be considered in a chronic disease like B-CLL. It is also possible that a formulation combining parthenolide with some other natural molecules like honokiol or magnolol, obtained indeed from the Magnoliaceae family of plants, or the classical treatments, might have a synergistically beneficial effect in B-CLL, being a potential promising strategy for the treatment of this hematological malignancy.

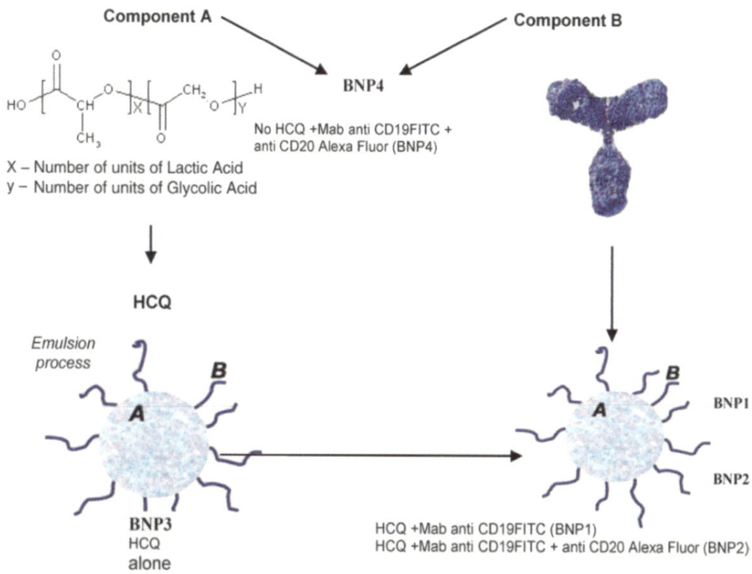

Fig. 1. Targeted biodegradable nanoparticle desing scheme.

Magnolia Grandiflora mainly contains Honokiol, Magnolol and Parthenolide (23) Honokiol and Magnolol are the major active constituents extracted from the bark of different Magnoliaceae species like Magnolia officinalis and Magnolia Grandiflora. They have a variety of pharmacological effects, such as anti-inflammatory, (21) antithrombotic, (25) anti-arrhythmic, (26)antioxidant (27)and anxiolytic effects, (28)and more recently, cytotoxic activity by inducing cell apoptosis in some cell lines (29). Magnolol and Honokiol-triggered apoptotic process is accompanied with down-modulation of Bcl-XL molecules (30) or through Caspase cascades activation (31) We have also shown that an aqueous Magnolia extract displayed a strong apoptotic effect on untreated as well as in heavily CLB treated B-CLL cells in vitro. We have published that Magnolia's extracts have efficacy in apoptosis and cytotoxicity induction and that these properties are exhibited mainly in tumors and not in normal cells, suggesting that an increase in NF-kappa B inhibitory protein and a decrease in NF-kappa B DNA binding activity or EGFR/PI3K/Akt signaling pathway or inhibition of telomerase activity might be involved in apoptosis induction (32). Phenylethyl-isothiocyanate (PEITC) is abundant in cruciferous vegetables, has potent preventing antineoplastic properties as well as pro-apoptotic activities against a large variety of cancers, it is also a ROS-generating agent capable to kill B-CLL cells in vitro and probably in vivo.

6. Hydroxychloroquine for CLL

Concerning HCQ, it could be say that it is an anti malarial and a Disease-Modifying Antirheumatic Drug (DMARD), very active against rheumatoid arthritis and lupus erythematosus which operates by inhibiting lymphocyte proliferation, antigen presentation in dendritic cells, release of enzymes from lysosomes, release of reactive oxygen species from macrophages, and production of IL-1 (33). Also it has demonstrated to be active as an antiviral agent, since it impedes the completion of the viral life cycle by inhibiting some processes occurring within intracellular organelles and requiring a low pH. For HIV-1, chloroquine and hydroxychloroquine also inhibit the glycosylation of the viral envelope glycoprotein gp120, which occurs within the Golgi apparatus (34). For all of this HCQ, that has been used in the clinic for decades with good results and a very safe profile (35) is a very interesting option to be loaded in nanoparticles with the intention to treat B-CLL and autoimmune diseases and maybe also some viral infections like HIV. Recently HCQ by itself has demonstrated an interesting pro-apoptotic effect and has been selected by the NIH as an anti-cancer drug that deserves further testing. Its antineoplastic properties in vitro depend on its concentration but this cannot routinely be obtained in vivo by the usual oral route of administration (3). HQC, induces a decrease in B-CLL cell viability in a dose- and time-dependent manner when tested in vitro. The mean LC50 calculated for the cells of 20 patients was 32 +/- 7 microg/ml (range, 10-75 microg/ml). A large increase in apoptotic cell numbers after 24 h of incubation with 50 microg/ml HCQ (55 +/- 6 vs. 23 +/- 3% in medium alone, $p < 0.001$). Indeed, HCQ in leukemic cells induced the features of apoptosis (cell shrinkage, decrease in mitochondrial transmembrane potential, phosphatidylserine externalization, chromatin condensation and DNA fragmentation). HCQ had marked selective cytotoxicity when compared with normal blood mononuclear cells, in which the LC50 was >100 microg/ml at 24 h. HCQ induced the proteolytic cleavage of poly(ADP(adenosine 5'-diphosphate)ribose) polymerase (PARP) and increased the activity of caspase-3. The expression of bcl-2 and bax proteins was significantly modified after incubation with the drug and HCQ activity against CLL cells occurred independently of the presence of IL-4, sCD40L and bone marrow stromal cells (36). The mechanisms behind the effects of HCQ on cancer are currently being investigated. The best- known effects (investigated in clinical and pre-clinical studies) include radiosensitizing effects through lysosome permeabilization, and chemosensitizing effects through inhibition of drug efflux pumps (ATP-binding cassette transporters) or other mechanisms like those of a lysosomotropic agent, meaning that it accumulates preferentially in the lysosomes of cells and in this way promotes apoptosis (37)

7. New treatments

7.1 Monoclonal antibodies

At present, there are mainly two antibodies with great clinical value for patients with CLL. The first is rituximab (Rituximab, Mabthera) that targets the CD20 antigen(38). This CD20 molecule is expressed on almost all B-cells of patients with B-CLL, but the intensity of expression appears to be lower than in patients with non Hodgkin lymphoma (NHL) (39,40). The second approved mAb is alemtuzumab (Campath-1H), a humanized therapeutic mAb that recognizes the CD52 antigen expressed on normal and neoplastic lymphoid cells. Alemtuzumab is an effective drug in CLL patients with poor risk cytogenetics, such as deletions in 17p. However, alemtuzumab is ineffective in patients with bulky nodal disease (>5 cm) (41-43). Both these "gaps" of these two mAbs, low CD20 expression and bulky nodal disease, could be overcome by nanoparticles technology. Ofatumumab (HuMax-CD20; Arzerra), is a second-generation, fully human, anti-CD20, IgG1 mAb. Ofatumumab recognizes a different CD20 epitope to rituximab (44,45). Compared with rituximab, ofatumumab has similar antibody- dependent cellular cytotoxicity (ADCC) but stronger complement-dependent cytotoxicity (CDC) and does not induce cell death by apoptosis. Ofatumumab potentially represents an active treatment option with clinical benefit for patients with very poor prognosis who have exhausted standard treatment options but also is a very interesting option for the construction of our particles. Lumiliximab is a genetically primatized, macaque human chimeric anti-CD23 IgG1; mAb investigated for the treatment of relapsed CLL. It induces ADCC and CDC, and enhances apoptosis when combined with current or emerging CLL therapies including CLB, fludarabine, alemtuzumab and rituximab. TRU-016 is an intravenously administered anti-CD37 IgG fusion protein for the potential treatment of B-cell malignancies, including CLL and non-Hodgkin's lymphoma. In addition, several other mAbs directed against lymphoid cells have been recently developed and investigated in preclinical studies and clinical trials. These treatments include epratuzumab, galiximab and anti-CD40 mAbs (46).

7.2 Phenethyl isothiocyanate-PEITC

Epidemiological studies support the evidence that the consumption of cruciferous vegetables has long been associated with a reduced risk in the occurrence of cancer at various sites, including the prostate, lung, breast, and colon (47).1 The anticarcinogenic effect of cruciferous vegetables is attributed to organic isothiocyanates (ITCs), which are present in a variety of edible cruciferous vegetables such as broccoli, watercress, cabbage, and so on (47). Phenethyl isothiocyanate (PEITC) is one of the ITC family of compounds that has attracted a great deal of attention owing to its remarkable cancer chemopreventive activity (48). In one study samples tested for genetic abnormalities, with deletion of 17p., and exhibiting resistance to F-ara-A (IC_{50} > 10 μM), consistent with the crucial effect of p53 on sensitivity to fludarabine remained sensitive to PEITC. The loss of p53 is known to promote genetic instability and mitochondrial dysfunction (49), which not only confers drug resistance but may also promote ROS production (50). In this way it is conceivable that the p53-null CLL cells may have elevated ROS generation and would be highly sensitive to PEITC. Since the loss of p53 is prevalent in cancer and associated with resistance to many standard therapeutic agents (51), the novel ROS-mediated strategy using agents such as PEITC may have potentially broad clinical implications. The increase in ROS generation in CLL cells may render them highly sensitive to PEITC, whereas normal lymphocytes with low ROS output are less vulnerable to this compound. CLL cells from patients in advanced stages refractory to fludarabine-based therapy still remain highly sensitive to PEITC due to their increased ROS generation (52).

To improve their efficacy, HDACi have been paired with other antitumor agents. There are several combination therapies, such as ROS-generating agents, that together may provide a therapeutic advantage over single-agent vorinostat (53).

This last combination of Vorinostat and a ROS generating agent like, Phenylethyl-isothiocyanate (PEITC), has already been tested by us in nanoparticles systems with very good results, and so, it would be a best to associate them in this way for the production of the next generation of BNPs.

7.3 Histone deacetylase inhibitors (HDACi)

Histone acetylation is another recent alternative for CLL treatment that consists in a posttranslational modification that plays a role in regulating gene expression.

More recently, other non-histone proteins have been identified to be acetylated which can regulate their function, stability, localization, or interaction with other molecules. Modulating acetylation with histone deacetylase inhibitors (HDACi) has been validated to have anticancer effects in preclinical and clinical cancer models. This has led to development and approval of the first HDACi, Vorinostat, for the treatment of cutaneous T cell lymphoma. The impressive anticancer activity observed in both in vitro and in vivo cancer models, together with their preferential effect on cancer cells, have led to a huge effort into the identification and development of HDACi with different characteristics. To date, several clinical trials of HDACi conducted in solid tumors and hematological malignancies have shown a preferential clinical efficacy of these drugs in hematological malignancies and in particular in cutaneous T-cell lymphoma (CTCL), peripheral T-cell lymphoma (PTCL), Hodgkin lymphoma (HL) and myeloid malignancies. Several agents are also beginning to be tested in combination therapies, either as chemo-sensitizing agents in association with standard chemotherapy drugs or in combination with DNA methyltransferase inhibitors (DNMTi) in the context of the so-called "epigenetic therapies", aimed to revert epigenetic alterations found in cancer cells. Vorinostat has demostrated also efficacy in Hodgkin and Non-Hodgkin Lymphomas (53-56). However, to date, targeting acetylation with HDACi as a monotherapy has shown modest activity against other cancers including B-CLL.

7.4 New biodegradable nanoparticle systems for the treatment of B-chronic lymphocytic leukemia and lymphomas

The pharmaceutical industry as well as the scientific community has been dedicating a big effort as well as a large financial investment in the generation of promising targeted new therapeutic approaches for the treatment of all types of cancers including B-CLL and other Non-Hodgkin lymphomas. These attempts have been design mainly to overcome the challenges associated with the development of drug resistance. Also novel strategies are urgently needed to by-pass the adverse side effects of standard and new chemo and biologic therapeutic agents given by oral, IV or IM routes. In this way, we and others, have proposed to use monoclonal coated and drug loaded biodegradable nanoparticles (BNPs) specially to promote cell epitope specific delivery, and an increased sensitivity to anti-neoplastic drugs. Nanoparticle-based systems are already a real possibility to treat B-CLL. This innovative strategy will generate a pipeline of products in the near future, which will change the way we will treat these patients as well as others with different but also complex and severe diseases. There will probably be no big differences between products of this kind but this little varieties will also not be trivial. The best available products such as those non-traditional pro-apoptotic compounds or its combinations, will be the substances to be selected and loaded in these particles, and this will be one of the clues for these particles to work. HCQ is one of the best candidates as seen in all our research studies. It will be important for the hematologist to completely understand the mechanisms of action of this substance when delivered inside BNPs. Many drugs as well as other biologic agents have poor cellular bioavailability (56). At low or suboptimal concentrations these compounds are not pro-apoptotic at all or their effects could be very different to those we are looking for. Consistent with this, HCQ in clinical trials for B-CLL given orally like for malaria or rheumatic disease, might not be provoking the desired effects or even some, that could be not good at all for the patients, specially considering that its apoptotic effects are only reach at very high concentrations that are impossible to obtained by the oral route. Combining HCQ with CLB will probably be synergistic especially for those patients with already resistant disease or with bad prognosis gene mutations (57). Also PEITC associated with Vorinostat as well as Parthenolide with Honokiol/Magnolol seem to be interesting combinations to try. In relation to the monoclonal antibodies that will coat the first generation of BNPs for B-CLL treatment, those that target the anti-CD20 receptor alone or in combination with the anti-CD19 antibody are surely the best candidates to begin. Then the anti-CD52 and anti-CD23 would also be good possibilities to be used. There are some biological needs for these treatments to succed: (i) they must exhibit "stealth" qualities to evade macrophage attack and the immune response; (ii) be nontoxic, traceable and biodegradable following systemic administration through any route; (iii) display effective pharmacokinetic properties; (iv) the polymer must protect the embedded therapeutics; and (v) they must be selective in their targeting to specific tissue sites. All these qualities are fulfilled by our BNPs. Regulatory changes are needed also at the FDA. FDA must provide clear regulatory/safety guidelines for therapeutic nanoparticles including those related to environmental and health issues, but must help to accelerate the introduction of these technologies as soon as possible in the market.

8. Production and characterization of the first generation of biodegradable nanoparticles and its use in the treatment of B-CLL

We have already described that almost all FDA approved antineoplastic drugs in clinical use today are not selective to cancer cells and can produce very toxic side effects (58). In order to obtain better results and tolerability other therapeutic strategies should be developed, specially those that could carry drugs in new delivery systems designed to specifically target cell receptors or epitopes an introduce the desired therapeutic agents loaded in a carrier such as a nanoparticle. These systems are a new technology for cancer therapy (59). Receptor-targeted nanoparticles like the ones presented here (200~300 nm) are good drug carriers and can transport large amounts of drugs, while having a prolonged circulation time (specially when surface PEGylated), as well as a very selective tumor penetration when coated with monoclonal antibodies such as the anti-CD20 Rituximab. These nanoparticles can release enough amounts of drugs inside the cancer cells and in this way overcome multidrug resistance (MDR) mechanisms which are over-expressed in many B-CLL cells (60). Other nanoparticles (e.g., liposomes, micelles, polymers, dendrimers) have demonstrated efficacy both in vitro and in vivo (61). Nanoparticles systems have emerged as important tools to modify the release profile for a large number of drugs including inhibitors, protein and peptide molecules. They are produced from biocompatible and biodegradable FDA approved materials, making them a promising therapeutic strategy for drug targeting and delivery, and surmounting the inherent limitations of regulation acceptance. Additional advantages include reduction of drug toxicity and increase of drug bioavailability . Several previous studies have already demonstrated the goal, and it is well known that when used to deliver chemotherapeutics to cancer models, nanoparticles have a higher maximum tolerated dose than free drug. Nanoparticles for example provide a promising carrier for cisplatin administration avoiding its side effects without a reduction of the efficacy, which was consistent with a higher activation of apoptosis than free-drug. Moreover, this simple strategy can promote co-assembly of drugs, imaging agents and targeting moieties into multifunctional nano-pharmaceutics. Most current anticancer agents do not greatly differentiate between cancerous and normal cells, leading to systemic toxicity and adverse effects. This lack of differentiation greatly limits the maximum drug allowable dose, but the overexpression of receptors or antigens in human cancers lends itself to efficient uptake by receptor mediated endocytosis. There is some previous but limited published experience with nanoparticles in lymphomas, including in vivo studies in lympho-proliferative diseases. We have already published (3) the possibility of using these pharmaceutical new systems to overcome drug resistance of B-Chronic Lymphocytic Leukemia cells. We used for this purpose, PEG-PLGA polymers based BNPs specially designed to be loaded with HCQ and coated with specific monoclonal antibodies. These BNPs induced apoptosis of malignant B-CLL cells at low concentrations. HCQ-BNPs with mAbs induced a decrease in cell viability in a dose and time-dependent manner. In leukemic cells, the nanoparticles reduced cell viability in doses and times significantly lower than in normal lymphocytes. In vitro treatment of drug-resistant B-CLL cells with these HCQ-loaded BNPs was shown to be significantly more effective ($P<0.001$) than BNPs without drug, indicating that treatment with empty BNPs had little impact on cell viability. BNPs encapsulated with HCQ, but without mAbs, had significantly less impact on in vitro cell viability ($P<0.001$). Anti-CD19 and anti-CD20 antibodies suspended in PBS with 10% BSA in AIM V medium alone without BNPs produced no significant apoptoticeffect in B-CLL or normal lymphocytes. Active targeting is based on specific interactions with receptors on target cells that may promote enhanced internalization of nanoparticles through receptor mediated endocytosis. In addition, a common method for reducing the recognition of nanoparticles by the RES is to coat their surfaces with polyethylene glycol (PEG). In addition to specific interactions between the ligands on the surface of nanoparticles and receptors expressed on the tumor cells, this may trigger receptor mediated endocytosis. Furthermore, active targeting has shown the potential to suppress multidrug resistance (MDR) via bypassing of P-glycoprotein-mediated drug efflux. The targeting ligands may not play a role until the targeted nanoparticles find the tumor sites. This is very easy for our particles as the targeted cells reside mainly inside the vascular compartment or in tissues with high accessibility to the vasculature, such as in the case of B-CLL. In this situation, targeting occurs relatively quickly and easily. When BNPs were coated with human anti-CD19 and anti-CD20 antibodies the apoptotic effect was more pronounced and enhanced. Confirming the idea that nano-constructs such as these ones targeting B-CLL cells should serve as customizable, targeted drug delivery vehicles capable of ferrying large doses of chemotherapeutic agents into malignant cells while sparing healthy ones. Our nanoparticles beside the original idea of loading them with an anti-malarial immune modifying drug such as HCQ, have the advantage of their special production process in which nano core shells of a median diameter of 250 nm can be obtained by a non-emulsion-polymerization method, and in which several different drugs or petides can be easily encapsulated while one or more monoclonal antibodies can be coated in their surface. We also tried a similar kind of nanoparticles, both, in-vitro and in-vivo, in a mice living model of human lymphoma, but

HCQ was combined this time with CLB in order to potentiate its effects, and Rituximab, the first anti-human CD20 monoclonal antibody approved by the FDA for the treatment of lymphomas (62), was attached to the surface of the BNPs. We have developed a special type of biodegradable targeted nanoparticles with demonstrated efficacy in vitro and in vivo in animal studies for B-CLL, lymphomas and autoinmune diseases. The rational design of these nanoparticles considered the possibility of delivering high concentrations of HCQ and its combination with CLB loaded in biodegradable (PLGA) nanoparticles and coated with the mentioned antibody. Ordinarily, CLB-resistant B-CLL lymphocytes are 5- to 6-fold more resistant in vitro, using the MTT assay, as compared to sensitive lymphocytes (IC50 CLB of _61.0 mmol=L can be considered sensitive). This is why delivering CLB in nanoparticle systems seems to be a good idea indeed in resistant phenotypes. Loss of viability in human CLL cells correlated with the early induction of apoptosis.

9. Encapsulation of CLB and HCQ sulfate in BNPs containing anti-human-CD20 monoclonal antibody rituximab functional groups on their outer shells

BNPs with an average diameter in the range of 250 nm (measured by Dyamic Light Scattering) were produced by a non-emulsion-polymerization proprietary technology (Bio-Target Inc. USA). The particles had a -0.05 mV surface potential, measure by its zeta potential. The nano- capsules used in this study included a shell region and a core region. The shell was made of three biocompatible biodegradable polymers: PEG-PLA (polyethylene-glycol-poly-lactic-acid) and PCL (polycaprolactone). The monoclonal antibody Rituximab was coated in their surface.

The core included two therapeutic agents: HCQ and CLB. In this way a capsule including two encapsulated anti-neoplastic agents were produced by this methodology. One specific aspect of these BNPs, was an anti human CD20 functional group (Rituximab) dispersed on the outer surface of the shell region. Three different kinds of BNPs were specially designed. BNP0: only polymer-BNPs (PEG-PLA-PCL) at a concentration of 1.66 mg/ml. BNP1: Polymer (PEG-PLA- PCL) at a concentration of 1.66mg/ml coated with the anti human-CD20 monoclonal antibody, Rituximab, at a concentration of 8.824 ug/ml, combined with a cyanine 5.5 (CY5.5) dye, a fluorescent molecular beacon that emits photons in the near-IR, at 0.465 ug/ml. BNP2: antihuman- CD20-BNPs + (HCQ + CLB) with polymer (PEGPLA- PCL) at 1.66mg/ml, Rituximab at 8.824 ug/ml, CY5.5 dye at 0.465 ug/ml, and CLB at 5mg/ml-HCQ at 5mg/ml. The particles were produced under class 100 clean room conditions and the CY5.5 dye was chemically attached after preparation of the base BNPs as described below. B-CLL Cells and Cell Culture with BNPs Heparinized blood was obtained after informed consent from 3 B-CLL (median age 64.4 years old) Rai-IV, p-53 mutated, patients. The mononuclear cell fractions were isolated by centrifugation on Ficoll-Hypaque gradients. Primary tumor B cells positive for CD5, CD19, CD23, CD20, CD38 and ZAP70, with unmutated Ig genes and p53 mutations were isolated from the B-CLL patient's mononuclear cell fractions respectively using a B-Cell Isolation Kit. Briefly, 2 x 105 freshly isolated cells, from the CLL patients, were incubated in triplicate for all experiments at 37°C and 5% CO2 at various concentrations of BNPs in RPMI 1640 serum-free medium. All BNPs were suspended at the time of use in PBS with 10% Bovine Serum Albumin (BSA) at a final total mass concentration of 900 ug/ml. Aliquots of 0.2, 0.5, 1, and 2 ul from these solutions were used for experiments. After 24 and 48 hours of incubation at 37°C, the number of residual viable cells was estimated in each BNPs system using Ethidium Bromide/Acridine Orange staining and immune-fluorescent microscopy counting as well as measurement of cell apoptosis using annexin-V and propidium-iodide by FACS analysis. Direct Tumor Cell Cytotoxicity Assays using BJAB and MEC-1 cells were also done. The procedure was modified from Macor et al. (63) in order to evaluate the effect of BNPs on BJAB cells, a human Burkitts lymphoma cell line already used to characterize Rituximab activity and on MEC-1, a cell line derived from a patient with chronic lymphocytic leukemia. 2x105 cells of each class were incubated in triplicate in RPMI 1640 serum-free medium (Sigma-Aldrich Italy) with various amounts of BNPs. All BNPs were suspended at the time of use in PBS with 10% Bovine Serum Albumin (BSA) at a final total mass concentration of 900 ug/ml. Aliquots of 0.2, 0.5, 1, and 2 ul from these solutions were used for experiments. After 48 hours of ncubation at 37°C, the number of residual viable cells was estimated using the MTT assay and percentage of dead cells was calculated. For toxicology Studies, 4 groups of 4 C57/Bl mice each were treated intraperitoneally with different amounts of BNP2 in order to evaluate their effects on healthy animals: Group 1 received 10 ul of BNP2 for 4 times (50 ug HCQ + 50 ug CLB). Group 2 received 20 ul BNP2 for 4 times (100 ug HCQ + 100 ug CLB) and Group 3 received 40 ul BNP2 for 4 times(200 ug HCQ+ 200 ug CLB). Group 4: 80 ul BNP2 for 4times(400 ug HCQ + 400 ug CLB). Each animal was treated on days 0, 2, 4 and 7 and followed up to day 21. Therapeutical tudies using a Human/Mouse Model of Burkitt´s Lymphoma were performed. Female severe combined immunodeficiency (SCID) mice (4-6 weeks of age) were purchased from Charles River and maintained under pathogen- free conditions. A SCID xenograft model of Human Lymphoma specially developed to investigate the in vivo distribution and therapeutic effects of monoclonals antibodies was used to analyze the effects of BNPs after the toxicology studies. BJAB cells were expanded in vitro and then implanted intraperitoneally (2x106 cells/mouse) in 15 SCID mice (day 0). Ten of these mice were used as controls and the other 5 mice were treated i.p. with 80 ul BNP2 (400 ug HCQ + 400 ug CLB) at days 4, 7, 10, 13. We analyzed survival of controls and treated mice for more than 120 days (end of experiment). Histological and immunohistochemicals analysis were done. Tumor peritoneal masses and liver were collected from sacrificed mice (for ethic reasons) and maintained in buffered- formaline for 16 hours. Samples were first washed in EtOH 70% for 2 hours and then in EtOH 100%. Histological and immunohistochemicals analysis were performed. Results obtained from the prior assays shown that BNPs2 formulated with the human anti-CD20 monoclonal antibody Rituximab, and drugs (HCQ and CLB) efficiently induced apoptosis of malignant human B-CLL cells in vitro. At 0.5 ul concentration, and 24 hs of cuture, these BNPs2 induced 4-fold more apoptosis in malignant B-CLL cells compared to BNPs0 and BNPs1, reaching at 48 hs of culture almost a 95% cell killing effect. Reductions of living B-CLL cells were observed in vitro at 24 and 48 hours for injections of all concentrations of BNPs2. Loss of viability correlated with early induction of apoptosis as confirmed by monitoring the B-CLL cells after Annexin V/propidium iodide staining. BNPs2 with Rituximab and drugs induced a decrease in cell viability in a dose and time dependent manner. In vitro treatment of these B-CLL cells with BNPs2 showed to be more effective than BNPs without drugs (BNP0) indicating that treatment with empty BNPs had little impact on cell viability. BNPs1 encapsulated with HCQ and CLB but without monoclonal antibody had almost no impact on in vitro cell viability. The killing effect of the different BNPs on the B-CLL derived cell line MEC-1 was also analysed. BNPs0 and BNPs1 had 0% cell killing effect after 48 hs in culture, while BNPs2 had 94% killing effect using 0,5 ul. One or 2ul concentrations added little killing effect in the assays. The same experiments performed with BNPs and the Burkitt´s lymphoma cell line (BJAB) showed similar results, obtaining levels of 94% cell killing with 1 ul of BNPs2. In vivo studies start analyzing BNP2 toxicity in healthy mice. C57/Bl mice were treated intraperitoneally with different amounts of BNP2 (10 ul, 20 ul, 40 ul or 80 ul) for 4 injection on days 0, 2, 4 and 7 and followed up to day 21 in order to see possible adverse effects. No side effects have been detected in all the study period in any of the animals injected with BNPs. Histological and immunochemical studies performed on survival animals do not produce information about the distribution of the BNPs because the analysis was performed several weeks after BNPs injections. The in vivo therapeutic effect study was concluded 120 days after the administration of the tumor cells to the animals. Control mice died within day 63 after tumor cell injection. Three treated mice died between day 72 and 98 and tumor mass and liver were collect from these animals. At day 120 only 2 treated mice appeared healthy even at the end of the study. Histological studies were performed on samples derived from tumor masses developed in the peritoneum of treated and untreated mice. The peritoneal masses observed in all untreated animals were mainly composed of sheets of homogeneous round- shaped, medium-sized malignant lymphoid elements showing cohesive growth. However, necrotic areas were seen in peritoneal histological masses derived from all BNPs2-treated mice.

10. Final discussion

We have studied and described a new kind of therapeutic BNPs with a functional specific group attached to their outer shell, the first human anti-CD20, FDA approved for Lymphoma treatment, monoclonal antibody Rituximab. We have also combined in these BNPs an antimalarial agent, Hydoxychloroquine, known to have pro-apoptotic properties, with the old anti-leukemic drug Chlorambucil. This last agent has been the gold standard treatment for B- CLL for many decades until the general acceptance of Fludarabine as first line choice treatment (64). Both drugs have been used alone or in combination with Rituximab and other agents for the treatment of many B cell malignancies (65). After initial good responses, these hematological neoplasias usually mutate, and become resistant to all modalities of standard treatments. B-CLL and Lymphomas seem to be different sides of the same coin. Their malignant cells have the same potential to kill the patients, but also the same potential to dye by apoptosis under similar targeted therapies, like the one we propose here. With the use of these BNPs we were able to specifically target a variety of B malignant cells such as those from B-CLL patients, as well as BJAB and MEC-1 cell lines, with outstanding cell killing efficiency by apoptotic mechanisms. These BNPs induced high levels of responses beside having some of those cells, like the ones from CLL patients, bad prognostic markers such as mutation of the p- 53 gen. Then, a BNP coated with Rituximab and loaded with HCQ and CLB could be an interesting therapeutic strategy in which the antimalarial drug with pro-apoptotic activity seems to have a synergistic effect when associated with a cytotoxic agent. Those mechanisms of drug resistance usually found in Lymphomas after several treatment modalities could be overcome by the use of these BNPs and this drug combination. We did not see any adverse effect related to the use of BNPs when tested in living mice models. This could be a good evidence of the safety of this kind of treatment. The survival advantage of those animals implanted with human lymphoma cells when treated with BNPs is provocative, but in some way it was expected after the good results obtained in our in vitro assays. This prolonged overall survival of the treated animals probably correlates well with some of the histological findings, in which cell apoptosis and necrosis were seen only in B cell tumor areas after injecting the mice models with BNP2. For all of this, it seems reasonable to do more animal studies of the same kind in order to accelerate a possible introduction of this promising technology into a first human clinical trial. Maybe changing at last, the high mortality associated with B-CLL and other indolent lymphomas.

11. References

[1] Raphael B, Andersen JW, Silber R, et al. Comparison of chlorambucil and prednisone versus cyclophosphamide, vincristine, and prednisone as initial treatment for chronic lymphocytic leukemia: long-term follow-up of an Eastern Cooperative Oncology Group randomized clinical trial. J Clin Oncol. 1991;9(5):770-6.

[2] Lagneaux L, Delforge A, Carlier S, Massy M, Bernier M, Bron D. Early induction of apoptosis in B-chronic lymphocytic leukaemia cells by hydroxychloroquine: activation of caspase-3 and no protection by survival factors.Br J Haematol.2001;112(2):344-52.

[3] Mansilla E, Marin GH, Nuñez L, et al. The lysosomotropic agent, hydroxychloroquine,delivered in a biodegradable nanoparticle system, overcomes drug resistance of B-chronic lymphocytic leukemia cells in vitro. Cancer Biother Radiopharm. 2010Feb;25(1):97-103.

[4] Marin GH, Mansilla E, Mezzaroba N. Exploratory study on the effects of biodegradablenanoparticles with drugs on malignant B cells and on a human/mouse model ofBurkitt lymphoma. Curr Clin Pharmacol. 2010;5(4):246-50.

[5] Bawa R. Nanoparticle-based Therapeutics in Humans: A Survey. Nanotechnology Law & Business. 2008; 5,2:135-155.

[6] Deglesne PA, Chevallier N, Letestu R. et al. Survival response to B-cell receptor ligation is restricted to progressive chronic lymphocytic leukemia cells irrespective of Zap70 expression. Cancer Res. 2006;66(14):7158-66.

[7] Zucchetto A, Bomben R, Dal Bo M et al. A scoring system based on the expression of sixsurface molecules allows the identification of three prognostic risk groups in B-cell chronic lymphocytic leukemia. J Cell Physiol. 2006;207(2):354-63.

[8] Ricky W. Johnstone, Erika Cretney, and Mark J. Smyth. P-Glycoprotein ProtectsLeukemia Cells Against Caspase-Dependent, but not Caspase-Independent, Cell Death. Blood 1999; 93,3: 1075-1085.

[9] Turgut B, Vural O, Pala FS, et al. 17p Deletion is associated with resistance of B-cell chronic lym- phocytic leukemia cells to in vitro fludarabine- induced apoptosis. Leuk Lymphoma. 2007;48: 311-220.

[10] Grever MR, Lucas DM, Dewald GW, et al. Com- prehensive assessment of genetic and molecular features predicting outcome in patients with chronic lymphocytic leukemia: results from the US Intergroup Phase III Trial E2997. J Clin Oncol. 2007; 25:799-804.

[11] Zhou Y, Hileman EO, Plunkett W, Keating MJ, Huang P. Free radical stress in chronic lympho- cytic leukemia cells and its role in cellular sensitivity to ROS-generating anticancer agents. Blood 2003;101:4098-4104.

[12] Kalil N, Cheson BD. Management of chronic lymphocytic leukaemia. Drugs Aging. 2000;16(1):9-27
[13] Silvennoinen R, Malminiemi K, Malminiemi O, Seppälä E, Vilpo J. Pharmacokinetics of chlorambucil in patients with chronic lymphocytic leukaemia: comparison of different days, cycles and doses.Pharmacol Toxicol. 2000;87(5):223-8.
[14] Tam KY, Leung KC, Wang YX. Chemoembolization agents for cancer treatment. Eur J Pharm Sci. 2011;44(1-2):1-10.
[15] Ren D, Kratz F, Wang SW. Protein nanocapsules containing doxorubicin as a pH-responsive delivery system. Small. 2011;7(8):1051-60
[16] Bergmann MA, Goebeler ME, Herold M, et al. Efficacy of bendamustine in patients with relapsed or refractory chronic lymphocytic leukemia: results of a phase I/II study of the German CLL Study Group. Haematologica. 2005;90(10):1357-64.
[17] Fischer K, Cramer P, Busch R. Bendamustine Combined With Rituximab in Patients With Relapsed and/or Refractory Chronic lymphocytic Leukemia: A Multicenter Phase II Trial of the German Chronic Lymphocytic Leukemia Study Group. J Clin Oncol. 2011 ; 8(1):38-47 .
[18] Cavalli R, Bisazza A, Bussano R. Poly(amidoamine)-Cholesterol Conjugate Nanoparticles Obtained by Electrospraying as Novel Tamoxifen Delivery System. J Drug Deliv. 2011;2011:587604.
[19] Magrone T, Jirillo E. Potential application of dietary polyphenols from red wine to attaining healthy ageing. Curr Top Med Chem. 2011;11(14):1780-96.
[20] Chow HH, Hakim IA. Pharmacokinetic and chemoprevention studies on tea in humans. Pharmacol Res. 2011 Aug;64(2):105-12.
[21] Song WZ, Cui JF, Zhang GD. Studies on the medicinal plants of the Magnoliaceae tuhoupo of Manglietia. J Chin Herbs 1989;24:295-9.
[22] Ross JJ, Arnason JT, Birnboim HC. Low concentrations of the fever few component parthenolide inhibit in vitro growth of tumor lines in a cytostatic fashion. Planta Med 1999;65:126-9.
[23] Yip-Schneider MT, Nakshatri H, Sweeney CJ, Marshall MS, Wiebke EA, Schmidt CM. Parthenolide and sulindac cooperate to mediate growth suppression and inhibit the nuclear factor-kappa B pathway in pancreatic carcinoma cells. Mol Cancer Ther 2005;4:587-94.
[24] Sweeney CJ, Mehrotra S, Sadaria MR, Kumar S, Shortle NH, Roman Y, *et al.* The sesquiterpene lactone parthenolide in combination with docetaxel reduces metastasis and improves survival in a xenograft model of breast cancer. Mol Cancer Ther 2005;4:1004-12.
[25] Marin GH, Mansilla E. Apoptosis induced by Magnolia Grandiflora extract in chlorambucil-resistant B-chronic lymphocytic leukemia cells.J Cancer Res Ther. 2010; 6(4):463-5.
[26] Marin G.H., Mansilla E. Parthenolide has apoptotic and cytotoxic selective effect on B-chronic lymphocytic leukemia cells. J. Appl. Biomed.2006; 4: 135–139.
[27] Yang SE, Hsieh MT, Tsai TH, Hsu SL. Inhibitory effect of magnolol and honokiol from Magnolia obovata on human fibrosarcoma HT-1080. Invasiveness in vitro. Planta Med 2001;67:705- 8.
[28] Sweeney CJ, Mehrotra S, Sadaria MR, Kumar S, Shortle NH, Roman Y, et al. The sesquiterpene lactone parthenolide in combination with docetaxel reduces

metastasis and improves survival in a xenograft model of breast cancer. Mol Cancer Ther 2005;4:1004-12.

[29] Battle TE, Castro-Malaspina H, Gribben JG, Frank DA. Sustained complete remission of CLL associated with the use of a Chinese herbal extract: Case report and mechanistic analysis. Leuk Res 2003;27:859-63.

[30] Wiedhopf RM, Young M, Bianchi E, Cole JR. Tumor inhibitory agent from Magnolia grandiflora (Magnoliaceae). I. Parthenolide. J Pharm Sci 1973;62:345.

[31] Clark AM, El-Feraly FS, Li WS. Antimicrobial activityof phenolic constituents of Magnolia grandiflora L. J Pharm Sci 1981;70:951-2.

[32] Yang SE, Hsieh MT, Tsai TH, Hsu SL. Down-modulation of BCl-XL, release ofcytochrome c and sequential activation of caspases during honokiol-inducedapoptosis in human squamous lung cancer CH27 cells. Biochem Pharmacol 2002; 63:1641-51.

[33] Ross JJ, Arnason JT, Birnboim HC. Low concentrations of the feverfew component parthenolide inhibit in vitro growth of tumor lines in a cytostatic fashion. Planta Med 1999;65:126-9.

[34] Kanno S, Kitajima Y, Kakuta M, Osanai Y, Kurauchi K, Ujibe M, et al. Costunolide-induced apoptosis is caused by receptor-mediated pathway and inhibition of telomerase activity in NALM-6 cells. Biol Pharm Bull 2008;31:1024-8

[35] Amaravadi RK, Lippincott-Schwartz J, Yin XM et al.Principles and current strategies for targeting autophagy for cancer treatment. Clin Cancer Res. 2011 Feb 15;17(4):654-66.

[36] Aguirre-Cruz L, Torres KJ, Jung-Cook H, Fortuny C, Sánchez E, Soda-Mehry A, Sotelo J, Reyes-Terán G Preferential concentration of hydroxychloroquine in adenoid tissue of HIV-infected subjects. AIDS Res Hum Retroviruses. 2010;26(3):339-42.

[37] Das SK, Pareek A, Mathur DS, Efficacy and safety of hydroxychloroquine sulphate in rheumatoid arthritis: a randomized, double-blind, placebo controlled clinical trial--an Indian experience. Curr Med Res Opin. 2007 Sep;23(9):2227-34.

[38] Lagneaux L, Delforge A, Dejeneffe M, Massy M, Bernier M, Bron D Leuk Hydroxychloroquine-induced apoptosis of chronic lymphocytic leukemia involves activation of caspase-3 and modulation of Bcl-2/bax/ratio.Lymphoma. 2002;43(5):1087-95.

[39] Rahim R, Strobl JS. Hydroxychloroquine, chloroquine, and all-trans retinoic acid regulate growth, survival, and histone acetylation in breast cancer cells. Anticancer Drugs. 2009;20(8):736-45.

[40] Robak T. Monoclonal antibodies in the treatment of chronic lymphoid leukemias. Leuk. Lymphoma.2004;45:205–19.

[41] Onrust SV, Lamb HM, Balfour JA. Rituximab. Drugs. 1999;58:79–88.

[42] O'Brien SM, Kantarjian H, Thomas DA, et al. Rituximab dose-escalation trial in chronic lymphocytic leukemia. J. Clin. Oncol. 2001;19:2165–70.

[43] Robak T. Alemtuzumab for B-cell chronic lymphocytic leukemia. Expert Rev. Anticancer Ther. 2008;8:1033–51

[44] Robak T. Novel monoclonal antibodies for the treatment of chronic lymphocytic leukemia. Curr Cancer Drug Targets. 2008;8:156–71.

[45] Coiffier B, Lepretre S, Pedersen LM, et al. Safety and efficacy ofofatumumab, a fully human monoclonal anti-CD20 antibody, in patients with relapsed or refractory B-cell chronic lymphocytic leukemia. A phase I–II study. Blood. 2008;11:1094–1100

[46] Robak T. Novel drugs for chronic lymphoid leukemias: mechanism of action and therapeutic activity.Curr Med Chem. 2009;16:2212–34.

[47] Conaway CC, Yang YM, Chung FL. Isothiocyanates as cancer chemo-preventive agents: their biological activities and metabolism in rodents and humans. Curr Drug Metab. 2002;3:233–255.

[48] Stoner GD, Morrissey DT, Heur YH, Daniel EM, Galati AJ, Wagner SA. Inhibitory effects of phenethyl isothiocyanate on N-nitrosobenzylmethylamine carcinogenesis in the rat esophagus. Cancer Res. 1991; 51:2063–2068.

[49] Matoba S, Kang JG, Patino WD, et al. p53 regulates mitochondrial respiration. Science 2006;312:1650-1653.

[50] Achanta G, Sasaki R, Feng L, et al. Novel role of p53 in maintaining mitochondrial genetic stability through interaction with DNA Pol gamma. EMBO J 2005;24: 3482-3492.

[51] Gasco M, Crook T. p53 family members and chemoresistance in cancer: what we know and what we need to know. Drug Resist Updat 2003;6:323-328.

[52] Trachootham D, Zhang H , Zhang W, Feng L, Du M, Zhou Y, Chen Z, Pelicano H, Plunkett W, Wierda W, Keating M, and Huang P. Effective elimination of fludarabine-resistant CLL cells by PEITC through a redox-mediated mechanism. Blood 2008; 112, 5: 1912-1922.

[53] Kirschbaum M, Frankel P, Popplewell L et al. Phase II study of vorinostat for treatment of relapsed or refractory indolent non-Hodgkin's lymphoma and mantle cell lymphoma. J Clin Oncol. 2011;29(9):1198-203.

[54] Miller CP, Singh MM, Rivera-Del Valle N, Manton CA, Chandra J. Therapeutic strategies to enhance the anticancer efficacy of histonedeacetylase inhibitors. J Biomed Biotechnol. 2011;20:5142-61.

[55] Robak T. Application of New Drugs in Chronic Lymphocytic Leukemia. Mediterr J Hematol Infect Dis.2010; 2(2): e2010011.

[56] Mercurio C, Minucci S, Pelicci PG. Histone deacetylases and epigenetic therapies of hematological malignancies.Pharmacol Res. 2010 ;62(1):18-34.

[57] Krystof V, Uldrijan S. Cyclin-dependent kinase inhibitors as anticancer drugs. Curr Drug Targets. 2010;11(3):291-302.

[58] Meng-Dan Z, Fu-Qiang H, Yong-Zhong D. Coadministration of glycolipid-like micelles loading cytotoxic drug with different action site for efficient cancer chemotherapy .Nanotechnology 2009; 20,5: 55-9. Jønsson V, Gemmell CG, Wiik A. Emerging concepts in the management of the malignant haematological disorders. Expert Opin Pharmacother. 2000;1(4):713-35.

[59] Islam T, Josephson L.Current state and future applications of active targeting in malignancies using superparamagnetic iron oxide nanoparticles. Cancer Biomark. 2009;5(2):99-107.

[60] Rao DA, Forrest ML, Alani AW, Kwon GS, Robinson JR. Biodegradable PLGA based nanoparticles for sustained regional lymphatic drug delivery. J Pharm Sci. 2010; 99(4):2018-31.

[61] Luo G, Yu X, Jin C, Yang F, et al LyP-1-conjugated nanoparticles for targeting drug delivery to lymphatic metastatic tumors. Int J Pharm. 2010; 385(1-2):150-6.

[62] Schulz H, Rehwald U, Morschhauser F et al. Rituximab in relapsed lymphocyte-predominant Hodgkin lymphoma: long-term results of a phase 2 trial by the German Hodgkin Lymphoma Study Group (GHSG). Blood. 2008;111(1):109-11.

[63] Macor P, Tripodo C, Zorzet S, et al. In vivo targeting of human neutralizing antibodiesagainst CD55 and CD59 to lymphoma cells increases the antitumor activity ofrituximab. Cancer Res 2007; 67(21): 10556-63.

[64] Rai K, Peterson BL, Appelbaum FR. Fludarabine compared with chlorambucil as primary therapy for chronic CLL. N. Engl. J Med 2000; 343: 1750-8.

[65] Huhn D., von Schilling C., Wilhelm M. Rituximab therapy of patients with B-cell CLLL. Blood 2001; 5: 1326-31